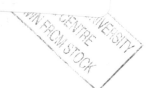

Listeria,

Listeriosis, and Food Safety

FOOD SCIENCE AND TECHNOLOGY

A Series of Monographs, Textbooks, and Reference Books

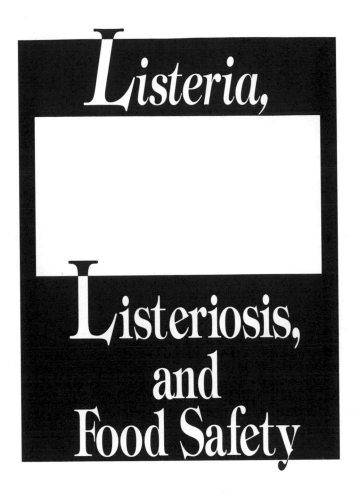

Listeria, Listeriosis, and Food Safety

Elliot T. Ryser
Elmer H. Marth
University of Wisconsin–Madison
Madison, Wisconsin

Marcel Dekker, Inc.   **New York • Basel • Hong Kong**

Library of Congress Cataloging-in-Publication Data

Ryser, Elliot T.
    Listeria, listeriosis, and food safety / Elliot T. Ryser, Elmer H.
Marth.
        p.   cm.
    Includes bibliographical references and index.
    ISBN 0-8247-8480-4 (alk. paper)
    1. Listeriosis. 2. Listeria monocytogenes. 3. Foodborne
diseases. 4. Food--Microbiology.   I. Marth, Elmer H. II. Title.
QR201.L7R9   1991   91-13461
615.9'52995--dc20   CIP

This book is printed on acid-free paper.

MARCEL DEKKER, INC.
270 Madison Avenue, New York, New York 10016

Current printing (last digit):
10 9 8 7 6 5 4 3 2 1

PRINTED IN THE UNITED STATES OF AMERICA

Preface

Interest in the occurrence of *Listeria* in food, particularly *Listeria monocytogenes*, escalated rapidly during the 1980s and continues unabated as a result of several major outbreaks of foodborne listeriosis. The first of these occurred during 1981 and involved consumption of contaminated coleslaw. In 1983, the reputation of the American dairy industry for producing safe products suffered when epidemiological evidence showed that 14 of 49 people in Massachusetts died after consuming pasteurized milk that was supposedly contaminated with *L. monocytogenes*. Two years later, consumption of contaminated Mexican-style cheese manufactured in California was directly linked to more than 142 cases of listeriosis, including at least 40 deaths.

Heightened public concern regarding the prevalence of *L. monocytogenes* in food prompted the United States Food and Drug Administration to initiate a series of *Listeria* surveillance programs. Subsequent discovery of this pathogen in many varieties of domestic and imported cheese, in ice cream, and in other dairy products prompted numerous product recalls, which in turn have led to staggering financial losses for the industry, including several lawsuits. These listeriosis outbreaks, together with a subsequent epidemic in Switzerland involving consumption of Vacherin Mont d'Or soft-ripened cheese and discovery of *L. monocytogenes* in raw and ready-to-eat meat, poultry, seafood, and vegetables, have underscored the need for additional information concerning foodborne listeriosis.

In 1961 Professor H. P. R. Seeliger, now retired from the University of Würzburg, published his time-honored book entitled *Listeriosis*. While his monograph has provided scientists, veterinarians, and the medical profession with much-needed information regarding *Listeria* and human/animal listeriosis as well as pathological, bacteriological, and serological methods to diagnose this disease, documented cases of foodborne listeriosis were virtually unknown 30 years ago. Although much information in his book is still valid today, some of the knowledge regarding media and/or methods used to isolate, detect, and identify *L. monocytogenes* in clinical and, particularly, nonclinical specimens is now largely out of date. The emergence of *L. monocytogenes* as a serious foodborne pathogen together with the virtual flood of *Listeria*-related papers that have appeared in scientific journals, trade journals, and numerous conference proceedings prompted us to review and summarize the current information so that food industry personnel, public health and regulatory officials, food microbiologists, veterinarians, and academicians have a ready source of information regarding this now fully emerged foodborne pathogen.

This book consists of 15 chapters which address the following topics: (a) *L. monocytogenes* as the causative agent of listeriosis; (b) occurrence and survival of this pathogen in various natural environments; (c) human and animal listeriosis; (d) characteristics of *L. monocytogenes* that are important to food processors; (e) conventional and rapid methods for isolating, detecting, and identifying *L. monocytogenes* in food; (f) recognition of cases and outbreaks of foodborne listeriosis; (g) incidence and behavior of *L. monocytogenes* in fermented and unfermented dairy products, meat, poultry (including eggs), seafood, and products of plant origin; and finally (h) incidence and control of this pathogen within various types of food-processing facilities. It is evident that major emphasis has been given to information that is directly applicable to food processors. Since information concerning the bacterium and the disease has been admirably reviewed by Professor Seeliger and others, our discussion of these topics should not be considered exhaustive. Thus the first four chapters of this book supply only pertinent background information to complement our discussion of foodborne listeriosis.

While many in the scientific community must be commended for the extraordinary progress made since 1985 toward understanding foodborne listeriosis, the continuing "explosion" of information concerning *Listeria* and foodborne listeriosis has made the 3-year task of compiling an up-to-date review of this subject quite difficult. Therefore, to produce as current a document as possible, we have included a bibliography of references that have appeared since the writing of the book was completed.

We acknowledge with gratitude the many investigators whose findings made this book both necessary and possible. Special thanks go to those individuals who shared unpublished information with us so that we could make the book as up to date as possible. Our thanks also go to those scientists who provided photographs or drawings; each person is acknowledged where the appropriate figure appears in the book. We thank Barbara Kamp, Pat Gustafson, Beverly Scullion, and Judy Grudzina for typing various parts of the manuscript. Illustrations were prepared by Jennifer Blitz and Suzanne Smith—their help is acknowledged and appreciated. Special thanks go to Dr. Ralston B. Read, Jr., formerly director of the Microbiology Division of the Food and Drug Administration and now deceased, who in 1984 encouraged development of a research program on foodborne *Listeria* at the University of Wisconsin—Madison, and to Dr. Joseph A. O'Donnell, formerly with Dairy Research, Inc. and now director of the California Dairy Foods Research Center, for his early interest in and support of research on behavior of *L. monocytogenes* in dairy foods.

Research done in the Department of Food Science at the University of Wisconsin—Madison and described in this book was supported by the U.S. Food and Drug Administration; the National Dairy Promotion and Research Board; the Wisconsin Milk Marketing Board; Kraft, Inc. (now Kraft General Foods); Carlin Foods; Chr. Hansen's Laboratory, Inc.; the Aristotelian University of Thessaloniki, Greece; the Cultural and Educational Bureau of the Egyptian Embassy in the U.S.; the Malaysian Agricultural Research and Development Institute; the Korean Professors Fund; and the College of Agricultural and Life Sciences, the Center for Dairy Research, and the Food Research

Institute, all of the University of Wisconsin. We thank all of these agencies for their interest in and support of research on *L. monocytogenes.*

Our book is dedicated to all persons who have contributed to a better understanding of foodborne listeriosis so that control of this disease is facilitated.

Elliot T. Ryser
Elmer H. Marth

Contents

1

Listeria monocytogenes: Characteristics and Classification

INTRODUCTION

In 1924, Murray et al. (63) isolated a small gram-positive bacillus from blood of infected rabbits. During the illness, a typical monocytosis was observed in the diseased animals. Hence, the organism was named *Bacterium monocytogenes*. Although Murray et al. (63) are generally credited with the first accurate description of the causative agent of listeriosis (known today as *Listeria monocytogenes*), numerous reports suggest that the organism was encountered in "listeric-like" infections as early as 1891 (34). In 1911, the Swedish worker Hülphers (41) isolated an organism from necrotic foci of a rabbit liver. The description of this isolate, which he named *Bacillus hepatis*, closely resembles the present-day description of *L. monocytogenes*. Probable isolations of *L. monocytogenes* also were reported by Atkinson (4) in 1915 and Dick (20) in 1919 in conjunction with clinical cases of human meningitis. In addition, Dumont and Cotoni (21) isolated a diphtheroid organism from cerebrospinal fluid in 1918 and deposited the culture at the Pasteur Institute in Paris. In 1940 this organism was identified by Paterson (67) as *L. monocytogenes*, thus making this isolate the oldest known strain of *L. monocytogenes*.

Three years after Murray et al. (63) provided the first accurate description of *L. monocytogenes*, Pirie (71) isolated a bacterium from a gerbille (African jumping mouse) in South Africa, which he named *Listerella hepatolytica* in honor of Lord Lister, who discovered antisepsis. After learning that *B. monocytogenes* and *L. hepatolytica* were the same organism, the name was changed to *Listerella monocytogenes*, and this designation was used for the next 12 years. In 1939, it was discovered that the name *Listerella* had been applied to a group of slime molds in 1906. Hence, in 1940, the proposed name change by Pirie (71) from *Listerella monocytogenes* to *Listeria monocytogenes* was accepted. This name change was later adopted in the sixth edition of *Bergey's Manual of Determinative Bacteriology* (10) and approved in 1954 by the Judicial Commission on Bacteriological Nomenclature and Taxonomy (1).

TAXONOMY

The genus *Listeria*, presently classified among "genera of uncertain affiliation" (90), was originally described by Pirie (71) as monotypic and contained only *L. monocytogenes*. However, in 1985 eight *Listeria* spp.—*L. monocytogenes, L. ivanovii, L. innocua, L.*

1

welshimeri, L. seeligeri, L. denitrificans, L. murrayi, and *L. grayi*—were recognized in the Approved Lists of Bacterial Names (5). Although these eight *Listeria* spp. also can be found in the ninth edition of *Bergey's Manual of Systematic Bacteriology,* three *Listeria* spp.—namely *L. grayi, L. murrayi,* and *L. denitrificans*—have been categorized as species *incertae sedis* (species of uncertain position) (46). According to results of a DNA/DNA hybridization study completed in 1974 by Stuart and Welshimer (98), *L. grayi* and *L. murrayi* have lower DNA homology values than do the six other *Listeria* spp. Based on these results, a proposal was made to place *L. grayi* and *L. murrayi* in a newly created genus, *Murraya*; however, this change has not been widely accepted.

The taxonomic position of these organisms is further complicated by recent numerical taxonomic and chemical (i.e., cell wall, cytochrome, fatty acid) studies, which indicate that *L. grayi* and *L. murrayi* are not distinctly different from *L. monocytogenes* (90). To further investigate the degree of relatedness between these organisms, the catalog of the RNAse T1-resistant oligonucleotides of the 16S RNA of *L. murrayi* was determined by Rocourt (74) and compared to those of *L. monocytogenes*. The high degree of similarity between these organisms suggested that *L. grayi* and *L. murrayi* should remain in the genus *Listeria* (83). Thus, until such time as the apparent conflicts in results between DNA hybridization and numerical taxonomic/chemical studies are resolved, these two organisms are probably best treated as species of uncertain affiliation.

In contrast to *L. grayi* and *L. murrayi*, at least four taxonomic studies completed since 1966 (13,45,96,98) indicate that *L. denitrificans* [of which only one isolate is presently recognized (82)] is more closely related to the genera *Corynebacterium* (98), *Cellulomonas* (13), or *Arthrobacter* (45) than to *Listeria*. Studies using DNA/DNA hybridization technology also suggest a low degree of relatedness between *L. denitrificans* and other *Listeria* spp. (97). After analyzing the 16S ribosomal RNA content, Rocourt concluded that *L. denitrificans* is not a member of the genus *Listeria* and proposed that the organism be transferred to a new genus *Jonesia* as *Jonesia denitrificans* (82). Although this organism is now appearing in the scientific literature as *J. denitrificans*, to our knowledge this name has not yet been formally approved. All evidence from morphological, biochemical, serological, chemical, and nucleic acid studies indicates that *L. denitrificans* is not a member of the genus *Listeria*; however, until the name *J. denitrificans* is formally approved, this organism will likely be retained as *L. denitrificans* in *Bergey's Manual of Systematic Bacteriology* and listed as a species of uncertain position.

MORPHOLOGY

Listeria monocytogenes is a gram-positive, non–spore-forming, non–acid fast, pleomorphic rod-shaped bacterium with rounded ends (34). When observed microscopically, fresh isolates are in the smooth, pathogenic form and appear as short diphtheroid-like rods measuring 1.0–2.0 μm × 0.5 μm (Figs. 1.1 and 1.2). Cells of young *Listeria* isolates may appear to be diplococci or cocci. The organism also can exhibit typical palisade formation, along with some V and Y forms. In contrast to the smooth form, long rods measuring 6–20 μm are typically observed in rough strains, which develop after 3–5 days of incubation (2). Initially, young cultures are without exception gram-positive;

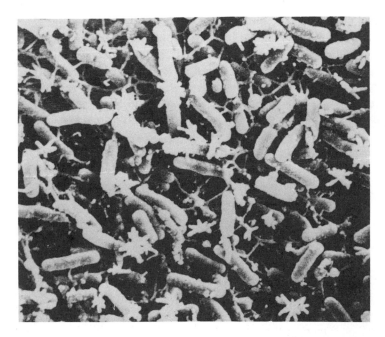

Figure 1.1   Electron micrograph of *L. monocytogenes*. (Courtesy of Dr. G. Comi, formerly of the University of Piacenza and now with the University of Udine, Italy.)

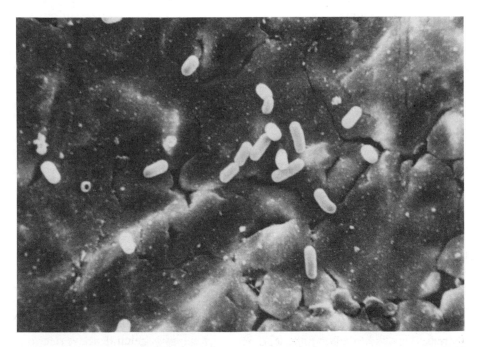

Figure 1.2   Electron micrograph of *L. monocytogenes* on a pitted stainless steel chip after treatment with 200 ppm sodium hypochlorite solution. (Courtesy of Dr. M. B. Liewen, formerly of the University of Nebraska and now with General Mills, Minneapolis, MN.)

however, examination of 2- to 5-day-old cultures often reveals gram-negative cells which resemble those of *Haemophilus influenzae* (34).

In addition to the typical morphological characteristics, *L. monocytogenes* is motile via flagella and exhibits a characteristic tumbling motility which can aid in identifying the organism (86). Tumbling motility is best observed in Tryptose Broth cultures incubated at 20°C. It is important that the culture for the motility test be incubated at or near room temperature since incubation at 37°C can either reversibly damage the one to six peritrichous flagella present on the bacterium or lead to development of a single flagellum (51). In either event, cultures incubated at 37°C are, at best, only weakly motile.

CULTURAL CHARACTERISTICS

Listeria monocytogenes grows at temperatures between 1 and 45°C, with optimal growth occurring between 30 and 37°C. Although isolation of *Listeria* may prove difficult at times, once isolated, the organism grows readily on common bacteriological media such as Tryptose Agar. This medium is excellent for maintaining and storing stock cultures at 3°C (34). When cultures grown on a clear medium (i.e., Tryptose Agar) are viewed under magnification using obliquely transmitted light as described by Henry (37), colonies of *L. monocytogenes* appear bluish-green and have a finely textured surface (see Fig. 6.3). With practice, this method, developed by Henry (37), can be used quite successfully to identify probable colonies of *L. monocytogenes* isolated from contaminated material. After 24 hours of incubation at 37°C, typical colonies are round, translucent, slightly raised with a finely textured surface, watery in consistency, bluish-gray under normal illumination, and have an entire margin. Colonies will vary in diameter between 0.3 and 1.5 mm, depending on the number of colonies present on the agar surface. After 5–10 days of incubation, well-separated colonies may reach 3–5 mm in diameter. Following repeated transfer, colonies representing the smooth virulent form of *L. monocytogenes* just described may revert to a rough avirulent form characterized by a coarsely textured surface, undulating border, and striations radiating toward the periphery of the colony (86).

Listeria monocytogenes also grows on blood agar. After 48 hours of incubation at 37°C, colonies on blood agar may reach 0.2–1.5 mm in diameter and be surrounded by a narrow zone of β-hemolysis. If β-hemolysis is particularly weak, the zone of clearing may only be observed after the colony is wiped off the agar surface (86). Prolonged incubation typically enhances the degree of β-hemolysis.

After inoculating Tryptose Broth with *L. monocytogenes*, the medium becomes turbid following 18–24 hours incubation at 37°C. Profuse growth is always observed slightly below the clear area near the surface of the medium, indicating a propensity for the organism to grow better with a reduced oxygen tension than in air (9,86). Excellent growth also occurs after partial replacement of oxygen with carbon dioxide; however, *ogenes* fails to grow under strict anaerobic conditions. Although isolation of *ogenes* reportedly is somewhat easier after incubating plates in an atmosphere sed levels of carbon dioxide, *L. monocytogenes* is generally accepted to be ally growing, mesophilic organism (86).

BIOCHEMICAL CHARACTERISTICS

Listeria spp. possess the following biochemical traits: catalase +, oxidase –, urease –, and Methyl Red/Voges–Proskauer (VP) test +/+ (except +/– for *L. denitrificans*). Esculin and sodium hippurate are hydrolyzed and acid (primarily lactic, acetic, isobutyric, isovaleric, and phenylacetic acid), but no gas is produced from fermentation of glucose (19,70). Of particular importance to food microbiologists is the fact that these organisms fail to hydrolyze gelatin, casein, or milk.

The eight *Listeria* spp. previously mentioned can be identified according to the biochemical tests listed in Tables 1.1 and 1.2. The CAMP test is particularly useful for differentiating species of *Listeria* (81). This test is done by streaking cultures of β-hemolytic *Staphylococcus aureus* and *Rhodococcus equi* vertically on a plate of sheep blood agar (Fig. 1.3). *Listeria* test cultures are then streaked at right angles to the two other cultures. After 48 hours of incubation at 35°C, β-hemolysis by *L. monocytogenes* is enhanced in the vicinity of the *Staphylococcus* streak, whereas β-hemolysis by *L. ivanovii* is enhanced near the *Rhodococcus* streak. *Listeria seeligeri* becomes hemolytic near the *Staphylococcus* streak, whereas the other species remain nonhemolytic. In addition, most strains of *L. monocytogenes* produce acid from maltose, rhamnose, salicin, levulose, and trehalose and are unable to produce acid from mannitol, xylose, melibiose, dulcitol, adonitol, inositol, arabinose, raffinose, sucrose, and inulin. Delayed or irregular acid production also has been observed with lactose, galactose, melezitose, sorbitol, and dextrin (90).

LISTERIA CAMP TEST

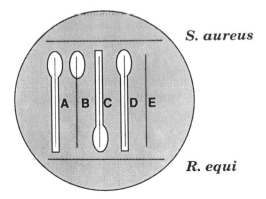

Figure 1.3 Diagram of CAMP test reactions for *Listeria* spp. The white areas within the dark circle represent β–hemolysis. Enlargement of the ends of the white areas represents enhanced hemolysis resulting from presence of *S. aureus* or *R. equi*. A: *Listeria monocytogenes* (typical hemolysis); B: *Listeria monocytogenes* (atypical hemolysis); C: *Listeria ivanovii*; D: *Listeria seeligeri*; E: *Listeria innocua*. (Courtesy of D. A. Jurick, Silliker Laboratories, Chicago Heights, IL.)

Table 1.1 Abbreviated Biochemical Identification of *Listeria* spp.

Listeria sp.	β-hemolysis	Nitrates reduced	CAMP test		Production of acid from		
			Staphylococcus aureus[a]	*Rhodococcus equi*[b]	Mannitol	Rhamnose	Xylose
L. monocytogenes	+	–	+	–	–	+	–
L. ivanovii	+	–	–	+	–	–	+
L. innocua	–	–	–	–	–	v[d]	–
L. welshimeri	–	–	–	–	–	v	+
L. seeligeri	v	–	+	–	–	–	v
L. denitrificans	–	+	ND[c]	ND	+	–	+
L. murrayi	–	+	ND	ND	+	v	–
L. grayi	–	–	ND	ND	–	–	–

[a]*S. aureus* NCTC 1803.
[b]*R. equi* NCTC 1621.
[c]Not determined.
[d]Variable.
Source: Adapted from Ref. 60.

Table 1.2 Traditional Differentiation of *Listeria* species

Biochemical test	*monocytogenes*	*ivanovii*	*innocua*	*welshimeri*	*seeligeri*	*grayi*	*murrayi*	*denitrificans*[a]
				Listeria sp.				
Dextrose	+	+	+	+	+	+	+	+
Esculin	+	+	+	+	+	+	+	+
Maltose	+	+	+	+	+	+	+	+
Mannitol	−	−	−	−	−	−	+	+
Rhamnose	+	−	V[b]	V	−	−	V	−
Xylose	−	+	−	+	+	−	−	+
Hippurate hydrolysis	+	+	+	+	+	−	−	−
Voges-Proskauer	+	+	+	+	+	+	+	−
Methyl red	+	+	+	+	V	+	+	+
Beta-hemolysis	+	+	−	−	V	−	−	−
Urea hydrolysis	−	−	−	−	−	−	−	−
Nitrate reduction	−	−	−	−	−	−	+	+
Catalase	+	+	+	+	+	+	+	+
H$_2$S on TSI	−	−	−	−	−	−	−	−
H$_2$S by lead acetate strip	−	−	−	−	−	+	+	−
CAMP positive/*S. aureus*	+	−	−	−	+	−	−	−
CAMP positive/*R. equi*	−	+	−	−	−	−	−	−

[a] Reclassified as *Jonesia denitrificans*.
[b] V = variable.
Source: Adapted from Ref. 33.

NUTRITIONAL REQUIREMENTS

Listeria monocytogenes is a nonfastidious organism that can reproduce in simple synthetic media (34,73,86). The bacterium will grow in common casein or gelatin-hydrolysate media containing glucose. The ideal carbohydrate for growth of *L. monocytogenes* is glucose (103), which cannot be replaced as an energy or carbon source by gluconate, xylose, arabinose, or ribose. Intermediate compounds of the pyruvate and citrate cycles also appear to be unsuitable as carbon and energy sources for *L. monocytogenes* (103). Blood and serum are not strict requirements for growth; however, both will enhance growth of the organism in media low in growth factors. Strains of *L. monocytogenes* differ in their need for B vitamins with some strains requiring both pyridoxine and riboflavin. A minimal growth medium for 15 strains of *L. monocytogenes* was developed by Ralovich (73), and included glucose, riboflavin, and biotin together with four amino acids—isoleucine, leucine, valine, and cysteine. Presence of Fe^{2+}, Mg^{2+}, Ca^{2+}, K^+, and PO_4^{3-} also was required for growth. Thioglycolate was added to ensure a low redox potential. Citrate was necessary as a chelating agent. Although not a strict growth requirement, increased levels of thiamine were needed to obtain colonies of reasonable size. In 1989, Chau and Shelef (14) also reported that while riboflavin alone or particularly in combination with biotin stimulated growth of *Listeria* in a different synthetic medium, addition of iron enhanced growth of listeriae only in the presence of riboflavin.

SEROLOGY

Using the serological methods of Kauffmann and White, Paterson (66,67) described four serological types of *L. monocytogenes* based on somatic (O) (from the German *ohne Hauch*) and flagellar (H) (from the German *Hauch*) antigens. Serotypes 1, 3, and 4 were differentiated on the basis of O antigens; whereas identification of serotype 2 was based on a unique H antigen. After additional O antigens were identified, Seeliger split serotype 4 into serotypes 4a and 4b, and Donker-Voet added serotypes 4c, 4d, and 4e to the list of recognized *L. monocytogenes* serotypes (86). Slight differences in H antigens also were observed in some cultures of serotypes 1 and 3, which led to creation of serotypes 1a and 3a (86).

Further studies have demonstrated that the O and H antigens of *Listeria* are complex carbohydrate-containing proteins with partially overlapping and partially specific fractions. The O antigens are heat stable and will survive for 1 hour in phosphate-buffered saline solution at 100°C, whereas the H antigens are heat labile and will not survive such a treatment.

Table 1.3 indicates all presently recognized serotypes of *Listeria* spp. as defined by their O and H antigenic structure. It should be noted that *L. innocua*, *L. ivanovii*, *L. seeligeri*, and *L. welshimeri* can share one or more somatic antigens with *L. monocytogenes*; however, *L. grayi* and *L. murrayi* can be differentiated from the remaining *Listeria* spp. on the basis of the flagellar H antigen (73). Commercial types 1, 4, and polyvalent antisera (Difco Laboratories, Inc., Detroit, MI) are currently available for serotyping *Listeria* isolates using either a slide or tube agglutination test. However, serotyping alone, without thorough biochemical characterization, is inadequate for identifying *L. monocytogenes*

Table 1.3   Serotypes of *Listeria* spp.

Listeria sp.	Serotype	Somatic (O) antigenic structure	Flagellar (H) antigenic structure
L. monocytogenes[a]	1/2a	I II (III)[b]	A B
	1/2b	I II (III)	A B C
	1/2c	I II (III)	B D
	3a	II (III) IV	A B
	3b	II (III) IV (XII) (XIII)	A B C
	3c	II (III) IV (XII) (XIII)	B D
	4a	(III) (V) VII IX	A B C
	4ab	(III) V VI VII IX X	A B C
	4b	(III) V VI	A B C
	4c	(III) V VII	A B C
	4d	(III) (V) VI VIII	A B C
	4e	(III) V VI (VIII) (IX)	A B C
	7	(III) XII XIII	A B C
L. ivanovii	5	(III) (V) VI (VIII) X	A B C
L. innocua	6a ("4f")	(III) V (VI) (VII) (IX) XV	A B C
	6b ("4g")[c]	(III) (V) (VI) (VII) IX X XI	A B C
L. grayi		(III) XII XIV [XVI][d]	E
L. murrayi		(III) XII XIV [XVII][d]	E

[a]*L. seeligeri* cannot be differentiated serologically from *L. monocytogenes*.
[b]( ) = not always present.
[c]*L. welshimeri* cannot be differentiated serologically from *L. innocua* serotype 6b.
[d][ ] = proposed in 1988 by J. Vazquez-Boland et al. (106).
Source: Ref. 88.

since this organism can share many of the same O and H antigens found in other *Listeria* spp. Although serotyping is a valuable tool for identifying isolates of *L. monocytogenes*, the procedure is of only limited value in epidemiological studies of listeriosis since generally about 90% of the isolates belong to only three (1/2a, 1/2b, and 4b) of 13 serotypes as demonstrated by McLauchlin in a survey of 722 clinical isolates in England (60).

PHAGE-TYPING

Phage-typing is based on lysis or destruction of a bacterial cell, which occurs as a result of infection with a highly specific bacteriophage (virus). Traditionally, phage-typing has been done on a solid medium which contains the bacteriophage along with a heavy inoculum of the test organism. After incubation, the extent of cell lysis is determined by counting the number of plaques (clearing zones), which, in turn, provides a quantitative assessment of the specificity of the bacteriophage toward the test organism in question. Successful application of phage-typing to other bacteria such as *S. aureus* prompted development of a phage-typing system for *L. monocytogenes*, which has proven useful in studying transmission and spread of the organism in outbreaks of listeriosis.

Currently, research in this area is focused on developing a comprehensive set of bacteriophages that can be used to phage-type *L. monocytogenes* as well as *L. innocua*, *L. ivanovii*, *L. seeligeri*, and *L. welshimeri* (79). Using various sets of bacteriophages, Rocourt et al. (80), Taylor et al. (101,102), and McLauchlin et al. (61) were able to phage-type 645 of 823 (78%), 131 of 186 (70%), 147 of 249 (59%), and 78 of 112 (64%) of the *L. monocytogenes* strains tested, respectively. Further examination of their data indicates that 5.7–37.0% and 75.5–87.2% of the strains belonging to serotypes 1 and 4, respectively, could be phage-typed. Using a set of 27 bacteriophages (six derived from serotypes 1/2a and 1/2b, eight from serotype 4b and 13 from serotypes 3c, 4ab, 5, 6a, and 7), Audurier et al. (5) determined that 108 of 186 (58.1%) isolates of *L. monocytogenes* serotype 4b obtained from a listeriosis outbreak in France belonged to a single phage type.

An international collaborative study has since been initiated to characterize, evaluate, and exchange phages to produce a more useful phage set for routine use. An international center has been established at the Pasteur Institute for identification and/or phage-typing of *Listeria* strains primarily of European origin submitted to this center for analysis since 1987. With this recent progress, phage-typing is likely to become a powerful investigative tool in future listeriosis outbreaks.

DNA RESTRICTION ANALYSIS

Despite recent successes in phage-typing and serotyping, epidemiological investigations frequently uncover *L. monocytogenes* strains that cannot be typed. Difficulties in phage-typing approximately 36% of the *L. monocytogenes* strains isolated in Britain led McLauchlin et al. (62) to develop a typing system based on DNA probe methodology. In their preliminary study, electrophoretically separated DNA fragments from 24 epidemiologically unrelated strains of *L. monocytogenes* were probed with biotin-labeled DNA sequences from *L. monocytogenes* and gave rise to eight different DNA hybridization patterns. Later, 15 different hybridization patterns were observed among 26 strains of *L. monocytogenes* that belonged to serotype 1/2 (85). In 1988 Facinelli et al. (22) attempted to characterize 45 *Listeria* cultures isolated from human, animal, and environmental sources according to serotype, phage-type, and the pattern obtained after treating chromosomal DNA with restriction endonucleases (Bam H1, Eco R1, and Hind III). Their results indicate that treatment of DNA with restriction enzymes could be used to type previously nontypeable strains of *Listeria*. Following further investigations, DNA probe assays and restriction endonuclease analysis may both become important epidemiological tools for tracking the spread of foodborne listeriosis.

ELECTROPHORETIC ENZYME TYPING

Multilocus enzyme electrophoresis (a method by which bacterial strains are differentiated according to electrophoretic motility of numerous metabolic enzymes) has been
used to study the genetic relatedness and epidemiology of several bacterial pathogens,
including *L. monocytogenes*. Piffaretti et al. (69) identified 45 distinctive electrophoretic
enzyme types of *L. monocytogenes* among 145 isolates obtained from human, animal,
and environmental sources in Europe, North America, and New Zealand. Cluster analysis
showed that all *Listeria* isolates could be grouped into one of two phylogenetic divisions
where divisions I and II contained only those strains belonging to serotypes 1/2b, 4a
and 4b, or 1/2a and 1/2c, respectively. Furthermore, both divisions included clinical and
environmental isolates, which is consistent with current evidence indicating that strains
responsible for human illness can be acquired from animal and environmental sources.
These researchers later identified 17 and 11 distinctive electrophoretic enzyme types
among 77 *L. monocytogenes* and 20 *L. innocua* isolates from clinical and environmental
sources, respectively (50). All *L. monocytogenes* isolates again belonged to one of two
distinctive phylogenetic divisions.

In 1988, CDC officials in Atlanta reported electrophoretically typing 309 *L.
monocytogenes* strains obtained from clinical specimens and various foods (31). Overall,
53 different electrophoretic enzyme types were discovered with 28, 12, and 9 enzyme
types identified among strains belonging to serotypes 1/2a, 1/2b, and 4b, respectively.
Furthermore, only two enzyme types contained strains belonging to more than one
serotype. Thus, as was true for phage-typing and DNA restriction analysis, electrophoretic
enzyme-typing also is likely to become increasingly important to investigators of
listeriosis outbreaks.

PATHOGENICITY AND PATHOGENESIS

Three of eight *Listeria* spp.—*L. monocytogenes*, *L. ivanovii*, and *L. seeligeri*—can cause
human and/or animal infections (40,91); however, cases involving the latter organism
are exceedingly rare, with only two cases of animal (76) and one case of human listeriosis
(84) thus far recorded. Despite one report that a single strain of *L. innocua* (strain 5-12
Welshimer) produced localized encephalitis in suckling mice (87), this bacterium is
universally accepted as being nonpathogenic as implied by the species name *innocua*
(from innocuous). Human infections by *L. ivanovii* also are rare, with only three
documented cases (12,76). Although *L. ivanovii* reportedly accounted for approximately
10% of the cases of animal listeriosis in Bulgaria (42), this organism is generally
considered far less virulent than *L. monocytogenes* (91). Since *L. monocytogenes* is
currently responsible for virtually all cases of human listeriosis and approximately 90%
of the listeriosis cases involving animals, the following discussion of virulence will focus
almost exclusively on *L. monocytogenes*.

Although the pathogenic nature of *L. monocytogenes* has been recognized for more
than 60 years, the mechanism by which this organism causes illness is highly complex and
remains poorly understood. For this discussion, the process by which *L. monocytogenes*
causes disease has been divided into three general steps—(a) penetration of the host,

(b) survival and multiplication of the organism within the host, and (c) invasion of target tissue.

Recently, Gaillard et al. (26) suggested that the intestinal tract may well be the primary site of entry for *L. monocytogenes*. The frequent occurrence of gastrointestinal symptoms at the onset of illness and the firmly established link between consumption of contaminated food and at least four outbreaks of listeriosis leads one to believe that listeriosis may be predominantly a foodborne infection. However, since approximately 5% of the general population harbors *L. monocytogenes* in its gastrointestinal tract, it is difficult to explain the extremely low incidence of human listeriosis. While still a topic of considerable debate, Seeliger (89) recently suggested that numerous subclinical infections that are thought to occur may lead to a state of immunity in large segments of the general population.

Once ingested, *L. monocytogenes* penetrates the intestinal lining and begins to multiply within the host. Hence, *L. monocytogenes* can be classified as an enteroinvasive pathogen. At least two distinct theories have been proposed concerning the site of penetration and replication once the organism has entered the intestinal tract. According to Racz et al. (72), epithelial cells lining the intestine serve both as a site of entry and as a site for bacterial multiplication before phagocytosis of the organism by macrophages lying within the lamina propria of the intestine. In contrast, MacDonald and Carter (57) suggested a two-stage process in which *L. monocytogenes* first crosses the intestinal barrier in M cells (specialized cells found in Peyer's patches in the intestine) and then begins replicating after being phagocytized by macrophages.

In the final step of the infectious process, *L. monocytogenes* lyses the macrophage and crosses the capillary epithelium to produce a septicemia. The pathogen then gains access to target organs (i.e., placenta and central nervous system including the brain) to cause an abortion or produce symptoms in the host that are characteristic of meningioencephalitis.

VIRULENCE FACTORS

Bacterial virulence (or pathogenicity) factors include all bacterially produced substances that allow an organism to cause illness or infection. As previously noted, *L. monocytogenes* must survive the acidity of the stomach, penetrate the intestinal lining, and grow in the host before the organism can produce illness. Like other enteroinvasive pathogens, *L. monocytogenes* possesses a variety of virulence factors that damage the host's tissue, thus allowing the organism to invade the bloodstream and produce illness. Those virulence factors that contribute to the disease-causing capability of *L. monocytogenes* include one or more hemolysins, a monocyte-promoting agent, various cell wall/cell membrane constituents, toxic oxygen species, and several undefined toxins.

The ability of *L. monocytogenes* to hemolyze blood was first recognized by Anton (2) in 1934; however, hemolysin production was not associated with virulence until 1962. In that year, Liu and Bates (54) reported that mice died following exposure to a filtrate from a culture of *L. monocytogenes* that contained hemolysin. Two years later, Njoku-Obi et al. (64) characterized this water-soluble hemolysin as a heat-labile protein inactivated by filtration but reactivated by addition of sodium thiosulfate. Hemolytic activity also was optimal at pH 5.5 but was greatly reduced at pH 7. Later work showed that this hemolysin reacted with antibody to streptolysin o (the β-hemolysin produced by *Streptococcus pyogenes*) (44) and, like streptolysin o, also possessed cardiotoxic activity (48). In addition, lytic activity of this hemolysin was reportedly suppressed by exposure to cholesterol (36) and enhanced at refrigeration temperatures (7) and in the presence of reducing agents (64). Although the molecular weight (MW) of this hemolysin was reported to range between 10,000 (92) and 170,000 (47), a lipolytic material of MW approximately 52,500 later was found to be associated with the hemolysin identified in the latter report (43).

Currently, *L. monocytogenes* hemolysin, also known as listeriolysin o, is generally recognized as a sulfhydral-activated, cholesterol-inhibited cytolysin that is antigenically similar to streptolysin o (16,32) and is composed of a single polypeptide chain of MW approximately 60,000. However, several reports indicate that *L. monocytogenes* produces one or more hemolysins that are immunologically (53,65), genetically (107), and presumably molecularly distinct from listeriolysin o. Recently, Parrisius et al. (65) proposed that the streptolysin o–related toxin (listeriolysin o) be designated as α-listeriolysin and that the remaining hemolysin(s) that does not cross-react with streptolysin o be designated as β-listeriolysin. In fact, β-hemolytic activity in 26 of 28 *L. monocytogenes* strains appeared to result from production of β-listeriolysin rather than streptolysin o–related α-listeriolysin. Present findings indicate that β-listeriolysin also may be responsible for the positive CAMP reaction typical of *L. monocytogenes*.

Secretion of hemolysin has been proposed as an important factor for promoting virulence of *L. monocytogenes*. This hypothesis is strongly supported by the fact that all *L. monocytogenes* strains isolated from natural infections have been both β-hemolytic and virulent in animal models (35,38,64,78,94), whereas atypical nonhemolytic strains isolated from environmental sources are invariably avirulent (35,38). [Although nonvirulent β-hemolytic strains of *L. monocytogenes* have been occasionally isolated from food and environmental samples (15,56), the apparent lack of pathogenicity has not yet been explained.] Furthermore, Gaillard et al. (25) found that loss of the gene coding for hemolysin in a virulent strain of *L. monocytogenes* led to production of a nonvirulent mutant with virulence being restored in a hemolysin-producing revertant strain. These and other findings (16) indicate that the gene coding for hemolysin in *L. monocytogenes* is at least partly responsible for the organism's virulence. However, while Rocourt and Seeliger (77) reported that hemolysin produced by *L. seeligeri* (another β-hemolytic *Listeria* spp. of which all but one known isolate is avirulent) is biologically and structurally distinct from hemolysin produced by *L. monocytogenes*, other researchers (49,52) later showed that listeriolysins produced by *L. monocytogenes*, *L. seeligeri*, and/or *L. ivanovii* are immunologically related. Nonetheless, it appears that while all β-hemolytic strains of *L. monocytogenes* are virulent, production of hemolysin by other *Listeria* spp. does not necessarily attest to an organism's virulence.

Current findings concerning the action of hemolysin in vivo agree with a model developed by Armstrong and Sword (3,99) over 20 years ago which explains intracellular growth of *L. monocytogenes*. The sequence of events after *L. monocytogenes* has penetrated the host begins with rapid phagocytosis of the invading bacterium (58) in an iron-poor environment (11), which in turn stimulates secretion of hemolysin (17,18). The acidic environment within phagosomes of macrophages also serves to increase hemolysin production. Irreversible binding of hemolysin to membrane cholesterol is followed by lysis of the intracellular membrane and release of listeriae into the cytoplasm, which in turn provides a more favorable environment (increased iron availability and higher pH) for bacterial growth. Following dissemination of *L. monocytogenes* within the host, local production of hemolysin associated with further bacterial growth also has been linked to formation of infective foci which appear in the spleen and liver during later stages of infection.

Several in vitro tests based on hemolysin production have been proposed for routine differentiation of pathogenic and nonpathogenic strains of *L. monocytogenes*. Equi-factor, a purified extracellular substance produced by *R. equi*, has been used in the CAMP test to enhance β-hemolysis of various pathogenic (to mice and guinea pigs) *L. monocytogenes* strains grown on agar containing 5% (w/v) sheep (93,94), horse (93), or human blood. A positive result for the CAMP test which suggests pathogenicity also was frequently associated with fermentation of rhamnose and nonfermentation of xylose (17).

In addition to hemolysin, cell wall components including peptidoglycan, lipoteichoic acid, and teichoic acid (23,105) also appear to play a role in virulence of *L. monocytogenes*. In fact, peptidoglycan is directly responsible for resistance of *L. monocytogenes* to lysozyme (an enzyme secreted by macrophages that degrades bacterial cell walls), which in turn contributes to the organism's survival within macrophages (27). For many years it was recognized that so-called rough strains of *L. monocytogenes* are far less virulent than smooth strains of the same organism. Although the reason for cell roughness is not yet fully understood, protein composition of the cell wall of rough strains appears to be altered from that of smooth strains (39). Loss of particular cell wall proteins may enhance the vulnerability of *L. monocytogenes* to the bactericidal action of macrophages.

Other cell wall constituents that may influence the virulence of *L. monocytogenes* are poorly understood. While lipids may increase intracellular survival of *L. monocytogenes*, the location of these lipids on the cell surface has not yet been determined (39). Several additional potentially toxic cell wall components of *L. monocytogenes* have been listed by Ralovich (73) and include (a) a water-soluble polysaccharide that induces lymphopenia and granulocytosis, (b) protein- and carbohydrate-containing extracts that are antigenic, pyrogenic, and able to induce lymphopenia and granulocytosis, and (c) a fractionated glycine lysate that was pyrogenic and able to induce granulocytosis. In addition, Wexler and Oppenheim (89) isolated an endotoxin lipopolysaccharide-like substance (similar to endotoxins produced by gram-negative bacteria) that was both pyrogenic and lethal to rabbits.

In 1924 Murray et al. (63) observed a pronounced monocytosis in rabbits infected with *L. monocytogenes* from which the organism derived its name. After considerable research, which was summarized by Ralovich (73), an anionic material possessing monocytosis-producing activity (MPA) was extracted from the cell membrane of *L. monocytogenes* (29,100). MPA reportedly has a MW of approximately 1000 and does not contain amino acids or carbohydrates. Regarding its biological activity, MPA stimulates monocyte but not lymphocyte or macrophage activity. While MPA is nontoxic to mice, macrophages become nonviable in vitro following 24 hours of incubation with MPA (28). In addition to MPA, extracts of heat-killed *L. monocytogenes* cells possess immunosuppressive activity (27). This active substance which induces suppressor macrophages and granulocytosis is composed of amino acids, carbohydrates, phosphorus, and glycerol and has a MW of approximately 150,000.

Research has shown that other biochemical markers also may be related to virulence. In 1962, *L. monocytogenes* was found to produce a lipolysin in an egg yolk medium (24). Although at the time only virulent strains consistently demonstrated lipolytic activity, lipolytic and hemolytic activity were since found to be independent of each other (73).

Virulence of *L. monocytogenes* also may be related to production of various toxic oxygen species. Godfrey and Wilder (31) demonstrated that two virulent strains of *L. monocytogenes* producing high levels of hydrogen peroxide and superoxide anion survived longer in macrophages obtained from mice than did an avirulent strain that produced only low levels of these two oxygen species. These findings suggest that pathogenic strains of *L. monocytogenes* may produce sufficient quantities of catalase (degrades hydrogen peroxide) and superoxide dismutase (degrades superoxide anion) to detoxify similar bactericidal factors produced within phagocytes (27). In addition, specific activity of superoxide dismutase increases in the presence of iron—a substance which has already been shown to increase susceptibility of mice to listeric infections.

Finally, Tysganova et al. (104) reported that virulent strains of *L. monocytogenes* exhibit higher levels of adenosine triphosphatase activity than do weakly virulent strains. In addition, lactate dehydrogenase activity was higher in weakly virulent than in virulent strains. Although many of these results appear interesting, further research is needed to more clearly define these proposed virulence factors using a larger number of *L. monocytogenes* strains.

PATHOGENICITY TESTING

As previously noted, all β-hemolytic strains of *L. monocytogenes* isolated from natural infections can be assumed to be pathogenic. While pathogenicity testing of typical β-hemolytic strains of *L. monocytogenes* isolated from food is listed as "optional" in identification procedures recommended by the FDA (55) and USDA (59), such a recommendation complies with public health concerns by removing contaminated product from the marketplace as quickly as possible. Nonetheless, it appears that virulence testing of *L. monocytogenes* isolates may be advisable, particularly if such a situation is likely to prompt legal action by the parties involved.

The only currently acceptable way of determining pathogenicity of an isolate of *L. monocytogenes* is by inoculating an animal with the test organism. Beginning in 1934, the Anton test was used to determine virulence of isolates suspected to be *L. monocytogenes* (73). In this procedure, one loopful of a 24-hour-old *L. monocytogenes* culture is inoculated into the conjunctival sac of a rabbit or guinea pig. If the organism is pathogenic, the test animal will develop purulent conjunctivitis 1–5 days after inoculation.

The other classical means of determining virulence is by inoculating the chorio-allantoic membrane of a chicken embryo with *L. monocytogenes* (73). After several days of incubation, pathogenic strains produce lesions in the liver, heart muscle, and central nervous system that closely resemble those of naturally occurring listeriosis.

Today these classical virulence tests have largely been replaced by the mouse pathogenicity assay. In this test, *L. monocytogenes* is grown in Trypticase Soy Broth-Yeast Extract at 35°C for 24 hours and then subcultured in duplicate in the same medium under the same conditions. Ten milliliters of the 24-hour-old culture are then centrifuged at $1600 \times g$ for 30 minutes. After resuspending the pellet in 1 ml of 0.85% saline solution

($\sim 10^{10}$ *Listeria* cells/ml), each of five 16–18-g Swiss white mice are injected inter-peritoneally with 0.1 ml of the suspension ($\sim 10^9$ *Listeria* cells/mouse). Pathogenic strains normally kill all five mice within 7 days (often within 5 days), whereas nonpatho-genic isolates are not fatal to the mice. This test should always be accompanied by use of known pathogenic (*L. monocytogenes*) and nonpathogenic (*L. innocua*) *Listeria* strains as controls.

While results from the mouse pathogenicity assay are widely accepted by the scientific community, maintaining sufficient numbers of mice for routine testing is expensive and time-consuming. Hence, a need exists for other types of *Listeria* patho-genicity models. Among the more promising models is the chick embryo, which was first proposed by Paterson in 1940 (68). According to the author, all chick embryos died within 72 hours after *L. monocytogenes* was inoculated onto exposed egg membranes or injected into the allantoic sac. Equally important, one nonvirulent and three rough *Listeria* strains failed to establish infection. Many years later, Basher et al. (6) found that 120–160 viable *L. monocytogenes* cells killed half of the chick embryos examined when the pathogen was inoculated onto the allantoic sac of fertile hens' eggs.

In response to recent public health concerns, Steinmeyer et al. (95) have attempted to revive interest in the chick embryo as a model for pathogenicity testing. For each strain tested, the chorioallantoic membrane of each of five 10-day-old chick embryos was inoculated with 0.1 ml of a *Listeria* culture diluted in Ringer solution (100–30,000 *Listeria* cells/egg). While all embryos inoculated with pathogenic strains died within 72 hours, embryos in eggs inoculated with nonpathogenic strains survived.

Even though chick embryos are more economical to use than mice, researchers are continuing to develop other types of pathogenicity assays using chick embryo fibroblast cells (8) as well as more conventional types of cell cultures and protozoa. If successful, such assays will be simpler and even more economical to use than the proposed chick embryo assay.

REFERENCES

1. Anonymous. 1954. Opinion 12. *Intern. Bull. Bacteriol. Nomencl. Taxon.* 4:150–151.
2. Anton, W. 1934. Kritisch-experimenteller Beitrag zur Biologie des *Bacterium monocytogenes*. Mit besonderer Berücksichtigung seiner Beziehung zur infektiösen Mononucleose des Menschen. *Zbl. Bakteriol. I Abt. Orig. 131*:89–103.
3. Armstrong, B. A., and C. P. Sword. 1966. Electron microscopy of *Listeria monocytogenes*-infected mouse spleen. *J. Bacteriol. 91*:1346–1355.
4. Atkinson, E. 1917. Meningitis associated with gram-positive bacilli of diphtheroid type. *Med. J. Australia 1*:115–118.
5. Audurier, A., A. G. Taylor, B. Carbonnelle, and J. McLauchlin. 1984. A phage typing system for *Listeria monocytogenes* and its use in epidemiological studies. *Clin. Invest. Med.* 7:229–232.
6. Basher, H. A., D. R. Fowler, F. G. Rodgers, A. Seaman, and M. Woodbine. 1984. Pathogenesis and growth of *Listeria monocytogenes* in fertile hens' eggs. *Zbl. Bakteriol. Hyg. A 256*:497–509.
7. Basher, H. A., D. R. Fowler, F. G. Rodgers, A. Seaman, and M. Woodbine. 1984. Role of haemolysin and temperature in the pathogenesis of *Listeria monocytogenes* in fertile hens' eggs. *Zbl. Bakteriol. Hyg. A 258*:223–231.
8. Basher, H. A., D. R. Fowler, A. Seaman, and M. Woodbine. 1985. Intra-cellular and extra-cellular growth of *L. monocytogenes* in chick embryo fibroblast cell culture. *Zbl. Bakteriol. Hyg. A 260*:51–56.

9. Bojsen-Møller, J. 1972. Human listeriosis—diagnostic, epidemiological and clinical studies. *Acta Pathol. Microbiol. Scand. Section B.* (Suppl.) *229*:1–157.

10. Breed, R. S., E. G. D. Murray, and A. P. Hitchens. 1948. *Bergey's Manual of Determinative Bacteriology*, 6th ed., Williams and Wilkins Co., Baltimore.

11. Bullen, J. J. 1981. The significance of iron in infection. *Rev. Infect. Dis. 3*:1127–1138.

12. Busch, L. A. 1971. New from the Center for Disease Control—human listeriosis in the United States, 1967–1969. *J. Infect. Dis. 123*:328–332.

13. Chatelain, R., and L. Second. 1976. Taxonomie numérique de quelques *Brevibacterium. Ann. Inst. Pasteur. 111*:630–644.

14. Chau, M. Y., and L. A. Shelef. 1989. Nutritional requirements of *Listeria* spp. Abst. Ann. Mtg. Amer. Soc. Microbiology, New Orleans, LA, May 14–18, Abst. I-133.

15. Conner, D. E., V. N. Scott, and D. T. Bernard. 1988. Pathogenicity of foodborne, environmental, and clinical isolates of *Listeria monocytogenes*. Ann. Mtg. Inst. Food Technol., New Orleans, LA, June 19–22, Abst. 322.

16. Cossart, P. 1988. The listeriolysin o gene: A chromosomal locus crucial for the virulence of *Listeria monocytogenes*. *Infection 16* (Suppl. 2):157–159.

17. Cowart, R. E. 1987. Iron regulation of growth and haemolysin production by *Listeria monocytogenes. Ann. Inst. Pasteur Microbiol. 138*:246–249.

18. Cowart, R. E., and B. G. Foster. 1985. Differential effects of iron on the growth of *Listeria monocytogenes*: Minimum requirements and mechanism of acquisition. *J. Infect. Dis. 151*:721–730.

19. Daneshvar, M. I., J. B. Brooks, G. B. Malcolm, and L. Pine. 1989. Analysis of fermentation products of *Listeria* species by frequency-pulsed electron-capture gas-liquid chromatography. *Can. J. Microbiol. 35*:786–793.

20. Dick, G. F. 1920. A case of cerebrospinal meningitis due to a diphtheroid bacillus. *J. Amer. Med. Assoc. 74*:84.

21. Dumont, J., and L. Cotoni. 1921. Bacille semblable au bacille du rouget du porc recontré dans le liquide céphalo-rachidien d'un méingitique. *Ann. Inst. Pasteur 35*:625–633.

22. Facinelli, B., C. Casolari, and V. Fabio. 1988. Restriction endonuclease analysis of the chromosomal DNA of *Listeria monocytogenes* and other species of the genus *Listeria*. Abstr. Annu. Mtg. Amer. Soc. Microbiol., Miami Beach, FL, May 8–13, Abstr. C-176.

23. Fiedler, F. 1988. Biochemistry of the cell surface of *Listeria* strains: A locating general view. *Infection 16* (Suppl. 2):92–97.

24. Füzi, M., and T. Pillis. 1962. Production of opacity in egg-yolk medium by *Listeria monocytogenes. Nature 196*:195.

25. Gaillard, J.-L., P. Berche, and P. Sansonctti. 1986. Transposon mutagenesis as a tool to study the role of hemolysis in the virulence of *Listeria monocytogenes. Infect. Immun. 52*:50–55.

26. Gaillard, J.-L., P. Berche, J. Mounier, S. Richard, and P. Sansonetti. 1987. Penetration of *Listeria monocytogenes* into the host: A crucial step of the infectious process. *Ann. Microbiol. 138*::259–264.

27. Galsworthy, S. B. 1987. Role of the cell surface in virulence of *Listeria monocytogenes. Ann. Inst. Pasteur Microbiol. 138*:273–276.

28. Galsworthy, S. B., and D. Fewster. 1988. Comparison of responsiveness to the monocytosis-producing activity of *Listeria monocytogenes* in mice genetically susceptible or resistant to listeriosis. *Infection 16* (Suppl. 2):118–122.

29. Galsworthy, S. B., S. M. Gurofsky, and R. G. E. Murray. 1977. Purification of a monocytosis-producing activity from *Listeria monocytogenes. Infect. Immun. 15*:500–509.

30. Gellin, B., W. Bibb, R. Weaver, and C. V. Broome. 1988. Enzyme typing clarifies the epidemiology of listeriosis. *Interscience Conf. Antimicrobial. Agents Chemotherapy*, Los Angeles, CA, Oct. 23–26, Abst. 1109.

31. Godfrey, R. W., and M. S. Wilder. 1985. Generation of oxygen species and virulence of *Listeria monocytogenes. Infect. Immun. 47*:837–839.

32. Goebel, W., S. Kathariou, M. Kuhn, Z. Sokolovic, J. Kreft, S. Köhler, D. Funke, T. Chakraborty,

and M. Leimeister-Wächter. 1988. Hemolysin from *Listeria*—biochemistry, genetics and function in pathogenesis. *Infection 16* (Suppl. 2):149–156.

33. Gray, M. L., and A. H. Killinger. 1966. *Listeria monocytogenes* and listeric infections. *Bacteriol. Rev. 30*:309–382.

34. Gray, M. L. 1960. Isolation of *Listeria monocytogenes* from oat silage. *Science 132*:1767–1768.

35. Groves, R. D., and H. J. Welshimer. 1977. Separation of pathogenic from apathogenic *Listeria monocytogenes* by three in vitro reactions. *J. Clin. Microbiol. 5*:559–563.

36. Hayes, P. S., J. C. Feeley, L. M. Graves, G. W. Ajello, and D. W. Fleming. 1986. Isolation of *Listeria monocytogenes* from raw milk. *Appl. Environ. Microbiol. 51*:438–440.

37. Henry, B. S. 1933. Dissociation in the genus *Brucella. J. Infect. Dis. 52*:374–402.

38. Hof, B. 1984. Virulence of different strains of *Listeria monocytogenes* serovar 1/2a. *Med. Microbiol. Immunol. 173*:207–218.

39. Hof, H., and S. Chatzipanagiotou. 1987. The role of surface structures of *Listeria* spp. for pathogenicity. *Ann. Inst. Pasteur Microbiol. 138*:268–273.

40. Hof, H., and P. Hefner. 1988. Pathogenicity of *Listeria monocytogenes* in comparison to other *Listeria* species. *Infection 16* (Suppl. 2):141–144.

41. Hülphers, G. 1911. Lefvernekros has kanin orsakad af en ej förut beskrifven bacterie. *Sven. Vet. Tidskr. 16*:265–273. Reprinted: 1959, *Medlemsbl. Sverge. Bet. Förb. 11*(Suppl.):10–16.

42. Ivanov, I., and N. Massalaski. 1979. Listeriosis in Bulgaria. In I. Ivanov (ed.), *Problems of Listeriosis.* National Agroindustriol Union, Sofia. Quoted in McLauchlin, J. 1987. A review— *Listeria monocytogenes*, recent advances in the taxonomy and epidemiology of listeriosis in humans. *J. Appl. Bacteriol. 63*:1–11.

43. Jenkins, E. M., and B. B. Watson. 1971. Extracellular antigens from *Listeria monocytogenes.* I. Purification and resolution of hemolytic and lipolytic antigens from culture filtrates of *Listeria monocytogenes. Infect. Immun. 3*:589–594.

44. Jenkins, E. M., A. N. Njoku-Obi, and E. W. Adams. 1964. Purification of the soluble hemolysins of *Listeria monocytogenes. J. Bacteriol. 88*:418–424.

45. Jones, D. 1975. A numerical taxonomic study of coryneform and related bacteria. *J. Gen. Microbiol. 87*:52–96.

46. Jones, D., and H. P. R. Seeliger. 1986. International committee on systematic bacteriology subcommittee on the taxonomy of *Listeria* and related bacteria. *Int. J. Syst. Bacteriol. 36*:117–118.

47. Kingdon, G. C., and C. P. Sword. 1970. Biochemical effects of *Listeria monocytogenes* hemolysin. *Infect. Immun. 1*:363–372.

48. Kingdon, G. C., and C. P. Sword. 1970. Cardiotoxic and lethal effects of *Listeria monocytogenes* hemolysin. *Infect. Immun. 1*:373–379.

49. Leifson, E., and M. I. Palen. 1955. Variations and spontaneous mutations in the genus *Listeria* in respect to flagellation and motility. *J. Bacteriol. 70*:233–240.

50. Kreft, J., D. Funke, A. Haas, F. Lottspeich, and W. Goebel. 1989. Production, purification and characterization of hemolysin from *L. ivanovii* and *L. monocytogenes* serovar 4b. *FEMS Microbiol. Lett. 57*:197–202.

51. Kressebuch, H., M. Aeschbacher, J. Bille, E. Bannerman, J. Rocourt, and J. C. Piffaretti. 1988. Genetic analysis of populations in the genus *Listeria.* Ann. Mtg. Amer. Soc. Microbiol., Miami Beach, FL, May 8–13, Abst. D-65.

52. Leimeister-Wächter, M., and T. Chakraborty. 1989. Detection of listeriolysin, the thiol-dependent hemolysin in *Listeria monocytogenes*, *Listeria ivanovii*, and *Listeria seeligeri. Infect. Immun. 57*:2350–2357.

53. Leimeister-Wächter, M., T. Chakraborty, and W. Goebel. 1987. Detection and presence of two haemolytic factors in *Listeria* spp. *Ann. Inst. Pasteur Microbiol. 138*:252–256.

54. Liu, P. V., and J. L. Bates. 1961. An extracellular haemorrhagic toxin produced by *L. monocytogenes. Can. J. Microbiol. 7*:107–108.

55. Lovett, J., and A. D. Hitchins. 1988. Listeria isolation—revised method of analysis (Oct. 13). In *Bacteriological Analytical Manual*, Food and Drug Administration, Washington, DC.

56. Lovett, J., D. W. Francis, and J. M. Hunt. 1987. *Listeria monocytogenes* in raw milk: Detection, incidence, and pathogenicity. *J. Food Prot. 50*:188–192.
57. MacDonald, T. T., and P. B. Carter. 1980. Cell-mediated immunity to intestinal infection. *Infect. Immun. 28*:516–523.
58. Mackaness, G. B. 1962. Cellular resistance to infection. *J. Exp. Med. 116*:381–406.
59. McClain, D., and W. H. Lee. 1988. Development of USDA-FSIS method for isolation of *Listeria monocytogenes* from raw meat and poultry. *J. Assoc. Off. Anal. Chem. 71*:660–664.
60. McLauchlin, J. 1987. A review—*Listeria monocytogenes*: Recent advances in the taxonomy and epidemiology of listeriosis in humans. *J. Appl. Bacteriol. 63*:1–11.
61. McLauchlin, J., A. Audurier, and A. G. Taylor. The evaluation of a phage-typing system for *Listeria monocytogenes* for use in epidemiological studies. *J. Med. Microbiol. 22*:357–365.
62. McLauchlin, J., N. A. Saunders, A. M. Ridley, and A. G. Taylor. 1988. Listeriosis and food-borne transmission. *Lancet i*:177–178.
63. Murray, E. G. D., R. A. Webb, and M. B. R. Swann. 1926. A disease of rabbits characterised by a large mononuclear leucocytosis, caused by a hitherto undescribed bacillus *Bacterium monocytogenes* (n. sp.). *J. Pathol. Bacteriol. 29*:407–439.
64. Njoku-Obi, A. N., E. M. Jenkins, J. C. Njoku-Obi, J. Adams, and V. Covington. 1963. Production and nature of *Listeria monocytogenes* hemolysins. *J. Bacteriol. 86*:1–8.
65. Parrisius, J., S. Bhakdi, M. Roth, J. Tranum-Jensen, W. Goebel, and H. P. R. Seeliger. 1986. Production of listeriolysin by beta-hemolytic strains of *Listeria monocytogenes. Infect. Immun. 51*:314–319.
66. Paterson, J. S. 1939. Flagellar antigens of organisms of the genus *Listerella. J. Pathol. Bacteriol. 48*:25–32.
67. Paterson, J. S. 1940. Antigenic structure of organisms of the genus *Listerella. J. Pathol. Bacteriol. 51*:427–436.
68. Paterson, J. S. 1940. Experimental infection of the chick embryo with organisms of the genus *Listerella. J. Pathol. Bacteriol. 51*:437–440.
69. Piffaretti, J.-C., H. Dressebach, M. Aeschbacher, J. Bille, E. Bannerman, J. M. Musser, R. K. Selander, and J. Rocourt. 1989. Genetic characterization of clones of the bacterium *Listeria monocytogenes* causing epidemic listeriosis. *Proc. Nat. Acad. Sci. USA 86*:3818–3822.
70. Pine, L., G. B. Malcolm, J. B. Brooks, and M. I. Daneshvar. 1989. Physiological studies on the growth and utilization of sugars by *Listeria* species. *Can. J. Microbiol. 35*:245–254.
71. Pirie, J. H. H. 1940. *Listeria*: Change of name for a genus of bacteria. *Nature 145*:264.
72. Racz, P., K. Tennar, and E. Mérö. 1972. Experimental *Listeria* enteritis. I. An electron microscopic study of the epithelial phase in experimental *Listeria* infection. *Lab. Invest. 26*:694–700.
73. Ralovich, B. 1984. *Listeriosis Research—Present Situation and Perspective*. Akademiai Kiado, Budapest.
74. Rocourt, J. 1987. Identification of *Listeria* isolates. In A. Schönberg (ed.), *Listeriosis—Joint WHO/ROI Consultation on Prevention and Control*, West Berlin, December 10–12, 1986, pp. 134–135. Institut für Veterinärmedizin des Bundesgesundheitsamtes, Berlin.
75. Rocourt, J., and B. Catimel. 1988. International phage typing center for *Listeria*: Report for 1987. 10th International Symposium on Listeriosis, Pecs, Hungary, Aug. 11–26, Abst. no. 40.
76. Rocourt, J., and H. P. R. Seeliger. 1985. Classification of different *Listeria* species. *Zbl. Bakteriol. Hyg. A 259*:317–330.
77. Rocourt, J., and H. P. R. Seeliger. 1987. Is haemolysin an *in vitro* marker of the pathogenic strains of the genus *Listeria? Ann. Inst. Pasteur Microbiol. 138*:277–279.
78. Rocourt, J., J.-M. Alonso, and H. P. R. Seeliger. 1983. Comparative virulence toward the five genomic groups of *Listeria monocytogenes* (*sensu lato*). *Ann.. Inst. Pasteur Microbiol. 134 A*:359–364.
79. Rocourt, J., B. Catimel, and A. Schrettenbrunner. 1985. Isolation of *Listeria seeligeri* and *L. welshimeri* phages: Phage-typing of *L. monocytogenes, L. ivanovii, L. innocua, L. seeligeri* and *L. welshimeri. Zbl. Bakteriol. Hyg. A 259*:341–350.
80. Rocourt, J., A Schrettenbrunner, and H. P. R. Seeliger. 1982. Isolation of bacteriophages from

Listeria monocytogenes serovar 5 and *Listeria innocua. Zbl. Bakteriol. Hyg., I Abt. Orig. A 251*:505–511.

81. Rocourt, J., A. Schrettenbrunner, and H. P. R. Seeliger. 1983. Biochemical differentiation of the *Listeria monocytogenes* (*sensu lato*) genomic group. *Ann. Inst. Pasteur Microbiol. 134 A*:64–71.

82. Rocourt, J., U. Wehmeyer, and E. Stackebrandt. 1987. Transfer of *Listeria denitrificans* to a new genus, *Jonesia* gen. nov. as *Jonesia denitrificans* comb. nov. *Int. J. Syst. Bacteriol. 37*:266–270.

83. Rocourt, J., U. Wehmeyer, P. Cossart, and E. Stackebrandt. 1987. Proposal to retain *Listeria murrayi* and *Listeria grayi* in the genus *Listeria. Int. J. Syst. Bacteriol. 37*:298–300.

84. Rocourt, J., H. Hof, A. Schrettenbrunner, R. Malinverni, and J. Bille. 1986. Méingite purulente aiguë à *Listeria seeligeri* chez un adulte immunocompétent. *Schweiz. med. Wschr. 116*:248–251.

85. Saunders, N. A., A. M. Ridley, J. McLauchlin, and A. G. Taylor. 1988. Typing of *L. monocytogenes* for epidemiological studies using DNA probes. 10th International Symposium on Listeriosis, Pecs, Hungary, Aug. 22–26, Abst. 36.

86. Seeliger, H. P. R. 1961. *Listeriosis*, Hafner Publishing Co., New York.

87. Seeliger, H. P. R. 1981. Nonpathogenic listeriae: *L. innocua* sp. n. *Zbl. Bakteriol. Hyg., I Abt. Orig. A 249*:487–493.

88. Seeliger, H. P. R. 1987. Classification of pathogenicity of *Listeria*. In A. Schönberg (ed.), *Listeriosis—Joint WHO/ROI Consultation on Prevention and Control*, West Berlin, December 10–12, 1986, pp. 56–62. Institut für Veterinärmedizin des Bundesgesundheitsamtes, Berlin.

89. Seeliger, H. P. R. 1988. Listeriosis—history and actual developments. *Infection 16*(Suppl. 2):80–84.

90. Seeliger, H. P. R., and D. Jones. 1987. *Listeria*. In J. G. Holt (ed.), *Bergey's Manual of Systematic Bacteriology*, 9th ed., Williams and Wilkins, Baltimore, pp. 1235–1245.

91. Seeliger, H. P. R., J. Rocourt, A. Schrettenbrunner, P. A. D. Grimont, and D. Jones. 1984. *Listeria ivanovii* sp. nov. *Int. J. Syst. Bacteriol. 34*:336–337.

92. Siddique, I. H., I. Fong Lin, and R. A. Chung. 1974. Purification and characterization of hemolysin produced by *Listeria monocytogenes. Amer. J. Vet. Res. 35*:289–296.

93. Skalka, B., J. Smola, and K. Elischerova. 1982. Different haemolytic activities of *Listeria monocytogenes* strains determined on erythrocytes of various sources and exploiting the synergism of equi-factor. *Zbl. Vet. Med. B 29*:642–649.

94. Skalka, B., J. Smola, and K. Elischerova. 1982. Routine test for *in vitro* differentiation of pathogenic and apathogenic *Listeria monocytogenes* strains. *J. Clin. Microbiol. 15*:503–507.

95. Steinmeyer, S. von, R. Schoen, and G. Terplan. 1987. Zum Nachweis der Pathogenität von aus Lebensmitteln isolierten Listerien am bebrüteten Hühnerei. *Arch. Lebensmittelhyg. 38*:95–99.

96. Stuart, M. R., and P. E. Pease. 1972. A numerical study on the relationships of *Listeria* and *Erysipelothrix. J. Gen. Microbiol. 73*:551–565.

97. Stuart, S. E., and H. J. Welshimer. 1973. Intrageneric relatedness of *Listeria* Pirie. *Int. J. Syst. Bacteriol. 23*:8–14.

98. Stuart, S. E., and H. J. Welshimer. 1974. Taxonomic reexamination of *Listeria* Pirie and transfer of *Listeria grayi* and *Listeria murrayi* to a new genus, *Murraya. Int. J. System. Bacteriol. 24*:177–185.

99. Sword, C. P. 1966. Mechanisms of pathogenesis in *Listeria monocytogenes*. I. Influence of iron. *J. Bacteriol. 92*:536–542.

100. Tadayon, R. A., K. K. Carroll, and R. G. E. Murray. 1970. Purification and properties of biologically active factors in lipid extracts of *Listeria monocytogenes. Can. J. Microbiol. 16*:535–544.

101. Taylor, A. G., J. McLauchlin, and A. Audurier. 1982. Phage-typing and serological studies in perinatal listeriosis. *J. Med. Microbiol. 15*:28.

102. Taylor, A. G., J. McLauchlin, H. T. Green, M. B. Macaulay, and A. Audurier. 1981. Hospital cross-infection with *Listeria monocytogenes* confirmed by phage-typing. *Lancet ii*:1106.

103. Trivett, T. L., and E. A. Meyer. 1971. Citrate cycle and related metabolism of *Listeria monocytogenes. J. Bacteriol. 107*:770–779.

104. Tysganova, A. A., A. V. Teterina, and V. M. Kotlyarov. 1979. Lactate dehydrogenase and adenosine triphosphate activity in weakly virulent and virulent strains of *Listeria. Sov. Agric. Sci. 5*:42–43.

105. Uchikawa, K-I., I. Sekikawa, and I. Azuma. 1986. Structural studies on teichoic acids in cell walls of several serotypes of *Listeria monocytogenes. J. Biochem. 9*:315–327.

106. Vazquez-Boland, J. A., L. Dominguez Rodriguez, J. F. Fernandez Garayzabal, J. L. Blanco Cancelo, E. Gomez-Lucia, V. Briones Dieste, and G. Suarez Fernandez. 1988. Serological studies on *Listeria grayi* and *Listeria murrayi. J. Appl. Bacteriol. 64*:371–378.

107. Vicente, M. F., F. Baquero, P. Cossart, and J. C. Perez-Diaz. 1987. Cloning of two possible haemolysin determinants from *Listeria monocytogenes. Ann. Inst. Pasteur. Microbiol. 138*:385–387.

2

Occurrence and Survival of *Listeria monocytogenes* in Natural Environments

INTRODUCTION

Listeria monocytogenes is widely distributed in the environment and has been isolated from a variety of sources including soil, vegetation, fecal material, sewage, and water. Improperly fermented silage is another important niche for this organism and has been cited as the source of infection in numerous cases of listeriosis involving domestic farm animals. *Listeria monocytogenes* also can survive longer under adverse environmental conditions than most other non–spore-forming bacteria of importance in foodborne disease, which makes this organism a particular threat to the food industry. Table 2.1 summarizes results from some of the studies which will now be discussed regarding survival of *L. monocytogenes* in soil, fecal material, sewage, water, and animal feed.

SOIL AND VEGETATION

Although much of the epidemiology concerning *L. monocytogenes* remains obscure, reports suggest that the primary habitat of the organism is in soil and decaying vegetation where the bacterium leads a saprophytic existence. Presence of *L. monocytogenes* in soil and vegetation is well documented (69,72,73). Weis and Seeliger (69) isolated *L. monocytogenes* from plant samples taken from 9.7% of cornfields, 13.3% of grainfields, 12.5% of cultivated fields, 44% of uncultivated fields, 15.5% of meadows/pastures, 21.3% of forests, and 23.1% of wildlife feeding grounds tested in southern West Germany. When from the same location, recovery of *L. monocytogenes* from plant and surface soil samples was similar. In contrast, analysis of soil samples taken at a depth of 10 cm from grainfields, uncultivated fields, meadows/pastures, and forest yielded 62.6, 35.2, 57.5, and 78.9% fewer positive samples, respectively, than did surface samples taken from the same locations.

Relatively large numbers of *L. monocytogenes* also were isolated from samples of mud, which suggests that a moist environment favors growth of the organism. Welshimer and Donker-Voet (73) could not isolate *L. monocytogenes* from soil or dead green vegetation collected in early fall; however, the organism was detected in virtually all samples of soil and decayed vegetation the following spring.

Survival of *L. monocytogenes* in soil depends on type of soil and its moisture content (71). After inoculating a series of cotton-plugged test tubes containing clay and a fertile

Table 2.1   Survival of *L. monocytogenes* in Various Environmental Samples

Sample	Storage temperature (°C)	Survival (days)
Soil		
Sterile soil (I)[a]	Outside—Winter/Spring	154
Clay soil (I)		
sealed tubes	24–26	225
cotton-plugged tubes	24–26	67
Fertile soil (I)		
sealed tubes	24–26	295
cotton-plugged tubes	24–26	67
Top soil (I)		
exposed to sunlight	NG[b]	12
not exposed to sunlight	NG	182
Moist soil	NG	ca. 497
Dry soil	NG	>730
Soil	4–12	240–311
Soil	18–20	201–271
Fecal material		
Cattle feces (NC)[c]	5	182–2190
Moist horse/sheep feces (I)	Outside	347
Dry horse/sheep feces (I)	Outside	730
Sheep feces	Outside	242
Liquid manure	Summer	36
Liquid manure	Winter	106
Sewage		
Sewage sludge cake (NC)		
surface	28–32	35
interior	48–56	49
sprayed on field	Outside	>56
Water		
Sterilized pond water (I)	Outside	7
Unsterilized pond water (I)	Outside	<7–63
Pond water	35–37	346
Pond water	15–20	299
Pond water/ice	2–8	790–928
Pond/river water	37	325
Pond/river water	2–5	750
Water	Outside	140–300
Distilled water (I)	4	<9
Animal feed		
Silage (NC)	4	450
Silage (NC)	5	180–2190
Mixed feed (I)	Outside	188–275
Oats (I)	Outside	150–300
Hay (I)	Outside	145–189
Straw (NC/I)	ca. 22	365
Straw (I)	Outside	47–207
Straw	Outside–Summer	23
Straw	Outside –Winter	135

[a]Inoculated.
[b]Not given.
[c]Naturally contaminated.
Source: Adapted from Refs. 4,5,49.

soil, populations of *L. monocytogenes* decreased approximately seven orders of magnitude after 67 days of storage at 24–26°C. Decreases in numbers of listeriae were directly related to moisture loss by the samples during extended storage. When the same experiment was repeated using properly sealed tubes which prevented evaporation, *Listeria* populations decreased by approximately two and more than seven orders of magnitude in fertile and clay soil, respectively.

In another study (14), samples of autoclaved soil were inoculated to contain ~5 × 10^2 *L. monocytogenes* CFU/g and were stored outside during winter at average high and low temperatures of 8°C and −15°C, respectively. The organism began to grow in sterile soil after an 84-day lag period and reached a population of ~1 × 10^7 CFU/g in May, following 154 days of storage.

These data support the hypothesis that the primary habitat for *L. monocytogenes* is decaying vegetation and surface soil. Furthermore, growth of the organism appears to be favored in early spring during "cold-enrichment," particularly in moist environments.

FECAL MATERIAL

Presence of *L. monocytogenes* in fecal material collected from infected as well as healthy sheep (36,37,62), cattle (42,59,62,66), goats (48,66), pigs (21,43,57), chickens (11,33,50,51,55,61), turkeys (12,41,52,61), and pheasants (61) is well documented. Excretion rates can vary widely among healthy animals. Ralovich (58) found that although 6 of 12 (50%) sheep flocks and 8 of 10 (80%) cattle herds were infected with *L. monocytogenes*, only 14.0% of sheep and 27.6% of cattle excreted the organism in their feces. He also observed that a flock of 40 nonexcreting sheep became excreters of the bacterium after being housed under stressful conditions. Reports suggest that between 2 and 16% of healthy cattle can excrete *L. monocytogenes* in their feces (18,58).

The bacterium has been detected in fecal material from other animals, some of which include seagulls (24), rooks (24), house sparrows (47), fish (9), and crustaceans (9). Since naturally occurring listeriosis has been reported in many other animals including mice (63), voles (52), rats (62), rabbits (52,62,68), guinea pigs (58), chinchillas (28), lemmings (56), hyraxes (56), mink (47), skunks (58), horses (70), dogs (47,63), cats (52), foxes (52), deer (23,52), buffalo (21), giraffes (17), bats (43), ducks (56), pigeons (56), partridges (56), eagles (56), parrots (56), canaries (56), owls (56), starlings (47), frogs (13), turtles (13), ticks (9), flies (9), and other forms of wildlife, it is reasonable to suspect that these animals also carry the bacterium in their feces.

Human feces collected from symptomatic and asymptomatic individuals also can contain *L. monocytogenes*. Ralovich (58) summarized data, primarily of European origin, which generally indicate that between 1.8 and 9.0% of the normal healthy human population (differing by age, sex, and profession) carries *L. monocytogenes* in its feces.

SEWAGE

Considering the frequency with which *L. monocytogenes* appears in human and animal feces, it is not surprising that the organism is often encountered in sewage and water. Watkins and Sleath (67) reported finding *L. monocytogenes* at levels between 700 and

>18,000 CFU/L in effluent from primary tanks of sewage treatment plants in England. No clear correlation was observed between populations of listeriae and *Escherichia coli*, fecal streptococci, *Clostridium perfringens*, or salmonellae. Preliminary work on survival of *L. monocytogenes* in sewage sludge sprayed onto land also indicated that numbers of the bacterium (ca. 200 CFU/g of soil) remained unaltered over an 8-week period. While investigating a West German sewage treatment plant, Geuenich and Müller (30) detected *Listeria* spp., including *L. monocytogenes*, in untreated waste water as well as in biologically treated (via oxidation) effluent at levels ranging between 10^3 and 10^5 CFU/ml. Since *Listeria* populations were generally only about 10 times lower in clear filtered waste water than in incoming sludge, biological oxidation does not appear to be highly effective in reducing populations of viable listeriae in sewage effluent.

After recovering *L. monocytogenes* from sewage sludge cake produced at a municipal sewage treatment plant in Iraq (2), Al-Ghazali and Al-Azawi (3) investigated behavior of this pathogen in sewage during processing. Although settling, aeration activation, digestion, and drying all were detrimental to survival of listeriae in sewage during processing, activation and digestion appeared to be most effective with each of these two processing steps accounting for 85 to 99.7% reductions in viable numbers of listeriae. Nonetheless, small numbers of *L. monocytogenes* were recovered from fully processed effluent (<3–15 CFU/ml) and sewage sludge cake (<3–7 CFU/ml), the latter of which is frequently dried and used as fertilizer in developing countries. These authors (4) subsequently demonstrated that listeriae could be eliminated from large piles of sewage sludge cake by storing the product in direct sunlight for at least 8 weeks under subtropical conditions. Since *L. monocytogenes* was inactivated somewhat faster in sludge from the surface than from the interior of the pile, it appears that moisture loss was largely responsible for elimination of the pathogen from this material during extended storage. Although use of such sewage sludge cake as fertilizer is not recommended, persons in developing countries and elsewhere who have no other alternative should be certain that the processed sludge cake has been properly stored a minimum of 8 weeks before use to produce as safe a fertilizer as possible.

WATER

According to Dijkstra (20), *L. monocytogenes* occurred in 21% of the surface water samples obtained from canals and lakes in northern Holland. Even though the lakes were frequented by swimmers, no case of human listeriosis was reported. In the same study, *L. monocytogenes* also was detected in 67% of the samples of sewage effluent. Although samples of sea water were negative, the bacterium was still found in a canal 25 miles downstream from the sewage treatment plant at the point where the canal emptied into the sea.

Currently, the literature contains no reports of human listeriosis resulting from contact with contaminated drinking water. However, using frogs that were inoculated orally with *L. monocytogenes*, Botzler (15) found that large numbers of listeriae were shed in feces 3–6 days after inoculation. Botzler (16) went on to demonstrate that the bacterium could be transmitted to other noninfected frogs by ingestion of fecally contaminated drinking water. Gray et al. (35) also successfully infected two sheep, four goats, and one cow by supplying the animals with drinking water inoculated with *L.*

monocytogenes. These studies raise a legitimate concern over the possibility of humans contracting listeriosis through contact with contaminated water.

ANIMAL FEED

An association between silage consumption and listeriosis in ruminants was observed as early as 1922 when results of an investigation in Iceland warned against a disease resembling listeriosis (known in Iceland as *votheysveiki* or silage sickness) which was relatively common in silage-fed animals. However, the apparent relationship between silage feeding and listeriosis was not clarified until 1960. In that year, Gray (34) reported isolating *L. monocytogenes* from the viscera of a female mouse and the fetuses of a pregnant mouse fed poor-grade silage which was thought to have caused death and abortion in cattle because it was contaminated with *L. monocytogenes*. Identical serotypes of *L. monocytogenes* were isolated post-mortem from the mice and cow, thus supporting the link between silage feeding and listeriosis (34). Today, numerous reports exist of listeriosis outbreaks in sheep and cows resulting from consumption of contaminated silage (24,26,27,31,38,39,74).

High-grade silage of good keeping quality is normally prepared from maize, grass, rye, oats, or leguminous plants that sometimes are wilted before ensiling (5). During silage manufacture, sugars present in plant materials are converted to primarily lactic acid by homofermentative lactobacilli and/or streptococci. After anaerobic fermentation has been completed, high quality silage generally has a pH ≤ 4.5, which prevents growth of most spoilage organisms (50).

Listeria monocytogenes has most frequently been associated with poor-quality silage which had a pH > 4.5 (24,26,31,38). In a survey of 291 grass silage samples collected from 113 farms with recent outbreaks of listeriosis, Grønstøl (38) isolated *L. monocytogenes* from 22, 37, and 56% of silage samples with pH values <4.0, 4.0–5.0, and >5.0, respectively. In another survey (27), the bacterium was isolated from 11 of 31 silages of excellent quality which had pH values between 3.6 and 4.0. Gouet et al. (32) showed that *L. monocytogenes* failed to grow at pH < 5.0 in gnotobiotic silage manufactured with a defined flora of lactic acid bacteria. Not only did *L. monocytogenes* fail to grow, but the organism was supposedly eliminated from the silage after 30 days of storage at 20°C. However, Dijkstra (19) demonstrated that *L. monocytogenes* can survive 4–6 years in naturally contaminated silage stored at 5°C.

Although detection of *L. monocytogenes* is often difficult when silage has a pH $\leq$ 5.0, Irvin (44) found that growth of the organism in silage resumed if the pH was adjusted to above 5.5. Fenlon (24) demonstrated that exposure of silage to air led to mold growth and a subsequent increase in pH, which was followed by growth of naturally present *L. monocytogenes*. Listeriae were detected in 22.2% of good-quality and in 44.0% of moldy silage samples examined. The lowest incidence of *L. monocytogenes* was observed in rotten silage having a pH between 7.3 and 8.6. Samples of rotten silage were hot as a result of aerobic degradation of the material, which may account for the lower incidence of *Listeria* in rotten than in moldy silage. When grass was ensiled in plastic bags, Fenlon (25) detected *L. monocytogenes* at a level of 1.1×10^6 CFU/g in an area of moldy silage which was centered around the tie seal and had a pH of 7.0. In contrast, silage in the center of the bag had a pH of 3.8 and was free of listeriae. In another study in which silage was implicated in a suspected listeriosis outbreak in calves (26), *L. monocytogenes* was detected at levels $\geq 1.2 \times 10^4$ CFU/g in moldy aerobic portions surrounding a silage clamp, whereas few if any organisms were observed in samples taken 2.5 cm below the clamp. That only a small portion of silage was contaminated helps to explain why only 3 of 25 calves contracted listeriosis.

Lactic acid inhibits growth of *L. monocytogenes* in bacteriological media and is likely a major factor in preventing growth of the bacterium in silage. However, lactic acid affords no protection against yeasts and mold. Therefore, silage must be kept anaerobic to avoid mold growth, which will lead to an increase in pH along with possible growth of *Listeria*. Potassium sorbate is widely used as a food additive to prevent yeast and mold growth and also prevents growth of *L. monocytogenes* in Tryptose Broth, provided that the pH is ≤ 5.0 (22). Therefore, it is likely that potassium sorbate could be used effectively to increase the aerobic stability of silage and, in the process, limit growth of listeriae (76).

In addition to traditional silage and less typical varieties prepared from orange peels and artichokes (65), other types of animal feed have been linked to outbreaks of listeriosis. For more than 80 years, ranchers in Canada and the northwestern United States have recorded numerous cases of listeric-like abortion in cattle that grazed on ponderosa pine needles. Adams et al. (1) isolated *L. monocytogenes* from the blood of mice fed a chow diet consisting of ground ponderosa pine needles. Injection of the *Listeria* isolate into mice led to symptoms that mimicked listeriosis in cattle, which suggests a possible link between the bacterium and "pine needle abortion."

While not yet associated with an outbreak of animal listeriosis, fermented edible waste also can be used as feed for domestic livestock. Hence, in 1981 Talkington et al. (64) examined the fate of *L. monocytogenes* in food waste fermented with *Lactobacillus acidophilus*. After waste obtained from a local school was inoculated with *L. acidophilus*, the product also was inoculated to contain approximately 2×10^6 *L. monocytogenes* CFU/ml, fermented at 5, 10, 20, and 30°C and analyzed daily over a 4-day period for numbers of listeriae. Despite direct plating of dilutions on five different media, the authors failed to reisolate *L. monocytogenes* from any samples, regardless of incubation time or temperature. However, since none of the samples underwent enrichment, these findings do not preclude the possibility that *L. monocytogenes* was present at levels lower than could be detected by direct plating. Nevertheless, as was true for fermented silage, production of lactic acid during fermentation of the food waste along with a simultaneous decrease in pH values (i.e., pH <4–5), undoubtedly played a crucial role in reducing numbers of listeriae in this product.

MODES OF TRANSMISSION

As previously noted, *L. monocytogenes* is widely distributed in the environment. Thus humans can come into contact with this pathogen through a variety of sources including animals, meat, milk, dairy products, seafood, and plants as well as insects, air, dust, dirt, feces, and other humans. Although the origin and mode of transmission of all forms of listeric infection is complex, an attempt has been made to trace the various routes of infection using data in the literature (Fig. 2.1).

Early comparative studies revealed no differences in biological and biochemical

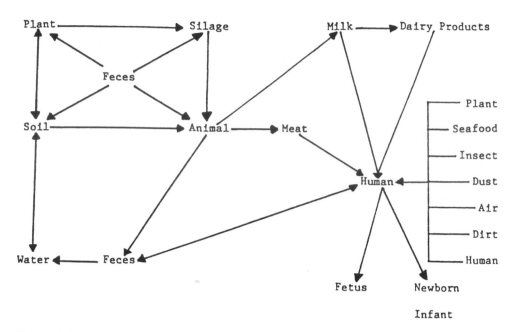

Figure 2.1 Routes for transmission of *L. monocytogenes* to humans.

properties of *L. monocytogenes* strains isolated from human and animal sources (62). Therefore, listeriosis traditionally has been recognized as a zoonosis—an infectious disease of animals that is transmissible to humans. In domestic animals such as cattle and sheep, listeriosis is most often associated with septicemia, encephalitis, and abortion. These same manifestations also are commonly observed in humans, which lends support to the zoonotic nature of listeriosis (62).

According to Ralovich (58), 24.8–76.2% of all listeric infections may result from human-to-human contact. Thus the direct or indirect spread of *L. monocytogenes* between humans appears to be a likely route of infection, particularly in cases of neonatal listeriosis.

In 1976, Kampelmacher et al. (46) studied the occurrence of *L. monocytogenes* in feces collected from pregnant women who did or did not have direct contact with farm or pet animals. Negligible differences in incidences of *Listeria* were observed in the three groups of fecal samples. Therefore, it may be concluded that contact with animals does not play a significant role in most cases of neonatal listeriosis.

The idea that listeriosis in humans can be spread from consumption of contaminated food is not new. As early as 1915, a group of people in Australia contracted a "listerio-sis-like" illness which suggested a possible foodborne route of infection (10). Between 1949 and 1957, consumption of raw milk was suspected as the cause of several massive listeriosis outbreaks in Germany and Czechoslovakia (62). Recent outbreaks in the United States resulting from consumption of Mexican-style cheese (45) and, presumably, pasteurized milk (29) have resulted in approximately 350 cases of listeriosis, including 100 deaths, and have reinforced the importance of listeriosis as a foodborne illness.

Milk and cheese are not the only food-related vehicles from which listeriosis can be acquired. In 1981, a large listeriosis outbreak occurred in the maritime provinces of Canada and resulted from consumption of coleslaw manufactured from contaminated cabbage (60). Investigators traced the cabbage to a farm where manure from *Listeria*-infected sheep was used to fertilize the cabbage field. Gudkova (40) reported isolating *L. monocytogenes* from pigs that were slaughtered and then consumed on a farm where several cases of listeriosis were diagnosed. Thus meat can also constitute a vehicle for transmission, especially if improperly cooked. Recently, *L. monocytogenes* was isolated from crabmeat (6,8) and shrimp (7), which suggests the possibility of contracting listeriosis from contaminated seafood. A detailed review of foodborne listeriosis has been reserved for Chapter 8.

Although oral infections presumably are the most common, listeriosis also can be acquired via respiratory, cutaneous, and ocular routes. In 1954, Ödegaard (53) reported the death of a farmer from listeric meningitis and bronchopneumonia following probable inhalation of contaminated fecal material while cleaning a sheep barn. Fatal pulmonary listeriosis also has been observed in cattle and has been traced to contaminated feed (75). Cases of cutaneous listeriosis also have been reported; one case occurred in a veterinarian following delivery of a fetus from an aborting cow that was infected with *L. monocytogenes* (54). Listeric infections occurring via the ocular route have been recognized for many years in both humans and animals (58). Anton's test for pathogenicity actually resulted from a laboratory accident in which a technician working with *Listeria* infected his face and developed conjunctivitis. Seeliger (62) also gave an account of an employee in a poultry shop who presumably developed conjunctivitis after handling infected chickens.

Finally, intermediate hosts may play a role in transmission of *L. monocytogenes*. A 42-year-old women reportedly died from listeric meningitis after being bitten by a tick. This tick was found feeding on several rodent species from which *L. monocytogenes* was previously isolated.

REFERENCES

1. Adams, C. J., T. E. Neff, and L. L. Jackson. 1979. Induction of *Listeria monocytogenes* infection by the consumption of ponderosa pine needles. *Infect. Immun. 25*:117–120.
2. Al-Ghazali, M. R., and S. K. Al-Azawi. 1986. Detection and enumeration of *Listeria monocytogenes* in a sewage treatment plant in Iraq. *J. Appl. Bacteriol. 60*:251–254.
3. Al-Ghazali, M. R., and S. K. Al-Azawi. 1988. Effects of sewage treatment on the removal of *Listeria monocytogenes*. *J. Appl. Bacteriol. 65*:203–208.
4. Al-Ghazali, M. R., and S. K. Al-Azawi. 1988. Storage effects of sewage sludge cake on the survival of *Listeria monocytogenes*. *J. Appl. Bacteriol. 65*:209–213.
5. Amtsberg, G. von. 1979. Epidemiologie und Diagnostik der Listeriose. *Dtsch. tierärztl. Wochenschr. 86*:253–257.
6. Anonymous. 1987. First confirmed finding in crabmeat confirmed by FDA. *Food Chem. News 29* (14):38.
7. Anonymous. 1987. Shrimp recalled because of *Listeria monocytogenes*. *Food Chem. News 29*(42):12–13.
8. Anonymous. 1988. Crabmeat undergoes class I recall because of *Listeria*. *Food Chem. News 29*(44):51.
9. Armstrong, D. 1985. *Listeria monocytogenes*. In G. L. Mandell, R. G. Douglas, Jr., and J. E. Bennett (eds.), *Principles and Practices of Infectious Diseases*, 2nd ed., John Wiley and Sons, New York, pp. 1177–1182.

10. Atkinson, E. 1917. Meningitis associated with gram-positive bacilli of diphtheroid type. *Med. J. Australia 1*:115–118.

11. Basher, H. A., D. R. Fowler, F. G. Rodgers, A. Seaman, and M. Woodbine. 1984. Pathogenicity of natural and experimental listeriosis in newly hatched chicks. *Res. Vet. Sci. 36*:76–80.

12. Belding, R. C., and M. L. Mayer. 1957. Listeriosis in the turkey—two case reports. *J. Amer. Vet. Med. Assoc. 131*:296–297.

13. Botzler, R. G. 1973. *Listeria* in aquatic animals. *J. Wildl. Dis. 9*:163–170.

14. Botzler, R. G. 1974. Survival of *Listeria monocytogenes* in soil and water. *J. Wildl. Dis. 10*:204–212.

15. Botzler, R. G. 1975. Rate of *Listeria monocytogenes* shedding from frogs. *J. Wildl. Dis. 11*:277–279.

16. Botzler, R. G., and A. B. Cowan. 1985. Transfer of *Listeria monocytogenes* between frogs. *J. Wildl. Dis. 21*:173–174.

17. Cranfield, M., M. A. Eckhaus, B. A. Valentine, and J. D. Strandberg. 1985. Listeriosis in Angolan giraffes. *J. Amer. Vet. Med. Assoc. 187*:1238–1240.

18. Dijkstra, R. G. 1966. Epidemiological investigations on listeriosis in cattle. 3rd Intern. Symp. Listeriosis, Bilthoven, The Netherlands, pp. 215–224.

19. Dijkstra, R. G. 1971. Investigations on the survival times of *Listeria* bacteria in suspensions of brain tissue, silage and faeces and in milk. *Zbl. Bakteriol. I. Abt. Orig. 216*:92–95.

20. Dijkstra, R. G. 1982. The occurrence of *Listeria monocytogenes* in surface water of canals and lakes, in ditches of one big polder and in the effluents of canals of a sewage treatment plant. *Zbl. Bakteriol. Hyg., I. Abt. Orig. B 176*:202–205.

21. Dutta, P. K., and B. S. Malik. 1981. Isolation and characterization of *Listeria monocytogenes* from animals and human beings. *Indian J. Animal Sci. 51*:1045–1052.

22. El-Shenawy, M. A., and E. H. Marth. 1988. Inhibition and inactivation of *Listeria monocytogenes* by sorbic acid. *J. Food Prot. 51*:842–847.

23. Eriksen, L., H. E. Larson, T. Christiansen, M. M. Jensen, and E. Eriksen. 1989. An outbreak of meningio-encephalitis in fallow deer caused by *Listeria monocytogenes*. *Vet. Rec. Mar. 19*:274–276.

24. Fenlon, D. R. 1985. Wild birds and silage as reservoirs of *Listeria* in the agricultural environment. *J. Appl. Bacteriol. 59*:537–543.

25. Fenlon, D. R. 1986. Growth of naturally occurring *Listeria* spp. in silage: A comparative study of laboratory and farm ensiled grass. *Grass Forage Sci. 41*:375–378.

26. Fenlon, D. R. 1986. Rapid quantitative assessment of the distribution of *Listeria* in silage implicated in a suspected outbreak of listeriosis in calves. *Vet. Rec. 118*:240–242.

27. Fensterbank, R., A. Audurier, J. Godu, P. Guerrault, and N. Malo. 1984. Study of *Listeria* strains isolated from sick animals and from the silage consumed. *Ann. Rech. Vet. 15*:113–118.

28. Finley, G. G., and J. R. Long. 1977. An epizootic of listeriosis in chinchillas. *Can. Vet. J. 18*:164–167.

29. Fleming, D. W., S. L. Cochi, K. L. Mac Donald, J. Brondum, P. S. Hayes, B. D. Plikaytis, M. B. Holmes, A. Audurier, C. V. Broome, and A. A. Reingold. 1985. Pasteurized milk as a vehicle of infection in an outbreak of listeriosis. *N. Engl. J. Med. 312*:404–407.

30. Geuenich, H.-H., and H. E. Müller. 1984. Isolation and quantitative determination of *Listeria monocytogenes* in raw and biologically treated waste water. *Zbl. Bakteriol. Hyg., I. Abt. Orig. B 179*:266–273.

31. Gitter, M., R. StJ. Stebbings, J. A. Morris, D. Hannam, and C. Harris. 1986. Relationship between ovine listeriosis and silage feeding. *Vet. Rec. 118*:207–208.

32. Gouet, P., J. P. Girardeau, and Y. Riou. 1977. Inhibition of *Listeria monocytogenes* by defined lactic microflora in gnotobiotic silages of lucerne, fescue, ryegrass and maize—influence of dry matter and temperature. *Anim. Feed. Sci. Technol. 2*:297–305.

33. Gray, M. L. 1958. Listeriosis in fowls—a review. *Avian Dis. 2*:296–314.

34. Gray, M. L. 1960. A possible link in the relationship between silage feeding and listeriosis. *J. Amer. Vet. Med. Assoc. 136*:205–208.

35. Gray, M. L., C. Singh, and F. Thorp. 1956. Abortion and pre- or postnatal death of young due to *Listeria monocytogenes*. III. Studies in ruminants. *Amer. J. Vet. Res. 17*:510–516.
36. Grønstøl, H. 1979. Listeriosis in sheep—*Listeria monocytogenes* excretion and immunological state in healthy sheep. *Acta Vet. Scand. 20*:168–179.
37. Grønstøl, H. 1979. Listeriosis in sheep—*Listeria monocytogenes* excretion and immunological state in sheep in flocks with clinical listeriosis. *Acta Vet. Scand. 20*:417–428.
38. Grønstøl, H. 1979. Listeriosis in sheep—isolation of *Listeria monocytogenes* from grass silage. *Acta Vet. Scand. 20*:492–497.
39. Grønstøl, H. 1980. Listeriosis in sheep—*Listeria monocytogenes* in sheep fed hay or grass silage during pregnancy. Immunological state, white blood cells, total serum protein and serum iron. *Acta Vet. Scand. 21*:1–10.
40. Gudkova, E. I., K. A. Mironova, A. S. Kus'minski, and G. O. Geine. 1958. A second outbreak of listeric angina in a single populated locality. *Zh. Mikrobiol. Epidemiol. Immunobiol. 35*:24–28.
41. Hatkin, J. M., and W. E. Phillips, Jr. 1986. Isolation of *Listeria monocytogenes* from an eastern wild turkey. *J. Wildlife Dis. 22*:110–112.
42. Hofer, E. 1983. Bacteriologic and epidemiologic studies on the occurrence of *Listeria monocytogenes* in healthy cattle. *Zbl. Bakteriol. Hyg. A 256*:175–183.
43. Höhne, K., B. Loose, and H. P. R. Seeliger. 1975. Isolation of *Listeria monocytogenes* in slaughter animals and bats of Togo (West Africa). *Ann. Inst. Pasteur Microbiol. 126A*:501–507.
44. Irvin, A. D. 1968. The effect of pH on the multiplication of *Listeria monocytogenes* in grass silage media. *Vet. Rec. 82*:115–116.
45. James, S. M., S. L. Fannin, B. A. Agree, B. Hall, E. Parker, J. Vogt, G. Run, J. Williams, L. Lieb, C. Salminen, T. Prendergast, S. B. Werner, and J. Chin. 1985. Listeriosis outbreak associated with Mexican-style cheese—California. *Morbid. Mortal. Weekly Rep. 34*:357–359.
46. Kampelmacher, E. H., D. E. Maas, and L. M. van Noorle Jansen. 1976. Occurrence of *Listeria monocytogenes* in feces of pregnant women with and without direct animal contact. *Zbl. Bakteriol. Hyg. I. Abt. Orig. A 234*:238–242.
47. Larsen, H. E. 1964. Investigation on the epidemiology of listeriosis—the distribution of *Listeria monocytogenes* in environments in which clinical outbreaks have not been diagnosticated. *Nord. Vet. Med. 16*:890–909.
48. Løken, T., E. Aspøy, and H. Grønstøl. 1982. *Listeria monocytogenes* excretion and humoral immunity in goats in a herd with outbreaks of listeriosis and in a dairy herd. *Acta Vet. Scand. 23*:392–399.
49. Mitscherlich, E., and E. H. Marth. 1984. *Microbial Survival in the Environment—Bacteria and Rickettsiae Important in Human and Animal Health*, Springer-Verlag, Berlin.
50. Moon, N. J. 1984. A short review of the role of lactobacilli in silage fermentation. *Food Microbiol. 1*:333–338.
51. Nagi, M. S., and J. D. Verma. 1967. An outbreak of listeriosis in chickens. *Ind. J. Vet. Med. 44*:539–543.
52. Nilsson, A., and K. A. Karlsson. 1959. *Listeria monocytogenes* isolations from animals in Sweden during 1948 to 1957. *Nord. Vet. Med. 11*:305–315.
53. Ödegaard, B., R. Grelland, and S. D. Henricksen. 1952. A case of *Listeria*—infection in man, transmitted from sheep. *Acta Med. Scand. 67*:231–238.
54. Owen, C. R., A. Meis, J. W. Jackson, and H. G. Stoenner. 1960. A case of primary cutaneous listeriosis. *N. Engl. J. Med. 262*:1026–1028.
55. Paterson, J. S. 1937. *Listerella* infection in fowls—preliminary note on its occurrence in East Anglia. *Vet. Rec. 49*:1533–1534.
56. Plagemann, O., and A. Weber. 1988. *Listeria monocytogenes* als Abortursache bei Klippschliefern (*Procavia capensis*). *Kleintierpraxis 33*:317–318.
57. Rahman, T., D. K. Sarma, B. K. Goswami, T. N. Upadhyaya, and B. Choudhury. 1985. Occurrence of listerial meningoencephalitis in pigs. *Ind. Vet. J. 62*:7–9.
58. Ralovich, B. 1984. *Listeriosis Research—Present Situation and Perspective*, Akademiai Kiado, Budapest.

59. Rodriguez, L. D., G. S. Fernandez, J. F. F. Garayzabal, and E. R. Ferri. 1984. New methodology for the isolation of *Listeria* microorganisms from heavily contaminated environments. *Appl. Environ. Microbiol. 47*:1188–1190.

60. Schlech, W. F., P. M. Lavigne, R. A. Bortolussi, A. C. Allen, E. V. Haldone, A. J. Wort, A. W. Hightower, S. E. Johnson, S. H. King, E. S. Nicholls, and C. V. Broome. 1983. Epidemic listeriosis—evidence for transmission by food. *N. Engl. J. Med. 303*:203–206.

61. Schwartz, J. C. 1969. Attempted isolations of *Listeria monocytogenes* from diagnostic accessions. *Am. J. Vet. Res. 30*:483–484.

62. Seeliger, H. P. R. 1961. *Listeriosis*, Hafner Publishing Co., New York.

63. Sturgess, C. P. 1989. Listerial abortion in the bitch. *Vet. Rec. 124*:177.

64. Talkington, D. D., E. B. Shotts, Jr., R. E. Wolley, W. K. Whitehead, and C. N. Dobbins. 1981. Introduction and reisolation of selected gram-positive bacteria from fermented edible waste. *Am. J. Vet. Res. 42*:1302–1305.

65. Vizcaino, L. L., M.-J. Cubero, and A. Contreras. 1988. Listeric abortions in ewes and cows associated to orange peel and artichoke silage feeding. Intern. Symposium on Listeriosis, Pecs, Hungary, Aug. 22–26, Abst. P29.

66. Von Winkenwerder, W. 1967. Das Vorkommen von *Listeria monocytogenes* bei Rindern in Niedersachsen. *Berl. Münch. tierärztl. Wschr. 23*:445–449.

67. Watkins, J., and K. P. Sleath. 1981. Isolation and enumeration of *Listeria monocytogenes* from sewage, sewage sludge and river water. *J. Appl. Bacteriol. 50*:1–9.

68. Watson, G. L., and M. G. Evans. 1985. Listeriosis in a rabbit. *Vet. Pathol. 22*:191–193.

69. Weis, J., and H. P. R. Seeliger. 1975. Incidence of *Listeria monocytogenes* in nature. *Appl. Microbiol. 30*:29–32.

70. Welsh, R. D. 1983. Equine abortion caused by *Listeria monocytogenes* serotype 4. *J. Am. Vet. Med. Assoc. 182*:291.

71. Welshimer, H. J. 1960. Survival of *Listeria monocytogenes* in soil. *J. Bacteriol. 80*:316–320.

72. Welshimer, H. J. 1968. Isolation of *Listeria monocytogenes* from vegetation. *J. Bacteriol. 95*:300–303.

73. Welshimer, H. J., and J. Donker-Voet. 1971. *Listeria monocytogenes* in nature. *Appl. Microbiol. 21*:516–519.

74. Wilesmith, J. W., and M. Gitter. 1986. Epidemiology of ovine listeriosis in Great Britain. *Vet. Rec. 119*:467–470.

75. Wohler, W. H., and C. L. Baugh. 1983. Pulmonary listeriosis in feeder cattle. *Mod. Vet. Pract. 64*:736–739.

76. Woolford, M. K. 1975. Microbiological screening of food preservatives, cold sterilants and specific antimicrobial agents as potential silage additives. *J. Sci. Food Agric. 26*:229–237.

3

Listeriosis in Animals

INTRODUCTION

The previous chapter indicated that numerous animal species are susceptible to listeric infection, with a large proportion of healthy animals shedding *L. monocytogenes* in their feces. Listeriosis in animals can occur either sporadically or as epidemics and often leads to fatal forms of encephalitis. Virtually all domestic animals are susceptible to listeriosis, with sheep (30,34,50,51,78,84), cattle (30,50,53,56,60,72,81), goats (44,45,67), and chickens (28,48,50,59) succumbing to infection most frequently. Unless properly treated, listeriosis in domestic livestock is usually fatal. However, milder infections in pregnant animals generally give rise to a damaged, dead, or aborted fetus (65).

INCIDENCE

Listeriosis in domestic livestock is being recognized with increasing frequency around the world. According to data for 1986 compiled by several branches of the United Nations (2), listeric infections in domestic animals were recognized in Afghanistan, Australia, Barbados, Benin, Canada, Chile, Cyprus, Ethiopia, Israel, Japan, Mozambique, New Zealand, Papua New Guinea, Senegal, Soviet Union, Swaziland, and the United States as well as all European nations except Malta and Luxembourg. Despite the increasing frequency with which listeriosis is being diagnosed in developed countries, the exact incidence of listeric infections in domestic livestock remains unknown.

According to Ralovich (58), annual numbers of listeriosis cases in animals have increased substantially since 1966 with about 2200, 1000, and 900 cases being reported in Bulgaria, East Germany, and Hungary in 1976, 1972, and 1980, respectively. Reports of listeriosis in domestic animals also have increased in New Zealand, West Germany, Greece, and England. During the early 1970s, the agricultural economies of Australia and Norway were adversely affected by the loss of approximately 1 million and 2000–2500 sheep, respectively, from listeric infection. Before a vaccine against listeriosis in sheep became available, the incidence of listeric infections in Norwegian livestock has remained relatively constant with approximately 1900–2300 sheep herds, 90–160 goat herds, and 3–17 cattle herds affected by listeriosis during the 10-year period between 1977 and 1986 (83). Dijkstra (18) also reported that 234–928 cases of listeric abortion occurred annually in cattle in The Netherlands between 1970 and 1985. During this same period, the annual percentage of abortions caused by *L. monocytogenes* in cattle ranged between 0.7 and 8.7% with an average of 3.2%.

In addition to relatively small numbers of acutely infected sheep, goats, and cattle, substantially larger proportions of animals within a herd may be asymptomatic carriers of *L. monocytogenes* and shed the organism in feces and milk (58,65). Sindoni et al. (69) conducted a serological survey in Italy on the frequency of anti-*Listeria* antibodies in sheep, cows, goats, and swine. Results from direct agglutination tests showed that 15 of 81 (18.5%) sheep, 17 of 154 (10.4%) cows, 27 of 156 (17.3%) goats, and 43 of 302 (13.3%) swine tested positive, suggesting previous exposure to *L. monocytogenes*. Using the complement fixation test, 5 of 81 (6.2%) sheep, 10 of 164 (6.1%) cows, 2 of 156 (1.3%) goats, and 16 of 324 (4.9%) swine tested positive for *Listeria*. The role of the symptomless carrier was clearly demonstrated in another report in which 30 of 44 listeriosis outbreaks on sheep farms involved introduction of clinically healthy animals from known infected herds (65). Thus these results indicate that a substantial pool of asymptomatic carriers exists to disseminate and perpetuate this disease.

Seasonal variation in the number of cases of animal listeriosis has often been observed. In the Northern Hemisphere (England, Bulgaria, Hungary, United States, France, and Germany), listeriosis in domestic animals generally occurs from late November to early May with the greatest incidence during February and March (29). Numbers of listeriosis cases increased when animals were fed silage during periods of extreme cold, whereas sharp decreases in numbers of reported cases were observed as soon as grass was available. Data from The Netherlands (18) indicate that most cases of listeric abortion in cattle occurred between December and May. Approximately 40% of these cases were linked to consumption of contaminated silage. Recent changes in production methods have reduced levels of *L. monocytogenes* in silage, which in turn has led to a considerable decrease in the incidence of listeriosis in silage-fed animals. Although in Norway listeriosis can be diagnosed year-round in sheep and goats, the illness is far more prevalent from October to June and also appears to be influenced by stable and feeding conditions (58).

Virtually all wild and domestic animals are susceptible to listeric infection. However, since the primary emphasis of this book is on foodborne listeriosis, the following discussion of symptomology will be limited to those animals that serve as important food sources for humans.

SYMPTOMOLOGY

Sheep

"Listeric-like" infections were observed in sheep as early as 1925 (65); however, Gill (24) is credited with the first isolation of *L. monocytogenes* from domestic farm animals. In 1929, he observed an illness in sheep which he called "circling disease." This name is still used today to describe listeric encephalitis, encephalomyelitis, and meningioencephalitis, which are the most common manifestations of listeriosis in ruminants, including sheep (65).

After an incubation period of not more than 3 weeks, clinical symptoms of ovine encephalitis may include elevated temperature and refusal to eat or drink. These initial symptoms are frequently followed by neurological disturbances, which include grinding of teeth, paralysis of masticatory muscles, and a stiff walk. At this point the animal moves in circles to the right or left, depending on the direction in which the head is bent. This characteristic movement accounts for the name "circling disease." Excessive salivation often occurs because of the animal's inability to swallow. In advanced stages, muscular incoordination develops and is followed by inability of the animal to walk. Death usually occurs within 2–3 days after onset of clinical symptoms, with the illness seldom lingering beyond 10 days (65).

Listeric infections in pregnant sheep often result in premature birth and infectious abortions (3,11,30,46). This illness seldom occurs concurrently with encephalitis (40). Initially, pregnant ewes contract purulent metritis, from which most recover. Intrauterine transmission of *L. monocytogenes* via the placenta leads to a septic infection of the fetus, which in turn gives rise to abortion or premature delivery with most fatalities occurring as stillbirths.

Listeriosis in young animals often assumes the form of a septicemia which is characterized by an elevated temperature, loss of appetite, and diarrhea. Although death may eventually occur as a result of extensive liver damage and focal pneumonia, the mortality rate is much lower for the septicemic than for the encephalitic form of listeriosis.

Goats

Manifestations of listeriosis in goats and sheep are essentially the same. Although meningioencephalitis predominates in goats, reports of listeric abortion are common. As is true for sheep, asymptomatic infections also have been noted in goats (65).

Cattle

In 1928, Matthews (47) reported an outbreak of encephalitis of unknown origin in cattle which, in retrospect, was probably bovine listeriosis. Several additional cases of bovine encephalitis were recorded during the early 1930s and also likely resulted from infection with *L. monocytogenes* (41). Listeric encephalitis has since been well documented (16,58,60,65) and accounts for about 90% of the total cases of bovine encephalitis in The Netherlands (77). This disease occurs more frequently in beef than dairy cattle. However, even in acute outbreaks, generally no more than 8–10% of a herd succumbs to infection.

Unlike listeric encephalitis in sheep and goats, most cattle survive at least 4–14 days after the initial onset of symptoms, with a few reports of spontaneous recovery (58). Clinical symptoms normally appear after an incubation period of 1–3 days and may include self-imposed segregation from other animals and neurological disturbances that result in circular movement ("circling disease"). Next, facial and throat muscles become paralyzed, which leads to refusal of feed because the animal cannot swallow. The body temperature is usually elevated, and some animals may develop conjunctivitis as well as various skin lesions. As the illness progresses, the tongue swells and protrudes from the mouth, which leads to increased secretion of viscous saliva and pronounced drooling. In the advanced stage, vision and locomotion are impaired and the animal becomes increasingly irritable. At this point, the illness may be confused with rabies. Finally, animals lapse into a coma and generally die within 1–2 days (65).

Infection of a pregnant cow with *L. monocytogenes* also can give rise to an aborted fetus, as first demonstrated by Graham et al. (27) in 1939. Today, listeriosis in cattle is frequently associated with abortion (53,58,65,70), which generally occurs during the second half of pregnancy. As was true for sheep, *L. monocytogenes* is transmitted to the fetus via the intrauterine/intraplacental route, which generally culminates in death of the fetus followed by abortion (65).

As with sheep (31–33) and goats (45), *L. monocytogenes* also can be shed in milk by dairy cattle. While not particularly common, generalized listeric infections can give rise to mastitis, which is a condition of great concern to the dairy industry. Beginning in 1938, Schmidt and Nyfeldt (61) postulated that a small outbreak of human listeriosis in Denmark may have been caused by drinking milk from mastitic cows; however, the role of *Listeria* in mastitic infections was not clearly identified until 1944. In that year, Wramby (82) isolated *L. monocytogenes* from milk and udders of mastitic cows in Sweden. Seven years later, *L. monocytogenes* was cultured from one sample of raw milk during an outbreak of human listeriosis in Halle, East Germany (65), which suggests that this organism can be a cause of atypical mastitis in dairy cows since the milk came from animals presumed to be healthy.

While far less common than *Listeria*-related abortion or encephalitis, documented cases in which *L. monocytogenes* was shed in milk as the result of mastitis can be found in the scientific literature (10,19,26,37,42,55,73,76,77). During one such outbreak, Kampelmacher (42) reported that dairy cattle shed *L. monocytogenes* at levels of 10,000–20,000 CFU/ml of milk. In 1956, de Vries and Strikwerda (77) described another case of bovine mastitis in which a penicillin-resistant strain of *L. monocytogenes* was cultured from one quarter of a 6-year-old dairy cow. Following acute onset, the condition soon became chronic with shedding of *L. monocytogenes* in the milk for 3 months.

The ability of *L. monocytogenes* to produce experimental mastitis in dairy cows was verified by Bryner et al. (8,9,79). Following reported intramammary inoculation of 34 Holstein cows with 10^3–10^7 *L. monocytogenes* cells, 75% of the animals became chronically infected and shed listeriae in milk leukocytes (ca. 10^3–10^5 *L. monocytogenes* CFU/ml of milk) for up to 8 months. Before infection, animals had serum agglutinin titers of ≤1:20–1:320; whereas 3 months postinfection, titers increased to as high as 1:20,480. Interestingly, injection of dexamethasone [a corticosteroid produced during stress (i.e., crowding, lactation, pregnancy) that decreases phagocytic activity and impairs the cellular immune system] led to a temporary 100- to 1000-fold increase in numbers of *L. monocytogenes* shed in milk. As part of a follow-up study (80), attempts are being made to correlate these titers to levels of *L. monocytogenes* shed in the milk.

Except for an elevated somatic cell count, the composition of milk from *Listeria*-mastitic cows generally appears normal. During an outbreak of mastitis in Yugoslavia (10), milk from a *Listeria*-infected dairy herd contained 18,000–400,000 (mean of 100,000) somatic cells/ml of milk. In such cases of naturally occurring listeric mastitis, *L. monocytogenes* normally exists as a facultative intracellular pathogen within somatic cells. Some researchers claim that the internalized position of *L. monocytogenes* may play a role in the organism's resistance to heat (see Chapter 9).

Listeric mastitis is not the only condition that allows for shedding of *L. monocytogenes* in milk. Excretion of this organism in milk (14,40,52,58) and colostrum (53) as a consequence of *Listeria*-related abortion and in milk (40,58) as a result of encephalitis also have been reported. In one such study, Osebold et al. (52) detected *L. monocytogenes* in milk and uterine discharges for up to 13 days following abortion. In another study, Dijkstra (15) found that 72 of 938 (7.7%) quarter milk samples from cows that had *Listeria*-related abortions were initially positive for *L. monocytogenes*. Following cold-enrichment at 5°C, positive samples increased to 40%.

Although milk associated with *Listeria*-related abortions or clinically severe cases of mastitis or encephalitis is unlikely to reach consumers, shedding of *L. monocytogenes* in milk from animals exhibiting only mild symptoms of listeriosis does constitute a significant risk to public health. Such concerns were raised by Hyslop and Osborne (40) during an outbreak of bovine listeriosis in 1958 when milk from a cow virtually without symptoms of listeriosis contained *L. monocytogenes*. Of even greater importance, however, are numerous reports indicating that this pathogen can be shed passively in milk from clinically normal cows (1,13,20,21,26,39,40,62,70). In 1967, Schultz (62) collected milk samples from 1004 cows and isolated *L. monocytogenes* from the milk of 10 animals, 7 of which appeared perfectly healthy. Shedding of listeriae in milk from these animals was intermittent, but continued for as long as 12 months.

Examination of dairy herds in Yugoslavia (69) also has demonstrated that clinically healthy cows can act as asymptomatic carriers of *L. monocytogenes* and secrete the organism in their milk for months comprising several lactation periods. In one such survey, *L. monocytogenes* was detected in milk from 3.2% of 845 clinically normal cows on seven farms in which listeriosis had been previously diagnosed (43). Working in Spain, Vizcaino and Garcia (75) also detected *L. monocytogenes* in milk collected from 13 of 36 seropositive albeit apparently healthy cows.

Numerous surveys of the raw milk supply prompted by dairy-related outbreaks of human listeriosis in 1983, 1985, and 1987 suggest that asymptomatic shedders are responsible for much of the *Listeria*-contaminated milk received at dairy-processing facilities. A detailed discussion of the incidence of *L. monocytogenes* in raw milk and related dairy products has been reserved for Chapters 9 and 10.

Swine

First described in 1940 (7), meningioencephalitis in swine begins with a sudden refusal to eat and is typically followed by various neurological disorders including trembling, partial paralysis, incoordination, circling movements, and convulsions. Infections during pregnancy may be followed by miscarriages and abortions. If untreated, death often occurs within 48 hours. Pathological findings from meningioencephalitis frequently include lesions and/or congestion in the brain as well as focal necrosis in the liver (29,65). While listerial meningioencephalitis in swine is considered rare, several such outbreaks have been reported including one in India (57) in which 27 of 75 pigs died during August and September of 1982.

Listeriosis in swine also can assume several other forms including septicemia, localized internal abscesses, and pox-like skin lesions (29); however, unlike sheep, goats, and cattle, all types of overt listeric infections are relatively rare in swine. In England, the Veterinary Investigation Center reported only 14 listeriosis cases in swine between

1975 and 1982 as compared to 666 cases in sheep and 472 cases in cattle (25). Listeriosis in pigs is also reported to be uncommon in The Netherlands (49). Widespread use of antibiotics in animal feed may be partly responsible for the low incidence of this disease in swine raised in developed countries.

Fowl

Avian listeriosis was first described in 1935 (64), 3 years after TenBroeck isolated *L. monocytogenes* (then *Bacterium monocytogenes*) from diseased chickens. While chickens have remained the most common avian host for this pathogen, listeric infections also have been observed in at least 22 other avian species, including such commonly consumed fowl as turkeys (6,38,50), ducks (28,65), geese (28,65), and pheasants (28). Interested readers are referred to a 1958 review article by Gray (28) which deals with all aspects of avian listeriosis, including 43 accounts of this disease in chickens. Despite the many sporadic cases of avian listeriosis that have been documented over the last 60 years, this disease is far less common in birds than in sheep, goats, and cattle. For example, listeric infections were discovered in only 13 of more than 38,000 chickens submitted for examination in Pennsylvania between 1960 and 1965 (63). Furthermore, large-scale outbreaks of listeriosis in chickens appear to be uncommon (48,54).

Recent reports suggest that up to 33% of all healthy chickens may asymptomatically shed *L. monocytogenes* in fecal material (16,17,71). Birds most likely become infected by pecking *Listeria*-contaminated soil, feces, or dead animals; however, contaminated fecal material also may pose a hazard to other livestock, as evidenced by one report (16) in which cattle developed listeric encephalitis after coming in contact with contaminated chicken litter. Thus while the true incidence of listeriosis in chickens and other forms of domestic livestock is undoubtedly much higher than published reports, listeriosis appears to be comparatively less common in domestic fowl.

While listeriosis in birds is often a secondary infection associated with viral infections (12) as well as salmonellosis, Newcastle disease, fowl pest, coryza, coccidiosis, worm infestations, mites, enteritis, lymphomatosis, ovarian tumors, and other immunocompromising conditions (29), listeric infections in previously healthy birds have also been observed. Septicemia, the most frequent manifestation of listeriosis in chickens and other domestic fowl, is characterized by focal necrosis within the viscera, particularly the liver and spleen (29). While not present in all cases (48), cardiac lesions frequently develop, which in turn lead to engorgement of cardiac vessels, pericarditis, and increased amounts of pericardial fluid (29,59). Other conditions produced by the septicemic form of avian listeriosis have included splenomeglia, nephritis, peritonitis, enteritis, ulcers in the ileum and ceca, necrosis of the oviduct, generalized or pulmonary edema, inflammation of the air sacs, and conjunctivitis. In acute cases, lesions resulting from these conditions may be partially obscured by congestion and hemorrhages throughout the viscera (29). Unfortunately, chickens and other domestic fowl that suffer from listeric septicemia normally exhibit few overt signs of disease other than progressive emaciation and usually die 5–9 days after infection.

Although far less common than the septicemic form of listeriosis, *L. monocytogenes* also can produce meningioencephalitis in domestic fowl. Unlike the septicemic form, domestic birds suffering from listeric meningioencephalitis exhibit several striking behavioral changes including incoordination, tremors, torticollis, unilateral/bilateral toe paralysis and dropped wings, all of which directly relate to disturbances of the central nervous system (5). Such infections are virtually always fatal. Post-mortem examination often reveals congestion and necrotic foci in the brain (5) along with many of the aforementioned conditions that are characteristic of listeric septicemia.

As is true for other newborn domestic farm animals, newly hatched chicks appear to be more susceptible to listeric infections than older birds (23,29). Following oral challenge of chickens with 10^2 or 10^6 *L. monocytogenes* cells, Bailey et al. (4) detected the pathogen more frequently in ceca, spleen, liver, and cloacal swab samples from 1- rather than 14- or 35-day-old chickens. Since avian listeriosis often appears as a secondary infection and adult birds are generally difficult to infect artificially (29), it appears that healthy birds possess a relatively high degree of resistance to listeric infections. These observations along with widespread use of antibiotics in poultry feed may help to explain the relatively low incidence of listeriosis in domestic fowl.

Fish and Crustaceans

Thus far occurrence of listeriosis in fish has been described in only one 1957 report from Romania (74). *Listeria monocytogenes* was isolated from the viscera of pond-reared rainbow trout that presumably became infected after consuming contaminated donkey meat. According to the investigators, the fish exhibited intermittent bouts of listlessness and agitation along with apparent blindness, loss of appetite, a blackened integument, and a bloody discharge from the anus, particularly females. Post-mortem examination revealed gross lesions throughout the viscera, serous fluid in the pericardial sac, and gas along with viscid liquid in the terminal portion of the intestinal tract as well as various histological changes relating to the liver, bile ducts, and kidneys. Although rainbow trout appear to be susceptible to listeriosis, absence of additional documented cases in fish since 1957 makes the significance of this single report difficult to interpret.

In 1959 *L. monocytogenes* also was detected in crustaceans gathered from a Russian stream (68). While this report confirms that crustaceans can harbor listeriae, the ability of these creatures to develop an actual *Listeria*-like illness remains questionable.

TREATMENT

The primary therapeutic goal in listeric encephalitis is to prevent the histopathological alterations that can lead to partial paralysis and permanent brain damage. Since these changes typically develop after the third or fourth day of infection, prompt antibiotic therapy of infected animals is crucial for their complete recovery. During early stages of bovine listeriosis, intramuscular administration of high doses of ampicillin or penicillin (40,000–44,000 IU/kg of body weight) has proven to be an effective treatment, provided the therapy is continued for 7–14 days. After 14 days, the dosage should be reduced by one-half and administered for an additional 7–14 days (18,60). Cases of septicemia and endometritis following abortion also have been successfully treated with antibiotics (56). In most cases of listeric infection, ampicillin is the antibiotic of choice (18,60).

In addition to administration of antibiotics, fluid therapy must be included to correct dehydration, acid-base imbalances, and electrolyte disturbances. Fluids must be forcibly given to animals that have lost the ability to swallow because of neurological disorders. Oral administration of fluids also aids in softening the extremely dry rumen contents which are painful to the animal. Lactated Ringer's solution can be given to correct electrolyte and acid-base imbalances. Acidotic animals require intravenous administration of bicarbonate, which should be continued until the blood pH returns to normal. Additional supportive therapy may include administration of vitamin E–selenium and analgesics in conjunction with transfer of rumen ingesta from healthy to infected animals as well as maintenance of good animal husbandry practices (18).

Listeriosis in sheep follows a hyperacute course with untreated animals seldom surviving beyond 4 days. Since irreparable neurological damage has already occurred at the first sign of symptoms, drug therapy is generally regarded as ineffective. Although sulfonamides and oxytetracycline have shown some promise, the overall prognosis remains poor (65,84).

A large increase in the incidence of listeric infections in Norway has prompted development of a vaccine against listeriosis in sheep (66). In field trials conducted in Norway (35), half of the sheep in 70 flocks (total of 3130 sheep) in which listeriosis had been a problem were vaccinated with a vaccine containing two attenuated strains of L. monocytogenes serotypes 1/2 and 4b, whereas the remaining half of the sheep served as unvaccinated controls. Both groups of animals were then housed together in the same pens. Results of this study showed listeriosis incidences of 1 and 3% in vaccinated and unvaccinated sheep, respectively. In 1984 a special license was issued to allow limited use of this vaccine in a 2-year field study (36). After vaccinating approximately 8% of all Norwegian sheep (ca. 145,000 head), the incidence of listeriosis reportedly decreased from approximately 4% before introduction of the vaccine to 1.5% after vaccination began. In addition, the percentage of listeric abortions was markedly lower in vaccinated than in unvaccinated sheep. While vaccination produced few adverse side effects, economic constraints suggest that vaccination of sheep should be confined to flocks that have exhibited recurrent listeric infections.

The outcome of listeriosis in goats is not quite as bleak. According to Løken and Grønstøl (44), 6 of 7 goats that exhibited moderate symptoms of listeric encephalitis recovered after daily intramuscular injections of penicillin (2.5 g) and dihydrostreptomycin (2.5 g) for 3 days. Two goats also recovered from listeric septicemia after being given penicillin (2.5 g) for 3 days. A relatively effective vaccine was developed recently to protect goats against listeric infections (22).

Since listeric encephalitis is a rapidly debilitating disease in ruminants, ampicillin and/or penicillin must be administered early during the course of infection if there is to be any reasonable hope of survival. Permanent neurological damage often occurs in ruminants, despite proper therapy. In view of the severe economic losses from listeric encephalitis in sheep, it may be prudent to consider vaccinating animals against listeriosis, particularly if they are being raised in areas prone to listeric infection.

REFERENCES

1. Amtsberg, G. von, A. Elsner, H. A. Grabbar, and W. Winkenwerder. 1969. Die epidemiologische und lebensmittelhygienische Bedeutung der Listerieninfektion des Rindes. *Dtsch. tierärztl. Wschr.* 76:497–501.

2. *Animal Health Yearbook.* 1986. Food and Agriculture Organization of the United Nations, World Health Organization and the International Office of Epizootics, Rome.
3. Arda, M. von, W. Bisping, N. Aydin, E. Istanbulluoglu, Ö. Akay, M. Izgür, Z. Karaer, S. Diker, and G. Kirpal. 1987. Ätiologische Untersuchungen über den Abort bei Schafen unter besonderer Berücksichtigung des Nachweises von Brucellen, Campylobacter, Salmonellen, Listerien, Leptospiren und Chlamydien. *Berl. Münch. tierärztl. Wschr. 100*:405–408.
4. Bailey, J. S., D. L. Fletcher, and N. A. Cox. 1990. *Listeria monocytogenes* colonization of broiler chickens. *Poultry Sci. 69*: 457–461.
5. Basher, H. A., D. R. Fowler, F. G. Rodgers, A. Seaman, and M. Woodbine. 1984. Pathogenicity of natural and experimental listeriosis in newly hatched chicks. *Res. Vet. Sci. 36*:76–80.
6. Belding, R. C., and M. L. Mayer. 1957. Listeriosis in the turkey—two case reports. *J. Amer. Vet. Med. Assoc. 131*:296–297.
7. Biester, H. E., and L. H. Schwarte. 1940. *Listerella* infection in swine. *J. Amer. Vet. Med. Assoc. 96*:339–342.
8. Bryner, J., R. Thornhill, I. Wesley, and M. van der Maaten. 1988. Experimental intramammary infection of dairy cows with *Listeria monocytogenes.* Abstr. Annu. Mtg. Amer. Soc. Microbiol., Miami Beach, FL, May 8–13, Abstr. P-20.
9. Bryner, J., M. van der Matten, and I. Wesley. 1988. Listeriosis in milk cows with intramammary inoculation of *Listeria monocytogenes.* Int. Symposium on Listeriosis, Pecs, Hungary, Aug. 22–26. Abst. 14.
10. Bunning, V. K., R. G. Crawford, J. G. Bradshaw, J. T. Peeler, J. T. Tierney, and R. M. Twedt. 1986. Thermal resistance of intracellular *Listeria monocytogenes* cells suspended in raw bovine milk. *Appl. Environ. Microbiol. 52*:1398–1402.
11. Carter, J. L., C. L. Chen, and S. M. Dennis. 1976. Serum levels of progesterone, estradiol and hydrocortisone in ewes after abortion due to *Listeria monocytogenes* type 5. *Amer. J. Vet. Res. 37*:1071–1073.
12. Cummins, T. J., I. M. Orne, and R. E. Smith. 1988. Reduced *in vivo* nonspecific resistance to *Listeria monocytogenes* infection during avian retrovirus-induced immunosuppression. *Avian Dis. 32*:663–667.
13. Dijkstra, R. G. 1966. Een studie over listeriosis bij runderen. *Tijdschr. Diergeneesk. 91*:906–916.
14. Dijkstra, R. G. 1971. Investigations on the survival times of *Listeria* bacteria in suspensions of brain tissue, silage and faeces and in milk. *Zbl. Bakteriol. I Abt. Orig. 216*:92–95.
15. Dijkstra, R. G. 1975. Recent experiences on the survival times of *Listeria* bacteria in suspensions of brain, tissue, silage, faeces and in milk. In M. Woodbine (ed.), *Problems of Listeriosis,* Leicester University Press, Leicester, pp. 71–73.
16. Dijkstra, R. G. 1976. *Listeria*-encephalitis in cows through litter from a broiler-farm. *Zbl. Bakteriol. Hyg., I Abt. Orig. B 161*:383–385.
17. Dijkstra, R. G. 1978. Incidence of *Listeria monocytogenes* in the intestinal contents of broilers on different farms. *Tijdschr. Diergeneesk. 103*:229–231.
18. Dijkstra, R. G. 1987. Listeriosis in animals—clinical signs, diagnosis and treatment. In A. Schönberg (ed.), *Listeriosis—Joint WHO/ROI Consultation on Prevention and Control,* West Berlin, December 10–12, 1986, pp. 68–76. Institut für Veterinärmedizin des Bundesgesundheitsamtes, Berlin.
19. Donker-Voet, J. 1962. My view on the epidemiology of *Listeria* infections. In M. L. Gray (ed.), *Second Symposium on Listeric Infection,* Montana State College, Bozeman, MT, pp. 133–139.
20. Donnelly, C. W. 1986. Listeriosis and dairy products: Why now and why milk? *Hoards Dairyman 121*(14):663, 687.
21. Farber, J. M., G. W. Sanders, and S. A. Malcom. 1988. The presence of *Listeria* spp. in raw milk in Ontario. *Can. J. Microbiol. 34*:95–100.
22. Fensterbank, R. 1987. Vaccination with a *Listeria* strain of reduced virulence against experimental *Listeria* abortion in goats. *Ann. Rech. Vét. 18*:415–419.
23. Guerden, L. M. G., and A. Devos. 1952. Listerellose bij pluimvee. *Vlaams Diergeneesk. Tschr. 21*:165–175.

24. Gill, D. A. 1931. Circling disease of sheep in New Zealand. *Vet. J. 87*:60–74.
25. Gitter, M. 1985. Listeriosis in farm animals in Great Britain. In C. H. Collins and J. M. Grange (eds.), *Isolation and Identification of Microorganisms of Medical and Veterinary Importance*, Academic Press, London.
26. Gitter, M., R. Bradley, and P. H. Blampied. 1980. *Listeria monocytogenes* infection in bovine mastitis. *Vet. Rec. 107*:390–393.
27. Graham, R. 1939. *Listerella* from a premature bovine fetus. *Science 90*:336–337.
28. Gray, M. L. 1958. Listeriosis in fowls—A review. *Avian Dis. 2*:296–314.
29. Gray, M. L., and A. H. Killinger. 1966. *Listeria monocytogenes* and listeric infections. *Bacteriol. Rev. 30*:309–382.
30. Gray, M. L., C. Singh, and F. Thorp. 1956. Abortion and pre- or postnatal death of young due to *Listeria monocytogenes*. III. Studies in ruminants. *Amer. J. Vet. Res. 17*:510–516.
31. Grønstøl, H. 1979. Listeriosis in sheep—*Listeria monocytogenes* excretion and immunological state in healthy sheep. *Acta Vet. Scand. 20*:168–179.
32. Grønstøl, H. 1979. Listeriosis in sheep—*Listeria monocytogenes* excretion and immunological state in sheep in flocks with clinical listeriosis. *Acta Vet. Scand. 20*:417–428.
33. Grønstøl, H. 1980. Listeriosis in sheep—*Listeria monocytogenes* in sheep fed hay or grass silage during pregnancy. Immunological state, white blood cells, total serum protein and serum iron. *Acta Vet. Scand. 21*:1–10.
34. Grønstøl, H. 1980. Listeriosis in sheep—isolation of *Listeria monocytogenes* from organs of slaughtered animals and dead animals submitted for post-mortem examination. *Acta Vet. Scand. 21*:11–17.
35. Gudding, R., H. Grønstøl, and H. J. Larsen. 1985. Vaccination against listeriosis in sheep. *Vet. Rec. 117*:89–90.
36. Gudding, R., L. L. Nesse, and H. Grønstøl. 1989. Immunisation against infections caused by *Listeria monocytogenes* in sheep. *Vet. Rec. 125*:111–114.
37. Hartwigk, H. von. 1958. Zum Nachweis von Listerien in der Kuhmilch. *Berlin Münch. tierärztl. Wochschr. 71*:82–85.
38. Hatkin, J. M., and W. E. Phillips, Jr. 1986. Isolation of *Listeria monocytogenes* from an eastern wild turkey. *J. Wildlife Dis. 22*:110–112.
39. Hyslop, N. St. G. 1975. Epdemiologic and immunologic factors in listeriosis. In M. Woodbine (ed.), *Problems of Listeriosis*, Leicester University Press, Leicester, pp. 94–105.
40. Hyslop, N. St. G., and A. D. Osborne. 1959. Listeriosis: A potential danger to public health. *Vet. Rec. 71*:1082–1091.
41. Jones, F. S., and R. B. Little. 1934. Sporadic encephalitis in cows. *Arch. Pathol. 18*:580–581.
42. Kampelmacher, E. H. 1962. Animal products as a source of listeric infection in man. In M. L. Gray (ed.), *Second Symposium on Listeric Infection*, Montana State College, Bozeman, MT, pp. 146–156.
43. Kovincic, I., B. Stajner, S. Zakula, and M. Galic. 1979. The finding of *L. monocytogenes* in the milk of cows from infected herds. In I. Ivanov (ed.), *Proceedings of the Seventh International Symposium on Listeriosis*, National Agroindustrial Union, Center for Scientific Information, Sofia, pp. 221–224.
44. Løken, T., and H. Grønstøl. 1982. Clinical investigations in a goat herd with outbreaks of listeriosis. *Acta Vet. Scand. 23*:380–391.
45. Løken, T., E. Aspøy, and H. Grønstøl. 1982. *Listeria monocytogenes* excretion and humoral immunity in goats in a herd with outbreaks of listeriosis and in a dairy herd. *Acta Vet. Scand. 23*:392–399.
46. Macleod, N. S. M., and J. A. Watt. 1974. *Listeria monocytogenes* type 5 as a cause of abortion in sheep. *Vet. Rec. 95*:365–367.
47. Mathews, F. P. 1928. Encephalitis in calves. *J. Amer. Vet. Assoc. 73*:513–516.
48. Nagi, M. S., and J. D. Verma. 1967. An outbreak of listeriosis in chickens. *Indian J. Vet. Med. 44*:539–543.
49. Narucka, V., and J. F. Westendorp. 1973. Het voorkomen van *Listeria monocytogenes* by slachtvarkens. *Tijdschr. Diergeneesk. 98*:1208.

50. Nilsson, A., and K. A. Karlsson. 1959. *Listeria monocytogenes* isolations from animals in Sweden during 1948 to 1957. *Nord. Vet. Med. 11*:305–315.
51. Ödegaard, B., R. Grelland, and S. D. Henricksen. 1952. A case of *Listeria*—infection in man, transmitted from sheep. *Acta Med. Scand. 67*:231–238.
52. Osebold, J. W., J. W. Kendrick, and A. Njoku-Obi. 1960. Cattle abortion associated with natural *Listeria monocytogenes* infections. *J. Amer. Vet. Med. Assoc. 137*:221–226.
53. Osebold, J. W., J. W. Kendrick, and A. Njoku-Obi. 1960. Abortion in cattle—experimentally with *Listeria monocytogenes. J. Amer. Vet. Med. Assoc. 137*:227–233.
54. Paterson, J. S. 1937. *Listerella* infection in fowls—preliminary note on its occurrence in East Anglia. *Vet. Rec. 49*:1533–1534.
55. Potel, J. 1953/1954. Ätiologie der Granulomatosis Infantiseptica. *Wiss. Z. Martin Luther Univ.-Halle, Wittenberg 3*:341.
56. Price, H. H. 1981. Outbreak of septicemic listeriosis in a dairy herd. *Vet. Med. Small Anim. Clin. 76*:73–74.
57. Rahman, T., D. K. Sarma, B. K. Goswami, T. N. Upadlhyaya, and B. Choudhury. 1985. Occurrence of listerial meningioencephalitis in pigs. *Indian Vet. J. 62*:7–9.
58. Ralovich, B. 1984. *Listeriosis Research—Present Situation and Perspective*, Akademiai Kiado, Budapest.
59. Ramos, J. A., M. Domingo, L. Dominguez, L. Ferrer, and A. Marco. 1988. Immunohistologic diagnosis of avian listeriosis. *Avian Pathol. 17*:227–233.
60. Rebhun, W. C., and A. deLahunta. 1982. Diagnosis and treatment of bovine listeriosis. *J. Amer. Vet. Med. Assoc. 180*:395–398.
61. Schmidt, V., and A. Nyfeldt. 1938. Über Mononucleosis Infectiosa und Meningoencephalitis. *Acta Oto-Laryng. 26*:680–688.
62. Schultz, G. 1967. Untersuchungen über das Vorkommen von Listerien in Rohmilch. *Monatsh. Veterinaermed. 22*:766–768.
63. Schwartz, J. C. 1967. Incidence of listeriosis in Pennsylvania livestock. *J. Amer. Vet. Med. Assoc. 151*:1435–1437.
64. Seastone, C. V. 1935. Pathogenic organisms of the genus *Listerella. J. Exp. Med. 62*:203–212.
65. Seeliger, H. P. R. 1961. *Listeriosis*, Hafner Publishing Co., New York.
66. Selbitz, H.-J. von. 1986. Immunological principles for control of listeriosis. *Monatsh. Veterinaermed. 41*:217–219.
67. Sharma, K. N., P. K. Mehrotra, and P. N. Mehrotra. 1983. Characterization of *L. monocytogenes* strains causing occulo-encephalitis in goats. *Ind. J. Anim. Sci. 54*:514–515.
68. Shlygina, K. N. 1959. Studies of variation in the causative organism of listeriosis. *Zh. Mikrobiol. Epidemiol. Immunobiol. 30*:68–75.
69. Sindoni, L., V. Ciano, I. Picerno, A. Di Pietro, and W. Farina. 1983. Ricerche sulla epidemiologia della listeriosi-Nota II: Ulteriori risultati di un' indagine sierologica sulla frequenza di anticorpi anti-*Listeria* in diverse specie animali dimoranti in alcune zone della Sicilia e della Calabria. *Arch. Vet. Ital. 34*:103–109.
70. Sipka, M., B. Stajner, and S. Zakula. 1973. Detection of *Listeria* in milk. *Wien. tierärztl. Monatsschr. 60*(2/3):50–52.
71. Skovgaard, N., and C. A. Morgen. 1988. Detection of *Listeria* spp. in faeces from animals, in feeds, and in raw foods of animal origin. *Int. J. Food Microbiol. 6*:229–242.
72. Smith, R. E., I. M. Reynolds, and R. A. Bennett. 1955. *Listeria monocytogenes* and abortion in a cow. *J. Amer. Vet. Med. Assoc. 126*:106–110.
73. Stajner, B. 1975. Excretion of *Listeria* through milk of infected cows. *Dairy Sci. Abstr. 37*:180.
74. Stamatin, N., C. Ungureanu, E. Constantinescu, A. Solnitzky, and E. Vasilescu. 1957. Infectia naturala cu *Listeria monocytogenes* la pastravul curcubeu *Salmo irideus. Annuar. Inst. Animal Pathol. Hyg. Bucuresti 7*:163–180.
75. Vizcaino, L. L., and M. A. Garcia. 1975. A note on *Listeria* milk excretion in sero-positive apparently healthy cows. In M. Woodbine (ed.), *Problems of Listeriosis*, Leicester University Press, Surrey, England, p. 74.

76. de Vries, J., and R. Strikwerda. 1957. Een geval van *Listeria*-mastitis bij het rund. *Tschr. Diergeneesk. 81*:833–838.
77. de Vries, J., and R. Strikwerda. 1957. Ein Fall klinischer Euter-Listeriose beim Rind. *Zbl. Bakteriol. Abt. I Orig. 167*:229–232.
78. Wardrope, D. D., and N. S. M. Macleod. 1983. Outbreak of *Listeria* meningioencephalitis in young lambs. *Vet. Rec. 113*:213–214.
79. Wesley, I. V., J. H. Bryner, and M. J. van der Maaten. 1989. Effects of dexamethasone on shedding of *Listeria monocytogenes* in dairy cattle. Ann. Mtg. Amer. Soc. Microbiol., New Orleans, LA, May 14–18, Abst. C-381.
80. Wesley, I., J. Warg, J. Bryner, and M. van der Maaten. 1988. Agglutination titers of serum and whey obtained from *Listeria monocytogenes*-infected dairy cattle. Abstr. Ann. Mtg. Amer. Soc. Microbiol., Miami Beach, FL, May 8–13, Abstr. E-91.
81. Wohler, W. H., and C. L. Baugh. 1983. Pulmonary listeriosis in feeder cattle. *Med. Vet. Pract. 64*:736–739.
82. Wramby, G. O. 1944. Om *Listerella monocytogenes* bakteriologi och om forekomst av *Listerella* infektioner has djur. *Skand. Vet. Tskr. 34*:278–290.
83. Yndestad, M. 1987. Personal communication.
84. Yousif, Y. A., B. P. Joshi, and H. A. Ali. 1984. Ovine and caprine listeric encephalitis in Iraq. *Trop. Anim. Health Prod. 16*:27–28.

4

Listeriosis in Humans

INTRODUCTION

Human listeriosis has likely been with us for many years. As mentioned earlier, at least seven cases of a listeriosis-like illness were recorded in the literature (48) before *L. monocytogenes* was first accurately described by Murray et al. (65) in 1926. In fact, Saxbe (83) theorized that this organism may have been responsible for changing the course of English history. In 1683, Princess Anne, the second daughter of King James II, married Prince George of Denmark, and she eventually became Queen of England in 1702. According to historical records, Queen Anne failed to produce an heir for the royal throne despite 17 pregnancies which included 12 miscarriages and/or stillbirths, four neonatal/infant deaths, and loss of a hydrocephalic son from meningitis at age 11. These events are strikingly similar to the present-day clinical picture of listeriosis to be described shortly. Following Queen Anne's death, the British Crown passed to the House of Hanover (King George I), which took advantage of the political situation to establish Sir Robert Walpole as the first Prime Minister of England.

While this historical account of a listeriosis-like illness within the British royal family is interesting and thought-provoking, the first case of listeriosis in humans was not confirmed until 1929. In that year, Nyfeldt (69) isolated *L. monocytogenes* from the blood of three patients who had contracted an infectious mononucleosis-like disease. [As fate would have it, the cultures isolated by Nyfeldt were unusual in that all belonged to serotype 3—a type so rare that it was not encountered again until 1954 (38).] During 1933 and 1934, *L. monocytogenes* was established as a cause of meningitis and perinatal infections in the United States (20). However, until 1945 the organism was only isolated sporadically from humans and resulted in fewer than 40 cases of human listeric infection recorded in the medical literature (48). The first recorded massive outbreak of human listeriosis occurred in East Germany between 1949 and 1957 and resulted in a dramatic increase in the number of stillborn infants. This outbreak caused an awareness of listeric infections in humans, which gradually spread from Europe to the United States (90).

Despite increased reports of listeric infection, human listeriosis remains a rare disease compared to other reportable illnesses. According to Ralovich (75) (Table 4.1), only 36 cases of listeriosis were recorded in Hungary between 1974 and 1985. During this 12-year period, listeric infections comprised only 0.01% of all cases of notifiable disease in Hungary, being dwarfed by scarlet fever, salmonellosis, and dysentery. Anthrax was the only notifiable illness with fewer reported cases than listeriosis.

Table 4.1 Notifiable Diseases in Hungary, 1974–1985

Disease	Number of cases	Number of deaths	Mortality (%)
Scarlet fever	137,006 (44.13)[a]	4(0.50)[b]	0.003
Salmonellosis	81,091 (26.12)	101(12.56)	0.12
Dysentery	74,727 (24.07)	52(6.47)	0.07
Dyspepsia coli	10,002 (3.22)	81(10.07)	0.81
Staphylococcosis	3,562 (1.15)	12(1.49)	0.34
Meningitis epidemica	848 (0.27)	84(10.45)	9.91
Tetanus	590 (0.19)	409(50.87)	69.32
Leptospirosis	580 (0.19)	18(2.23)	3.10
Brucellosis	576 (0.19)	3(0.37)	0.52
Tularemia	491 (0.16)	1(0.12)	0.20
Typhus abdominalis	439 (0.14)	11(1.36)	2.51
Pertussis	429 (0.14)	7(0.87)	1.63
Diphtheria	48 (0.02)	5(0.62)	10.42
Paratyphus	46 (0.01)	0(0.00)	0.00
Listeriosis	36 (0.01)	15(1.86)	41.67
Anthrax	10 (0.003)	1(0.12)	10.0
Total	310,481	804	

[a]Percent of the total number of cases.
[b]Percent of the total number of deaths.
Source: Adapted from Ref. 49.

Furthermore, listeriosis ranked seventh in overall numbers of fatalities and was responsible for 1.86% of the total number of deaths from notifiable diseases in Hungary (Table 4.1). However, in terms of mortality rate, listeriosis ranked second to tetanus with 41.67% of the cases ending in death. Thus, although numbers of listeriosis cases in the general population appear to be small, consequences of a listeric infection can be devastating.

INCIDENCE

The true incidence of human listeriosis is largely unknown because of (a) variable interest in investigating probable cases of listeriosis in different countries, (b) a general inability to detect mild listeriosis cases, and (c) a lack of uniform reporting of the disease in different countries (49). According to earlier literature, only 36 cases of human listeriosis were recorded up to 1945. Since that time, the number of cases reported worldwide increased to about 1000 in 1960 and 1500 in 1962. In 1972, Seeliger (75) estimated the total number of human listeriosis cases at about 5000. During the 1970s, slight increases in numbers of listeric infections were observed in England, France, and Spain; a similar trend occurred during the 1980s in Belgium, Denmark, France, and Switzerland (76).

Data collected from various sources (Table 4.2) show a dramatic increase in numbers of reported listeric infections in the United States during two periods—1933–1966 and 1970–1977. Incidences of listeriosis in California, New York, and Illinois were similar to the national average of 0.65 case/10^6 people for the period of 1970–1977.

Heightened awareness of *L. monocytogenes* fostered by major outbreaks of foodborne listeriosis in 1981 (86), 1983 (32), 1985 (47), and 1987 (4) has led to development of improved methods to detect the bacterium. This has led to a dramatic increase in the number of listeriosis cases reported since 1985. Consequently, there have been attempts to reevaluate the incidence of listeriosis in the United States. Compilation of all reported cases of listeriosis in New Jersey, Tennessee, Missouri, Oklahoma, Washington, and Los Angeles County during 1986 led Broome et al. (18) at the Centers for Disease Control to project that approximately 1600 cases of listeriosis occur annually in the United States with an annual incidence of ~6.7 cases/10^6 population. In addition, Mascola et al. (59,60) identified 94 listeriosis cases in Los Angeles County during the 12-month period between August 1985 and September 1986 and 64 cases during 1987, which in turn yielded an annual incidence rate of ~8.5 cases/10^6 population. Thus it appears that the incidence of listeriosis in the United States has risen approximately 10-fold during the last 15 years. However, in reality, this dramatic increase in incidence of listeriosis is almost certainly the result of increased awareness of *L. monocytogenes* prompted by the 1985 listeriosis outbreak in southern California which was linked to consumption of Mexican-style cheese. Data concerning prevalence of listeriosis in Canada between 1971 and 1982 (Table 4.2) reveal a disproportionately high incidence of listeric infections in Nova Scotia (2.68 cases/10^6 people) and Prince Edward Island (2.61 cases/10^6 people) as compared to the remaining Canadian provinces (average of 0.63 case/10^6 people). The higher incidence of listeriosis in Nova Scotia also is the direct result of a major foodborne outbreak in 1981 which was linked to consumption of contaminated coleslaw (27,86). Although this outbreak was officially responsible for only 41 cases of listeriosis, 83 cases were reported in 1981, 82 of which were traced to *L. monocytogenes* serotype 4b (27). If the 83 cases of listeriosis that occurred in 1981 are omitted, then an average of 2.40 listeriosis cases/10^6 people would have occurred annually in Nova Scotia between 1972 and 1982. Thus it appears this outbreak was responsible for at least 79 cases. Although the incidence of listeriosis was moderately higher in Canada during 1972–1982 than in the United States during 1970–1977, eliminating 79 cases of the 1981 outbreak in Nova Scotia from the calculations results in an incidence of 0.70 case/10^6 people in Canada as compared to 0.65 case/10^6 people in the United States. Thus there is essentially no difference between the incidences of listeriosis in the United States and Canada.

Early European data (Table 4.3) indicate that the prevalence of listeriosis varied widely among different countries with average annual incidence rates ranging from 0.04 to 3.70 cases/10^6 population during 1949 to 1986. Not surprisingly, inadequate or in most instances nonexistent reporting led to an underestimation of listeriosis cases in Europe. Increased reporting of listeriosis in Europe did not become evident until Vacherin Mont d'Or soft-ripened cheese was linked to a major outbreak of listeriosis in Switzerland near the end of 1987 (13,14,19). Western European data collected during and after this outbreak (Table 4.4) indicate an incidence rate of ~3.6–8.0 listeriosis cases/10^6 population in all countries except France with the latter rate being two to four

Table 4.2 Incidence of Human Listeriosis in the United States and Canada

Country	Year	Total number of cases	Average number of cases/year	Approximate median population ($\times 10^6$)	Average incidence /10^6 people	Ref.
United States	1933–1966	731	22.15	152.27	0.14	8
United States	1970–1977	1118	139.75	218.85	0.65	75
United States (31 states)	1971	104	104	—	—	40
California	1971	10	10	19.95	0.50	40
Illinois	1971	7	7	11.11	0.63	40
New York	1971	8	8	18.24	0.43	40
Tennessee	1971	7	7	3.92	1.79	40
United States	1978–1982	—	—	—	ca. 1.0	85
United States	1980–1982	ca. 2400	800	—	ca. 3.6	7, 87
United States	1985–1986	ca. 1600	1600	238.6	ca. 6.7	18, 87
California						
Los Angeles County	1985–1986	94	94	7.83	11.7	59
Los Angeles County	1987	64	64	7.83	8.5	60
Pennsylvania	1985	—	—	—	ca. 3.0	88
New Jersey	1985	—	—	—	ca. 5.0	88
United States	1986	ca. 1700	1700	229.6	ca. 7.4	73
Canada	1951–1982	362	11.3	19.68	0.57	49
Canada	1951–1971	101	4.81	17.91	0.27	9
Canada	1972–1982	258 (178)[a]	23.73 (16.18)	24.03	1.08 (0.70)	15
British Columbia	1972–1982	20	1.82	2.74	0.66	15
Alberta	1972–1982	10	0.91	2.24	0.40	15
Manitoba	1972–1982	6	0.54	1.03	0.53	15
Saskatchewan	1972–1982	7	0.64	0.97	0.66	15
Ontario	1972–1982	59	5.36	8.63	0.63	15
Quebec	1972–1982	34	3.09	6.44	0.48	15
New Brunswick	1972–1982	7	0.64	0.70	0.91	15
Nova Scotia	1972–1982	107 (28)[a]	9.72	0.85	11.43 (2.99)	15
Prince Edward Island	1972–1982	3	0.27	0.12	2.21	15
Newfoundland	1972–1982	5	0.45	0.57	0.79	15

[a]Estimated number of cases not including 79 cases presumed to be associated with the 1981 listeriosis outbreak in Nova Scotia.

Table 4.3 Incidence of Human Listeriosis in 15 European Countries, 1949–1986

Country	Years	Total number of cases	Average number of cases/year	Approximate median population ($\times 10^6$)	Average annual incidence per 10^6 people
Belgium[a]	1982–1985	145	36.25	9.83	3.70
Bulgaria	1955–1981	11	0.40	7.85	0.05
Denmark	1958–1974	164	10.25	4.78	2.14
East Germany	1949–1981	1924	58.30	17.30	3.37
Finland	1961–1977	15	0.93	4.61	0.20
France	1970–1975	1021	170.16	51.7	3.29
Greece	1967–1979	5	0.41	8.93	0.04
Hungary[a]	1965–1986	61	2.90	10.53	0.28
Netherlands	1958–1976	435	22.89	13.03	1.76
Slovakia	1960–1981	48	2.28	4.73	0.48
Sweden	1958–1981	289	12.04	7.26	1.66
Switzerland	1958–1980	118	5.13	2.51	2.04
United Kingdom	1967–1981	618	41.20	54.44	0.76
West Germany	1950–1966	832	52.00	59.04	0.88
Yugoslavia	1960–1977	35	1.94	20.37	0.09

[a]From Ref. 76.
Source: Adapted from Ref. 75.

Table 4.4 Incidence of Listeriosis in Western Europe, 1981–1988

Country	Year(s)	Total number of cases	Approximate population ($\times 10^6$)	Annual incidence 10^6 people	Ref.
Austria	1986	39	7.55	5.2	2
Denmark	1986	—	—	ca. 8.0	13
France	1984	—	—	ca. 11.3	37
	1986	811	55.81	14.7	35, 36
	1987	—	—	ca.15.0	13
Norway	1987	15	4.20	3.6	99
Sweden	1987	32	8.37	3.8	99
Switzerland	1988	—	—	ca. 6.0	13
United Kingdom	1987	—	—	ca. 5.0	13
England and Wales	1983	115	49.96	2.30	5, 39
	1984	113	49.96	2.26	5, 39
	1985	149	49.96	2.98	5, 39
	1986	134	49.96	2.68	5, 39
	1987	259	49.96	5.18	5, 39
	1988	ca. 290	49.96	5.12	5, 39
Scotland	1987	35	5.12	6.83	22
	1988	40	5.12	7.81	22

times higher. Thus, excluding France, the annual incidences of listeriosis in Austria, Denmark, Norway, Sweden, Switzerland, and the United Kingdom are generally similar to rates of illness observed in the United States and probably Canada.

According to results from a March 1989 survey of 24 member nations of the International Dairy Federation (44), all 14 European countries responding to the survey as well as the United States, Canada, Australia, New Zealand, and Japan agreed that *L. monocytogenes* is a current public health concern in each country. To our knowledge, listeriosis is presently a notifiable disease in only six European countries—East Germany, Iceland, Norway, Sweden, Switzerland (75,77), and West Germany (3), in which only neonatal and meningitis cases are reportable. However, the Public Health Laboratory Service in the United Kingdom is attempting to obtain food histories from all listeriosis victims via voluntary reporting to further define the significance of *L. monocytogenes* as a foodborne pathogen (5,39). Such persistence on the part of European public health officials will probably further confirm similar rates of listeric infection in Western Europe and North America as evidenced by recent increased rates of listeriosis in England/Wales and Scotland (Table 4.4).

SUSCEPTIBILITY AND RESISTANCE
TO LISTERIC INFECTION

Surveys generally have shown that between 1 and 9% of the human population carries *L. monocytogenes* in its feces, with most individuals remaining asymptomatic (75). Although listeriosis is of minimal concern to healthy individuals, certain segments of the population, including pregnant women, newborns, and adults suffering from an underlying illness that results in a compromised immune system, can develop life-threatening illness (8). The latter group includes adults who are undergoing treatment for malignancies such as lymphoma or leukemia, as well as carcinomas of the breast (40,63), stomach, adrenal glands, and liver (67). Individuals who have undergone organ transplants, particularly renal (17,40,63,72,94,97), and hemodialysis also are at increased risk of developing listeriosis as are patients suffering from collagen-vascular disease, rheumatoid arthritis, aplastic anemia, asthma, and ulcerative colitis since many of these conditions are treated with corticosteroids or other types of immunosuppressive therapy (40,67). Finally, patients suffering from various chronic diseases including alcoholism (16,17,40,63,72), sarcoidosis, diabetes (16), cirrhosis of the liver (16,72), and otitis also are predisposed to develop listeric infections (67).

The age distribution of reported cases of listeriosis is not uniform. Two surveys made in the United States during 1970–1971 and 1980–1981 indicate that most cases occur in the very young and the very old (1). Infants less than 1 year old comprised the largest group of individuals with listeric infections and accounted for at least 25% of all listeriosis cases. [In a Canadian survey, neonatal listeriosis accounted for approximately 45% of the total number of cases reported between 1951 and 1972 (27).] A bimodal age distribution was observed for listeriosis cases in newborn infants with mean ages of 1.3 and 14.0 days at the time of onset. Cases of early onset listeriosis normally acquire infection directly from the mother (89), whereas late onset cases may result from nosocomial transmission (7,62,93). Approximately 55% of listeriosis cases reported in this survey occurred in adults ≥45 years old, with approximately 30% of the cases occurring in individuals ≥65 years of age, most of whom were suffering from an underlying illness. Although the route of infection in adults is seldom known, nosocomial transmission has been reported (69). Normal healthy individuals between 1 and 44 years old comprised <20% of the total number of listeriosis cases reported in this survey, which suggests that most people are resistant to infection by *L. monocytogenes*.

Although many people come in contact with or carry *L. monocytogenes*, few individuals develop listeriosis. Thus far the phenomenon of resistance to listeric infection has been studied primarily in mice. Assuming that mice and the normal human population respond similarly to *L. monocytogenes*, then resistance to this bacterium can be divided into an early nonimmunologic phase of natural resistance which is under genetic control and a later phase of immunologically acquired specific cellular resistance (50).

These two distinct phases of resistance are related to growth of *L. monocytogenes* in the liver and spleen of mice. Within 10 minutes after injecting mice with a sublethal dose of *L. monocytogenes*, 90% of the organisms are captured by the liver, with most of the remaining organisms trapped in the spleen. Six hours later, 90% of the cells originally captured in the liver are destroyed through antibacterial activity expressed by resident tissue macrophages (large phagocytes) also known as Kupffer cells. However, any remaining viable cells begin to grow logarithmically within susceptible liver and spleen macrophages and reach a maximum population 2–3 days after infection was initiated. At this point, rapid bacterial inactivation begins through development of acquired cellular resistance. Recovery of the host normally occurs within a week (49,50).

Activation of T-lymphocytes leading to acquired cellular immunity is a three-stage process. The first stage that occurs in response to a listeric infection involves two significant events: (a) priming of prekiller T-cells and (b) generation of *Listeria* antigen–specific helper T-cells. During the second stage, helper T-cells are stimulated by *Listeria* antigens to release a soluble substance or lymphokine (interleukin-2). In the final phase interleukin-2 converts the prekiller T-cell into a *L. monocytogenes*–dependent cytotoxic T-lymphocyte which rapidly destroys the organism (23). Recently, Lu (54) demonstrated that newborn mice are more susceptible than older mice to listeric infections because of the absence of cell-surface immune-response-gene-associated (Ia) antigens which are needed to generate *Listeria* antigen–specific helper T-cells. Therefore, in the absence of Ia antigens, prekiller T-cells cannot be converted to killer T-cells and cellular resistance cannot be acquired.

Considering that the most striking feature of acquired immunodeficiency syndrome (AIDS) is the profound impairment of the patient's T-cell–mediated immune response, it is surprising to learn that even though approximately 5% of the general population harbors *L. monocytogenes* as part of its normal intestinal microflora, as of November 1989 only 11 AIDS patients in the United States and Western Europe have acquired listeric infections (11,15,29,34,41,51,55,58,59,71,80–82,84). Five of these 11 listeriosis cases occurred in Los Angeles County, California, between January 1, 1985, and January 1986, during which time 1909 cases of AIDS were reported. Thus the annual incidence of listeriosis among AIDS patients in Los Angeles County was ~2.6 cases/1000 patients. When compared to the incidence of listeriosis for all individuals residing in Los Angeles County, 0.0085 case/1000 population, it becomes evident that AIDS patients are about 305 times more likely than the general public to contract listeriosis. Using somewhat different figures, FDA officials (6) recently reported that individuals with AIDS or AIDS-related conditions are 670 times more likely to contract listeric infections than individuals with normal immune systems. Although these findings indicate that AIDS patients are many times more likely to contract listeriosis than the general public, the startling fact remains that thus far (early 1989) only 11 AIDS patients are known to have acquired listeric infections.

Knowing that AIDS produces an extreme form of immunosuppression, one would logically conclude that the incidence of listeriosis among AIDS patients should be much higher. While reasons behind the lower-than-expected incidence of listeriosis in AIDS patients are poorly understood, Jacobs and Murray (46) suggested that various epidemiological and genetic influences, as well as nonimmune and immune mechanisms, may be involved. Among these theories, one possibility is that rigorous antibiotic (i.e., trimethoprim/sulfamethoxazole) therapy used in treating Pneumocystis pneumonia in AIDS patients may decrease exposure to *L. monocytogenes* by eliminating the bacterium from the gastrointestinal tract. Genetic determinants of resistance to listeric infections also might be at least partially active in AIDS patients. Current evidence also suggests that the nonspecific host defense mechanism may remain active enough to ward off listeric infections in AIDS patients. Finally, although only T4+-cells are presently known to respond to microbial antigens, the lower-than-expected incidence of listeriosis in AIDS patients suggests that yet another type of T-cell may be able to activate an alternative antilisterial immune mechanism.

Although little information is available concerning the host defense mechanism in human newborns, Issekutz et al. (45) concluded that infected infants lack both a specific antibody response as well as a cell-mediated immune response to *L. monocytogenes*. Read and Williams (79), using interferon, increased the killing activity of natural killer T-cells from human infants, which shows that decreased cellular immunity to listeric infection at birth results from small numbers of natural killer T-cells rather than a poor functional capacity of these cells.

Natural resistance to listeric infection in mice is regulated by one major, autosomal, dominant gene. Genetic control of natural resistance becomes apparent during logarithmic growth of *L. monocytogenes*, during which time mice of a genotype susceptible to listeric infection fail to prevent growth of the bacterium to lethal levels and succumb to the illness before acquired cellular resistance can develop. In contrast, mice belonging to a resistant genotype can prevent growth of *Listeria* during the initial 2 days until acquired cellular resistance develops. In this instance, genetically determined natural resistance to listeriosis is correlated with an increased ability to promptly mobilize macrophages at an infective site (66). The importance of natural resistance cannot be overemphasized since the short generation time of *L. monocytogenes* would otherwise allow the organism to reach lethal levels before acquired cellular resistance could be developed.

Resistance of mice to listeric infection also is affected by factors other than genetic makeup. Although the mycotoxin designated as T-2 (synthesized by molds in the genus *Fusarium*) can suppress both cell-mediated and humoral immune systems in laboratory mice by destroying lymphocytes and lymphoid organs (i.e., thymus, spleen, and lymph nodes), Corrier and Ziprin (25) recently found that mice given multiple daily oral doses of T-2 toxin 5 days before intraperitoneal inoculation with *L. monocytogenes* were more resistant to listeric infections than were control mice. Substantial decreases in mortality rates also were observed for toxin-treated rather than nontreated mice. Further work demonstrated resistance to listeric infection when mice were given simultaneous oral or intraperitoneal doses of T-2 toxin and *L. monocytogenes* (26). Later Ziprin and McMurray (100) reported that T-2 toxin did not afford resistance when mice inhaled aerosols containing *L. monocytogenes*. Thus it appears the effect of T-2 toxin on the course of listeric infection is not determined by the toxin alone, but rather by the route of exposure to *L. monocytogenes*. While the mechanism by which T-2 toxin enhances resistance to listeric infections in certain situations remains unclear, several authors have postulated that ingestion of T-2 toxin may stimulate macrophage activity in mice in a manner similar to cyclophosphamide, which also increases resistance to listeric infection (12,96).

Inoculating mice with heat-killed or avirulent strains of bacteria in genera other than *Listeria* also appears to enhance resistance to listeric infections. Nomoto et al. (68) reported that intravenous injection of mice with heat-killed cells of *Lactobacillus casei* led to increased resistance to listeriosis which lasted at least 21 days. Similarly, Selbitz et al. (92) found that intraperitoneal injection of an avirulent strain of *Salmonella dublin* into mice enhanced their resistance to listeric infection. Resistance of both *L. casei*– and *S. dublin*–treated mice to listeriosis was associated with increased macrophage activity. These findings indicate that resistance in mice to *L. monocytogenes* infections can be enhanced by other microorganisms. Assuming that similarities exist between the response of mice and humans to listeric infection, numerous environmental factors yet to be discovered also may contribute to increased resistance or susceptibility to listeriosis in humans.

CLINICAL MANIFESTATIONS OF VARIOUS FORMS OF LISTERIOSIS

The clinical features of listeric infection vary widely and often are confused with other illnesses. However, human listeriosis is generally characterized by pus-forming, miliary granulomas (masses of inflamed tissue comprised of many small lesions) and focal necroses. Such granulomas associated with listeriosis are commonly referred to as

Table 4.5 Manifestations of Listeriosis in Humans

---

1. Listeriosis during pregnancy
2. Listeriosis of the newborn (granulomatosis infantiseptica)
3. Meningitis, meningioencephalitis, and encephalitis
4. Cutaneous form
5. Septicemia with pharyngitis and mononucleosis
6. Oculoglandular form
7. Cervicoglandular form
8. Granulomatosis septica and typhoid-pneumonic form
9. Other forms

"listeriomas." Size, number, and site of these lesions vary among cases and depend on the infectious dose and route of infection as well as age and immunological state of the individual. Based on the most prominent clinical symptoms, Seeliger and Finger (91) identified nine manifestations of listeric infection (Table 4.5). However, cases of human listeriosis cannot always be classified into one of these nine categories since combinations of two or more manifestations may occur simultaneously or in succession.

LISTERIOSIS DURING PREGNANCY

Infection of pregnant women commonly results in a variety of "flu-like" symptoms including fever, chills, headache, and backache. Pharyngitis, diarrhea, and pyelitis (inflammation of the pelvis of the kidney) have been noted, but meningitis is rare (89,91). However, infected pregnant women may be asymptomatic or exhibit only mild symptoms (90). During the appearance of symptoms that are an expression of listeric bacteremia, the bacterium can be isolated from maternal blood, umbilical cord blood, lochia (discharge from uterus and vagina following delivery), vaginal mucous, urine, and placental tissue (91).

Listeriosis in pregnant women most often develops after the fifth month of gestation and leads to infection of the fetus either via the transplacental route or during delivery (91). However, some listeriosis cases have developed before the fourth month of pregnancy and may have led to embryo damage.

The time interval between maternal and fetal infections is poorly defined. In some cases, abortion or stillbirth occurred immediately after the mother experienced "flu-like" symptoms, whereas in others these events were separated by several weeks. After recovery, the mother may carry *L. monocytogenes* in her feces and genital tract for a considerable time, which may lead to recurring problems in later pregnancies (90).

LISTERIOSIS OF THE NEWBORN
(GRANULOMATOSIS INFANTISEPTICA)

In 1961, Seeliger (90) firmly established granulomatosis infantiseptica as a listeric infection. Today, neonatal listeriosis is among the most dangerous forms of listeriosis and is a major cause of fetal damage and infant death, along with syphilis, erythroblastosis, and toxoplasmosis. As previously mentioned, listeric infection of the fetus normally occurs via the transplacental route as a result of maternal bacteremia, after which the organism is spread to all organs and eventually excreted in the urine. Since respiratory and gastrointestinal distress are commonly observed in newborn infants suffering from listeriosis, it has been postulated that the fetus becomes infected through aspiration of contaminated amniotic fluid into which *Listeria*-contaminated urine was discharged. Evidence suggests that not all listeric infections in newborn infants are acquired in utero; some have resulted from direct contact with vaginal mucous during delivery (91). Hence, attention should be given to disinfection of resuscitation equipment and proper handwashing to avoid cross-infection within delivery rooms and neonatal units. However, numerous reports also indicate that neonatal listeriosis can be acquired as a cross-infection within hospitals with approximately 42 such infections occurring in Britain between 1967 and 1985 (61).

Symptoms of neonatal listeriosis are somewhat variable, but generally include respiratory distress, heart failure, forced respiration, cyanosis, refusal to drink, vomiting, convulsions, soft whimpering, mucous stools, and early discharge of meconium (greenish mass that accumulates in the bowel during fetal life). Although examination of the pharynx is difficult in newborns, this step should never be omitted if listeriosis is suspected, since characteristic multiple granulomas (listeriomas) are routinely observed along the posterior pharyngeal wall. Temperature is of little diagnostic importance since cases with both hyper- and hypothermia have been observed. Histologic examination may reveal pronounced leukocytosis (increase in number of leukocytes) along with an increase in the number of immature red and white blood cells. Occasionally, monocytosis (increase in number of monocytes—large phagocytic leukocytes) also has been observed (90,91). Since few symptoms are unique to neonatal listeriosis, proper etiological diagnosis must rely on isolation of the bacterium from various specimens including meconium, amniotic fluid, infant and maternal blood, and the maternal genital tract (8).

Pathologically, neonatal listeriosis is characterized by development of small nodules on numerous internal organs. The widespread appearance of numerous grayish-yellow nodules on the liver is particularly common. Similar findings often have been observed in the spleen, adrenal glands, lungs, esophagus, posterior pharyngeal wall, and tonsils. Subepithelial granulomas often undergo necrosis with cutaneous nodules occurring most frequently on the back and lumbar region of the infant. Granulomas also have been detected in lymph nodes, thymus, bone marrow, myocardium, testes, and skeletal muscle. Occasional involvement of the intestinal tract is primarily confined to lymphatic structures of the small intestine and appendix (59).

In untreated cases of perinatal listeriosis, prospects for survival are poor with the mortality rate approaching 100%; however, prompt antibiotic therapy has resulted in many survivors. Long-term prognosis depends on whether or not the infection has spread to the central nervous system and resulted in meningitis. Complications of perinatal listeriosis may then include hydrocephalus and mental retardation. Degen and Goldenbaum (28) examined 29 of 43 children over a period of 1–8 years after being diagnosed as having neonatal listeriosis. Results showed that 5 of 29 children had neurological disorders, which included three cases of hydrocephalus (28) in which increased levels of cerebrospinal fluid (CSF) within the cranial cavity cause the cerebral ventricles to expand which, in turn, results in enlargement of the skull and forehead as well as atrophy of the brain (90). Compromised intellectual development was observed in 7 of 29 children, which included three cases of moderate to severe mental retardation. Evans et al. (31) examined eight 16-month-old survivors of fetal or neonatal listeriosis for long-term medical or developmental disabilities. Six of eight infants exhibited no evidence of neurological or developmental disabilities. Although 4 of 6 infants remained healthy after recovering from neonatal listeriosis, two infants developed critical postnatal infections. The remaining two infants were born prematurely with severe perinatal listeriosis, which included central nervous system complications (meningitis and/or intraventricular hemorrhage). Although intelligence of these two infants appeared normal, both suffered from spastic displagia (paralysis of the identical part on the right and left sides of the body).

In both cases, premature delivery was related to development of severe illness leading to a long-term handicap. However, in the absence of meningitis and other neurological complications, long-term prognosis of perinatal listeriosis survivors is very good.

MENINGITIS, MENINGIOENCEPHALITIS, AND ENCEPHALITIS

Meningitis, meningioencephalitis, and encephalitis comprise the most dangerous category of listeric infections and are usually a consequence of generalized bacteremia. However, lymphatic spread from localized infections of the nose, throat, eye, and ear also have been reported (91).

Although no age group is spared from listeric meningitis, this illness develops primarily in newborn infants and older adults, typically males over 50 years of age. Clinically, this illness cannot be differentiated from other forms of bacterial meningitis; hence, diagnosis rests solely on results from bacteriological tests. The course of the disease is often fulminant (sudden onset of great severity) and has a fatality rate of approximately 70% in untreated patients or patients that are treated too late in the course of infection (91). Finally, those individuals who survive listeric meningitis may be afflicted with various brain abnormalities including hydrocephalus, cerebral edema, and cerebellar atrophy (57).

At the onset of listeric meningitis in newborns and young infants, symptoms resemble those of an acute infection and may include shallow and rapid breathing, slight cyanosis, lethargy, fever, and anorexia. After appearance of convulsions, muscular twitching, interrupted breathing, severe cyanosis, and increased irritability, prognosis is no longer favorable with death an all too common occurrence (53,91).

Listeria monocytogenes is one of the most frequent causes of meningitis in immunocompromised adults. This illness begins less suddenly in adults than in infants with the appearance of "flu-like" symptoms, which are followed by development of headaches, leg pains, fever, chills, increasing rigidity of the neck, nausea, vomiting, and photophobia. Eventually, victims become somnolent with intermittent bouts of convulsions and dehydration and finally die in a coma. Symptoms may vary among individuals, with older children often experiencing respiratory and gastrointestinal distress before more typical symptoms of listeric meningitis (90).

Diagnosis of listeric meningitis can be aided by recognition of specific compositional changes of blood and CSF. Principal changes in blood composition include an increased sedimentation rate, granulocytosis (increased number of leukocytes having a granular cytoplasm), and occasional monocytosis. Changes in CSF include elevated pressure as well as increased and decreased concentrations of protein and glucose, respectively. In most instances, a high white blood cell count (predominantly neutrophils, monocytes, and macrophages) gives CSF a turbid appearance. In gram-stained smears of CSF, *L. monocytogenes* appears as a short gram-positive rod and is found both extra- and intracellularly. Unfortunately, *L. monocytogenes* is sometimes mistakenly identified as a Group B streptococcus. Such a misdiagnosis could result in administration of an inappropriate antibiotic and lead to disastrous consequences (91).

The remaining form of infection, listeric encephalitis, exhibits two phases; the first lasts about 10 days and is characterized by headache, backache, vomiting, conjunctivitis, and rhinitis. The second or acute phase begins about 10 days later with a high fever which is followed by disturbances of the central nervous system. Visible lesions are found almost exclusively in the pons and medulla oblongata of the brain; however, lesions in the ganglions of the brain stem, cerebellum, and spinal cord are relatively rare (10). Death normally ensues within 2–3 days if the victim is not appropriately treated with antibiotics.

CUTANEOUS FORM

In addition to skin lesions that can occur as a result of septic infections in neonates, cutaneous lesions also have been reported for adults, particularly farmers and others who come in direct contact with tissues (e.g., cow's placenta) from infected animals (21,70). Cutaneous listeriosis is characterized by development of pinhead-size nodules which increase to the size of a small pea after about 1 day. Then each nodule begins to produce pus and the periphery turns red. At this point, *L. monocytogenes* often can be isolated in pure culture from these pustules. Administration of sulfonamides generally leads to a rapid and complete cure (70); however, in one instance cutaneous infection of a Dutch farmer led to a fatal septicemia (90).

SEPTICEMIA WITH PHARYNGITIS AND MONONUCLEOSIS

In 1929, Nyfeldt (69) claimed that *L. monocytogenes* was the causative agent of infectious mononucleosis since the organism was isolated from the blood of patients who had an infectious mononucleosis-like disorder. However, Nyfeldt's claim could not be confirmed with other patients suffering from mononucleosis since *Listeria* did not stimulate production of heterophile antibodies. Although the Epstein-Barr virus is now accepted as the causative agent of infectious mononucleosis, *L. monocytogenes* can produce symptoms that closely mimic this illness. These symptoms include severe pharyngitis, fever, tonsilitis, lymphadenopathy, and leukocytosis accompanied by peripheral monocytosis. A positive diagnosis only can be made after isolating the organism from blood, lymph nodes, or throat washings of the victim (91). Prognosis for this form of listeric infection is generally good; however, fatalities have been reported, including a 35-year-old man who developed listeric pneumonia as a complication of the infection. Although conservative treatment generally results in a spontaneous cure within 3–4 weeks, several additional months may be required for complete recovery (90).

OCULOGLANDULAR FORM

Conjunctivitis sometimes accompanies the mononucleosis-like form of listeric infection just described. This disease also can develop independently of other forms of listeric infection through direct contamination of the eye. Symptoms of oculoglandular listeriosis normally include conjunctivitis and enlargement of the parotid and submandibular glands, accompanied by fever and lymphocytosis. The incubation period is assumed to be between 3 and 45 days with the illness generally lasting 1–3 months. Although listeric conjunctivitis normally heals spontaneously, one case complicated by meningitis ended fatally (90).

CERVICOGLANDULAR FORM

This relatively rare form of listeric infection occurs primarily in older adults as a complication of listeric septicemia and is characterized by inflammation of the neck and lymph glands. Sometimes the affected lymph nodes discharge pus freely, whereas in other instances lymph nodes must be surgically drained (91).

GRANULOMATOSIS SEPTICA AND TYPHOID PNEUMONIC FORM

In humans, listeriosis may take a septic course with variable clinical manifestations. This form of listeriosis may accompany listeric septicemia and can lead to central nervous system involvement. In some cases, this form of listeric infection has taken a course similar to granulomatosis infantiseptica of newborns. If high temperatures predominate, the infection resembles typhoid fever. Symptoms of pneumonia also have been noted, particularly after administration of cortisone (91), along with at least 35 cases of listeric endocarditis (33,82).

OTHER FORMS

Focal infections with *L. monocytogenes* can result in arthritis, osteomyelitis, spinal or brain abscesses, peritonitis (66), and cholecystitis (8). Individuals with disseminated listeriosis may exhibit acute hepatitis along with elevated levels of glutamic-oxaloacetic transaminase and alkaline phosphatase. Most of these focal infections occur in immunocompromised adults (8).

TREATMENT

Although some individuals may recover spontaneously from listeric infections, early antibiotic therapy is usually required to prevent permanent disabilities and possible death. Clinical results concerning susceptibility of *L. monocytogenes* to various antibiotics are somewhat conflicting.

Most clinical isolates of *L. monocytogenes* are sensitive in vitro to penicillin, ampicillin, tetracycline, erythromycin, chloramphenicol, and cephalothin; however, many of these antibiotics have adverse side effects when administered in vivo. Tetracycline is not recommended for use in neonates and children since the drug can stain teeth and alter bone growth. More important, this drug is generally only bacteriostatic; hence, subsequent relapses of illness can occur. Although chloramphenicol, streptomycin, and sulfonamides readily penetrate the blood-brain barrier, these antibiotics can be toxic to neonates and so are seldom used to treat cases of neonatal listeriosis. Cephalosporin is suitable for treating listeriosis in children; however, poor diffusion through the blood-brain barrier makes this drug unsuitable for treating meningitis (91). Armstrong (8) has promoted erythromycin as the drug of second choice for treating cases of listeriosis. However, in vitro tests conducted by Hawkins et al. (42) demon *L. monocytogenes* is relatively tolerant to erythromycin as compared to ampi

Not too many years ago, β-lactam antibiotics such as ampicillin or penic generally used to treat most forms of listeric infection. However, it is now widely recognized that the minimum concentration of ampicillin, penicillin, erythromycin, and many other antibiotics needed to kill *L. monocytogenes* (minimum bactericidal concentration) may be many times higher than the level needed to prevent growth (minimum inhibitory concentration) of the organism. Hence, antibiotic concentrations attained in listeriosis patients are frequently only high enough to prevent growth of *Listeria* rather than to eliminate the organism (30,56,95). This situation is further complicated by the intracellular nature of *L. monocytogenes* in that bactericidal concentrations of antibiotics are difficult to achieve intracellularly. While the current literature generally indicates that listeric infections are best treated with ampicillin (40,56,93), several ampicillin- (74,78) and penicillin-resistant (95) strains of *L. monocytogenes* have been reported.

Several attempts have been made to enhance the effectiveness of ampicillin in treating listeric infections. Use of various antibiotics in combination with ampicillin has been the most thoroughly investigated means of synergistically increasing bactericidal activity. The combination of ampicillin and an aminoglycoside antibiotic, of which gentamicin is the most common, prevented growth of *L. monocytogenes* and killed the pathogen sooner than when ampicillin was used alone (30,52). Several additional β-lactam/aminoglycoside antibiotic combinations also have proven useful (30,56) as well as the combination of trimethoprim and sulfamethoxazole, which was highly effective in vitro (98). Rifampin also appears promising in treating listeriosis since this antibiotic remains active against intracellular listeriae (43); however, the combination of rifampin and ampicillin decreases the effectiveness of ampicillin. Preliminary experiments with mice have shown that when used alone, encapsulation of ampicillin within liposomes can increase the intracellular concentration of the antibiotic to bactericidal levels (9). These findings may have important ramifications for treating human listeriosis in the future.

Despite development of many new antibiotics, the optimal antibiotic therapy for treating listeric infections is not yet known (56). Nevertheless, favorable results have been most frequently obtained using ampicillin either alone or in combination with gentamicin (40,56,93). Listeriosis patients, including newborn infants, are normally somewhat immunocompromised. Hence, relatively high doses of ampicillin must be given to obtain effective concentrations of the drug in the bloodstream and cerebrospinal fluid. Adults with septicemic or neurological forms of listeriosis should receive 6–12 g of ampicillin (i.v.) daily in three to four doses, whereas newborns suffering from similar disorders should be given 200–400 mg ampicillin/kg body weight/day. Therapy should be continued for a minimum of 4 weeks to obtain adequate antibiotic concentrations within granulomatous tissue of the liver and spleen. Expectant mothers with minor symptoms of listeriosis should receive 3–6 g of ampicillin daily, either i.v. or orally, for at least 2–3 weeks. Individuals with oculoglandular or cutaneous forms of listeriosis should be given 3–6 g of ampicillin daily until all clinical symptoms disappear. If a patient is allergic to β-lactam antibiotics, co-trimoxazole, rifampin, chloramphenicol, or erythromycin can be substituted for ampicillin.

REFERENCES

1. Albritton, W. L., S. L. Cochi, and J. C. Feeley. 1984. Overview of neonatal listeriosis. *Clin. Invest. Med. 7*:311–314.
2. Allerberger, F. 1988. Listeriosis in Austria—Report of an outbreak in Austria 1986. 10th International Symposium on Listeriosis, Pecs, Hungary, August–22–26, Abst. No. 20.
3. Anonymous. 1987. Empfehlungen zur Erkennung und Verhütung von Infektionen mit *Listeria monocytogenes. Bundesgesundhbl. 30*:369–370.
4. Anonymous. 1988. Foodborne listeriosis—Switzerland. *J. Food Prot. 51*:425.
5. Anonymous. 1988. Listeriosis surveillance. Communicable Dis. Report, May 20.
6. Anonymous. 1988. *Listeria* strain found to survive boiling of shrimp. *Food Chem. News 30*(1):34.
7. Anonymous. 1989. CDC estimates 800 listeriosis cases, 150 deaths annually in U.S. *Food Chem. News 30*(48):20.
8. Armstrong, D. 1985. *Listeria monocytogenes.* In G. L. Mandell, R. G. Douglas, Jr., and J. E. Bennet (eds.), *Principles and Practices of Infectious Diseases,* 2nd ed., John Wiley and Sons, New York, pp. 1177–1182.
9. Bakker-Woudenberg, I. A. J. M., A. F. Lokerse, J. C. Vink van den Berg, and F. H. Roerdink. 1988. Liposome-encapsulated ampicillin against *Listeria monocytogenes in vivo* and *in vitro. Infection 16*(Suppl. 2):165–170.
10. Békàssy, N. A., S. Cronqvist, S. Garwicz, and T. Wiebe. 1987. Arterial occlusion due to *Listeria* meningioencephalitis in an immunocompromised boy. *Scand. J. Infect. Dis. 19*:485–489.
11. Beninger, P. R., M. C. Savla, and C. E. Davis. 1988. *Listeria monocytogenes* meningitis in a patient with AIDS-related complex. *J. Infect. Dis. 158*:1396–1397.
12. Bennett, M., and E. E. Baker. 1977. Marrow-dependent cell function in early stages of infection with *Listeria monocytogenes. Cell. Immunol. 33*:203–210.
13. Bille, J. 1988. Epidemiology of human listeriosis in Europe with special reference to the Swiss outbreak. *Proceedings, Society for Industrial Microbiology—Comprehensive Conference on Listeria monocytogenes,* Rohnert Park, CA, Oct. 2–5.
14. Bille, J., J. Rocourt, F. Mean, M. P. Glauser, and the group "*Listeria*-Vaud." 1988. Epidemic food-born listeriosis in Western Switzerland. II. Epidemiology. Interscience Conference on Antimicrobial Agents and Chemotherapy, Los Angeles, CA, Oct. 23–26, Abst. 107.
15. Bizet, C., D. Mechali, J. Rocourt, and F. Fraisse. 1989. *Listeria monocytogenes* bacteremia in AIDS. *Lancet i*:501.
16. Bojsen-Møller, J. 1972. Human listeriosis—diagnostic, epidemiological and clinical studies. *Acta Pathol. Microbiol. Scand.* Section B, Suppl *29*:1–157.
17. Bowmer, E. J., J. A. Mckiel, W. H. Cockcroft, N. Schmitt, and D. E. Rappay. 1973. *Listeria monocytogenes* infections in Canada. *Can. Med. Assoc. J. 109*:125–135.
18. Broome, C. V., B. Gellin, and B. Schwartz. 1988. Epidemiology of listeriosis in the United States. *Proceedings, Society for Industrial Microbiology—Comprehensive Conference on Listeria monocytogenes,* Rohnert Park, CA, Oct. 2–5, Abstr. I-9.
19. Bula, Ch., J. Bille, F. Mean, M. P. Glauser, and the Group "*Listeria*-Vaud." 1988. Epidemic food-born listeriosis in Western Switzerland. I. Description of the 58 adult cases. Interscience Conference on Antimicrobial Agents and Chemotherapy, Los Angeles, CA, Oct. 23–26, Abst. 1106.
20. Burn, C. G. 1936. Clinical and pathological features of an infection caused by a new pathogen of the genus *Listerella. Amer. J. Pathol. 12*:341–348.
21. Cain, D. B., and V. L. McCann. 1986. An unusual case of cutaneous listeriosis. *J. Clin. Microbiol. 23*:976–977.
22. Campbell, D. M. 1989. Listeriosis in Scotland, 1988. *Lancet i*:492.
23. Chen-Woan, M., D. D. McGregor, and I. Goldschneider. 1984. Activation of *Listeria monocytogenes*-induced prekiller T cells by interleukin-2. *Clin. Invest. Med. 7*:287–295.
24. Ciesielski, C. A., A. W. Hightower, S. K. Parsons, and C. V. Broome. 1988. Listeriosis in the United States: 1980–1982. *Arch. Intern. Med. 148*:1416–1419.

25. Corrier, D. E., and R. L. Ziprin. 1986. Enhanced resistance to listeriosis induced in mice by preinoculation treatment with T-2 mycotoxin. *Amer. J. Vet. Res. 47*:856–859.
26. Corrier, D. E., and R. L. Ziprin. 1987. Immunotoxic effects of T-2 mycotoxin on cell-mediated resistance to *Listeria monocytogenes* infection. *Vet. Immunol. Immunopathol. 14*:11–21.
27. Davies, J. W., E. P. Ewan, P. Varughese, and S. E. Acres. 1984. *Listeria monocytogenes* infections in Canada. *Clin. Invest. Med. 7*:315–320.
28. Degen, R. von, and C. Goldenbaum. 1965. Katamnestische Untersuchungen von Kindern mit geheilter Neugeborenen-Listeriose. *Dtsch. med. Wschr. 90*:1898–1905.
29. de la Lande, Ph., Ph. Barthelemy, F. Goldstein, and G. Terris. 1988. Un cas de *Listeri* anale au cours d'un SIDA. *Gastroenterol. Clin. Biol. 12*:972–973.
30. Espaze, E. P., and A. E. Reynaud. 1988. Antibiotic susceptibilities of *Listeria: in vitro* studies. *Infection 16*(Suppl. 2):160–164.
31. Evans, J. R., A. C. Allen, R. Bortolussi, T. B. Issekutz, and D. A. Stinson. 1984. Follow-up study of survivors of fetal and early onset neonatal listeriosis. *Clin. Invest. Med. 7*:329–334.
32. Fleming, D. W., S. L. Cochi, K. L. MacDonald, J. Brondum, P. S. Hayes, B. D. Plikaytis, M. B. Holmes, A. Audurier, C. V. Broome, and A. L. Reingold. 1985. Pasteurized milk as a vehicle of infection in an outbreak of listeriosis. *N. Engl. J. Med. 312*:404–407.
33. Gallagher, P. G., and C. Watanakungkorn. 1988. *Listeria monocytogenes* endocarditis: A review of the literature 1950–1986. *Scand. J. Infect. Dis. 20*:359–368.
34. Gould, I. A., L. C. Belok, and S. Handwerger. 1986. *Listeria monocytogenes*: A rare cause of opportunistic infection in the acquired immunodeficiency syndrome (AIDS) and a new cause of meningitis in AIDS—A case report. *AIDS Res. 2*:231–234.
35. Goulet, V., and S. Brohier. 1989. La listériose en France en 1986: Recensement auprès de laboratoires hospitaliers. *Pathol. Biol. 37*:206–211.
36. Goulet, V., and E. Espaze. 1988. Epidemiological surveillance of human listeriosis in France. Intern. Symposium on Listeriosis, Pecs, Hungary, Aug. 22–26, Abst. 26.
37. Goulet, V., J. L. Leonard, and J. Celers. 1986. Etude epidemiologique de la listériose humaine en France en 1984. *Rev. Epidemiol. Sante Publique 34*:191–195.
38. Gray, M. L., and A. H. Killinger. 1966. *Listeria monocytogenes* and listeric infections. *Bacteriol. Rev. 30*:309–382.
39. Hall, S. M., N. Crofts, R. J. Gilbert, P. N. Pini, A. G. Taylor, and J. McLauchlin. 1988. Epidemiology of listeriosis, England and Wales. *Lancet i*:502–503.
40. Hansen, P. B., T. H. Jensen, S. Lykkegaard, and H. S. Kristensen. 1987. *Listeria monocytogenes* meningitis in adults: Sixteen consecutive cases 1973–1982. *Scand. J. Infect. Dis. 19*:55–60.
41. Harveyn, R., and P. Chandrasekar. 1988. Chronic meningitis caused by *Listeria* in a patient infected with human immunodeficiency virus. *J. Infect. Dis. 157*:1091.
42. Hawkins, A. E., R. Bortolussi, and A. C. Issekutz. 1984. *In vivo* and *in vitro* activity of various antibiotics against *Listeria monocytogenes* type 4b. *Clin. Invest. Med. 7*:335–341.
43. Hof, H., and P. Emmerling. 1984. Murine model for therapy of listeriosis in the compromised host. *Chemotherapy 30*:125–130.
44. International Dairy Federation. 1989. Pathogenic *Listeria*. Circular 5/89, Brussels, Belgium.
45. Issekutz, T. B., J. Evans, and R. Bortolussi. 1984. The immune response of human neonates to *Listeria monocytogenes* infection. *Clin. Invest. Med. 7*:281–284.
46. Jacobs, J. L., and H. W. Murray. 1986. Why is *Listeria monocytogenes* not a pathogen in the acquired immunodeficiency syndrome? *Arch. Intern. Med. 146*:1299–1300.
47. James, S. M., S. L. Fannin, B. A. Agree, B. Hall, E. Parker, J. Vogt, G. Run, J. Williams, L. Lieb, C. Salminen, T. Prendergast, S. B. Werner, and J. Chin. 1985. Listeriosis outbreak associated with Mexican-style cheese—California. *J. Amer. Med. Assoc. 254*:474.
48. Kaplan, M. M. 1945. Listerellosis. *N. Engl. J. Med. 232*:755–759.
49. Kaufmann, S. H. E. 1988. Listeriosis: New findings—current concerns. *Microb. Pathogenesis 5*:225–231.
50. Kongshavn, P. A. L., and E. Skamene. 1984. The role of natural resistance in protection of the murine host from listeriosis. *Clin. Invest. Med. 7*:253–257.

51. Koziol, K., K. S. Rielly, R. A. Borin, and J. R. Salcedo. 1986. *Listeria monocytogenes* meningitis in AIDS. *Can. Med. Assoc. J. 135:43–44.*

52. Larsson, S., M. H. Walder, S. N. Cronberg, A. B. Forsgren, and T. Moestrup. 1985. Antimicrobial susceptibilities of *Listeria monocytogenes* strains isolated from 1958 to 1982 in Sweden. *Antimicrob. Agents Chemother. 28:*12–14.

53. Levy, E., and E. Nassau. 1960. Experience with listeriosis in the newborn. An account of a small epidemic in a nursery ward. *Ann. Paediat. 194:*321–330.

54. Lu, C. Y. 1984. The delayed ontogenesis of Ia-positive macrophages: Implications for host defense and self-tolerance in the neonate. *Clin. Invest. Med. 7:*263–267.

55. Marchou, B., J. Ch. Auvergnat, and M. Armengaud. 1988. Listeriose au cours de l'infection par ie VIH; à propos d'un case de méningite purulente. *Médicine et Maladies Infecteuses 18:*779.

56. Marget, W., and H. P. R. Seeliger. 1988. *Listeria monocytogenes* infections—therapeutic possibilities and problems. *Infection 16*(Suppl. 2):175–177.

57. Marrie, T. J., M. Riding, and B. Grant. 1984. Computed tomographic scanning in *Listeria monocytogenes* meningitis. *Clin. Invest. Med. 7:*355–359.

58. Mascola, L., L. Lieb, J. Chiu, S. L. Fannin, and M. J. Linnan. 1988. Listeriosis: An uncommon opportunistic infection in patients with acquired immunodeficiency syndrome—a report of five cases and a review of the literature. *Amer. J. Med. 84:*162–164.

59. Mascola, L., F. Sorvillo, J. Neal, K. Iwakoshi, and R. Weaver. 1989. Surveillance of listeriosis in Los Angeles County, 1985–1986. *Arch. Intern. Med. 149:*1569–1572.

60. Mascola, L., L. Chun, J. Thomas, W. F. Bibe, B. Schwartz, C. Salminen, and P. Heseltine. 1988. A case-control study of a cluster of perinatal listeriosis identified by an active surveillance system in Los Angeles County. *Proceedings, Society for Industrial Microbiology— Comprehensive Conference on Listeria monocytogenes*, Rohnert Park, CA, Oct. 2–5, Abstr. P-10.

61. McLauchlin, J. 1987. *Listeria monocytogenes*, recent advances in the taxonomy and epidemiology of listeriosis in humans. *J. Appl. Bacteriol. 63:*1–11.

62. McLauchlin, J., and P. N. Hoffman. 1989. Neonatal cross-infection from *Listeria monocytogenes. Communicable Dis. Report 16:*3–4.

63. Medoff, G., L. J. Kunz, and A. N. Weinberg. 1971. Listeriosis in humans: An evaluation. *J. Infect. Dis. 123:*247–250.

64. Moore, R. M., and R. B. Zehmer. 1973. From the Center for Disease Control—listeriosis in the United States—1971. *J. Infect. Dis. 127:*610–611.

65. Murray, K. G. D., R. A. Webb, and M. B. R. Swann. 1926. A disease of rabbits characterized by a large mononuclear leucocytosis, caused by a hitherto undescribed bacillus *Bacterium monocytogenes* (n. sp.). *J. Pathol. Bacteriol. 29:*407–439.

66. Myers, J. P., G. Peterson, and A. Rashii. 1983. Peritonitis due to *Listeria monocytogenes* complicating continuous ambulatory peritoneal dialysis. *J. Infect. Dis. 148:*1130.

67. Nieman, R. E., and B. Lorber. 1980. Listeriosis in adults: A changing pattern. Report of eight cases and review of the literature, 1968–1978. *Rev. Infect. Dis. 2:*207–227.

68. Nomoto, K., S. Miake, S. Hashimoto, T. Yokokura, M. Mutai, Y. Yoshikai, and K. Nomoto. 1985. Augmentation of host resistance of *Listeria monocytogenes* infection by *Lactobacillus casei. J. Clin. Lab. Immunol. 17:*91–97.

69. Nyfeldt, A. 1929. Etiologie de la mononucléose infectieuse. *C. R. Soc. Biol. 101:*590.

70. Owen, C. R., A. Meis, J. W. Jackson, and H. G. Stoenner. 1960. A case of primary cutaneous listeriosis. *N. Engl. J. Med. 262:*1026–1028.

71. Patey, O., C. Nedelec, J. P. Emond, R. Mayorga, N. N. 'Go, and C. Lafaix. 1989. *Listeria monocytogenes* septicemia in an AIDS patient with a brain abscess. *Eur. J. Clin. Microbiol. Infect. Dis. 8:*746–748.

72. Pathak, N. I. 1976. The *Listeria monocytogenes* infection—a case report and review of the literature with special reference to the cases in Maine. *J. Maine Med. Assoc. 67:*196–198.

73. Pinner, R. W. 1989. Personal communication.

74. Pollock, S. S., T. M. Pollock, and M. J. Harrison. 1986. Ampicillin-resistant *Listeria monocytogenes* meningitis. *Arch. Neurol. 43*:106.
75. Ralovich, B. 1984. *Listeriosis Research—Present Situation and Perspective*, Akademiai Kiado, Budapest.
76. Ralovich, B. S. 1987. Epidemiology and significance of listeriosis in the European countries. In A. Schönberg (ed.), *Listeriosis—Joint WHO/ROI Consultation on Prevention and Control*, West Berlin, December 10–12, 1986, pp. 21–55. Institut für Veterinärmedizin des Bundesgesundheitsamtes, Berlin.
77. Ramsden, G. H., P. M. Johnson, C. A. Hart, and R. G. Farquharson. 1989. Fatal *Listeria* meningitis in immunosuppressed patient. *Lancet i*:794.
78. Rapp, M. F., H. A. Pershadsigh, J. W. Long, and J. M. Pickens. 1984. Ampicillin-resistant *Listeria monocytogenes* meningitis in a previously healthy 14-year-old athlete. *Arch. Neurol. 41*:1304.
79. Read, S. E., and B. R. G. Williams. 1984. The host defense system in the human newborn: The role of interferon and the natural killer cell. *Clin. Invest. Med. 7*:259–262.
80. Read, E. J., J. M. Orenstein, T. L. Chorba, A. M. Schwartz, G. L. Simon, J. H. Lewis, and R. S. Schulof. 1985. *Listeria monocytogenes* sepsis and small cell carcinoma of the rectum: An unusual presentation of the acquired immunodeficiency syndrome. *Amer. J. Clin. Pathol. 83*:385–389.
81. Real, F. X., J. W. M. Gold, S. E. Krown, and D. Armstrong. 1984. *Listeria monocytogenes* bacteremia in the acquired immunodeficiency syndrome (letter). *Ann. Intern. Med. 101*:883.
82. Riancho, J. A., S. Echevarria, J. Napal, R. Martin-Duron, and J. Gonzalez-Macias. 1988. Endocarditis due to *Listeria monocytogenes* and human immunodeficiency virus infection. *Amer. J. Med. 85*:737.
83. Saxbe, W. B. 1972. *Listeria monocytogenes* and Queen Anne. *Pediatrics 49*:97–101
84. Schattenkerk, J. K. M. E., C. Klöpping, J. D. Speelman, R. J. van Ketel, and S. A. Danner. 1986. Report of a listeric infection in an AIDS patient (letter). *Ann. Intern. Med. 104*:726.
85. Schlech, W. F., J. I. Ward, J. D. Band, A. Hightower, D. W. Fraser, and C. V. Broome. 1985. Bacterial meningitis in the United States, 1978 through 1981: The National Bacterial Meningitis Surveillance Study. *J. Amer. Med. Assoc. 253*:1749–1754.
86. Schlech, W. F., P. M. Lavigne, R. A. Bortolussi, A. C. Allen, E. V. Haldane, A. J. Wort, A. W. Hightower, S. E. Johnson, S. H. King, E. S. Nicholls, and C. V. Broome. 1983. Epidemic listeriosis—evidence for transmission by food. *N. Engl. J. Med. 303*:203–206.
87. Schwartz, B., C. V. Broome, G. R. Brown, A. W. Hightower, C. A. Ciesielski, S. Gaventa, B. G. Gellin, L. Mascola, and the Listeriosis Study Group. 1988. Association of sporadic listeriosis with consumption of uncooked hot dogs and undercooked chicken. *Lancet ii*:779–782.
88. Schwartz, B., D. Hexter, C. V. Broome, A. W. Hightower, R. B. Hirschhorn, J. D. Porter, P. S. Hayes, W. F. Bibb, B. Lorber, and D. G. Faris. 1989. Investigation of an outbreak of listeriosis: New hypothesis for the etiology of epidemic *Listeria monocytogenes* infections. *J. Infect. Dis. 159*:680–685.
89. Schwarze, R., C.-D. Bauermeister, S. Ortel, and G. Wichmann. 1989. Perinatal listeriosis in Dresden 1981–1986: Clinical and microbiological findings in 18 cases. *Infection 17*:131–138.
90. Seeliger, H. P. R. 1961. *Listeriosis*, Hafner Publishing Co., New York.
91. Seeliger, H. P. R., and H. Finger. 1976. Listeriosis. In J. S. Remington and J. O. Klein (eds.), *Infectious Diseases of the Fetus and Newborn Infant*, W. B. Saunders Co., Philadelphia, pp. 333–365.
92. Selbitz, H. J., H. Meyer, and G. Steinbach. 1988. Quantitative bakteriologische Untersuchungen und experimentell infizierten Labortieren. *Arch. Exper. Vet. Med.*, Leipzig *42*:83–91.
93. Sethi, S. K., M. A. Ghafoor, and J. Vandepitte. 1989. Outbreak of neonatal listeriosis in a regional hospital in Kuwait. *Eur. J. Pediatr. 148*:368–370.

94. Stamm, A. M., W. E. Dismukes, B. P. Simmons, C. G. Cobbs, A. Elliot, P. Budrich, and J. Harmon. 1982. Listeriosis in renal transplant recipients: Report of an outbreak and review of 102 cases. *Rev. Infect. Dis. 4*:665–682.

95. Trautmann, M., J. Wagner, M. Chahin, and T. Weinke. 1985. *Listeria* meningitis: Report of ten recent cases and review of current therapeutic recommendations. *J. Infect. 10*:107–114.

96. Tripathy, S. P., and G. B. Mackaness. 1969. The effect of cytotoxic agents on the primary immune response to *Listeria monocytogenes. J. Exp. Med. 130*:1–16.

97. Watson, G. W., T. J. Fuller, J. Elms, and R. M. Kluge. 1978. *Listeria* cerebritis. Relapse of infection in renal transplant patients. *Arch. Intern. Med. 138*:83–87.

98. Winslow, D. L., and G. A. Pankey. 1982. *In vitro* activities of trimethoprim and sulfamethoxazole against *Listeria monocytogenes. Antimicrob. Agents Chemother. 22*:51–54.

99. Yndestad, M. 1987. Personal communication.

100. Ziprin, R. L., and D. N. McMurray. 1988. Differential effect of T-2 toxin on murine host resistance to three facultative intracellular bacterial pathogens: *Listeria monocytogenes, Salmonella typhimurium*, and *Mycobacterium bovis. Amer. J. Vet. Res. 49*:1188–1192.

5

Characteristics of
Listeria monocytogenes
Important to Food Processors

INTRODUCTION

Today's food manufacturer relies on a variety of processing techniques to produce a safe and wholesome product with a suitable shelf life. The most common methods of food preservation involve heating, cooling, freezing, drying, or fermentation, which reduces survival of pathogenic and spoilage microorganisms through controlled lowering of pH. Chemical preservatives such as sodium chloride, sorbic, propionic, and lactic acid, sodium benzoate, and sodium nitrite, are frequently used in combination with one or more of the five basic food preservation methods. These additives may help reduce *Listeria* in food by creating unfavorable conditions for growth and/or survival of this bacterium. When used correctly, commercial sanitizers and cleaning compounds aid in controlling the spread of *L. monocytogenes* by inactivating the organism. In this chapter, the five processing methods just listed will be considered along with preservatives and sanitizers for their effects on growth and/or survival of *L. monocytogenes*. While the various methods available to control microbial growth will be dealt with individually, the reader is reminded that, in most instances, several preservation techniques are used concurrently to control growth and survival of pathogenic and spoilage organisms that may be present in food.

TEMPERATURE

Under laboratory conditions, *L. monocytogenes* was originally reported to grow at temperatures between 3 and 45°C (82), with optimal growth occurring between 30 and 37°C (121,141). In 1972, Wilkins et al. (165) examined the temperature range for growth of *L. monocytogenes* in a medium containing 1% tryptone, 1% yeast extract, 0.3% K_2HPO_4, and 0.1% glucose. Extrapolation of data from an Arrhenius plot of exponential growth rates collected at various temperatures indicated that the bacterium had maximum, optimum, and minimum growth temperatures of 45–50°C, 38°C, and 3°C, respectively, which generally agree with the growth temperatures most frequently mentioned in earlier textbooks. However, the current edition of *Bergey's Manual of Systematic Bacteriology* (142) gives the minimum growth temperature as 1°C. In support of this change from 3 to 1°C, Junttila et al. (97) found that growth of 78 *L. monocytogenes* strains on Tryptose Soy Agar occurred at a mean minimum temperature of 1.1 (±0.3)°C with 10 and 2 strains of *L. monocytogenes* serotype 1/2 growing at 0.8 and 0.5°C, respectively. In contrast, *L. innocua* (19 strains), *L. murrayi* (1 strain), and *L. grayi* (1 strain) failed to grow at temperatures below 1.7 (±0.4), 2.8, and 3.0°C, respectively. While researchers in Florida also observed slight growth of *L. monocytogenes* in laboratory media as low as 1°C, Walker et al. (163) confirmed the ability of this pathogen to multiply at even lower temperatures with three *L. monocytogenes* strains exhibiting generation times of 62 to 131 hours in chicken broth and pasteurized milk, respectively, during extended incubation at –0.1 to –0.4°C.

Growth of *L. monocytogenes* in laboratory media at 1°C is very slow; however, when incubated at higher temperatures, i.e., 3–6°C, the growth rate of the pathogen increases so the organism can attain a final population of approximately 10^8 CFU/ml after several weeks of incubation (65). In a study by Bojsen-Møller (21), flasks containing Tryptose Phosphate Broth were inoculated with one of several *L. monocytogenes* strains and incubated at 4, 10, or 15°C. *Listeria monocytogenes* exhibited average generation or doubling times of 12.02, 5.03, and 2.63 hours during incubation at 4, 10, and 15°C, respectively. Thus, increasing the incubation temperature a modest 6°C reduced the generation time nearly 60%, which is comparable to results obtained for other psychrotrophic bacteria. Since many other bacterial species fail to grow at refrigeration temperatures, extended incubation of clinical, environmental, and food samples previously diluted in a nonselective medium such as Tryptose Broth (TB) often was successful for isolating *L. monocytogenes*. This method, which forms the basis for cold enrichment, is still used today on a limited basis and will be discussed in detail in Chapter 6, which deals with isolation and detection methods for *Listeria*.

The ability of *L. monocytogenes* to initiate growth at low temperatures poses a serious threat to the food industry and particularly to manufacturers of dairy products. In 1987, Rosenow and Marth (131) examined growth of four *L. monocytogenes* strains in autoclaved samples of skim, whole, and chocolate milk and whipping cream that were incubated at 4, 8, 13, 21, and 35°C. *Listeria* growth rates were generally similar in all four products at a given temperature and increased with an increase in incubation temperature. Generation times in hours for listeriae in all four products ranged between 29.73 and 45.55 at 4°C, 8.66 and 14.55 at 8°C, 4.45 and 6.92 at 13°C, and 1.72 to 1.91 at 21°C, with a uniform 0.68 at 35°C. *Listeria monocytogenes* reached maximum populations of 10^7–10^9 CFU/ml in all products that were incubated 30–45 days at 4°C, 11–14 days at 8°C, 5.0–5.8 days at 13°C, 2.1 days at 21°C, and 1 day at 35°C. In addition, numbers of listeriae failed to decrease substantially in the four products during extended storage. Theoretical calculations based on these data indicate that *Listeria* populations could increase from 10 to 4.2×10^6 organisms/quart of milk during 10 days of storage at 8°C (46°F), a temperature that may be encountered in some home and commercial refrigeration units. Donnelly and Briggs (51) also reported rapid growth of five *L. monocytogenes* strains in inoculated samples of whole, skim, and reconstituted nonfat dry milk (11% total solids) during incubation at 4, 10, 22, and 37°C.

Beside the obvious effect of temperature on *Listeria* growth rates, several reports suggest that virulence of the bacterium is increased when it is grown at low rather than high temperatures. Durst (55) reported that 7 of 36 weakly virulent *L. monocytogenes* strains became markedly virulent to mice by intraperitoneal injection after maintaining the cultures on agar slants for 6 months at 4°C. Similarly, Wood and Woodbine (168) found one strain of *L. monocytogenes* that was more virulent to chick embryos when grown at 4 rather than 37°C. Thus the possibility exists that cold storage may enhance virulence of some *L. monocytogenes* strains isolated from refrigerated foods.

Even though *L. monocytogenes* is usually unable to grow below 0.5°C, this pathogen can readily survive at much lower temperatures. Such survival is not surprising since some cells of many bacterial stock cultures remain viable during extended frozen storage in skim milk or other suitable media.

Numerous reports of *Listeria*-contaminated ice cream in the United States and elsewhere have prompted several investigators to examine viability of *L. monocytogenes* in laboratory media during frozen storage. Using Tryptose Phosphate Broth, Hof et al. (86) found viable populations of *L. monocytogenes*, *L. ivanovii*, *L. innocua*, *L. seeligeri*, and *L. welshimeri* decreased 50, 90, 90, 40, and 50%, respectively, following 3 weeks of frozen storage at −20°C. These findings suggest that *L. monocytogenes* can remain viable as long or longer than most other *Listeria* spp. during extended storage at subzero temperatures.

In 1989, El-Kest and Marth (62) reported preliminary results concerning increased lethality and sublethal injury that resulted from freezing suspensions of *L. monocytogenes* in TB and phosphate buffer. Overall, slow freezing at −18°C was more lethal and injurious to this organism than rapid freezing at −198°C. While 85.2 and 69.8% of the population was inactivated and injured, respectively, when cell suspensions were frozen and stored in phosphate buffer at −18°C, addition of 2− 4% glycerol or 2% milk components (i.e., casein, milk fat, and lactose) was later found to markedly decrease the extent of cell death and injury during frozen storage (63). However, no evidence of cell injury or death was observed in corresponding samples stored at −198°C. When TB was used in place of phosphate buffer, the extent of cell injury increased for suspensions stored at −198°C, but decreased for similar suspensions stored at −18°C. In the latter instance, 52.3% of the population was sublethally injured as compared to 72–80% of *L. monocytogenes* cells in a virtually identical study (80). As expected, multiple freeze/thaw cycles were more detrimental to survival of listeriae than was a single such cycle. Such treatments were far more damaging to the pathogen when done at −18°C (100% lethal, 0% injury) rather than −198°C (16–34% lethal, 11–27% injury) with generally similar behavior observed using TB and phosphate buffer.

Thus far, most investigations have dealt with viability of *L. monocytogenes* in frozen laboratory media; however, two preliminary reports concerning viability of listeriae in frozen foods have recently appeared in the scientific literature. According to these reports (117,118), *L. monocytogenes* populations decreased only 1–3 orders of magnitude in inoculated samples of canned milk, 10% Karo corn syrup, ground beef, ground turkey, frankfurters, canned corn, and ice cream mix during 8 weeks of frozen storage at −18°C. A somewhat greater decrease in numbers of viable listeriae was observed for samples of frozen tomato soup, possibly because of the lower pH of the product. With the exception of tomato soup, no sublethally injured listeriae were recovered from any other frozen foods. Given the recent discovery of *L. monocytogenes* in frozen ready-to-eat foods (e.g., ice cream, frozen dairy products) and the apparent inability to positively link such foods to clinical cases of listeriosis, future investigations need to more clearly define how the viability and pathogenicity of this organism are affected in food during extended frozen storage.

ACIDITY (pH)

According to the ninth edition of *Bergey's Manual of Systematic Bacteriology* (142), *L. monocytogenes* can only grow at pH values from 5.6 to 9.6, with optimal growth occurring at neutral to slightly alkaline pH values; the latter was recently verified by Petran and Zottola (121). The minimum pH value for growth is based on the work of Seeliger (141), who in 1961 reported that *L. monocytogenes* failed to grow in dextrose broth at pH <5.6 after 2–3 days of incubation at 37°C. In addition, subcultures from the medium were no longer routinely successful.

Recent listeriosis outbreaks linked to consumption of fermented dairy products have reopened the issue of a minimum pH requirement for growth which has now been revised downward. During 1987, Lang et al. (104) examined growth at 13°C of *L. monocytogenes* (strain Ohio, isolated from recalled Liederkranz cheese) in TB adjusted to pH 5.0 and 5.6. Following lag periods of 2.0 days at pH 5.0 and 0.5 day at pH 5.6, the pathogen grew and reached maximum populations of 1.5×10^8 and 4×10^8 CFU/ml in TB adjusted to pH 5.0 and 5.6, respectively. During logarithmic growth, the organism exhibited generation times of 13.1 and 4.4 hours in media adjusted to pH 5.0 and 5.6, respectively. Thus, although *Listeria* failed to grow in TB at pH 5.0 during the initial 2 days of incubation, further incubation led to growth of the organism with maximum populations being reached after approximately 21 days at 13°C.

Subsequent investigations have shown that *L. monocytogenes* can proliferate in laboratory media adjusted to even lower pH values. When inoculated into Trypticase Soy Broth acidified with hydrochloric acid, according to George et al. (78), all 16 *L. monocytogenes* strains tested initiated growth at pH values as low as 4.39–4.63 during extended incubation at 20 or 30°C. While results from at least four independent studies (22,77,118,148) confirm the ability of *L. monocytogenes* to multiply in similar laboratory media adjusted to pH 4.4–4.6 with hydrochloric, citric, or malic acid, Farber et al. (74) recently observed growth of *L. monocytogenes* at 30°C in double-strength Brain Heart Infusion Broth acidified with hydrochloric acid to a pH value as low as 4.3. Furthermore, *L. innocua*, *L. seeligeri*, and *L. ivanovii* also were reported to grow in Brain Heart Infusion Broth acidified with hydrochloric acid to pH values as low as 4.53, 4.88, and 5.16, respectively (77). Thus the minimum pH at which *L. monocytogenes* and most other *Listeria* spp. can grow is well below pH 5.0, provided that these organisms are incubated at near-optimum temperatures and allowed sufficient time to overcome an extended lag phase.

As might be expected, the minimum pH at which *L. monocytogenes* can grow is markedly influenced by incubation temperature and the type of acid added to the medium, the latter of which will be discussed in some detail later in this chapter. In one study (168), TB previously adjusted to pH 5.0 and 5.6, was inoculated to contain ~1 × 10^3 *L. monocytogenes* CFU/ml and then incubated at 4 and 13°C. Although listeriae failed to grow in TB at pH 5.0 incubated at 4°C, bacterial populations decreased <10-fold during 67 days of storage. In contrast, increasing the incubation temperature to 13°C led to growth at pH 5.0 with the organism attaining a final population of ~1 × 10^8 CFU/ml. These results are similar to those of Lang et al. (104) described earlier. Two additional studies reported during 1988 and 1989 examined the relationship between incubation temperature and growth of *L. monocytogenes* in laboratory media acidified to low pH values. In the first of these investigations, George et al. (78) found that minimum pH values of 4.39–4.63, 4.39–4.62, 4.62–5.05, 4.62–5.05, and 5.23–5.45 permitted growth of 16 *L. monocytogenes* strains in Trypticase Soy Broth incubated at 30, 20, 10, 7, and 4°C, respectively. Subsequently, Sorrells et al. (148) reported that four different *L. monocytogenes* strains grew in Tryptic Soy Broth acidified to pH values as low as 4.40 following 7–28 days of incubation at 10°C, whereas previously growth of this organism at pH 4.4 was only observed at ≥20°C. Hence, some *L. monocytogenes* strains may be able to grow, albeit slowly, in laboratory media adjusted to pH 4.4 and incubated at near-refrigeration temperatures.

While growth of *L. monocytogenes* at pH < 4.3 has not yet been documented, this organism appears to be fairly acid tolerant under such conditions. According to Reimer et al. (129), *L. monocytogenes* was recovered from inoculated samples of citrate/phosphate buffer acidified to pH 3.3 and held 4 hours at 37°C. However, the pathogen was not found after 1 hour in a similar buffer adjusted to pH 1.4.

In addition to these findings, Ahamad and Marth (2) found that *L. monocytogenes* exhibited average D-values (i.e., time necessary to inactivate 90% of the population) of 13.3 and 11.3 days when the pathogen was held at 7°C in TB previously adjusted to pH values of 4.0–4.1 and 3.6–3.7, respectively, with citric acid. Since these authors obtained average D-values of only 2.2 and 1.4 days for corresponding cultures incubated at 35°C, it is evident that *L. monocytogenes* can tolerate exposure to acid far better at near-refrigeration than ambient temperatures. Such behavior raises concerns about the safety of refrigerated acid and low acid foods that may have been subjected to postprocessing contamination.

Of even greater importance to the food industry is the relationship between pH, temperature, and possible growth of *L. monocytogenes* under the less than optimal conditions found in many foods. In a study prompted by the listeriosis outbreak in Canada linked to consumption of contaminated coleslaw (140), Conner et al. (39) demonstrated that *L. monocytogenes* can tolerate, and in some instances grow in cabbage juice at pH values ≤ 5.6. Unclarified cabbage juice, obtained through chopping, grinding, and pressing fresh cabbage, was autoclaved (121°C/15 minutes), cooled and adjusted with sterile lactic acid to pH values of 3.8–5.6 in 0.2-unit increments. Samples of cabbage juice at various pH values were then inoculated with one of two *L. monocytogenes* strains at 10^4 CFU/ml and incubated at either 5°C for 63 days or 30°C for 21 days. These researchers found that after 3 days at 30°C, both *Listeria* strains reached maximum populations of ~10^9 CFU/ml in cabbage juice which had an initial pH ≥ 5.2. Rapid growth of listeriae during this period was followed by equally rapid destruction with the organism no longer detectable after ~15 days at 30°C. In cabbage juice adjusted to pH 5.0 and incubated at 30°C, both *Listeria* strains exhibited a 3-day lag period and then grew to maximum populations ≥10^8 CFU/ml after 7 days of incubation before numbers decreased. At pH ≤ 4.8, *L. monocytogenes* was inactivated in samples incubated at 30°C. Rates of inactivation increased as the pH decreased with listeriae no longer detectable after 3 days in samples at pH ≤ 4.2. Although incubation at 5°C prevented growth of *L. monocytogenes* in cabbage juice adjusted to pH ≤ 5.6, listeriae populations remained constant in samples at pH ≥ 5.2 during 22 days of storage. In contrast, numbers of *Listeria* gradually decreased in samples adjusted to pH ≤ 5.2 during this same 22-day period. Inactivation rates were inversely related to pH with the organism surviving 49 days at pH 5.0–4.8 as compared to <21 days in samples of cabbage juice adjusted to pH 4.6 and 4.4. Thus, as previously observed with laboratory media, refrigeration temperatures also appear to provide some protection to *L. monocytogenes* against the stressful effects of low pH in food.

Over 45% of the dairies in North America process frozen concentrated orange juice into orange juice for retail sale. Hence, Parrish and Higgins (118) investigated behavior of *L. monocytogenes* at 4°C in inoculated (~10^6 CFU/ml) samples of orange serum adjusted to pH values of 3.6–5.0. Survival of the pathogen ranged between 21 days at pH 3.6 and >90 days at pH 4.8 and 5.0 with growth of listeriae limited to orange serum adjusted to pH 5.0. As expected, *Listeria* was inactivated faster at higher than lower incubation temperatures with the pathogen eliminated after 5 and 8 days from orange serum at 30°C and adjusted to pH values of 3.6–4.0 and 4.2–5.0, respectively. Interestingly, *Listeria* populations increased approximately 10- and 100-fold in orange serum adjusted to pH values of 4.8 and 5.0, respectively, during the first 2 days of incubation at 30°C before decreasing to nondetectable levels 6 days later. While acidic fruit juices appear to be unlikely sources of *L. monocytogenes*, the fact that this pathogen survived well beyond the normal shelf life of nonsterile orange juice (orange serum) suggests that such products should not automatically be eliminated as possible vehicles of infection in future epidemiological investigations of human listeriosis.

In 1988, Ryser and Marth (138) examined growth of *L. monocytogenes* at different pH values in whey collected during manufacture of Camembert cheese. Samples of whey were adjusted to pH values between 5.0 and 6.8, filter-sterilized, inoculated to contain 5×10^2 to 1×10^3 *L. monocytogenes* (4 strains) CFU/ml and incubated at 6°C. Although no growth occurred in whey at pH ≤ 5.4, small numbers of the organism survived during the entire 35-day storage period. In contrast to the study involving cabbage juice (39), all four strains grew in whey at pH 5.6 after 3 days of incubation at 6°C. Under these conditions, the four *Listeria* strains had generation times ranging between 25.3 and 31.6 hours and attained maximum populations of ~1×10^7 CFU/ml after 24 days at 6°C. As expected, *L. monocytogenes* had significantly ($p < 0.05$) shorter generation times in whey samples at pH 6.2 (14.8–21.1 hours) and pH 6.8 (14.0–19.4 hours) than at pH 5.6. The organism also attained higher final populations in whey at pH 6.2 and 6.8 than at pH 5.6. Whey at pH 5.4 was cultured with *Penicillium camemberti* for 18 days, the mold was removed by filter-sterilization, and whey samples were inoculated separately with four strains of *L. monocytogenes*. Two of the four *Listeria* strains grew after a lag period of 10 days and reached maximum populations of ~1×10^4 CFU/ml after 35 days at 6°C. Generation times for *L. monocytogenes* were significantly ($p < 0.05$) shorter and final populations were consistently higher in whey previously cultured with *P. camemberti* than in uncultured whey at the same pH values.

Studies concerning the effect of pH on growth and/or survival of *L. monocytogenes* in various cheeses indicate that this bacterium can survive at least 28 days in creamed and uncreamed cottage cheese at pH 5.02–5.68 (134), 70 to ≥434 days in Cheddar cheese at pH 5.00–5.15 (135), >115 days in Colby cheese at pH 5.00–5.18 (169), ≥70 days in semi-hard Manchego-type cheese at pH 5.10–5.80 (47), ≥180 days in cold-pack cheese food without preservatives at pH 5.21–5.45 (137), ≥180 days or grow to levels of ~1×10^6 to 1×10^7 CFU/g in brick cheese at pH 6.9–7.3 (139), and grow to levels of ~10^6–10^7 CFU/g in 65-day-old, fully ripened Camembert cheese at pH 5.9–7.2 (136). Similar studies concerned with behavior of *L. monocytogenes* in fermented meats have shown that this bacterium can survive in hard salami at pH 4.3–4.5 during refrigerated storage (96). Although these and other studies will be discussed in greater detail in the chapters of this book dealing with behavior of *Listeria* in dairy and meat products, the data indicate that *L. monocytogenes* is unlikely to initiate growth in food products which have a pH ≤ 5.2. Thus, as will be shown later, active lactic starter cultures play an important role in preventing growth of *L. monocytogenes* in fermented foods during refrigerated storage.

ACIDIFYING AGENTS

As mentioned earlier, growth and inactivation rates for *L. monocytogenes* vary markedly in the presence of different acidifying agents. Antibacterial action of weak organic acids such as acetic, citric, lactic, malic, and tartaric acid is related to pH and the degree of dissociation (i.e., pKa) with the undissociated form being most bactericidal. For example, at pH 5.0, 34.9% of acetic (pKa 4.75) and 6.1% of lactic acid (pKa 3.08) will be undissociated. Therefore, under these conditions acetic acid would be expected to exhibit greater antibacterial activity than lactic acid.

Experiments to determine the effect of lactic acid on growth of *L. monocytogenes* were conducted by Bojsen-Møller (21). Polymyxin-Tryptose Phosphate Broth containing 0, 0.003, 0.03, and 0.3 M lactic acid was adjusted to pH 5.0, 6.0, and 7.0 using HCl or NaOH; inoculated to contain ~10^3 *L. monocytogenes* CFU/ml, and incubated at 35 and 4°C. When incubated at 35°C, *Listeria* populations decreased in broth at pH 5.0 that contained 0.3 and 0.03 M lactic acid, whereas rapid growth occurred with 0 and 0.003 M lactic acid after a prolonged lag period. Although *L. monocytogenes* grew at 35°C in broths at pH 6.0, numbers of listeriae increased only 100-fold when broth contained 0.3 M lactic acid. Rapid growth at pH 7.0 and 35°C was observed for all concentrations of lactic acid. When the incubation temperature was decreased to 4°C, *L. monocytogenes* was eliminated after 27–42 days from broth at pH 5.0 and containing 0.3 M lactic acid, whereas numbers of listeriae remained unchanged in the same medium containing the three lower concentrations of lactic acid. The combination of pH 6.0 and 0.3 M lactic acid led to a stationary *Listeria* population at 4°C. Following a lag phase of ~14 days, *L. monocytogenes* grew at 4°C and had generation times of 54 and 39 hours in broth with (0.03 and 0.003 M) and without lactic acid, respectively. Although the combination of pH 7.0 and 0.3 M lactic acid prevented growth of *L. monocytogenes* at 4°C, the organism grew at the three lower lactic acid concentrations after a lag phase of ~7 days and then had generation times of ~21 hours. These results indicate that *L. monocytogenes* did not behave uniformly in broth containing identical levels of undissociated lactic acid. Additionally, the antibacterial effect of lactic acid was markedly influenced by the incubation temperature.

More recently, Ahamad and Marth (1) investigated growth of *L. monocytogenes* at 35°C in TB adjusted to pH ≤ 5.0 with various acids. According to these authors, *L. monocytogenes* failed to grow in TB adjusted to pH < 5.0 with lactic or acetic acid. However, the organism grew in TB adjusted to pH 4.8 with HCl and attained a maximum population of ~1×10^8 CFU/ml after 36 hours at 35°C. In contrast, numbers of listeriae increased only ~10-fold in TB acidified to pH 4.8 with citric acid and held 72 hours at 35°C. Using an experimental design similar to that of Bojsen-Møller (21), Ahamad and

Marth (2) examined the ability of different acetic, citric, and lactic acid concentrations to prevent growth of *L. monocytogenes* in TB during extended incubation at temperatures from 7 to 35°C. As expected, the pathogen was markedly affected by type and concentration of acid as well as incubation temperature. Presence of as little as 0.05% acetic acid (pH 5.8–5.9) in TB caused noticeable inhibition of *Listeria* with deleterious effects of acetic as well as citric and lactic acid more evident at low rather than high incubation temperatures. Increasing the concentration of acetic, citric, or lactic acid to 0.2% (pH 4.4–4.6) completely suppressed growth of the organism at all incubation temperatures with death of the pathogen occurring in the presence of ≥0.3% (pH < 4.2–4.3) acetic, citric, or lactic acid. In contrast, citric acid was less inhibitory than acetic acid, with growth of listeriae occurring in all samples with 0.1% citric acid, regardless of temperature. The relationship between incubation temperature and inhibition of *L. monocytogenes* was particularly evident with lactic acid; the pathogen proliferated in the presence of 0.1% lactic acid at all temperatures except 7°C. However, unlike the other two acids tested, 0.3 and 0.5% lactic acid led to only partial inactivation of the pathogen during extended incubation. While acetic acid had most antilisterial activity followed by lactic and citric acid, results from a follow-up study (3) showed that during extended incubation at both 13 and 35°C, presence of 0.3 and 0.5% citric acid in TB was most injurious to *L. monocytogenes* followed in order by similar concentrations of lactic and acetic acid. Since acid-injured listeriae survived approximately nine times longer at 13 than 35°C, previously unforeseen public health problems may arise from our present inability to readily detect such injured cells in refrigerated foods.

In 1989, Sorrells et al. (148) published results from another study that examined the effect of pH, acidulant, time, and temperature on growth and survival of *L. monocytogenes* in Tryptic Soy Broth acidified to pH values of 4.4–5.2 with hydrochloric, acetic, lactic, malic, or citric acid. Based on average minimum pH values permitting growth of four *L. monocytogenes* strains at 10, 20, and 35°C, acetic acid was again most inhibitory (pH 5.04) followed by lactic (pH 4.73), citric (pH 4.53), malic (pH 4.46), and hydrochloric acid (pH 4.46). These findings generally agree with those of Ahamad and Marth (2) and several other investigators (20,66,74). As in the previous study by Ahamad and Marth (2), longest survival of listeriae occurred at lower rather than higher incubation temperatures. However, since the inhibitory activity of the various acids tested was markedly different when based on equal molar concentrations of acid rather than pH, these data again indicate that differences in antilisterial activity of acidulants depends on both type and concentration of acid rather than on pH alone.

SALT

Resistance of *L. monocytogenes* to sodium chloride is well documented. According to the ninth edition of *Bergey's Manual of Systematic Bacteriology* (142), *L. monocytogenes* can grow in Nutrient Broth supplemented with up to 10% (w/v) NaCl. While this viewpoint concerning tolerance of *Listeria* to NaCl is apparently based on results from Larsen (105), preliminary data from one investigative team (77) reported in 1988 indicate that one strain of *L. monocytogenes* grew at 8–30°C during extended incubation in Brain Heart Infusion Broth (pH ~5.0) that contained up to 12% NaCl. Under identical conditions, single strains of *L. ivanovii*, *L. seeligeri*, and *L. innocua* were only slightly less halotolerant, with growth ceasing in the presence of >10% NaCl. However, since these findings concerning *L. monocytogenes* are contrary to other reports, independent confirmation of the results is needed before the value for halotolerance of this newly emerged foodborne pathogen can be revised upward.

Studies by Brzin (28,29) during the mid-1970s demonstrated that *L. monocytogenes* undergoes various morphological changes when grown in media containing high levels of NaCl. *Listeria* cells were elongated (maximum length 55 μm) and filamentous when incubated at 37 or 30°C for 24 hours on 5% human serum agar containing 8–9% NaCl and 0.4–0.6% agar. Under these conditions, cell multiplication was inhibited without simultaneous inhibition of cell growth. Attempts to grow listeriae on the same medium containing 9% NaCl led to complete inhibition of cell division and either partial or total cessation of cell growth, which ultimately led to fewer elongated and deformed cells. Microscopic changes in *Listeria* cells grown on salt agar also were associated with changes in colonial morphology. When incubated at 30 or 37°C in the presence of 8–9% NaCl, *L. monocytogenes* produced star-like colonies characterized by a rough surface, irregular border, and longer than usual straight or coiled protrusions. Such colonies contained large numbers of elongated filamentous cells. In addition to long twisted filamentous forms, occasional fusiform and spheroplast-like forms also were observed, particularly for cells from small colonies. In contrast, when grown on the same media and incubated at 22 or 10°C, colonies became progressively smoother and tended to develop regular borders. Cells from these colonies were less elongated and filamentous with microscopic changes being most pronounced in cells from small rather than large colonies. Altered morphological forms of *L. monocytogenes* persisted only as long as the bacterium was grown on media containing 8–9% NaCl. Listeriae reverted back to their typical nonfilamentous, nonelongated form after 24 hours of incubation in salt-free media.

Extended survival of listeriae occurs at a wide range of salt concentrations. Studies at ambient temperatures demonstrated that *L. monocytogenes* can persist at least 150 days in pure salt (145) and 545 days in 0.85% NaCl (125). In 1955, Stenberg and Hammainen (153) reported that 10 *L. monocytogenes* strains survived >1 year at 20–24°C in Nutrient Broth containing 1% dextrose and 10% NaCl. Listeriae also survived 34–68 days and 24 days in the same medium containing 12 and 24% NaCl, respectively. In experiments by Shahamat et al. (144), *L. monocytogenes* was inactivated in Trypticase Soy Broth containing 10.5, 13.0, and 25.5% NaCl after 14, 9, and 4 days at 37°C, respectively. Survival times in media containing 25.5% NaCl increased from 3 days at 37°C to 24 days at 22°C and to >132 days at 4°C. These data indicate that the length of survival by *Listeria* in concentrated salt solutions can be increased dramatically by lowering the incubation temperature.

Lang et al. (104) found that growth of *L. monocytogenes* in TB containing 6% NaCl is markedly influenced by pH. In their study, TB containing either 0 or 6% NaCl (w/v) was adjusted to pH 5.0, 5.6, 6.2, and 6.8 with HCl, inoculated to contain ~500 *L. monocytogenes* CFU/ml and incubated at 13°C. When grown in salt-free media at pH 5.0, 5.6, 6.2, and 6.8, this organism had generation times of 13.1, 4.4, 3.5, and 2.9 hours, as compared to 77.8, 7.2, 5.0, and 6.3 hours in the same medium containing 6% NaCl, respectively. Thus the combination of pH 5.0 and 6% NaCl was most effective in inhibiting growth of *Listeria*. The slow growth rate of *L. monocytogenes* under these conditions was reflected in a final population of only 1×10^4 CFU/ml after 42 days at 13°C as compared to populations of 10^8–10^9 CFU/ml in all remaining samples after 7–14 days at 13°C. Borovian (22) recently reported that *L. monocytogenes* grew at 10°C in culture media adjusted to pH 4.5 and 6.0 and containing ≤ 4.0 and $\leq 7.0\%$ NaCl, respectively. These findings are in accord with those of Lang et al. (104).

Several studies have examined the fate of *L. monocytogenes* in salted food and food-related products. Conner et al. (39) determined growth patterns of *L. monocytogenes* in cabbage juice supplemented with $\leq 5\%$ NaCl. Two *Listeria* strains grew at 30°C and pH 6.1 in cabbage juice containing 1% NaCl, but failed to grow in the presence of $\geq 1.5\%$ NaCl. In cabbage juice at pH 6.1 and containing $\leq 5\%$ NaCl, populations of both strains of the pathogen decreased ~90% during 70 days at 5°C. Stenberg and Hammainen (153) placed organs (liver, heart, kidney) from *Listeria*-infected mice in solutions of 3, 6, or 12% NaCl and stored the specimens at 4°C. *Listeria monocytogenes* remained viable for 238–246 days, 88–112 days, and 27 days in solutions containing 3, 6, and 12% NaCl, respectively. In another study Kukharkova et al. (103) demonstrated that *L. monocytogenes* can survive >60 days in meat stored at 4°C in a 30% NaCl brine solution which also contained nitrate. According to Sielaff (145), *L. monocytogenes* was detected in infected beef that was immersed in a solution of 22% NaCl and stored 100 days at 15–20°C. Results just described indicate that this pathogen is likely to survive for long periods in salted foods, particularly meat. In addition, several studies to be discussed in the chapter dealing with behavior of *L. monocytogenes* in dairy products indicate that this organism can survive and/or grow in brine solutions used during cheese manufacture.

MOISTURE

The moisture requirement for microbial growth can best be expressed in terms of water activity (a_w), which is defined as the ratio of the water vapor pressure of a food substrate to the vapor pressure of pure water at the same temperature. Like most bacterial species, *L. monocytogenes* grows optimally at a_w ~ 0.97 (121). However, when compared to most spoilage organisms, this pathogen also has a rather unique ability to multiply at a_w values as low as 0.92. As previously mentioned, *L. monocytogenes* can grow in complex laboratory media containing up to 10% NaCl (142). Skovgaard (147) estimated the a_w of such a medium at ~0.93 and therefore predicted that *L. monocytogenes* would not grow at $a_w < 0.93$. The minimum a_w for growth of *L. monocytogenes* estimated by Skovgaard was recently confirmed by Sperber (150). Using liquid laboratory media adjusted with NaCl to various a_w values, growth of *L. monocytogenes* at 35°C was observed at an a_w of 0.943 but not at 0.935. Similarly, adjustment of a_w using sucrose and glycerol allowed growth of *L. monocytogenes* at minimum a_w values of 0.941 and 0.932, respectively. While this organism did not appear to grow at $a_w < 0.932$, Shahamat et al. (144) reported that the bacterium survived at least 132 days at 4°C in Trypticase Soy Broth containing 25.5% NaCl, which would be expected to have an a_w of ~0.83.

Using Trypticase Soy Broth containing 9.1–65% sucrose, Petran and Zottola (121) demonstrated that *L. monocytogenes* can grow at an a_w value as low as 0.92 (i.e., 39.4% sucrose) during 24 hours at 30°C with the pathogen surviving <48 hours in similar media having a_w values ≤ 0.88 (i.e., $\geq 50.0\%$ sucrose). Subsequently, when sucrose/phosphate buffer solutions were inoculated to contain $\sim 10^4$–10^5 L. monocytogenes CFU/ml and held at 140°C, Sumner et al. (155) reported that the pathogen was about four times more heat resistant in buffer having an a_w value of 0.90 as compared to 0.98. Thus, given the inverse relationship between a_w and thermal resistance along with the ability of L. monocytogenes to grow at an a_w value of 0.92 and ferment concentrated sucrose solutions, this organism also may be important to companies that manufacture foods containing high levels of sugar as has already been demonstrated for Karo corn syrup stored at refrigeration temperatures (117).

Of more practical importance to food processors, Johnson et al. (96) recently found that L. monocytogenes survived at least 84 days at 4°C in fermented hard salami which had an a_w between 0.79 and 0.86. Extended survival of listeriae in sausage occurred despite the presence of 5.0–7.8% NaCl, 156 ppm sodium nitrite, and a pH of 4.3–4.5. The authors suggested that L. monocytogenes might survive longer at an a_w of 0.91, which is occasionally found in commercial hard salami. However, they also predicted that growth of the bacterium in such sausage would be unlikely, given the combination of salt, sodium nitrite, low pH, and low storage temperature.

Additional information concerning the relationship between a_w and growth/survival of L. monocytogenes can be obtained from several dairy-related studies. Using pasteurized whole milk inoculated to contain ~ 500 L. monocytogenes CFU/ml, Ryser and Marth (135) manufactured Cheddar cheese which, according to Marcos and Esteban (109), had a_w values between 0.972 and 0.979. Although minimal growth of Listeria occurred during the initial 21 days of ripening, the organism survived as long as 224 and >434 days in Cheddar cheese (pH 5.0–5.1) ripened at 13 and 6°C, respectively. Since Listeria reportedly grows well within this a_w range, the combined effects of low pH and low ripening temperature probably played a dominant role in preventing substantial growth of listeriae.

Camembert cheese also prepared by Ryser and Marth (136), had a_w values between 0.959 and 0.984 (109), which should have allowed growth of L. monocytogenes. However, listeriae populations remained constant or decreased in cheese at pH 4.6 to ~ 5.5 during the first 20–30 days of ripening. Initiation of rapid Listeria growth in cheese at a pH between ~ 5.5 and 6.0 illustrates that pH rather than a_w is primarily responsible for determining growth characteristics of listeriae in Camembert cheese.

SURVIVAL ON FOOD AND NONFOOD CONTACT SURFACES

Present reports indicate that L. monocytogenes is a very hardy organism, being able to survive up to 21 years in refrigerated laboratory media (41) as well as 10 days in tap water incubated at 22°C and 6, 3, and 1 day in distilled water stored at 22, 30, and 40°C, respectively (44). Moreover, this pathogen is also relatively resistant to drying. These observations have led to questions concerning the ability of L. monocytogenes to survive on various types of materials common to food-processing facilities.

Herald and Zottola (85) examined the ability of a culture of L. monocytogenes grown at 10, 21, and 35°C in Trypticase Soy Broth at pH 5, 7, and 8 to attach to stainless steel. A small stainless steel chip was placed in a culture vial containing L. monocytogenes and then incubated at 21 or 35°C for 18–24 hours or at 10°C for 36–48 hours. Following incubation, analysis of the chips using scanning electron microscopy (SEM) revealed that the pathogen adhered to stainless steel at all pH values and temperatures studied; however, cells with fibrils were observed only at 21 and 10°C. Amounts of exopolymeric attachment material were greater when the organism was incubated at 10 rather than 35°C and increased with the length of incubation. Subsequent SEM work (114) has shown that these attachment fibrils are highly susceptible to the germicidal action of commonly used sanitizing agents including chlorine and quaternary ammonium compounds.

Since *L. monocytogenes* survives for long periods at low a_w values, it is not surprising that this organism also is remarkably resistant to drying. Pomanskaya (125) reported that after drying cells of *L. monocytogenes* on oats, the bacterium survived 1009 and 188 days when stored at <0°C and 15–20°C, respectively. According to Baranenkov (15), *L. monocytogenes* survived 90 days on the surface of intact eggs that were stored at 5°C. In a larger study, Durst and Sawinsky (56) moistened various inert materials with a 24-hour-old Nutrient Broth culture containing ~10^9 *L. monocytogenes* CFU/ml and stored the materials in sterile petri plates at ambient temperature. *L. monocytogenes* survived <24 hours on glass, iron, and aluminum, <48 hours on paper and plastic, 7 but not 42 days on porcelain, 182 but not 365 days on wood, and at least 365 days on gauze. Finally, *L. monocytogenes* also reportedly survived more than 1 day on stainless steel (133), 165 days on contaminated wool stored at 8–22°C (15), 105 days on dried threads stored at room temperature (160), 20–30 days on tiles (155), and at least 20 days on 250-μm-diameter glass beads (164). These findings attest to the tenacity of *L. monocytogenes* on many types of food contact and non–food contact surfaces commonly found in food-processing environments.

Of particular interest to the dairy industry is a 1987 study by Stanfield et al. (152) which examined survival of three *L. monocytogenes* strains on exterior surfaces of waxed cardboard and plastic milk containers. Both container types were contaminated by swabbing their surfaces with a heavy suspension of an 18- to 24-hour-old unstressed or stressed (heat-shocked at 56°C for 30 minutes) *L. monocytogenes* culture, and then containers were stored at –0.8 to 6.6°C for 14 days. Unstressed cells of *L. monocytogenes* were recovered after 14 days of storage from at least one site on the surface of plastic and waxed cardboard containers. Although heat-shocked cultures generally survived a maximum of 2 days on either type of carton, one strain was recovered from the surface of a plastic container after 4 days of storage. Results of this study demonstrate that both stressed and unstressed *L. monocytogenes* can survive on exterior surfaces of milk containers, provided that the initial inoculum is heavy. Hence, dairy processors need to prevent *L. monocytogenes* from contaminating milk cartons, which in turn could allow this pathogen to enter walk-in coolers.

THERMAL INACTIVATION

Thermal processing is the most widely used method to preserve food and to destroy harmful microorganisms, thus rendering food safe for human consumption. The established association of *L. monocytogenes* with raw milk in the 1950s gave rise to several early studies dealing with the possible resistance of this organism to pasteurization. In 1983, interest in this topic was revived as a result of a listeriosis outbreak in Massachusetts that was epidemiologically linked to consumption of pasteurized milk. The literature now contains a wealth of information on thermal resistance of *L. monocytogenes* in a variety of foods. While data concerning heat resistance of *L. monocytogenes* in fluid milk will be presented now, our discussion regarding thermal inactivation of listeriae in other foods has been reserved for Chapters 11, 12, 13, and 14, which deal with the incidence and behavior of *Listeria* spp. in meat, poultry, seafood, and products of plant origin, respectively.

Numerous conflicting reports concerning the unusual heat resistance of *L. monocytogenes* in milk can be found in the early literature. In 1951, Potel (126) demonstrated that *L. monocytogenes* died rapidly in milk held at 80°C. [Since this manuscript actually dealt with a determination of whether or not *L. monocytogenes* produced spores, many authors have misquoted the results of this study as indicating that *L. monocytogenes* survived heating at 80°C for 5 minutes (50).] However, the following year Ozgen (116) reported that *L. monocytogenes* survived 15 seconds at 100°C. In 1955, Stenberg and Hammainen (153) published results of a study which examined the heat resistance of five *L. monocytogenes* strains in milk at different pasteurization temperatures. Using small diameter capillary tubes filled with inoculated milk, these researchers demonstrated that *L. monocytogenes* was not completely inactivated until the milk was held at 65°C for 5 minutes, 75°C for 2 minutes, or 80°C for 3–5 minutes. Thermal resistance of *L. monocytogenes* also was studied by Stajner et al. (151). When milk contained approximately 5×10^5 *L. monocytogenes* CFU/ml, the organism survived heat treatments of 71 and 74°C for 42 seconds, but did not survive heating at 85 and 95°C for 15 and 5 seconds, respectively. In 1957, Dedie and Schulze (42) examined thermal resistance of 54 strains of *L. monocytogenes* in milk using 0.2–0.3-mm diameter capillary tubes. According to their results, *L. monocytogenes* survived 30–40 seconds at 65°C, 10 seconds at 75°C, and ~1 second at 85°C. Ikonomov and Todorov (93) used a pilot-plant–sized tubular glass pasteurizer to examine heat resistance of *Listeria* in milk obtained from ewes and cows. The milk was pasteurized (63–65°C/30 minutes), inoculated to contain ~10^7–10^8 *L. monocytogenes* CFU/ml, and then repasteurized at temperatures between 63 and 74°C. They found that the pathogen survived 20 minutes at 63°C, 10 minutes at 65°C, 3 minutes at 68°C, 1 minute at 70°C, 20 seconds at 72°C, and <20 seconds at 74°C. Thus results of virtually all these early studies indicate that *L. monocytogenes* can survive high-temperature short-time (HTST) pasteurization at 71.6°C for 15 seconds.

Several different approaches have been used to determine thermal resistance and have given rise to conflicting results. Findings from the early pasteurization study of Bearns and Girard (16) have recently become controversial. Their experimental approach involved inoculating 20×150-mm screw-capped test tubes of sterile skim milk with approximately 5×10^1 to 5×10^7 *L. monocytogenes* CFU/ml. All tubes were placed in a water bath at 61.7°C so that the milk surface was 3–4 cm below the water level in the water bath. Tubes were held in a wire test tube rack attached to a mechanical shaker and were allowed to bounce in the rack to aid in mixing. Results obtained from direct-plating of milk on Tryptose Agar indicate that *L. monocytogenes* survived 35 minutes at 61.7°C, provided that the organism was present at an initial level $\geq 5 \times 10^4$ CFU/ml. From these data, the authors calculated a $D_{61.7°C}$ value (i.e., the time necessary to decrease the population 90% at 61.7°C) of 10.9 minutes which indicates that *L.*

monocytogenes, if present at populations >10^3 CFU/ml, can survive vat pasteurization at 61.7°C for 30 minutes.

Using the method of Bearns and Girard (16), Donnelly et al. (52) demonstrated that complete inactivation of *L. monocytogenes* in milk with an initial population of 10^6–10^7 *Listeria* CFU/ml cannot be accomplished within 30 minutes at 62, 72, 82, or even 92°C. Extensive tailing of survivor curves was observed after initial 1000- to 10,000-fold decreases during the first 5 minutes of heating. These investigators concluded that the "open tube" method of Bearns and Girard (16) is unreliable to determine thermal inactivation rates of microorganisms and offered several explanations for their conclusion. One explanation is that condensate and splashed cells accumulated on the test tube cap, which was above the level of water in the water bath and, therefore, not exposed to thermal inactivation temperatures. Condensate containing listeriae would be expected to drip back into the heating menstruum, thus eventually establishing a constant low population of survivors. A more likely explanation is that the test tube walls were coated with cells of *Listeria* during initial mixing. The test tubes were not completely submerged in the water bath; therefore, cells on the test tube wall would not be exposed to thermal inactivation temperatures. Since a constant surface area is presumably coated with listeriae, low levels of survivors would likely be detected throughout the inactivation process. Concurrent studies by Donnelly et al. (52) using a "sealed tube" method demonstrated that *L. monocytogenes* was rapidly inactivated in milk at 62°C. The "sealed tube" method involved adding 1.5 ml of sterile whole milk inoculated to contain ~10^7 *L. monocytogenes* CFU/ml to a 2.0-ml vial, sealing it, and then submerging the vial in a water bath at the desired temperature for various times. In contrast to results of Bearns and Girard (16), thermal inactivation profiles obtained by the "sealed tube" method were linear for three strains of *L. monocytogenes* during the entire inactivation period and gave rise to $D_{62°C}$ values between 0.1 and 0.4 minute, depending on the strain of bacterium. From the aforementioned results, it is apparent that the inactivation rate for *L. monocytogenes* at pasteurization temperature depends on methodology used to study heat resistance of the bacterium.

In 1987, Beckers et al. (17) compared thermal resistance of *L. monocytogenes* in TB using an "open tube" and "sealed bag" method and obtained results similar to those of Donnelly et al. (52) just described. After inoculating TB to contain approximately 5 × 10^3 *L. monocytogenes* CFU/ml, the "open tube" method failed to eliminate listeriae from samples that were held at 60, 65, 70, 75, and 80°C for 30, 30, 15, 5, and 1 minute, respectively. In the "sealed bag" method, TB containing 10^3–10^4 *L. monocytogenes* CFU/ml was heated in sealed plastic bags by immersion in a water bath at the desired temperature. According to these investigators, 4 of 4, 1 of 4, and 0 of 4 *L. monocytogenes* strains survived 10 seconds at 64, 67, and 70°C, respectively. Results obtained by the "sealed bag" method were confirmed by inoculating milk with the same strains previously grown in TB and then heating the milk in a plate pasteurizer. Using this method, *L. monocytogenes* could not be detected after 10 seconds at 70°C. Thus this study also serves to negate the "open tube" method as an acceptable approach to determine thermal inactivation rates of bacteria such as *L. monocytogenes*.

Benedict (18) described a novel approach to estimate thermal death of *L. monocytogenes* in ionic media. Using a water-jacketed dialysis system, spectrophotometer, and flow cuvettes, release of cellular components from *L. monocytogenes* into various ionic media was monitored. The UV absorbance of the diffusate was recorded at 15-second intervals during heating in the test medium at 25, 55, 60, 65, and 70°C. Diffusion rates plotted from temperature profiles and spectra compared favorably to results from standard thermal death methods. In addition, rates of cellular leakage at various temperatures were initially parallel to the thermal death rate, but became more rapid as heating progressed.

As a result of the 1983 listeriosis outbreak in Massachusetts that was epidemiologically linked to consumption of pasteurized milk, Bradshaw et al. (26) investigated thermal resistance of *L. monocytogenes* in raw milk. A culture of *L. monocytogenes* strain Scott A (serotype 4b, clinical isolate associated with the outbreak in Massachusetts) was diluted in phosphate-buffered water and inoculated into raw milk to yield ~10^5 CFU/ml. Portions of 1.5 ml were dispensed into 13×100-mm borosilicate glass tubes, which were sealed and immersed in a water bath at temperatures ranging between 52.2 and 71.7°C. Inoculated samples of raw milk also were heated in a slug flow heat exchanger at 71.7 and 74.4°C. Thermal processing of inoculated milk samples at seven temperatures between 52.2 and 74.4°C led to D-values ranging between 28.1 minutes and 0.7 second, respectively, including a $D_{71.7°C}$ of 0.9 second and a $D_{63.3°C}$ of 19.9 seconds. These investigators also noted that the thermal resistance of strain Scott A remained unchanged over a 2-year period. Survivors from some heating trials also were tested and were no more heat resistant than the parent culture, which suggests that the extensive tailing observed by Bearns and Girard (16) cannot be explained on the basis of heat-resistant mutants.

Working in France, Lemaire et al. (107) used open vessels and sealed capillary tubes to assess resistance of *L. monocytogenes* strains to vat and high-temperature short-time (HTST) pasteurization, respectively. When samples of inoculated milk were held at 60°C in open vessels, $D_{60°C}$ values for 38 different *L. monocytogenes* strains ranged from 1.3 to 6.5 seconds. In contrast, $D_{72°C}$ values of 0.06–1.5 seconds were obtained when *L. monocytogenes* was heated in sealed capillary tubes, with strains of serotype 1 generally more heat resistant than those of serotype 4. These findings along with those of Bradshaw et al. (26) indicate that current minimum vat (61.7°C/30 minutes) and HTST (71.6°C/15 seconds) pasteurization requirements established by the Food and Drug Administration are probably adequate to destroy expected levels of *L. monocytogenes* in raw milk.

In 1986, Donnelly and Briggs (51) reported results of a study that examined the influence of milk composition and incubation temperature on thermal resistance of *L. monocytogenes*. Five *L. monocytogenes* strains were incubated at 37°C for 12 hours, 22 and 10°C for 24 hours, or 4°C for 48 hours in sterile whole milk, skim milk, and reconstituted nonfat milk with 11% solids. Following incubation, 1.5 ml of milk containing ~10^8 *L. monocytogenes* CFU/ml was transferred to a 2-ml glass vial which was crimp-sealed and immersed in a circulating ethylene glycol bath at temperatures between 55 and 65°C. Although $D_{62.7°C}$ values for the five *Listeria* strains ranged between 0.35 and 1.0 minute, all strains exhibited maximum heat resistance when previously incubated at 37°C for 12 hours. Additional thermal inactivation studies using the most heat-resistant strain resulted in $D_{55°C}$ and $D_{65°C}$ values of 24 and 0.1 minute, respectively, and a z-value of 4.3°C. After extrapolating the linear thermal inactivation plot through 71.7°C, the authors concluded that the most heat resistant strain used in their study would be unable to survive in whole milk during HTST pasteurization. In addition, thermal resistance of

L. monocytogenes was not significantly affected by prior growth in skim, whole, or reconstituted nonfat milk with 11% solids, regardless of incubation temperature before inactivation, which suggests that the organism would be unable to survive pasteurization in these products as well.

Going one step further, Bradshaw et al. (25) examined the thermal resistance of *L. monocytogenes* strain Scott A in raw, autoclaved, and commercially sterile whole milk (~3.25% milk fat), raw and autoclaved skim milk (≤0.5% milk fat), heavy cream (38% milk fat), and pasteurized ice cream mix (~10.6% milk fat). Thermal resistance was determined as in their previous study (26) by dispensing 1.5–2.0-ml portions of inoculated (~10^5 strain Scott A CFU/ml) milk, cream, or ice cream mix into 13 × 100-mm borosilicate glass tubes which were sealed and heated in a water bath at temperatures from 52.2 to 79.4°C. *Listeria* inactivation studies done with raw, autoclaved, and commercially sterile whole milk yielded $D_{71.7°C}$ values of 0.9, 2.0, and 2.7 seconds, respectively, indicating significantly ($p \leq 0.05$) greater survival in presterilized than in other samples of whole milk. The $D_{71.7°C}$ value for strain Scott A in presterilized skim milk was 1.7 seconds, whereas the organism had $D_{68.9°C}$ values of 6.0 and 7.8 seconds in raw and autoclaved cream, respectively. Thermal processing of pasteurized ice cream mix at 68.3, 73.9, and 79.4°C resulted in D-values of 231.0, 31.5, and 2.6 seconds, respectively. According to pasteurization guidelines developed by the Food and Drug Administration, all milk products (except chocolate milk) must be held at 71.7°C for a minimum of 15 seconds. If the product contains >10% fat, the pasteurization temperature must be increased by 2.9°C. These guidelines also stipulate that eggnog (and normally ice cream mix) must be heated to 79.4°C for a minimum of 25 seconds. Although their data indicate that *L. monocytogenes* should not survive in properly pasteurized raw whole milk or ice cream mix, their other findings raise serious questions concerning the adequacy of pasteurization to inactivate *L. monocytogenes* in reprocessed products.

Thermal inactivation of *L. monocytogenes* in reconstituted nonfat dry milk (NFDM) was investigated by El-Shenawy et al. (70). Suspensions of *L. monocytogenes* cells in reconstituted NFDM (10% solids) were placed in capillary tubes which were heated in a water bath at 50, 55, 60, 65, 70, and 75°C for various times. Overall, thermal inactivation rates for *L. monocytogenes* were linear throughout the entire course of heating with estimated $D_{62.8°C}$ and $D_{71.7°C}$ values of 20 and 0.94 second, thus reaffirming that pasteurization as defined by the FDA should inactivate freely suspended cells of *L. monocytogenes*.

Studies to this point have dealt with thermal inactivation of freely suspended cells of *L. monocytogenes* in milk and other fluid dairy products. However, in cases of naturally acquired bovine listeriosis, the pathogen is not normally freely suspended in milk, but rather exists as a facultative intracellular bacterium within phagocytic leukocytes (neutrophils and macrophages) typically present in milk of animals suffering from listeric mastitis. The facultative intracellular nature of *L. monocytogenes* has led some investigators to speculate that cells of the pathogen inside leukocytes are partially protected from thermal inactivation and thus are more able to survive pasteurization than are freely suspended cells of the bacterium.

Bunning et al. (34) determined thermal resistance of *L. monocytogenes* in parallel experiments using freely suspended bacteria in raw milk as well as *L. monocytogenes* cells that were inside of mouse peritoneal phagocytes. Phagocytes were elicited in mice by injecting 10^7 heat-killed *L. monocytogenes* (strain Scott A) cells into the peritoneum and then were harvested by peritoneal lavage. Differential staining indicated that the cell preparation was made up of 70% macrophages, 25% neutrophils, and 5% lymphocytes. Opsonized cells of *L. monocytogenes* (incubated in normal mouse serum at 37°C for 30 minutes) were incubated in the phagocytic suspension for 60 minutes to allow phagocytosis. Phagocytes containing listeriae (average of 2.7–19.1 organisms/cell) were washed three times by centrifugation and suspended in raw milk to obtain ~10^5 intracellular *Listeria*/ml. Thermal resistance determinations were done using the "sealed tube" method of Bradshaw et al. (25,26) described earlier in this chapter. Mean D-values for suspensions of intracellular *L. monocytogenes* in raw milk held at 52.2, 57.8, 63.3, and 68.9°C were 3170, 490, 33.3, and 7.0 seconds, respectively, as compared to D-values of 2290, 445, 33.4, and 7.2 seconds when freely suspended cells were held at 52.2, 57.8, 63.3, and 68.9°C, respectively. Extrapolation of the data led to $D_{71.7°C}$ values of 1.9 and 1.6 seconds for phagocytized and freely suspended listeriae, respectively. Under these experimental conditions, the intracellular position did not appreciably protect *L. monocytogenes* from thermal inactivation during pasteurization.

Subsequently, several methods were developed to obtain bovine phagocytes containing internalized cells of *L. monocytogenes*, and such phagocytes have proven useful in evaluating thermal resistance of intracellular listeriae. Briggs et al. (27) enhanced production of bovine phagocytes (93% neutrophils, 5% macrophages, and 2% lymphocytes) by infusing *Escherichia coli* endotoxin into the mammary gland. This procedure produced an average of 2.4×10^6 phagocytes/ml of milk of which 89% were viable. Although only 39% of the endotoxin-induced phagocytes ingested *L. monocytogenes* (average of 27 listeriae/phagocyte) as compared to 64% of normal bovine phagocytes, no difference in bactericidal activity was observed between endotoxin-induced and normal phagocytes. In another study, Donnelly et al. (53) developed an in vitro assay to analyze uptake of *L. monocytogenes* cells by bovine phagocytes. Somatic cells harvested from fresh mastitic milk were composed of 61% neutrophils, 20% macrophages, and 19% lymphocytes. Although 75% of the neutrophils ingested opsonized *L. monocytogenes* cells as compared to only 41% of the macrophages, both cell types contained an average of 19 listeriae per phagocyte. Maximum *Listeria* uptake by phagocytes occurred within 30 minutes of incubation at 37°C. Following ingestion, listeriae were resistant to the bactericidal activity of phagocytes.

In 1988, Bunning et al. (35) reported results of a study comparing thermal resistance of freely suspended and phagocytized cells of *L. monocytogenes*, the latter having been prepared as previously described using endotoxin-induced bovine phagocytes (27). Sterile whole milk was inoculated to contain ~10^6 intracellular (average of 26 bacteria/phagocyte) or freely suspended (obtained by sonicating phagocytes) *L. monocytogenes* cells/ml and heated at 57.8, 62.8, 66.1, and 68.9°C using the "sealed tube" method or at 66.1, 68.9, 71.7, and 74.4°C using a slug flow heat exchanger. Using the "sealed tube" method, the predicted $D_{62.8°C}$ value for intracellular *L. monocytogenes* was 53.8 seconds, indicating a safe 33.4-D margin of inactivation for vat pasteurization (62.8°C/30 min). Using the slug flow heat exchanger, $D_{71.7°C}$ values predicted from linear regression analysis were 4.1 seconds for intracellular and 2.7 seconds for freely suspended listeriae. Hence, the intracellular position of *L. monocytogenes* did not significantly (statistically) increase heat resistance under the defined parameters of this study. More important, these results indicate potentially unsafe 3.7- and 5.6-D margins of inactivation for intracellular and freely suspended listeriae, respectively, using the present minimum HTST pasteurization requirements (71.7°C/15 sec).

In 1988, Yugoslavian and American researchers (102) pooled their efforts to determine thermal resistance of *L. monocytogenes* in naturally infected cows' milk as well as in sterilized milk inoculated to contain ~10^2–10^3 *L. monocytogenes* CFU/ml. According to their preliminary report, no listeriae were recovered from naturally infected cows' milk (originally containing very low levels of listeriae) that was processed at 71.7°C for ≥2 seconds using a two-phase slug flow tubular heat exchanger. However, *L. monocytogenes* was detected after samples of inoculated milk were heated at 71.7°C for 2 and 4, but not 10 seconds, and then stored for 28 days at 4°C, thus suggesting a $D_{71.7°C}$ value for freely suspended cells of *L. monocytogenes* that is larger than that calculated by Bunning et al. (35) in the previous study.

With the exception of the collaborative study just discussed (102), most other results concerning heat resistance of intracellular *L. monocytogenes* were obtained using phagocytes that were artificially induced to engulf listeriae. The first study that examined heat resistance of *L. monocytogenes* in milk from a naturally infected cow was reported in 1962 by Donker-Voet (49). Milk from this cow contained 2×10^3 to 2×10^4 extracellular listeriae and >10^6 leukocytes/ml but otherwise appeared completely normal. Although no attempt was made to examine bovine phagocytes for intracellular listeriae, the organism was presumably present in some of the leukocytes. After pooling the milk for a week and holding it at 4°C, milk was heated in a plate-pasteurizer at 54–76.5°C for 15 seconds and then examined for surviving *Listeria* cells. Unfortunately, by the time enough milk was obtained for a pasteurization trial, the milk was heavily contaminated with other microorganisms, making isolation of listeriae from milk extremely difficult. Furthermore, leukocytes may have disintegrated, and the bacterial cells they may have contained were liberated and became freely suspended cells in the milk. In this study, *L. monocytogenes* survived a heat treatment of 59.0°C for 15 seconds, but did not survive in milk heated at ≥62.3°C for 15 seconds. This experiment was repeated using naturally contaminated milk from the same cow that was held for only 2 days at 4°C. Pasteurized milk was added to the contaminated milk to increase the volume of milk available for pasteurization. Although the initial *Listeria* population was not determined in the diluted milk before heating, *L. monocytogenes* was detected in milk processed at 63.7°C for 15 seconds. However, *L. monocytogenes* was not found in milk heated at 66.3, 68.0, 70.0, or 72.8°C for 15 seconds.

Pasteurization studies using *L. monocytogenes*–contaminated milk obtained from cows artificially infected with the bacterium were recently conducted by Doyle et al. (54). A laboratory culture of *L. monocytogenes* strain Scott A was inoculated into the udder of each of four Holstein cows. Once listeric mastitis had developed, milk from these animals was pooled and held 2 days (and in one instance 4 days) at 4°C until sufficient quantities were available to process in a pilot-scale plate pasteurizer (Cherry-Burrell, model 217SB-1) at 71.7–73.9°C for 16.4 seconds (nine trials) or 76.4–77.8°C for 15.4 seconds (three trials). Before pasteurization, milk contained <10^2 to 1.9×10^4 free *Listeria* cells and 4.5×10^5 to 2.4×10^6 somatic cells/ml. In addition, the milk generally contained 10^3–10^4 *L. monocytogenes* cells within polymorphonuclear leukocytes (PMNL)/ml (average of 1.5–9.2 listeriae/PMNL). During pasteurization, 100-ml samples of milk were taken after 2, 4, and 6 minutes of operation and analyzed for *L. monocytogenes* using two direct-plating and three enrichment procedures, all of which will be discussed in Chapter 6. Viable *L. monocytogenes* was isolated from milk in six of nine trials in which the milk was heated to 71.7–73.9°C for 16.4 seconds. In contrast, *L. monocytogenes* was not detected in milk from the remaining three trials in which the milk was processed at 76.4–77.8°C for 15.4 seconds. Additional studies on the fate of *L. monocytogenes* within PMNL indicated that the organism was no longer detectable in PMNL after 3 days of storage at 4°C. Disappearance of listeriae after 3 days was accompanied by partial degradation of PMNL, with complete breakdown occurring after 4 days. These findings suggest that holding raw milk at 4°C for 4 or more days would eliminate any thermoprotective effect for listeriae that might result from their engulfment by PMNL.

In the study just described, Doyle et al. (54) contended that phagocytized *L. monocytogenes* (<0.1% infectivity with 1.5–9.2 listeriae/PMNL) cells were protected during pasteurization of milk at 71.7–73.9°C for 16.4 seconds. In contrast, using an in vitro method of phagocytosis, Bunning et al. (35) reported that the intracellular position of *L. monocytogenes* (42% infectivity with 26 *Listeria*/phagocyte) did not augment heat resistance of the organism, despite much larger numbers of engulfed listeriae in this study than in that of Doyle et al. (54). Lack of agreement between these two studies might be the result of the bacterium being in different physiological states. It is well known that bacteria are generally more heat resistant during the stationary than the logarithmic phase of growth. Thus nongrowing listeriae within bovine phagocytes may be more heat resistant than actively growing cells that are engulfed by phagocytes or are freely suspended in milk.

While the aforementioned study by Doyle et al. (54) renewed concerns about the ability of *L. monocytogenes* to survive minimum requirements for HTST pasteurization of raw milk, many in the scientific community remained somewhat skeptical that this pathogen could survive such a treatment when naturally present in raw milk. Consequently, several research groups attempted to independently confirm the results obtained by Doyle et al. (54).

Working in Canada, Farber et al. (75) inoculated 1200 L of raw whole milk to contain 10^5 *L. monocytogenes* (a mixture of 10 strains including Scott A) CFU/ml. After heating milk at 60–72°C for 16.2 seconds in a pilot-plant–sized regenerative plate pasteurizer, *L. monocytogenes* was recovered from milk heated up to 67.5°C but was not recovered from milk processed at 69 or 72°C. In addition, raw milk containing 10^3–10^4 *L. monocytogenes* CFU/ml (~10^5 somatic cells/ml with 10–50% of macrophages containing ~1–20 listeriae/macrophage) was obtained from a naturally infected cow, pooled for 2–2.5 days, held at 4°C, and then heated in the pasteurizer. According to these authors, *L. monocytogenes* survived heat treatments of 64 and 66°C for 16.2 seconds, but failed to survive processing at ≥67°C for 16.2 seconds.

FDA officials conducted a similar study (115) in which listeric mastitis was produced in 22 cows through repeated inoculations with a pure culture of *L. monocytogenes*. Milk from these animals which contained ~10^3–10^4 *L. monocytogenes* CFU/ml (present both intra- and extracellularly) was then sent from Iowa to Cincinnati, Ohio, and pasteurized in a commercial-sized HTST pasteurizer that met minimum requirements for pasteurization, i.e., 71.7°C/15 seconds. As in the Canadian study by Farber et al. (75),

L. monocytogenes was never detected in 22 separate lots of milk that were minimally pasteurized.

In contrast to the two studies just described (75,115), Doyle et al. (54) reported that *L. monocytogenes* survived HTST pasteurization at 71.7–73.9°C for 16.4 seconds when the organism was present within phagocytes. Doyle et al. (54) and Farber et al. (75) both used comparable pasteurization as well as *Listeria* detection methods and even reported similar numbers of intracellular listeriae per phagocyte. However, Doyle et al. (54) used a pure culture of *L. monocytogenes* strain Scott A, which is among the most heat resistant strains known, whereas Farber et al. (75) employed a mixed culture containing numbers of strain Scott A approximately equal to each of nine other strains of previously unknown thermal resistance properties. Given that heat resistance of *L. monocytogenes* was recently reported to vary among strains (17,26), with strains identified as serotype 1 supposedly more heat resistant than those identified as serotype 4 (107) (strain Scott A is an exception), strain differences in thermal resistance may help explain the different outcomes obtained in those two pasteurization studies. As previously noted, differences in the physiological state of the organism when tested also might play a role in increased thermal resistance. Results of Knabel et al. (100) illustrate the point. They found that strict anaerobic incubation markedly increased recovery of thermally injured *L. monocytogenes* cells. Use of this technique yielded results suggesting the pathogen could survive vat pasteurization. However, since only one *L. monocytogenes* strain was used in this study, the findings need to be interpreted with some caution.

After weighing all of the foregone evidence, the answer to the question of whether or not *L. monocytogenes* can survive pasteurization still appears to be partly obscured by conflicting results. Although Doyle et al. (54) reported viable *L. monocytogenes* present in naturally contaminated milk following minimum required HTST pasteurization, one must remember that the strain of *L. monocytogenes* used in their study was among the most heat-resistant strains known and that the milk to be pasteurized contained ~10^3–10^4 *L. monocytogenes* CFU/ml, i.e., levels at least 100–1000 times higher than would be expected to occur in commingled raw milk entering any dairy factory. Hence, with this information, the inability of Farber et al. (75) and FDA workers (115) to recover *L. monocytogenes* from similarly pasteurized milk, and the failure of anyone to conclusively prove that this pathogen has ever survived proper pasteurization in any commercially produced dairy product, we conclude along with the CDC (8,9,13), FDA officials (115), and the World Health Organization (166) that "pasteurization is a safe process which reduces the number of *L. monocytogenes* occurring in raw milk to levels that do not pose an appreciable risk to human health." Furthermore, a recent report (24) indicates that *L. ivanovii*, *L. seeligeri*, and *L. welshimeri* are even less heat resistant than *L. monocytogenes*; consequently proper pasteurization also should eliminate these *Listeria* spp. from milk, thus producing a *Listeria*-free product.

IRRADIATION

Since the character and composition of most raw agricultural products are adversely affected by thermal processing, considerable effort has been spent on developing alternative methods to rid such foods of harmful microorganisms. While use of electromagnetic radiation to inactivate both pathogenic and spoilage microorganisms in food did not receive serious attention until shortly after World War Two, today such use is gaining widespread acceptance.

The entire electromagnetic spectrum consists of at least six distinct forms of radiation that differ according to wavelength, frequency, and penetrating power; however, only ultraviolet and ionizing radiation (i.e., gamma radiation) are of practical importance to food manufacturers. Ultraviolet radiation, i.e., a nonionizing form of radiation ranging in wavelength from 136 to 4000 angstroms, is strongly bactericidal to vegetative cells. Unfortunately, the poor penetrating power of ultraviolet radiation restricts its use to eradication of airborne contaminants and treatment of food contact and non–food contact surfaces as well as surfaces of foods such as fruit cakes and related products during packaging. Ionizing forms of radiation such as gamma radiation have wavelengths of ≤ 2000 angstroms. Unlike ultraviolet radiation, the excellent penetrating power of gamma radiation (wavelength = 0.1–1.4 Å) makes this form of radiation far better suited for external and internal decontamination of foods. While exposing food to gamma radiation doses of 10–50 kiloGrays (kGy) [i.e., a unit of absorbed radiation dose equivalent to 10^5 rads (10^7 erg/kg or 1000 joules/kg)] generally produces a commercially sterile product, current FDA regulations do not permit exposure of most foods to >3 kGy. Nevertheless, such doses are sufficient to inactivate populations of *L. monocytogenes* that one would normally encounter in most raw foods.

Ultraviolet Radiation

In 1971 Collins (38) determined the susceptibility of *L. monocytogenes* to ultraviolet radiation emitted from a 14 w cold cathode mercury vapor lamp. Tryptone Soy agar plates containing $\sim 10^9$ *L. monocytogenes* were exposed to a radiation output of 40 w/cm^2 at 40 cm from the source for 30, 60, 90, and 120 seconds and then incubated for 3 days at 37°C. Populations of *L. monocytogenes* decreased 10-fold during the first 60 seconds of irradiation (D-value of 60 seconds) after which the rate of inactivation increased sharply with a D-value of ~15 seconds. *Listeria monocytogenes* was markedly more resistant to radiation than *E. coli* or *Serratia marcescens*, which are commonly used to test effectiveness of ultraviolet lamps.

Seventeen years later, Yousef and Marth (170) also reported that *L. monocytogenes* was inactivated by exposing the bacterium to ultraviolet energy. Following 4 minutes of exposure to short-wave (254 nm) ultraviolet energy (100 µw/cm^2), the number of *L. monocytogenes* (strain Scott A) decreased approximately seven orders of magnitude on Tryptose Agar plates that were previously spread with a 24- or 48-hour-old culture of the test organism. In contrast, *L. monocytogenes* numbers remained constant after 10 minutes of exposure to long-wave (364 nm) ultraviolet energy. Increasing the intensity of short-wave ultraviolet radiation to 550 µw/cm^2 nearly doubled the rate at which *L. monocytogenes* was inactivated. These investigators also found that dry rather than moist *Listeria* cells were more resistant to radiation. Exposing a dried film of *L. monocytogenes* cells in a petri plate to short-wave ultraviolet energy (100 µw/cm^2) decreased the population by two rather than the seven orders of magnitude obtained with moist cells on Tryptose Agar. Fortunately, when present in food-processing environments, numbers of listeriae appear to be relatively low. Hence, results from the aforementioned study suggest that ultraviolet energy may be of some practical importance in reducing airborne contaminants, including listeriae, in food production and storage areas.

Gamma Irradiation

Its superior penetrating power prompted recent investigations to largely focus on defining sensitivity of *L. monocytogenes* to gamma irradiation in TB or similar culture media. Unlike the aforementioned controversy concerning thermal resistance, results from five gamma irradiation studies conducted in the United States (37,71,77,92) and Hungary (156) are strikingly similar with reported D-values ranging from 0.28 to 0.61 kGy for 12 different *L. monocytogenes* strains. In addition, exposure to a gamma radiation dose of ~1.7–4.0 kGy was generally sufficient to reduce numbers of *L. monocytogenes* as well as of *L. ivanovii* and *L. seeligeri* by six to seven orders of magnitude. Overall, these findings suggest that *Listeria* spp. are likely to be at least equally, if not slightly more, resistant to gamma irradiation in culture media than are other commonly encountered non–spore forming foodborne pathogens such as *Salmonella typhimurium* (D-value = 0.28 kGy) (161), *Staphylococcus aureus* (D-value = 0.24 kGy) (161) and *Yersinia enterocolitica* (D-value = 0.11 kGy) (72).

While differences between *L. monocytogenes* strains likely account for most of the observed variation in D-value, irradiation sensitivity of *L. monocytogenes* is also affected by age of the culture, irradiation menstruum, and the type of medium used to enumerate the pathogen after irradiation. According to Huhtanen et al. (92), 1.5- and 2.5-hour-old cultures of *L. monocytogenes* were somewhat more resistant to gamma irradiation than those incubated 5 and 18 hours before exposure. Surviving cells previously exposed to high radiation doses also were subsequently found to be no more resistant than the parent culture. Consequently, observed differences between sensitivity of young and old cultures probably resulted from innate differences between strains rather than from development of radiation-resistant mutants. These authors also reported that 12-hour-old centrifuged cultures of *L. monocytogenes* were most resistant to 1.0 kGy gamma radiation when resuspended in fresh culture media or the original culture supernatant liquid followed in order by phosphate buffer and distilled water. Inability of distilled water to effectively scavenge cell-damaging free radicals produced during irradiation is likely responsible for decreased resistance of the pathogen in water than in culture media that contain high concentrations of free radical–quenching organic compounds. It is not surprising that *L. monocytogenes* is more resistant to gamma irradiation when present in foods than in culture media. (Results from several studies that examined the ability of gamma irradiation to eliminate this pathogen from meat and poultry products are discussed in Chapters 11 and 12, respectively.) Finally, two independent investigations (71,119) have shown that D-values for irradiation resistance are markedly affected by type of plating media used to enumerate the pathogen after irradiation. In both studies, a significantly higher ($p < 0.05$) D-value resulted from increased recovery of the pathogen with nonselective or semi-selective rather than highly selective plating media. These findings indicate that substantial numbers of listeriae were sublethally injured during exposure to gamma irradiation. Since repair and subsequent growth of injured cells is frequently inhibited by some of the selective agents used in highly selective media, D-values for organisms exposed to irradiation or any other potentially injurious treatment always should be determined using the least selective plating media possible. The topic of sublethal injury will be explored in greater detail in the following chapter.

HYDROSTATIC PRESSURE

While most microorganisms except certain ocean-dwelling species grow best under normal atmospheric pressure, exposure to hydrostatic pressure >600 atmospheres often induces cellular changes that can be lethal to non–spore forming organisms. Hence, exposure to increased hydrostatic pressure has been suggested as another means of inactivating certain spoilage and pathogenic organisms in raw and pasteurized milk as well as meat, poultry, seafood, fruits, and vegetables.

Recognizing the proven ability of high hydrostatic pressure to inactivate *Salmonella* spp. in laboratory media, Hoover (87) and Styles et al. (154) examined the behavior of *L. monocytogenes* strains Scott A and CA in phosphate buffered saline solution during exposure to pressures of 2380–3400 atmospheres (i.e., 35,000–50,000 psi) at ambient temperatures. Strains Scott A and CA were fairly baro-tolerant, exhibiting D-values of 597 and 73 minutes, respectively, in the presence of 2380 atmospheres. However, populations of strains Scott A and CA decreased five and three orders of magnitude, respectively, following only 15 minutes of exposure to 3400 atmospheres. When these experiments were repeated using ultra-high temperature processed milk, 80 minutes at 3400 atmospheres were required to inactivate an *L. monocytogenes* population of 1×10^7 CFU/ml. Thus both *Listeria* strains were more resistant to high hydrostatic pressure when suspended in milk than in buffer.

Unfortunately, large numbers of listeriae were only sublethally injured in milk held under 3060 atmospheres for 40 minutes. Incubating pressure-treated milk samples at 37°C for 6 hours led to numbers of strain Scott A that were only 10-fold lower than the original population before treatment. Hence, high hydrostatic pressure probably will have to be used with other food-preservation methods such as thermal processing to ensure complete elimination of listeriae from processed foods. Readers interested in this topic are referred to a 1989 review article by Hoover et al. (89) in which potential applications of high hydrostatic pressure to food preservation are discussed at greater length.

POTASSIUM SORBATE

Since their approval in the United States during the 1950s, potassium sorbate and sorbic acid have been widely used to extend the shelf life of many foods including butter, cheese, meat, cereals, and bakery items. While most effective against yeasts and molds, these antimicrobial agents also inhibit a wide range of bacteria, particularly aerobic catalase-positive organisms. Hence, several investigators have assessed the ability of potassium sorbate and sorbic acid to inhibit *L. monocytogenes* in laboratory media and several foods.

According to data collected by El-Shenawy and Marth (65), the ability of potassium sorbate to prevent growth of *L. monocytogenes* is related to temperature and pH. In the absence of potassium sorbate, generation times for *L. monocytogenes* in TB at pH 5.6

decreased from 1.13 days to 49 minutes as the incubation temperature increased from 4 to 35°C. Addition of 2500 ppm potassium sorbate to the medium prevented growth of *Listeria* at 4°C and led to complete demise of the organism after 66 days, whereas listeriae grew with a generation time of 9 hours in the same medium incubated at 35°C. Potassium sorbate was more effective at lower pH values at 4°C with *L. monocytogenes* surviving 48 days at pH 5.0 rather than 66 days at pH 5.6 in a medium containing 2500 ppm potassium sorbate and incubated at 35°C. *Listeria* populations reached a maximum of 5×10^6 CFU/ml at pH 5.6 in a medium containing 2500 ppm potassium sorbate and incubated at 35°C; however, the organism failed to grow in the same medium adjusted to pH 5.0.

When working with food, Ryser and Marth (137) found that four strains of *L. monocytogenes* were eliminated faster from cold-pack cheese food at pH 5.45 that contained 3000 ppm sorbic acid (4100 ppm potassium sorbate) rather than from cheese food at pH 5.2 manufactured without preservative. After inoculating cheese food containing sorbic acid with one of four *L. monocytogenes* strains at a level of $\sim5 \times 10^2$ CFU/g, the pathogen survived an average of 142 days during storage at 4°C. Although *L. monocytogenes* failed to grow in cheese food with a pH of 5.21 and made without sorbic acid, the pathogen survived during the normal 6-month shelf life of the product at potentially hazardous numbers of $\sim1 \times 10^2$ CFU/g. Since potassium sorbate works best at pH < 6.0 and is generally ineffective at pH > 6.5, it is not surprising to learn that Dje et al. (46) found potassium sorbate to be of little use in inactivating *L. monocytogenes* in samples of reconstituted NFDM.

SODIUM PROPIONATE

Although markedly less effective than potassium sorbate, El-Shenawy and Marth (65) recently demonstrated that >2000 ppm sodium propionate can inhibit growth of *L. monocytogenes* in TB at pH 5.0. As in their study with sorbate (67), generation times for *L. monocytogenes* in TB at pH 5.6 and without sodium propionate decreased from 1.13 to 49 minutes as the incubation temperature increased from 4 to 35°C. In TB at pH 5.6 and containing 3000 ppm sodium propionate, generation times decreased from 3.0 days to 4.5 hours as the incubation temperature increased from 4 to 35°C. Using TB at pH 5.0 and containing 3000 ppm sodium propionate, *Listeria* populations decreased 10-fold during 67 days of incubation at 4°C. When the same medium was incubated at 35°C, numbers of *L. monocytogenes* decreased $\sim$1000-fold with the organism no longer being detected after 78 days. At pH 5.0 and incubation temperatures of 13, 21, and 35°C, growth was inhibited to various degrees when the medium contained 500–3000 ppm sodium propionate. Final numbers of *L. monocytogenes* depended on concentration of sodium propionate in the medium and ranged between 10^3 and 10^8 CFU/ml.

In 1987, Lang et al. (104) found that *L. monocytogenes* grew at 13°C in TB at pH 5.0 and containing 0 and 6% NaCl; however, growth was prevented by addition of 5000 ppm propionic acid at both salt concentrations as well as by the combination of 6% NaCl and 0.1% propionic acid. Using TB at pH 5.6 and containing 0, 1000, or 5000 ppm propionic acid, *L. monocytogenes* grew to final populations of 10^7–10^8 and 10^4–10^5 CFU/ml in the presence of 0 and 6% NaCl, respectively. Generation times calculated for listeriae in the salt-free medium at pH 5.6 and containing 0, 1000, and 5000 ppm propionic acid were

4.4, 10.3, and 16.1 hours, respectively, rather than 7.2, 18.1, and 42.1 hours, respectively, in the same medium containing 6% NaCl. Similar behavior by *L. monocytogenes* was subsequently noted during extended incubation at 4 to 30°C in Brain Heart Infusion Broth (pH 5.9) containing 4.0% NaCl and 0.15% potassium sorbate (77).

When used at 3000 ppm, Ryser and Marth (137) found sodium propionate was less effective than sorbic acid in eliminating four strains of *L. monocytogenes* from cold-pack cheese food at pH 5.20–5.45. Cheese food was inoculated to contain ~5 × 10^2 *L. monocytogenes* CFU/g and stored at 4°C; the pathogen survived an average of 142 and 130 days in product that contained sodium propionate and sorbic acid, respectively. In contrast, the pathogen was present in cheese food made without preservatives at levels of ~1 × 10^2 CFU/g after 6 months of refrigerated storage.

SODIUM BENZOATE

In 1988, El-Shenawy and Marth (64) reported that sodium benzoate is more inhibitory to *L. monocytogenes* than is either potassium sorbate or sodium propionate. As in their other studies (65,67), TB was used and was supplemented with 0–3000 ppm sodium benzoate in increments of 500 ppm, adjusted to pH 5.0 and 5.6 with hydrochloric acid, inoculated to contain ~10^3 *L. monocytogenes* CFU/ml and incubated at 4, 13, 21, or 35°C. At pH 5.6, *L. monocytogenes* was inactivated in the presence of ≥2000 ppm sodium benzoate after 60 days of incubation at 4°C. At pH 5.0, the organism was completely nonviable in TB containing ≥1500 ppm sodium benzoate after 24–30 days of incubation at 4°C, whereas lower concentrations of sodium benzoate led to gradual decreases in numbers of listeriae during 66 days at 4°C. At pH 5.6, the pathogen grew in TB containing ≤ 2000 ppm sodium benzoate during incubation at 13°C, but did not grow in the medium containing ≥ 2500 ppm sodium benzoate. Reducing the pH to 5.0 led to decreased growth of *Listeria*, particularly at higher concentrations of sodium benzoate. At 21 and 35°C, the organism grew only in TB containing ≤ 2000 sodium benzoate. Reducing the pH to 5.0 led to limited growth of the pathogen at 21 and 35°C in TB containing 500 or 1000 ppm sodium benzoate, whereas higher concentrations of preservatives caused complete or partial inhibition or inactivation of *L. monocytogenes*.

Inhibition and inactivation of *L. monocytogenes* in the presence of sodium benzoate is affected by (a) temperature (i.e., more rapid at higher than lower incubation temperatures), (b) concentration of benzoic acid (i.e., more rapid at higher than lower concentrations), and (c) pH (i.e., more rapid at lower than higher pH values) as well as the type of acid used to adjust the growth medium. When TB was acidified to pH values of 5.0 and 5.6 with acetic, tartaric, lactic, or citric rather than hydrochloric acid, El-Shenawy and Marth (66) found the antilisterial activity of sodium benzoate was greatly enhanced. For example, 1500 ppm sodium benzoate led to complete inactivation of *L. monocytogenes* after 96 hours at 35°C when acetic or tartaric acid were used to adjust the pH of the medium to 5.0; under the same conditions the pathogen remained viable at least 78 hours longer when the pH of the medium was adjusted with hydrochloric acid. Similarly, 3000 ppm sodium benzoate completely inactivated the pathogen within 48 hours at 35°C when the medium was acidified to pH 5.0 with lactic or citric acid, whereas 60 hours were required when the medium was adjusted to the same pH with hydrochloric acid. Overall, 1500 to 3000 ppm sodium benzoate inactivated *L. monocytogenes* within 24–40 and 24–96 hours when the pathogen was inoculated into TB acidified to pH 5.0 with acetic or tartaric acid and incubated at 35 and 13°C, respectively. In contrast, inactivation of listeriae in TB acidified to pH 5.0 with lactic or citric acid occurred only in the presence of 3000 ppm sodium benzoate with the pathogen no longer detectable in samples following 1 and 12–15 days at 35 and 13°C, respectively. *Listeria monocytogenes* also survived and/or grew during 4 and 15 days at 35 and 13°C, respectively, in all samples containing 500–3000 ppm sodium benzoate that were adjusted to pH 5.6 with any of the four organic acids. Overall, the authors concluded that acetic and tartaric acid were most effective in enhancing the antilisterial effects of sodium benzoate followed by lactic and citric acid.

Using a minimal glucose-citrate medium (lacking a nitrogen source) adjusted to pH 5.5 with sodium hydroxide, Yousef et al. (172) demonstrated that death rates for *L. monocytogenes* were affected far more by incubation temperature than by presence of 1000–3000 ppm benzoic acid in the medium with D-values decreasing ~100-fold as the incubation temperature was increased from 4 to 35°C. Injured listeriae also were detected after plating samples on restrictive and nonrestrictive media. Although the extent of cell injury was somewhat greater at lower than higher incubation temperatures, addition of 3000 ppm benzoic acid to the medium did not increase recovery of sublethally injured cells. Hence, benzoic acid at concentrations of ~1000–3000 ppm exhibited strong bacteriostatic but only modest bactericidal activity. These data along with the recent isolation of an apparent sodium benzoate–resistant strain of *L. monocytogenes* from an animal-based dairy ingredient (58), suggest that use of benzoic acid alone to control *Listeria* in food is questionable. However, Emme et al. (73) recently found that repeated exposure of *L. monocytogenes* to 1000 ppm benzoic acid did not increase resistance of the organism to this widely used food additive.

SODIUM NITRITE

Studies undertaken by Shahamat et al. (143) during the 1970s examined effects of various concentrations of sodium nitrite and sodium chloride on growth of *L. monocytogenes* in Trypticase Soy Broth at different temperatures and pH values. When incubated at 37, 22, and 4°C in broth at pH 7.4, *L. monocytogenes* grew at nitrite concentrations as high as 25,000, 30,000, and 10,000 ppm, respectively. Inhibitory effects of nitrite were enhanced at pH 6.5, particularly at lower incubation temperatures, with complete inhibition caused by 1500 ppm nitrite at 4°C. Minimum inhibitory concentrations of nitrite were further reduced at all three incubation temperatures and at pH 5.5, with 600 ppm nitrite being sufficient to inhibit growth at 4°C. However, bacteriostatic activity of nitrite was greatest at pH 5.0 and at 22 and 37°C, with no growth reported at nitrite concentrations of >800 and 400 ppm, respectively. Addition of 3.0% sodium chloride to the medium failed to increase the bacteriostatic action of sodium nitrite. Although minimum inhibitory nitrite concentrations were only slightly lower with 5.5 or 8.0% sodium chloride at pH 7.4 or 6.5, the combination of 5.5 or 8.0% sodium chloride and pH values of 5.0 or 5.5 led to minimum inhibitory concentrations of nitrite that were generally 8- to 20-fold lower than controls prepared without sodium chloride. Inhibitory effects of nitrite were again most pronounced at 4°C when the chemical was combined with sodium chloride.

As mentioned earlier, behavior of *L. monocytogenes* in food and culture media depends on the interactive effects of temperature, pH, type of acidulant, salt content, a_w, and types and concentrations of food additives that may be present in the system. The effectiveness of sodium nitrite as an antilisterial agent also is strongly influenced by these same factors.

Following emergence of *L. monocytogenes* as a serious foodborne pathogen, Buchanan et al. (31) used a factorial design to determine the effect of sodium nitrite (0–1000 ppm) in combination with incubation temperature (5–37°C), initial pH (6.0–7.5), sodium chloride (0.5 vs. 4.5%), and atmosphere (aerobic vs. anaerobic) on growth of *L. monocytogenes* in Tryptose Phosphate Broth. While lag periods, generation times, and maximum populations were all affected by these five interacting variables, sodium nitrite was most listeriostatic when used in conjunction with low pH, increased sodium chloride, refrigeration temperatures, and anaerobic conditions that simulated vacuum packaging.

Continuing the work just described, Buchanan et al. (32) used a factorial/supplemental central composite design to quantitatively assess the effects of temperature (5, 10, 19, 28, 37°C), pH (4.50, 5.25, 6.00, 6.75, 7.50), sodium chloride (0.5, 1.5, 2.5, 3.5, 4.5%), sodium nitrite (0, 50, 100, 150, 200, 1000 ppm), and atmosphere (aerobic vs. anaerobic) on the growth kinetics of *L. monocytogenes* strain Scott A in Tryptose Phosphate Broth. After growth curves were constructed for each of the experimental cultures using regression analysis to obtain "best fit" Gompertz Equation curves, results were analyzed by response surface analysis to generate a polynomial model that could mathematically predict lag periods, exponential growth rates, generation times, and maximum populations for *L. monocytogenes* in association with any of the five variables examined. Overall, changes in response of the organism to the five environmental factors were most evident as altered experimental growth rates and lag periods. *Listeria monocytogenes* also achieved similar maximum populations in all instances except those that involved growth of the pathogen under environmental extremes in the presence of high concentrations of sodium nitrite.

These equations were subsequently used to develop a Lotus 1-2-3 computer-based program to predict growth kinetics of *L. monocytogenes* in association with any combination of the five variables previously mentioned. While they encountered some irregularities in the first-generation program designated Pathogen Modelling Program Version 2.0, these problems were reportedly corrected by the developers in Version 2.1 (30). Although this latter program should provide the first useful "round number" estimates of *Listeria* growth kinetics, users must keep in mind that this program is based on growth of one *L. monocytogenes* strain in a laboratory medium. Hence, there is no assurance that these values will match those that would be observed in various foods.

Working with food, Johnson et al. (96) found that growth of *L. monocytogenes* was suppressed at 4°C in hard salami sausage that had a pH of 4.3–4.5 and contained 5.0–7.8% NaCl plus 156 ppm sodium nitrite. Although their findings agree with those of Shahamat et al. (143), the combination of low water activity (a_w 0.79–0.86) and low pH were probably more important in preventing growth of listeriae than was the 156 ppm sodium nitrite. Findings of Glass and Doyle (79) also indicate that 3.5% sodium chloride plus 156 ppm sodium nitrite in meat at pH 6.2 controlled growth of *L. monocytogenes* in sausage held at 90°F. Under these conditions, additional acid development through fermentation is essential to prevent growth of listeriae.

FATTY ACIDS

Recently, Pfeiffer et al. (121) investigated the effects of 100 ppm each of butyric, caprylic, and caproic acids on growth of four *L. monocytogenes* strains in TB at pH 5.6 during incubation at 13°C. Butyric and caproic acid failed to inhibit growth of *L. monocytogenes* as evidenced by average generation times of 4.5, 4.0, and 4.4 hours in TB with butyric, with caproic, and without fatty acids, respectively. In these three cultures, *L. monocytogenes* grew to a population of $\sim3 \times 10^8$ CFU/ml after 7 days of incubation. In contrast, the average generation time for *L. monocytogenes* was about twice as long (9.40 h) in TB containing caprylic rather than caproic or butyric acid or in the control without fatty acids. Along with the slower growth rate, slightly lower *Listeria* populations ($\sim1 \times 10^8$ CFU/ml) were observed after 14 rather than 7 days for butyric and caproic acid.

SULFUR COMPOUNDS

In limited studies by Ryser and Marth (139), growth of four *L. monocytogenes* strains in TB at 10°C was not inhibited by 10 ppm methyl sulfide, dimethyl disulfide, or methyl trisulfide. Yousef et al. (173) reported that growth of *L. monocytogenes* was not adversely affected by addition of 5% dimethyl sulfoxide to TB during incubation at 35°C, but increasing the concentration of dimethyl sulfoxide to 10% led to significant reductions both in growth rate and maximum population.

ANTIOXIDANTS

Antioxidants such as butylated hydroxyanisole (BHA), butylated hydroxytoluene (BHT), tertiary butylhydroquinone (TBHQ), and propyl gallate comprise an important category of food additives. While primarily used to prevent oxidation of fat, some of these antioxidants also possess antimicrobial activity.

Limited trials on destruction of *L. monocytogenes* by BHA were initiated by Al-Issa et al. (4) during the early 1980s. Tryptone Soy Broth containing 50 ppm BHA was inoculated to contain $\sim10^5$ *L. monocytogenes* CFU/ml and examined for numbers of the bacterium. The *Listeria* population decreased ~1000-fold during the first 12 hours at 37°C and remained at a level of $\sim10^2$ CFU/ml after 24 hours of incubation. The same authors also found that successive subculturing of *L. monocytogenes* in a medium containing glycerol followed by inoculation into Tryptone Soy Broth containing 50 ppm BHA led to rapid *Listeria* growth with populations reaching 10^8–10^9 CFU/ml after 24 hours at 37°C. Development of BHA resistance correlated with a high lipid content in the cell wall and membrane as a result of prior growth in a medium containing glycerol. Supporting evidence indicates that fattened cells of *L. monocytogenes* become susceptible to BHA when grown in a glycerol-free medium.

In response to recent concerns about foodborne listeriosis, Payne et al. (120)

investigated the potential of BHA, BHT, TBHQ, and propyl gallate to inhibit growth of *L. monocytogenes* on Tryptose Phosphate Agar during 18 hours of incubation at 35°C. Using an agar dilution method, TBHQ proved to be the most effective with a minimum inhibitory concentration of 64 ppm followed by BHA, propyl gallate, and BHT with minimum inhibitory concentrations of 128, 256, and 512 ppm, respectively.

While these findings may at first appear promising for the food industry, *L. monocytogenes* is far more likely to encounter sublethal rather than minimum inhibitory concentrations of antioxidants in food. Consequently, Yousef et al. (173) examined the growth kinetics of *L. monocytogenes* strain Scott A in TB containing BHA (100–300 ppm), BHT (300–700 ppm), and TBHQ (10–30 ppm) during 54 hours of incubation at 35°C. Overall, these findings agreed with those of Payne et al. (120) in that TBHQ again was the most inhibitory to *L. monocytogenes* followed by BHA and BHT. According to the authors, *L. monocytogenes* exhibited increasingly longer lag periods and generation times as well as lower maximum populations in the presence of BHA at 100–200 ppm with concentrations ≥300 ppm proving to be lethal. Since all three growth parameters were increasingly affected as the sublethal concentrations of BHA increased, it appears that the organism was unable to metabolically detoxify this antioxidant. Therefore, addition of up to 200 ppm BHA to food as permitted by the FDA will likely contribute to overall keeping quality and safety of some products. Unlike BHA, *L. monocytogenes* was unaffected by presence of ≤300 ppm BHT; however, poor solubility of BHT in TB prevented critical analysis of this antioxidant at concentrations >300 ppm. Interestingly, increasing the concentration of TBHQ from 10 to 30 ppm led to an exponentially longer lag period for *L. monocytogenes*, but did not appreciably affect generation times or maximum populations. Hence, unlike BHA, these observations suggest that *L. monocytogenes* can metabolically detoxify sublethal concentrations of TBHQ to safe levels and initiate growth thereafter. From this evidence, it appears that BHA may be of greater benefit than TBHQ for inhibiting growth of listeriae in food.

Since TBHQ appeared potentially useful, Payne et al. (120) examined the antilisterial activity of this antioxidant in milk. Reconstituted NFDM (10% solids) was inoculated to contain 10 *L. monocytogenes* CFU/ml; addition of 150 ppm TBHQ prevented growth of and variably inactivated the pathogen during 24 hours at 35°C. Although numbers of listeriae increased nearly 100-fold in similar samples inoculated to contain ~10^3 *L. monocytogenes* CFU/ml, maximum populations were still approximately three orders of magnitude lower than those observed in TBHQ-free control samples. Results obtained by repeating these experiments at refrigeration temperatures were more encouraging (46) with original *Listeria* inocula of 10^1 and 10^3 CFU/ml being reduced to nondetectable levels or remaining constant, respectively, during 10 days at 4°C. While these preliminary findings suggest that addition of TBHQ to foods at FDA-permissible levels of ≤ 200 ppm may be of some benefit in inhibiting and/or inactivating *L. monocytogenes*, present FDA regulations (10) stipulate that TBHQ and all other such additives can only be used as antioxidants and cannot be added indiscriminately to foods for other purposes.

Two phenolic antioxidants that exhibit antimicrobial activity, namely methyl paraben and propyl paraben, also have been approved for limited use in certain foods manufactured in the United States. Consequently, Payne et al. (120) examined the ability of methyl and propyl paraben as well as several nonapproved phenolic antioxidants (caffeic acid, coumaric acid, ferulic acid, gallic acid, quercetin, and tannic acid) to inhibit growth of *L. monocytogenes* on Tryptose Phosphate Agar plates during 18 hours of incubation at 35°C. With eight different strains of the pathogen, propyl and methyl paraben yielded minimum inhibitory concentrations of 512 and >512 ppm, respectively. [Preliminary results from another study (77) indicate that *L. monocytogenes*, *L. ivanovii*, and *L. seeligeri* are all about equally sensitive to methyl paraben.] Results for the nonapproved phenolic antioxidants showed that tannic acid was most listericidal (minimum inhibitory concentration of 256 ppm) with all remaining antioxidants yielding minimum inhibitory concentrations of >512 ppm.

With this information in hand, these researchers went on to determine the antilisterial activity of propyl paraben in milk. Using reconstituted NFDM (10% solids) inoculated to contain 10 or 10^3 *L. monocytogenes* CFU/ml, populations of listeriae were approximately three to four orders of magnitude lower in samples containing 1000 rather than 0 ppm propyl paraben following 24 hours at 35°C. When these experiments were repeated at refrigeration temperatures (46), *Listeria* counts in milk samples containing 1000 ppm propyl paraben remained constant during 10 days at 4°C.

Going one step further, Dje et al. (46) investigated behavior of *L. monocytogenes* in 10% (w/v) aqueous suspensions of raw chicken meat and frankfurters to which 1000 ppm propyl paraben was added. While *L. monocytogenes* attained maximum populations of ~10^8 CFU/ml in propyl paraben-free chicken suspensions following 24 hours at 35°C, numbers of listeriae increased only approximately 10-fold to a maximum of 10^5 CFU/ml in similar suspensions containing 1000 ppm propyl paraben. Thus, as was true for samples of reconstituted NFDM incubated at 35°C, propyl paraben was marginally effective in inhibiting growth of this pathogen in chicken suspensions. However, unlike these samples, addition of 1000 ppm propyl paraben to frankfurter suspensions failed to prevent growth of *L. monocytogenes* with similar growth rates and maximum populations of ~10^8 CFU/ml appearing after 24 hours of incubation at 35°C in samples prepared both with and without propyl paraben. Since *L. monocytogenes* and propyl paraben are primarily present in the water and lipid phases of these suspensions, respectively, the higher percentage of fat in frankfurter than in chicken suspensions likely accounts for increased growth of listeriae in the former. Even though propyl paraben appears to be only minimally listericidal in high fat foods, this antioxidant reportedly remains relatively bactericidal at pH values ≤7.0. Hence, this antioxidant may eventually prove to be useful in various low fat foods.

LIQUID SMOKE

Many commercially available liquid smoke products used in processed meats and sausages also can inactivate common foodborne organisms including *E. coli*, *S. aureus*, and *Lactobacillus viridescens*. These artificial liquid smoke flavorants owe their activity to presence of phenolic compounds and acetic acid, both of which are bactericidal at relatively low concentrations.

After *L. monocytogenes* was recognized as a possible health hazard in ready-to-eat meat and sausage products, several investigators examined the potential of various liquid smoke compounds to inactivate *L. monocytogenes* in phosphate buffer and culture media commonly used to isolate this pathogen from meat products. Using sterile phosphate buffer at pH 5.64 and inoculated to contain 1×10^5 *L. monocytogenes* CFU/ml (111), three of five liquid smoke compounds (CharSol-10, Aro-Smoke P-50, and CharDex Hickory) tested at a concentration of 0.5% reduced the pathogen to nondetectable levels after 4 hours at ambient temperature. When the concentration of liquid smoke products was decreased to 0.25%, numbers of listeriae were still reduced to nondetectable levels within 4 hours using either CharSol-10 or Aro-Smoke P-50. However, CharDex Hickory was far less effective at the lower concentration with 24 hours of incubation required to completely inactivate the pathogen. Listericidal activity of these liquid smoke compounds also appeared to be at least partially related to levels of acetic acid present in the various preparations.

Subsequently, Wendorf (165) found that the same liquid smoke compounds were far less listericidal when added to USDA-recommended Listeria Enrichment Broth rather than phosphate buffer. Interactions between liquid smoke constituents and protein in the enrichment broth were probably at least partially responsible for the observed decrease in listericidal activity.

While three of five liquid smoke compounds were effective against *L. monocytogenes* in buffer and to a lesser extent in culture media, recent work by Wendorf (165) has shown that concentrations of liquid smoke needed to inactivate *L. monocytogenes* in processed meats are well above organoleptically acceptable limits. The practicality of using liquid smoke to inactivate *L. monocytogenes* in processed meat and sausage will be discussed at greater length in Chapter 12, which deals with the incidence and behavior of *Listeria* in meat products.

SPICES

Although primarily used as flavoring and seasoning agents, many spices contain specific chemicals and/or essential oils that can inactivate or inhibit various pathogenic and spoilage organisms. Consequently, two independent surveys were made to identify spices that might be useful in inhibiting growth of *L. monocytogenes* in food.

In 1989, Ting and Deibel (159) reported preliminary results from one such survey in which a concentration gradient method was used to study the effect of 14 different spices on *L. monocytogenes*. While the pathogen remained completely viable in the presence of 3% (w/v) black pepper, chili pepper, cinnamon, garlic, mustard, paprika, parsley, and red pepper during extended storage at 4 and 25°C, *Listeria* was sensitive at 25°C to oregano, cloves, sage, rosemary, nutmeg, and thyme, with calculated minimum inhibitory concentrations of 0.70, 0.72, 1.29, 1.54, 2.72, and 2.75%, respectively. The latter six spices also were inhibitory to *L. monocytogenes* at 4°C. When added to culture media, growth of the pathogen at both incubation temperatures was prevented by as little as 0.5% oregano. However, when exposed to 0.5% cloves, *Listeria* populations decreased only 2.4 orders of magnitude after 1 and 14 days of incubation at 25 and 4°C, respectively. Unfortunately, further experiments showed that cloves and oregano were both no longer active against listeriae when present in a meat slurry at a level of 1.0%.

The ability of commercially available spices to prevent growth of *L. monocytogenes* in TB also was investigated by Bahk et al. (14). With the exception of an increased lag phase, behavior of listeriae during extended incubation at 35 and 4°C was relatively unaffected by the presence of 0.5% ginger, onion, garlic, or mustard as well as ginseng saponin or mulberry extract at concentrations ≤0.3%. However, unlike the previous study, addition of 0.5% cinnamon was somewhat inhibitory to *L. monocytogenes* with the pathogen attaining maximum populations that were 1.5–2.6 orders of magnitude lower than in controls. Growth of listeriae at 35°C also was partly suppressed by presence of 0.5% cloves, with the pathogen attaining a maximum population 1.6 orders of magnitude lower than that observed in the control. However, *Listeria* populations decreased steadily in TB containing 0.5% cloves during extended incubation at 4°C. The germicidal action of cinnamic aldehyde in cinnamon and euginol in cloves is well recognized, and so one can speculate that these compounds also may be at least partly responsible for the inhibitory activity of these spices toward *Listeria*.

MICROBIAL COMPETITION

Many foods subjected to postprocessing contamination with *L. monocytogenes* are also likely to contain psychrotrophic pseudomonads. Thus Farrag and Marth (76) investigated associative growth of *L. monocytogenes* [strain Scott A and California (CA)] with *Pseudomonas fluorescens* or *Pseudomonas aeruginosa* in TB incubated at 7 and 13°C. While growth of both *Listeria* strains was slightly retarded by the presence of viable, nongrowing cells of *P. fluorescens* during the first 7 days of incubation at 7°C, extended incubation led to *Listeria* populations that were similar ($\sim10^8$ CFU/ml) to those observed in cultures without *P. fluorescens*. When the incubation temperature was increased to 13°C, strain Scott A attained similar maximum populations of $\sim10^9$ CFU/ml, regardless of whether or not *P. fluorescens* was present. However, *P. fluorescens* was somewhat detrimental to survival of strain Scott A with the *Listeria* population 1.3 orders of magnitude lower in mixed rather than pure cultures following 56 days of incubation. In contrast, growth of strain CA was somewhat enhanced in the presence of *P. fluorescens,* with the pathogen attaining relatively stable maximum populations of 9.1–9.5 $\log_{10}$ CFU/ml after 42 days at 13°C. According to these researchers, presence of viable, nongrowing cells of *P. aeruginosa* had little if any effect on growth or survival of either *Listeria* strain during extended incubation at 7°C. When the incubation temperature was increased to 13°C, *P. aeruginosa* failed to appreciably affect the behavior of strain Scott A. However, this pseudomonad adversely affected survival of strain CA with populations 1.8 orders of magnitude lower in mixed than in pure cultures after 56 days of incubation. In general, growth of *P. fluorescens* and *P. aeruginosa* at both incubation temperatures was unaffected by presence of either *Listeria* strain.

BACTERIOCINS

Successful use of antibiotics to control bacterial pathogens in domestic livestock prompted interest in the potential application of antibiotics to food preservation. However, because of widespread fears that routine use of medically important antibiotics may increase the antibiotic resistance of bacterial pathogens, only one small group of nonmedically important antibiotics, namely bacteriocins, are currently permitted in food. Nisin, by far the most important polypeptide bacteriocin, is produced by certain strains of *Streptococcus lactis* (*Lactococcus lactis* subsp. *lactis*) and has proven to be extremely useful in preventing outgrowth of *Clostridium* spp., including *Clostridium botulinum*, in certain foods including fermented dairy and meat products.

Nisin

In 1980, Mohamed et al. (112) reported results from a series of experiments that were designed to determine the effectiveness of nisin against *Listeria*. When Nutrient Broth at pH 7.4 contained 4–16 International Units (IU) of nisin/ml, populations of *L. monocytogenes* decreased $>10^5$/ml during 28 hours at 37°C. After this initial decrease, *Listeria* grew rapidly and attained final populations of $\sim10^8$ CFU/ml. *Listeria monocytogenes* strains 4379 and 10357 required 32 and 256 IU of nisin/ml, respectively, for complete inhibition. At 22°C, strain 4379 was somewhat less sensitive to nisin and required 64 IU of nisin/ml for complete inhibition. Decreasing the pH of the medium from 7.4 to 5.5 led to a 16-fold decrease in level of nisin required to inhibit both strains. Greater stability and solubility of nisin at pH 5.5 rather than 7.4 is most likely responsible for the increased antilisterial activity.

The current association between *L. monocytogenes* and foodborne illness prompted renewed interest in the apparent antilisterial activity of nisin. Using Trypticase Soy Agar, Benkerroum and Sandine (19) reported that six *L. monocytogenes* strains were variably resistant to nisin with minimum inhibitory concentrations ranging from 1.4×10^2 to 1.18×10^5 IU/ml. Similar degrees of nisin resistance also were observed for two strains of *L. ivanovii* and one of *L. seeligeri*. Several additional studies also have demonstrated various degrees of nisin resistance for *L. monocytogenes*. According to preliminary data collected by Taylor (158), several *L. monocytogenes* strains were resistant to 500 IU of nisin/ml, with strain Scott A able to multiply in laboratory media containing 2000 IU of nisin/ml. Although Tatini (157) found that 512–1024 ppm nisin was required to inhibit growth of 12 *L. monocytogenes* strains in laboratory media, *Salmonella typhimurium* and *E. coli* remained viable in the presence of up to 10,000 ppm nisin. While these findings suggest that *L. monocytogenes* may be less resistant to nisin than some other potentially hazardous microorganisms, one must keep in mind that some unusually resistant strains of *L. monocytogenes* do exist.

In 1989, Harris et al. (83) examined sensitivity and resistance of *L. monocytogenes* to nisin. According to these authors, populations of listeriae decreased 6–7 orders of magnitude when nisin levels in Brain Heart Infusion Agar were increased from 0 to 10 µg/ml. However, a relatively stable population of nisin-resistant mutants ($\sim$100–1000 CFU/ml) developed on agar plates containing 10–50 µg nisin/ml with nisin-resistant mutants occurring at a frequency of 10^{-6}–10^{-8} in media containing 50 µg nisin/ml. Although all nisin-resistant mutants selected from agar plates were more resistant than their parent strains, further testing revealed that nisin resistance was related to ability of nisin-resistant strains to bind nisin rather than to specific genes coding for nisin resistance in plasmid DNA.

As indicated by the earlier findings of Mohamed et al. (112), antilisterial activity of nisin is strongly influenced by various environmental factors, including pH. After recognizing that a pH of 7.4 is less than optimal for nisin activity, Benkerroum and Sandine (19) determined the sensitivity of one *L. monocytogenes* strain to nisin in Tryptose Soy Broth adjusted to pH values of 3.5–7.0. Overall, *Listeria* populations decreased from ~10^3 CFU/ml to nondetectable levels in broth containing 3.7×10^2 IU nisin/ml after 24 hours of incubation at 37°C. However, population increases of approximately 10-fold that occurred in broth cultures at pH 7.0 and 6.48 during the first 12 hours of incubation were no longer observed in similar samples adjusted to pH ≤ 5.94. This enhancement of antilisterial nisin activity at lower pH values also has been observed by Harris et al. (83). Furthermore, preliminary data from Tatini (156) indicate that average minimum nisin concentrations of 512, 1365, 2560, and 2496 ppm were required to inhibit growth of several *L. monocytogenes* strains on Trypticase Soy-Yeast Extract Agar adjusted to pH values of 5.0, 5.5, 6.0, and 6.5, respectively. Thus increased susceptibility of *L. monocytogenes* to nisin at pH values ≤ 6.0 appears to be fairly well established.

The antilisterial action of nisin is further complicated by incubation temperature and presence of sodium chloride. According to Tatini (157), minimum concentrations of nisin necessary to inhibit growth of *L. monocytogenes* were typically two to four times greater at 35 than at 4°C. In addition, when *L. monocytogenes* was incubated at 4°C in broth containing ≤400 ppm nisin, lag periods for the various strains tested increased from 16 to 69 days as the nisin concentration increased from 0 to 400 ppm. In 1989, Harris et al. (83) also reported that addition of 2% sodium chloride enhanced the listericidal activity of nisin in laboratory media, particularly at levels of <10 μg/ml.

Nisin-producing strains of *S. lactis* have been used legally inside and outside the United States to manufacture certain cheeses and other dairy products that call for a mesophilic fermentation. While many European countries have allowed direct addition of nisin to food for some time, this practice was not permitted in the United States until 1989 when FDA officials amended the food standard for pasteurized process cheese to allow addition of not more than 250 ppm nisin to the finished product (6,11,12). However, since the information in this discussion suggests that allowable levels of nisin may not completely inhibit *L. monocytogenes* in pasteurized process cheese spreads that have been subjected to postpasteurization contamination, incorporation of nisin in such products should not preclude use of proper sanitary practices.

Other Bacteriocins

In addition to nisin, additional plasmid or chromosomally determined bacteriocins produced by *S. lactis* (36,149) and other bacterial species including certain strains of *Lactobacillus acidophilus* (112,84,128), *Lactobacillus helveticus* (84,94), *Lactobacillus plantarum* (84), *Pediococcus acidilactici* (45,84,88,127), *Pediococcus pentosaceus* (40,45,84,88,149), and *Bacillus* spp. (14,105,170) also can inactivate selected spoilage and pathogenic organisms, with several of these bacteriocins effective against *L. monocytogenes*. While many of these bacteriocins are poorly characterized and have not yet been approved as direct food additives, the lactic acid bacteria that produce most of these antimicrobial agents can be used commercially in starter cultures to manufacture a variety of fermented dairy, meat, and vegetable products. Hence, the potential exists for such bacteriocins to be used as natural food preservatives.

During 1989 results from two survey-type studies were reported in which different strains of lactic acid bacteria were screened for antilisterial metabolites. Using an agar lawn method, Raccach et al. (128) found that 1 of 2, 3 of 3, 2 of 3, and 1 of 1 strains of

L. acidophilus, P. acidilactici, P. pentosaceus, and *S. lactis* subsp. *diacetylactis*, respectively, were somewhat inhibitory to at least 1 of 4 *L. monocytogenes* strains tested, with greater activity observed during incubation at 25 rather than at 10 or 32°C. More important, only one of these seven strains of lactic acid bacteria that was antagonistic toward *Listeria* failed to produce a recognized bacteriocin with four additional strains of non–bacteriocin producing lactic acid bacteria failing to inhibit the pathogen. In the second of these investigations, Harris et al. (84) used an agar-based deferred antagonism assay and found that 1 of 2, 2 of 2, 1 of 1, 1 of 1, and 2 of 2 bacteriocin-producing strains of *Lactobacillus* spp. (unidentified), *S. lactis, Leuconostoc* sp. (unidentified), *P. acidilactici*, and *P. pentosaceus* exhibited various degrees of inhibitory activity toward seven strains of *L. monocytogenes* and one of *L. innocua*. Since listericidal activity was drastically reduced by inclusion of protease in the test medium, the bacteriocins produced by these lactic acid bacteria appear to be proteinaceous in nature. Subsequent work revealed that cell-free supernatant liquids from only one strain each of *Lactobacillus* sp., *Leuconostoc* spp., and *P. acidilactici* inhibited both *L. monocytogenes* and *L. innocua* in a well diffusion assay. Although different findings obtained in these two assays may reflect the ability of listeriae to overcome finite levels of bacteriocin present in the well diffusion assay by proteolysis of the inhibitor or by outgrowth of a mutant population resistant to the bacteriocin, these two hypotheses were not evaluated further.

In a more in-depth study, Carminati et al. (36) noted that culture extracts from 7 of 7 bacteriocin-producing strains of *S. lactis* were listericidal to 6 strains of *L. monocytogenes* on agar media. While partial characterization of these bacteriocin-like compounds showed that they were all proteinaceous in nature, listericidal action was not related to cell lysis. Instead, the authors speculated that inhibitory activity of these compounds may be dependent on presence of specific bacteriocin receptors on the cell wall of the pathogen. Subsequently, Spelhaug and Harlander (149) found that one nisin-producing strain of *S. lactis* inhibited growth of *L. monocytogenes* (14 strains), *L. innocua* (4 strains), *L. ivanovii* (1 strain), *L. seeligeri* (1 strain), and *L. welshimeri* (2 strains) on common laboratory media. Normally nisin is not affected by proteolytic enzymes, and since all of the bacteriocin-like compounds examined in these two studies were partially or completely inactivated by one or more proteases, it is likely that substances other than nisin were responsible for at least some of the observed listericidal activity.

Certain bacteriocin-producing strains of pediococci used to manufacture fermented sausage also can inhibit growth of listeriae in laboratory media. In conjunction with the aforementioned study, Spelhaug and Harlander (149) identified two strains of *P. pentosaceus* (formerly classified as *P. cerevisiae*) that prevented growth on Brain Heart Infusion Agar of the 22 *Listeria* strains just described as well as single strains of *Bacillus cereus, Clostridium perfringens*, and *S. aureus*. Further testing confirmed that the observed listericidal activity resulted from production of bacteriocin-like substances rather than excessive levels of hydrogen peroxide or acid, both of which can influence growth of listeriae.

The number of reports describing listericidal activity associated with bacteriocin-producing strains of *P. acidilactici* is even larger. In 1988, Hoover et al. (88) used agarose gel electrophoresis to identify a 5.5-megadalton plasmid that encoded for the same bacteriocin in three different strains of *P. acidilactici* designated PO_2, B5627, and PC. While the bacteriocin associated with this DNA plasmid was inhibitory to three of five

L. monocytogenes strains on agar media, loss of the plasmid directly correlated with loss of listericidal activity. However, at least two distinct bacteriocins produced by strain PO_2 were effective against listeriae. According to Dishart et al. (45), one of these bacteriocins had a molecular weight > 10,000 and could extend the lag phase of *L. monocytogenes* in liquid media.

Demonstrated listericidal activity of one specific plasmid-mediated bacteriocin, namely PA-1, produced by *P. acidilactici* strain PAC 1.0 is also attracting considerable interest. After cultures of *P. acidilactici* PAC 1.0 and cell-free supernatant culture fluid from this organism were found to inhibit growth of eight different *L. monocytogenes* strains in agar media, Pucci et al. (127) conducted a series of experiments to determine the potential use of bacteriocin PA-1, the listericidal agent produced by this particular strain of *P. acidilactici*. According to the authors, a dry milk-fortified powder prepared from PAC 1.0 supernatant culture fluid contained ~16,000 active units (AU) of bacteriocin PA-1 powder/g with an average minimum inhibitory concentration of 54.7 AU/ml calculated for one strain of *L. monocytogenes* in APT broth. Subsequent experiments showed that as little as 12 minutes of exposure to APT broth containing 200 AU of PA-1 powder/ml was sufficient to lyse about half of the *Listeria* cells present. Furthermore, rapid inactivation of listeriae in similar media over a pH range of 5.5–7.0 occurred during incubation at both 4 and 32°C.

The potential benefits of this bacteriocin to the food industry were recognized, and commercial samples of cottage cheese (pH 5.1), cheese sauce (pH 6.0), and half-and-half (pH 6.6) were inoculated to contain 10^2–10^4 *L. monocytogenes* CFU/g or ml and 100 AU of PA-1 powder/g or ml, except cottage cheese, which received 10–50 AU of PA-1 powder/g. According to these authors (127), viable numbers of *L. monocytogenes* decreased rapidly in all foods during the first day of refrigerated storage. While the pathogen attained populations of 10^3–10^5 CFU/ml or g in cheese sauce and half-and-half following 7–14 days of refrigerated storage, these levels were still approximately two to five orders of magnitude lower than those observed in corresponding samples prepared without PA-1 powder. These results demonstrate the ability of bacteriocin PA-1 to retard and/or inhibit growth of *L. monocytogenes* in high protein/high fat dairy products. A United States patent covering production and use of bacteriocin PA-1 as a potential food preservative has been issued (81).

In addition to the aforementioned species of lactic acid bacteria, other bacteriocin-producing organisms including *Bacillus* spp. also have been investigated for their potential to inhibit *L. monocytogenes*. As early as 1965, Larsen and Gundstrup (106) reported that certain strains of *Bacillus subtilis* and *Bacillus pumilus* prevented growth of *L. monocytogenes* in Tryptose Agar and TB during incubation at 37 and 4°C, respectively. Using the agar well diffusion method, sterile culture filtrates from both *Bacillus* spp. also produced various sized *Listeria* inhibition zones, thus attesting to production of one or more bacteriocin-like compounds. Further experiments showed that three of five *Bacillus* culture filtrates retained their listericidal activity during 60 or more days of refrigerated storage. In addition, one of these culture filtrates exhibited considerable thermal tolerance with the apparent bacteriocin-like compound remaining listericidal even after 5 minutes of heating at 100°C.

Nearly 25 years later, Bahk et al. (14) isolated another *Bacillus* sp. from mulberry extract that exhibited pronounced inhibitory activity against *L. monocytogenes* on agar media. In a follow-up study (170), supernatant culture fluid from this *Bacillus* sp. prevented growth of three different *L. monocytogenes* strains on Tryptose Agar. Listericidal activity also was reportedly greater using supernatant culture fluid obtained from this *Bacillus* sp. during late rather than early logarithmic or stationary growth. Since cell-free extracts of this *Bacillus* sp. were far less inhibitory to the pathogen than supernatant culture fluid, the apparent bacteriocin-like compound(s) associated with listericidal activity appears to have been produced extracellularly. However, unlike the previous study (105), these inhibitory compounds were sensitive to heat with complete inactivation caused by autoclaving. Hence, this particular bacteriocin appears to be different from that previously described by Larsen and Gundstrup (106). While present laws do not permit direct addition of *Bacillus* spp. to food, further work regarding antimicrobial agents produced by nonpathogenic *Bacillus* spp. may eventually lead to inclusion of these organisms and/or the bacteriocins produced by these organisms in the list of permitted food additives.

LYSOZYME

Lysozyme is an important natural enzyme which prevents bacterial growth (particularly gram-positive organisms) in foods of animal origin, including hen's eggs and milk. Lysozyme is particularly attractive as a food preservative since the enzyme is active between 4 and 95°C, stable over a wide range of pH values, specific for bacterial cell walls, and is not harmful to humans. Although not yet approved as a food additive in the United States, lysozyme has been used successfully in Europe to prevent "blowing" caused by *Clostridium* spp. in Gouda, Edam, and other brine-salted cheeses.

In 1987, Hughey and Johnson (90) evaluated four *L. monocytogenes* strains isolated during foodborne listeriosis outbreaks for their susceptibility to lysozyme. After non-growing cells of *L. monocytogenes* in the stationary growth phase were suspended in phosphate buffer containing 10 mg of lysozyme/L, 70–80% of the cells were lysed after 6 hours as determined by optical density measurement. In contrast, all four strains grew in Brain Heart Infusion Broth containing 20–200 mg of lysozyme/L. Similarly, actively growing cultures of *L. monocytogenes* in the logarithmic growth phase were not lysed after 12 hours of exposure to 100 mg of lysozyme/L. Various chemicals also were examined for their ability to potentiate lysis of growing cells of *L. monocytogenes* in the presence of lysozyme. Addition of 0.85% lactic acid stopped growth of *L. monocytogenes* and led to slow lysis of cells by lysozyme. Ethylenediamine tetra-acetic acid (EDTA) was the most effective potentiator of cell lysis, whereas 0.05% potassium sorbate, 0.25% glycine, 5 mM sodium acetate, 0.95% ethanol, 0.01% sodium dodecyl sulfate, 5 mM thioglycolate, 5 mM dithiothreitol, and 10 mM ascorbic acid were relatively ineffective. The effectiveness of EDTA and lysozyme for inhibition of *Listeria* growth also was tested using Brain Heart Infusion Agar. Although 100 mg of lysozyme/L or 1 mM EDTA failed to inhibit growth of two of four *L. monocytogenes* strains, the combination of EDTA and lysozyme led to substantial growth inhibition as compared to the control without these two additives.

Johnson (95) also found that lysozyme inhibited growth of *L. monocytogenes*, particularly when the organism was incubated at refrigeration temperatures. Adjusting the pH of the medium to 5.6 led to a decreased *Listeria* growth rate, which in turn resulted in complete inhibition of *L. monocytogenes* in the presence of lysozyme with or without EDTA. Since iron also is important for *Listeria* growth, addition of conalbumin (which specifically binds iron) also potentiated the inhibitory effect of lysozyme at pH 5.5 and 7.0.

Preliminary experiments (91) also demonstrated increased lysis of *L. monocytogenes* when cells were heated before or during exposure to lysozyme. These findings prompted Hughey et al. (91) to examine the effect of EDTA and lysozyme on growth of *L. monocytogenes* in Camembert cheese, bratwurst, and various fresh vegetables during extended refrigerated storage. Discussion of these results will be deferred until Chapters 11, 12, and 14 which deal with the incidence and behavior of *Listeria* in cheese, meat, and products of plant origin, respectively.

HYDROGEN PEROXIDE

Hydrogen peroxide is of limited use as a food preservative. While most effective when combined with heat (i.e., milk pasteurization, sugar processing), hydrogen peroxide was approved by the FDA for sterilizing multilayer packaging materials used in aseptic processing systems.

According to Dominguez et al. (48), *L. monocytogenes* was eliminated from autoclaved milk that was inoculated to contain 9.5×10^7 *L. monocytogenes* CFU/ml, treated with 0.0495% hydrogen peroxide and held for 24 hours at 15°C. In another experiment, samples of autoclaved milk containing ≤0.0495% hydrogen peroxide were inoculated to contain a mixed culture of *L. monocytogenes*, *S. aureus*, and *Streptococcus faecalis* (each organism at ~1×10^7 CFU/ml) and examined for numbers of each bacterial species during 48 hours of incubation at 4, 15, and 22°C. Although *L. monocytogenes* populations decreased approximately 10-, 16-, and 40-fold during the first 24 hours of incubation at 4, 15, and 22°C, respectively, the organism grew during the second 24 hours and reached populations ≥ 1×10^7 CFU/ml. Thus hydrogen peroxide was generally ineffective in decreasing numbers of listeriae in milk containing equal numbers of *S. aureus* and *S. faecalis*. Similar studies using raw milk treated with 0.0495% hydrogen peroxide, inoculated to contain ~2×10^5 *L. monocytogenes* CFU/ml and incubated at 4°C demonstrated that numbers of listeriae increased slightly as compared to the natural microflora. While addition of hydrogen peroxide to refrigerated raw milk contaminated with *L. monocytogenes* could create a selective enrichment for listeriae, preliminary results from another recent study (99) showed that hydrogen peroxide markedly reduced thermal resistance of *L. monocytogenes* in laboratory media. Hence, hydrogen peroxide may eventually prove useful in increasing the thermal destruction of this pathogen in milk.

LACTOPEROXIDASE SYSTEM

The lactoperoxidase (LP) system, a naturally occurring antimicrobial system in milk, has been proposed as a means for extending the shelf life of raw milk when extended storage at refrigeration temperatures is not possible as in certain developing countries. Proper functioning of this system is dependent upon adequate levels of lactoperoxidase, thiocyanate, and hydrogen peroxide with concentrations of the latter two constituents normally present in milk at levels below those needed to activate the system. In the LP system, lactoperoxidase catalyzes oxidation of thiocyanate (SCN⁻) by hydrogen peroxide to hypothiocyanous acid (HOSCN) and hypothiocyanate (OSCN⁻), these end-products are responsible for inactivating many microorganisms that are common to milk including *S. aureus*, *Salmonella typhimuruim*, psychrotrophic pseudomonads, and some strains of lactic acid bacteria.

In 1987, Siragusa and Johnson (146) reported preliminary results of a study which examined inhibition of *L. monocytogenes* by the LP system. Their model LP system contained equimolar concentrations (0.3 mM) of potassium thiocyanate and hydrogen peroxide in Tryptic Soy Broth fortified with 0.5% yeast extract. After addition of 0.4 IU of lactoperoxidase/ml, flasks were inoculated with a 12-hour-old culture of *L. monocytogenes* and monitored spectrophotometrically (A_{650}) for listeriae. Except for a prolonged lag period of 4 rather than 1–2 hours for controls, the LP system failed to inhibit growth of *L. monocytogenes* at 37°C. In contrast, growth of *Listeria* was markedly inhibited by the LP system at 20°C with a lag period of 41 hours rather than 4–8 hours for the control. The pathogen grew after the lag phase and had growth rates of 0.16 h⁻¹ and 0.46 h⁻¹ with and without the LP system, respectively. Maximum *Listeria* populations also were lower with the LP system than in controls. Thus in this particular study the LP system was bacteriostatic rather than bactericidal to *L. monocytogenes* at 20°C.

Following this initial report, several additional studies were done to determine the ability of the LP system to temporarily inhibit growth of *L. monocytogenes* in laboratory media. Using similar model broth systems to those just described, two investigative teams (69,98) also found that the LP system lengthened the lag period for relatively large initial inocula of *L. monocytogenes* during incubation at 10–35°C, but did not appreciably affect growth rates once the pathogen overcame the inhibitory effects of the LP system.

Kamau et al. (98) showed that *L. monocytogenes* behaved similarly in the presence of the LP system whether or not the pathogen was in the logarithmic or stationary growth phase, and El-Shenawy et al. (69) found that initial *L. monocytogenes* populations of 30–50 CFU/ml decreased to nondetectable levels following 2 hours of exposure to the LP system at 35°C. Thus efficacy of the LP system as an antilisterial agent appears to be more closely related to initial numbers of listeriae exposed to the LP system than the physiological state of the organism. Using selective and nonselective plating media, El-Shenawy et al. (69) also demonstrated that the pathogen was not sublethally injured during exposure to the LP system. However, since Kamau et al. (99) reported that the LP system significantly reduced thermal resistance of *L. monocytogenes* in similar laboratory media held at 52.2–57.8°C (mean $D_{57.8°C}$-values of 0.73 and 2.08 minutes with and without exposure to the LP system, respectively), use of the LP system in conjunction with thermal processing may prove useful in enhancing destruction of listeriae in raw milk.

In contrast to the findings just discussed, Denis and Ramet (43) reported that the LP system completely eliminated *L. monocytogenes* (initial populations ~10¹–10³ CFU/ml) from Trypticase Soy Broth with 0.65% yeast extract following ≤1, 2–6, and 4–10 days of incubation at 30, 15, and 4°C, respectively, depending on the initial inoculum. However, unlike the previously described model broth systems, these authors added glucose oxidase to their LP system. Since this enzyme oxidizes glucose to gluconic acid, the resulting lowering of pH likely increased the bactericidal effect of the LP system beyond what would have been observed in similar model systems having pH values near neutrality. Furthermore, *L. monocytogenes* is also reportedly inhibited and/or inactivated in TB and milk containing ≥0.75% gluconic acid during extended incubation at 13 and 35°C (68). (Similar results were observed using glucono-delta-lactone which readily hydrolyzes to free gluconic acid in laboratory media and milk.) Hence, these findings likely reflect the combined effects of the LP system, pH and gluconic acid rather than that of the LP system alone.

Results from two additional investigations dealing with antilisterial activity of the LP system in ultra-high-temperature–treated (UHT) milk rather than broth also have appeared in the scientific literature. Using two different UHT milk-based LP systems containing lactoperoxidase (30 mg/L), potassium thiocyanate (84 mg/L), glucose (10 g/L), and glucose oxidase (2 mg/L) both with and without urea peroxide (376 mg/L) as a hydrogen peroxide-generating mechanism, Earnshaw and Banks (57) found that initial *L. monocytogenes* populations of ~10^4 CFU/ml decreased to 10^2 CFU/ml in both LP systems during 6 days of incubation at 10°C. Since the pH of both UHT milk-based systems decreased from 6.5 to <6.0 during incubation, the antilisterial activity observed in both of these systems once again probably resulted from the combined effects of acid production and the LP system rather than the LP system alone. Denis and Ramet (43) also found that *L. monocytogenes* populations decreased in a similar UHT milk-based LP system containing lactoperoxidase, potassium thiocyanate, and glucose oxidase. However, unlike the study just described, their LP system completely eliminated the pathogen (initial populations of 10^1–10^4 CFU/ml) from UHT milk following 6–21 and 7–30 days of incubation at 15 and 4°C, respectively, with estimated D-values of approximately 5 and 8 days at these same temperatures. Thus as expected, the LP system was more detrimental to listeriae at higher rather than lower temperatures. In contrast, the pathogen attained populations of ~10^8 and 10^4 CFU/ml following 7 days of incuba-tion at 15 and 4°C, respectively. While no mention was made of the probable pH changes that occurred during incubation with the LP system (i.e., inclusion of glucose oxidase likely decreased the pH), results presented thus far suggest that the LP system is far less useful in fresh than in slightly acidified milk.

In the only study reported thus far in which an LP system was used in raw milk containing naturally occurring levels of lactoperoxidase along with 0.25 mM thiocyanate anion and 0.25 mM hydrogen peroxide, El-Shenawy et al. (69) found that *L. monocytogenes* was often only slightly inhibited. In samples inoculated to contain ~10^4 and 10^7 *L. monocytogenes* CFU/ml, the pathogen attained maximum populations of ≥10^8 CFU/ml after overcoming an extended lag phase. However, this LP system was far more effective in raw milk inoculated to contain *Listeria* populations (i.e., 10^2 CFU/ml) similar to those that have been observed in cases of naturally occurring listeric mastitis. Under these conditions, the pathogen was completely inactivated after 2–4 and 12–24 hours of incubation at 35 and 4°C. Thus, as was true for microbiological media and UHT milk, the LP system was again more effective in raw milk stored at higher than lower temperatures. Since *L. monocytogenes* was susceptible to the LP system under conditions used in this study, it appears that the activated LP system would likely prove useful for decreasing numbers of naturally occurring listeriae in raw milk before milk-processing facilities receive the product.

CHLORINE COMPOUNDS

Sodium hypochlorite and other chlorine-containing compounds have been widely used by the food industry to decrease populations of most common pathogenic and spoilage organisms in food production and processing facilities. In the absence of organic debris, chlorine rapidly inactivates most non–spore forming bacteria even when used at the very low concentrations found in chlorinated drinking water. While the actual mechanism of disinfection is not fully understood, germicidal activity of chlorine has generally been attributed to hypochlorous acid (HOCl), which is generated in aqueous solutions of sodium hypochlorite and other chlorine-containing compounds. While HOCl can in turn dissociate to form the hypochlorite ion (OCl^-) and hydrogen ion (H^+), depending on the pH of the solution, the neutral electric charge of the former suggests that HOCl can more easily penetrate the bacterial cell wall than OCl^-. Thus, it is not surprising that the germicidal activity of HOCl is 80 times that of OCl^-. After diffusing into the cell, HOCl is thought to inactivate the organism by inducing formation of toxic oxygen species or combining with proteins, which may in turn inhibit key enzymatic reactions and alter cell membrane permeability.

Numerous studies have dealt with the lethal effects of various chlorinated sanitizing agents on *L. monocytogenes*. Beginning in 1969, Baranenkov (15) found that hypochlorite could effectively control *L. monocytogenes* on the surface of hen's eggs. Chloramine also was later shown to be listericidal when used under acidic conditions at concentrations of 0.1–0.2% (110). More recently, Lopes (108) reported that two chlorine-based sanitizers (one containing 8.5% sodium hypochlorite with 8% active chlorine and the other containing 25.8% sodium dichloro-*s*-triazinetrione) solutions containing 100 ppm active chlorine both reduced *L. monocytogenes* populations by more than five orders of magnitude 30 seconds after exposure to either sanitizer solution. These findings were subsequently confirmed by Rossmoore and Drenzek (133). Further tests by Lopes (108) revealed that the organic chlorine-based sanitizer was slightly more effective against *L. monocytogenes* than the sodium hypochlorite–based sanitizer; the former had a lower pH, which would, in turn, lead to higher concentrations of HOCl, the most bactericidal form of chlorine. A new chlorine dioxide-based sanitizing agent with the proprietary name of Anthium Dioxide also has been approved by the FDA for use in the food industry. According to the manufacturer (7), the unusual effectiveness of this formula against *L. monocytogenes* and other microorganisms results from a special activator which converts large quantities of stabilized chlorine dioxide to the free form.

Following the published report by Lopes (108), Brackett (23) determined the germicidal effect of reagent-grade sodium hypochlorite and household bleach on two *L. monocytogenes* strains (Scott A and LCDC 81-861) previously associated with outbreaks of foodborne listeriosis. After 20 seconds of exposure to ≥50 ppm available chlorine, both compounds led to substantial reductions in numbers of viable *L. monocytogenes* in phosphate buffer. However, *Listeria* populations remained relatively stable for an additional 4.6 minutes and in several instances listeriae survived ≥5 minutes with free residual chlorine levels that approached 40 ppm. Since 10 ppm available chlorine was ineffective, results of this study indicate that the minimum chlorine concentration needed to kill *L. monocytogenes* lies between 10 and 40 ppm.

Effectiveness of chlorine as a germicide against *L. monocytogenes* also was examined in depth and later reviewed by El-Kest and Marth (59,60,61). Cells of *L. monocytogenes* strain Scott A were harvested from 24- and 48-hour-old slants or broth cultures, washed by centrifugation in 20 mM phosphate buffer solution or 0.312 mM phosphate buffer dilution water, and then exposed at 25°C to sodium hypochlorite solutions at pH 7.0 (25°C) that contained 0.5–10 ppm available chlorine. Using a solution containing 5 ppm available chlorine, numbers of survivors decreased approximately six orders of magnitude after only 30 seconds with the organism no longer detectable by direct-plating on Tryptose Agar after 1 hour. [Preliminary results from Rosales et al. (130) also showed that populations of *L. monocytogenes*, *L. ivanovii*, and *L. seeligeri* decreased more than five orders of magnitude following 30 seconds of exposure to distilled water (pH ~ 7.0) containing $\geq$25 ppm hypochlorite (i.e., $\geq$23.8 ppm available chlorine).] Exposing *L. monocytogenes* to 0.5, 1, 2, 5, and 10 ppm available chlorine resulted in corresponding D-values of 61.7, 11.3, 6.7, 4.9, and 4.7 seconds. While germicidal activity clearly increased with increasing concentrations of available chlorine, the effectiveness of sodium hypochlorite also was affected by several additional factors. Increased resistance of *L. monocytogenes* to chlorine was observed using (a) 24- rather than 48-hour-old cultures, (b) cells harvested from broth rather than agar slants, and (c) cultures exposed to solutions containing 20 mM rather than 0.312 mM phosphate. Five and 10 ppm of available chlorine was also partially neutralized in the presence of 0.05 and 0.1% peptone (nitrogenous compound). Given a recent report (130) indicating that hypochlorite concentrations of up to 400 ppm were of little use against *L. monocytogenes*, *L. ivanovii*, or *L. seeligeri* when these organisms were suspended in reconstituted NFDM (10% solids), it is clear that germicidal activity of chlorine can only be maintained if organic material is effectively removed before exposure.

Additional work by El-Kest and Marth (61) demonstrated that populations of *L. monocytogenes* decreased most rapidly in sodium hypochlorite solutions at 5 followed by 35 and 25°C. Increased permeability of *L. monocytogenes* cells at lower rather than higher temperatures may account for these observed differences in listericidal activity. Marked variation in chlorine sensitivity also was observed among the three *L. monocytogenes* strains tested. However, since dissociation of HOCl to OCl⁻ and H⁺ increases with increasing pH, resistance and/or survival of *L. monocytogenes* in the presence of chlorine compounds ultimately depends on the pH of the suspending medium. For example, exposing the pathogen to 1 ppm available chlorine for 30 seconds led to population decreases of ~10,000-, 1000-, and 5-fold at pH 5, 7, and 9, respectively. Hence, for chlorine to be effective against listeriae and other microorganisms, it is imperative that such solutions have pH values < 7.0.

While the work of El-Kest and Marth (59–61) clearly indicates that the minimum listericidal concentration of free chlorine lies between 1 and 5 ppm (similar to that observed for many other non–spore forming bacteria) depending on pH, temperature, presence of organic material, and bacterial strain, earlier studies (23,57) conducted under less controlled conditions showed minimum listericidal concentrations of free chlorine that were markedly higher. Similar problems also were probably encountered by Mustapha and Liewen (114) who found that a minimum of ~100 ppm sodium hypochlorite was required to reduce *L. monocytogenes* populations $\geq$10,000-fold in sterile distilled water during 2–5 minutes of exposure.

Since *L. monocytogenes* can adhere to stainless steel, these researchers (114) also investigated the ability of sodium hypochlorite to reduce numbers of listeriae on both smooth and pitted stainless steel chips. While destruction of the pathogen was greater on smooth than pitted stainless steel surfaces, cells incubated on either surface for 1 hour were more resistant to the lethal action of sodium hypochlorite than those remaining on such surfaces 24 hours before exposure. Lower moisture levels on steel surfaces incubated 24 rather than 1 hour were likely at least partially responsible for enhancing the listericidal effect of sodium hypochlorite. In contrast to these findings, Rossmoore and Drenzek (133) recently reported that *L. monocytogenes* populations decreased five orders of magnitude on relatively moist surfaces of glazed and unglazed ceramic tile as well as stainless steel chips following exposure to 100 ppm sodium hypochlorite as directed by the manufacturer. Furthermore, in no instance was *L. monocytogenes* more resistant than single cultures of *Pseudomonas* or *Serratia*. Although surfaces that are free of the latter two nonpathogenic organisms should also be free of listeriae, the same does not apply to surfaces that have not been thoroughly cleaned before being sanitized. When the same three surfaces were treated with 1 and 10% solutions of milk and blood, *Listeria* populations decreased one to four orders of magnitude in the presence of 100 ppm sodium hypochlorite. Hence, while all current evidence indicates that sodium hypochlorite concentrations of ≥100 ppm are sufficient to eliminate *L. monocytogenes* and most other non–spore forming organisms from food contact and non–food contact surfaces of equipment, it is imperative that users of such sanitizing agents follow the manufacturer's recommendations and thoroughly remove all organic debris from surfaces before treatment.

OTHER SANITIZING AGENTS

In addition to chlorine compounds, other chemical sanitizers are available for controlling microbial contaminants in food-processing facilities. Most of these sanitizing agents belong to one of three remaining categories: (a) iodophors, (b) quaternary ammonium compounds frequently called "quats," and (c) acid sanitizers. Iodophors, water-soluble complexes of elemental iodine, and nonionic surface-active agents owe their bactericidal activity to release of free elemental iodine and hypoiodous acid, which is enhanced under acidic conditions. In contrast, quaternary ammonium compounds are best classified as noncorrosive germicidal cationic detergents that remain active at relatively high pH values. Finally, acid sanitizers such as phosphoric and citric acid–containing compounds are frequently used in conjunction with rinsing agents in automated cleaning systems better known as clean-in-place or CIP systems. Unlike iodophors, acid sanitizers are nonvolatile and retain their bactericidal activity at temperatures below 100°C. As is true for chlorine compounds, these other sanitizing agents must also generally reduce populations of a given test organism at least five orders of magnitude during 30 seconds of exposure at ambient temperatures before the particular agent is deemed effective.

Interest in the listericidal activity of non–chlorine based sanitizers dates back to at least 1969 when Baranenkov (15) reported that iodine monochloride could effectively eliminate *L. monocytogenes* from the surface of hen's eggs. Shortly thereafter, creosote (33), phenol (110,123), formaldehyde (123), and sodium hydroxide (110) were added to the list of listericidal agents along with mercuric (110) and quaternary ammonium compounds (e.g., cetylpyridinium bromide) (110). Sodium hydroxide at concentrations of 1–2% solubilizes the cytoplasmic membrane of *Listeria* (124), whereas bactericidal concentrations of ethyl alcohol, phenol, and formaldehyde inhibit certain key enzymes including succinic and xanthine dehydrogenase (123).

During the 1970s, several sanitizing agents were evaluated for treating soil samples inoculated with *L. monocytogenes*. According to Vranchen et al. (162) 5 days of exposure to 5 liters of 3% formaldehyde solution was required before *L. monocytogenes* was eliminated from one square meter of soil. In a later study (5), one square meter of soil was *Listeria*-free 3 hours after treatment with 0.5 liter of an aqueous solution containing 3% quaternary ammonium compound. While sanitization of soil has little direct bearing on the food industry, such practices may be useful in decreasing *Listeria* populations on farms that have experienced cases of listeriosis in domestic livestock.

Following recent reports of foodborne listeriosis, a series of studies were done to determine the listericidal activity of non–chlorine based sanitizers that are routinely used by the food industry. According to experimental evidence presented in 1986 by Lopes (108), acid anionic, iodophor, and quaternary ammonium compounds are effective against *L. monocytogenes* when used at concentrations recommended by manufacturers. Numbers of *L. monocytogenes* were reduced more than five orders of magnitude after 30 seconds of exposure to two different acid anionic sanitizers that contained 200 ppm of active ingredients (5% dodecyl benzene sulfonic acid and 30% orthophosphoric acid or 2.6% sulfonated oleic acid and 15% orthophosphoric acid). Similar reductions in *Listeria* populations were obtained with a quaternary ammonium compound diluted to contain 200 ppm of the active ingredient *n*-alkyl dimethyl benzyl ammonium chloride (12–16 carbon atoms in the alkyl group). An iodophor sanitizer diluted to contain 12.5 ppm titratable iodine was equally effective against the test organism. Thus all sanitizers tested showed effective antilisterial activity when used at concentrations recommended by the manufacturer.

Two years later, Rosales et al. (130) found that populations of *L. monocytogenes*, *L. ivanovii*, and *L. seeligeri* decreased more than five orders of magnitude following exposure to aqueous solutions containing 12.5–100 ppm (pH 2.7–5.0) iodophor, 12.5–100 ppm (pH 4.9–6.8) quaternary ammonium compound, 100–400 ppm (pH 2.4–3.1) acid sanitizer, 400 ppm (pH 7.9) phenolic compound, and 50–100 ppm (pH 2.8–3.0) of a combined quaternary ammonium compound/acid sanitizer preparation. When these experiments were repeated using 10% reconstituted nonfat dry milk (10% solids) rather than aqueous solutions of sanitizers, reductions in *Listeria* populations of more than five orders of magnitude only were observed for two of three iodophors, one of three quaternary ammonium compounds, and one of one quaternary ammonium compound/acid sanitizer preparations at concentrations of 200–400, 400, and 400 ppm, respectively. Although all aqueous solutions proved to be listericidal at concentrations recommended by the manufacturer, only one iodophor, quaternary ammonium compound, and phenolic sanitizer were listericidal at recommended concentrations when the test organism was suspended in milk.

Information from two additional investigations dealing with listericidal effects of various non–chlorine based sanitizing agents also became available in 1989. In the first such study, Mustapha and Liewen (114) reported that aqueous solutions containing 100–800 ppm of one quaternary ammonium compound (i.e., *n*-alkyl dimethyl dichlorobenzyl ammonium chloride) exhibited greater listericidal activity than similar solutions of sodium hypochlorite when *L. monocytogenes* was exposed to these sanitizing agents in vitro. Moreover, a 50 ppm aqueous solution of the quaternary ammonium compound was equally effective when the pathogen was present on smooth as well as pitted surfaces of stainless steel chips with populations decreasing more than four orders of magnitude following short-term exposure.

In the second of these two investigations, Rossmoore and Drenzek (133) examined the ability of four quaternary ammonium compounds as well as peroxyacetic acid, glutaraldehyde, MCI (5-chloro 2-methyl 4-isothiazolin 3-one and 2-methyl 4-isothiazolin 3-one), dodecyl benzene sulfonic acid/orthophosphoric acid, and sulfonated oleic acid/orthophosphoric acid to inactivate *L. monocytogenes, Pseudomonas,* and *Serratia* on glazed/unglazed ceramic tile and stainless steel. When used according to the manufacturer's instructions, peroxyacetic acid, glutaraldehyde, MCI, and one of four quaternary ammonium compounds reduced numbers of listeriae more than five orders of magnitude, regardless of the type of surface tested, and population decreases of three to five orders of magnitude were noted for the three remaining quaternary ammonium compounds. Since *L. monocytogenes* was consistently more sensitive to these sanitizers than the other two organisms tested, destruction of *Pseudomonas,* i.e., a frequently used group of indicator organisms for general sanitation, also should guarantee elimination of listeriae from properly treated surfaces.

To better simulate conditions that are likely to exist in dairy- and meat-processing facilities, these researchers repeated the study just described (133) using surfaces that were precoated with 1 and 10% solutions of milk or blood before exposure to the same sanitizing agents. Not surprisingly, destruction of listeriae by most sanitizers decreased one to four orders of magnitude in the presence of increasing concentrations of milk and blood, with the latter being most detrimental to germicidal activity. However, since peroxyacetic acid and glutaraldehyde maintained peak listericidal activity in the presence of up to 10% milk and blood, these two sanitizers appear to be best suited for controlling listeriae within milk- and meat-processing facilities.

Since water-based chain conveyor lubricants also may serve as a potential source for spoilage and pathogenic microorganisms, including *L. monocytogenes,* incorporation of sanitizing agents into lubricants has been suggested as one means of minimizing spread of microbial contaminants in food-processing facilities. Although *L. monocytogenes* populations in inoculated samples of sanitizer-free lubricant (pH 9.5) decreased only two orders of magnitude during 14 days of storage at ambient temperatures (133), numbers of listeriae decreased more than five orders of magnitude following 30 minutes of exposure to lubricant containing as little as 25 ppm glutaraldehyde (132). Furthermore, data collected during a field investigation (133) showed that addition of 85 ppm glutaraldehyde to a conveyor chain lubricant reduced general bacterial contamination along a dairy floor conveyor belt by an average of 4.4 $\log_{10}$ CFU/60 cm^2. While *L. monocytogenes* was not directly used in the latter study, this pathogen still appears to be equally if not more sensitive to glutaraldehyde than *Pseudomonas* and other microbial contaminants. Hence, if *L. monocytogenes* was present initially, this bacterium was likely eliminated during exposure to glutaraldehyde.

As is true for steel and tile surfaces, conveyor lubricants also come in contact with various organic materials in food-processing facilities. Hence, Rossmoore and Drenzek (133) recently examined behavior of *L. monocytogenes* in lubricants containing 25–50 ppm glutaraldehyde, 5–10 ppm MCI, and 500–1000 ppm parachlorometaxylenol in combination with 1% added milk and blood. In the presence of 1% milk, 50 ppm glutaraldehyde was most effective with numbers of listeriae decreasing more than five orders of magnitude following 3 hours of exposure. However, in samples containing 1% blood rather than 1% milk, only 1000 ppm parachlorometaxylenol retained sufficient germicidal activity to reduce *Listeria* populations more than five orders of magnitude within 24 hours. While parachlorometaxylenol exhibited similar activity in the presence of milk, addition of 5–10 ppm MCI was of little value in decreasing numbers of listeriae in lubricant containing 1% milk or blood.

In addition to lubricants, several water-based cooling system fluids used in the dairy and meat industry also are subject to sporadic contamination with pathogenic microorganisms including *L. monocytogenes*. Consequently, Rossmoore and Drenzek (133) examined the potential benefit of adding low concentrations of glutaraldehyde, parachlorometaxylenol, and MCI to sweet water (i.e., potable refrigerated water containing a corrosion inhibitor) and an aqueous solution of 35% propylene glycol, both of which are commonly used in the cooling section of pasteurizers and other types of heat exchangers. According to this report, *L. monocytogenes* populations in inoculated samples of sweet water (pH 9.3) and 35% propylene glycol (pH 8.8) decreased only approximately one and three orders of magnitude, respectively, following 14 days of storage at 3.5°C. In sharp contrast, addition of 25 ppm glutaraldehyde to sweet water and propylene glycol containing 1% milk completely inactivated *L. monocytogenes* populations of 10^5 CFU/ml in less than 1 hour as did addition of 100 ppm parachlorometaxylenol to propylene glycol. Inclusion of 100 ppm parachlormetaxylenol in sweet water and 10 ppm MCI in both coolants was at best only marginally effective with the pathogen surviving at least 48 hours in several instances. Thus, while a low concentration of glutaraldehyde can be effectively used to inactivate *L. monocytogenes* in sweet water and propylene glycol, use of parachlorometaxylenol for such a purpose should be limited to solutions of propylene glycol.

ANTISEPTIC SOAPS

In contrast to the sanitizing agents just discussed, information about antilisterial activity of antiseptic soaps is presently confined to two preliminary reports. According to one investigative team (130), full strength solutions of three commercially available antiseptic soaps, namely Mikro-x, Ioderm, and Zerobac, were strongly listericidal with populations of *L. monocytogenes*, *L. ivanovii*, and *L. seeligeri* decreasing seven orders of magnitude following 30 seconds of exposure. Isoderm (a chlorine/quaternary ammonium compound-based soap) remained almost equally effective when diluted 1:4, whereas Zerobac (an iodophor-based soap) retained strong listericidal activity at a dilution of 1:8.

In the second such study from which data are now available (101), fingers of human volunteers were inoculated to contain 10^5 or 10^9 *L. monocytogenes* CFU/finger to test the effectiveness of moist soap and a commercially produced finger wipe containing isopropyl alcohol and citric acid as active ingredients. Overall, numbers of listeriae on fingers were generally reduced no more than 100- or 10,000-fold after 5 seconds of rubbing in phosphate buffer and moist soap, respectively. Therefore, a population decrease of approximately 100-fold can be attributed to physical removal of the pathogen during rubbing. In contrast, *L. monocytogenes* populations consistently decreased ≥10,000-fold after rubbing the fingers with finger wipes for 5 seconds. Thus, strong listericidal activity of these particular finger wipes and the ease with which they can be applied should make such products useful to food handlers in the food service industry.

REFERENCES

1. Ahamad, N., and E. H. Marth. 1988. Unpublished data.
2. Ahamad, N., and E. H. Marth. 1989. Behavior of *Listeria monocytogenes* at 7, 13, 21, and 35°C in tryptose broth acidified with acetic, citric or lactic acid. *J. Food Prot.* 52:688–695.
3. Ahamad, N., and E. H. Marth. 1990. Acid injury of *Listeria monocytogenes. J. Food Prot.* 53:26–29.
4. Al-Issa, M., D. R. Fowler, A. Seaman, and M. Woodbine. 1984. Role of lipid in butylated hydroxyanisole (BHA) resistance of *Listeria monocytogenes. Zbl. Bakteriol. Hyg. A* 258:42–50.
5. Andryunin, Y. I. 1980. Study of the disinfectant activity of the preparation nitran. *Ir. VNIIVS* (Dezinfects. Prom. Zhivotrov.): 30–34.
6. Anonymous. 1988. Nisin preparation affirmed as GRAS for cheese spreads. *Food Chem. News* 30(6):37–38.
7. Anonymous. 1988. Listeriacide. *Food Prot. Rep.* 4(5):1A.
8. Anonymous. 1988. Proper pasteurization procedures should control *Listeria*, CDC says. *Food Chem. News* 30(4):10.
9. Anonymous. 1988. Update—listeriosis and pasteurized milk. *Morbid. Mortal. Weekly Rep.* 37:764–766.
10. Anonymous. 1988. Code of Federal Regulations. Title 21, Sections 172.110, 172.115 and 172.185. Office of Federal Regulations, National Archives Record Services, General Service Administration, Washington, DC.
11. Anonymous. 1989. Pasteurized process cheese spread: Amendment of standard identity. *Fed. Reg.* 54:6120–6121.
12. Anonymous. 1989. Cheese spread standard amended to ok nisin preparation. *Food Chem. News* 30(5):58–59.
13. Anonymous. 1989. Update—listeriosis and pasteurized milk. *Dairy Food Environ. Sanitat.* 9:150.
14. Bahk, J. A. E. Yousef, and E. H. Marth. 1989. Behaviour of *Listeria monocytogenes* in the presence of selected spices. *Lebensm. Wiss. Technol.* 22:66–69.
15. Baranenkov, M. A. 1969. Survival rate of *Listeria* on the surface of eggs and the development of methods for disinfecting them. *Tr. Vses. Nacuh - Issled. Inst. Vet. Sanit.* 32:453–458.
16. Beams, R. E., and K. F. Girard. 1958. The effect of pasteurization on *Listeria monocytogenes. Can. J. Microbiol.* 4:55–61.
17. Beckers, H. J., P. S. S. Soentoro, and E. H. M. Delfgour-van Asch. 1987. The occurrence of *Listeria monocytogenes* in soft cheeses and raw milk and its resistance to heat. *Int. J. Food Microbiol.* 4:249–256.
18. Benedict, R. C. 1987. A spectrophotometric diffusion-rate method to estimate thermal death of *Listeria monocytogenes* in ionic media. Ann. Mtg. Inst. Food Technol., Las Vegas, NV, June 16–19, Abstr. 120.
19. Benkerroum, N., and W. E. Sandine. 1988. Inhibitory action of nisin against *Listeria monocytogenes. J. Dairy Sci.* 71:3237–3245.
20. Berry, E. D., and M. B. Liewen. 1988. Survival and growth of *Listeria monocytogenes* in the presence of food preservatives and acids. Ann. Mtg. Inst. Food Technol., New Orleans, LA, June 19–22, Abstr. 317.
21. Bojsen-Møller, J. 1972. Human listeriosis—diagnostic, epidemiological and clinical studies. *Acta Pathol. Microbiol. Scand. Sec. B. Suppl.* 229:1–157.

22. Borovian, G. E. 1989. Control of *Listeria monocytogenes* in comparison to other food pathogens using food preservatives. Proc. Ann. Mtg. Amer. Soc. Microbiol., New Orleans, LA, May 14–18, Abstr. 167.

23. Brackett, R. E. 1987. Antimicrobial effect of chlorine on *Listeria monocytogenes*. *J. Food Prot. 50*:999–1003.

24. Bradshaw, J. G., J. T. Peeler, and J. Lovett. 1988. Thermal resistance of *Listeria* species in whole milk. Ann. Mtg. Inst. Food Technol., New Orleans, LA, June 19–22, Abstr. 167.

25. Bradhaw, J. G., J. T. Peeler, J. J. Corwin, J. M. Hunt, and R. M. Twedt. 1987. Thermal resistance of *Listeria monocytogenes* in dairy products. *J. Food Prot. 50* :543–544, 546.

26. Bradshaw, J. G., J. T. Peeler, J. J. Corwin, J. M. Hunt, J. T. Tierney, E. P. Larkin, and R. M. Twedt. 1985. Thermal resistance of *Listeria monocytogenes* in milk. *J. Food Prot. 48*:743–745.

27. Briggs, E. H., C. W. Donnelly, C. M. Beliveau, and W. L. Beeken. 1987. Comparison of uptake of *Listeria monocytogenes* by normal and endotoxin-induced phagocytes of bovine origin. Proc. Ann. Mtg. Amer. Soc. Microbiol., Atlanta, GA, March 1–6, Abstr. P-26.

28. Brzin, B. 1973. The effect of NaCl on the morphology of *Listeria monocytogenes*. *Zbl. Bakteriol. Hyg., I Abt. Orig. A 225*:80–84.

29. Brzin, B. 1975. Further observations of changed growth of *Listeria monocytogenes* on salt agar. *Zbl. Bakteriol. I. Abt. Orig. A 232*:287–293.

30. Buchanan, R. L. 1989. Pathogen modelling program—Version 2.1. Microbial Food Safety Research Unit, USDA/ARS Eastern Regional Research Center, Philadelphia, PA.

31. Buchanan, R. L., H. G. Stahl, and R. C. Whiting. 1989. Effects and interactions of temperature, pH, atmosphere, sodium chloride and sodium nitrite on growth of *Listeria monocytogenes*. *J. Food Prot. 52*:844–851.

32. Buchanan, R. L., H. G. Stahl, and J. G. Phillips. 1989. Response surface model for predicting the effects of various environmental parameters on the growth of *Listeria monocytogenes*. Ann. Mtg. Inst. Food Technol., Chicago, IL, June 25–29, Abstr. 471.

33. Buchnev, K. N., and T. F. Omarov. 1972. Resistance of *Listeria* to some physical and chemical factors. *Tr. Alma-At. Zoovet. Inst. 20*:142–145.

34. Bunning, V. K., R. G. Crawford, J. G. Bradshaw, J. T. Peeler, J. T. Tierney, and R. M. Twedt. 1986. Thermal resistance of intracellular *Listeria monocytogenes* cells suspended in raw bovine milk. *Appl. Environ. Microbiol. 52*:1398–1402.

35. Bunning, V. K., C. W. Donnelly, J. T. Peeler, E. H. Briggs, J. G. Bradshaw, F. G. Crawford, C. M. Beliveau, and J. T. Tierney. 1988. Thermal inactivation of *Listeria monocytogenes* within bovine milk phagocytes. *Appl. Environ. Microbiol. 54*:364–370.

36. Carminati, D., G. Giraffa, and M. G. Bossi. 1989. Bacteriocin-like inhibitors of *Streptococcus lactis* against *Listeria monocytogenes*. *J. Food Prot. 52*:614–617.

37. Cirigliano, M. C., and C. L. Hartman. 1989. Sensitivity of *Listeria monocytogenes* to gamma irradiation. Ann. Mtg. Amer. Soc. Microbiol., New Orleans, LA, May 14–18, Abstr. P-2.

38. Collins, F. M. 1971. Relative susceptibility of acid-fast and non-acid-fast bacteria to ultraviolet light. *Appl. Microbiol. 21*:411–413.

39. Conner, D. E., R. E. Brackett, and L. R. Beuchat. 1986. Effect of temperature, sodium chloride, and pH on growth of *Listeria monocytogenes* in cabbage juice. *Appl. Environ. Microbiol. 52*:59–63.

40. Daeschel, M. A., and T. R. Klaenhammer. 1985. Association of a 13.6 megadalton plasmid in *Pediococcus pentosaceus* with bacteriocin activity. *Appl. Environ. Microbiol. 50*:1538–1541.

41. Darie, P., and I. Constantina. 1988. Studies on *Listeria monocytogenes* resistance under laboratory conditions. *Proc. Int. Symp. Listeriosis*, Pecs, Hungary, August 22–26, Abstr. 50.

42. Dedie, K., and D. Schulze. 1957. Die Hitzeresistenz von *Listeria monocytogenes* in Milch. *Berliner Münchener tierärztl. Wschr. 70*:231–232.

43. Denis, F., and J.-P. Ramet. 1989. Antibacterial activity of the lactoperoxidase system on *Listeria monocytogenes* in trypticase soy broth, UHT milk and French soft cheese. *J. Food Prot. 52*:706–711.

44. Dickgiesser, N. 1980. *Listeria monocytogenes* as a cause of nosocomial infections: A study of the survival of pathogenic microorganisms in the environment. *Infection 8*:199–201.

45. Dishart, K. J., M. A. Hermes, and D. G. Hoover. 1988. Antilisterial activity of pediococci. Proc. Ann. Mtg. Inst. Food Technol., New Orleans, LA, June 19–22, Abstr. 169.
46. Dje, Y., K. D. Payne, and P. M. Davidson. 1989. Unpublished data.
47. Dominguez, L., J. F. F. Garayzabal, J. A. Vazquez, J. L. Blanco and G. Suarez. 1987. Fate of *Listeria monocytogenes* during manufacture and ripening semi-hard cheese. Lett. Appl. Microbiol. *4*:125–127.
48. Dominguez, L., J. F. F. Garayzabal, E. R. Ferri, J. A. Vazquez, E. Gomez-Lucia, C. Ambrosio, and G. Suarez. 1987. Viability of *Listeria monocytogenes* in milk treated with hydrogen peroxide. *J. Food Prot. 50*:636–639.
49. Donker-Voet, J. 1962. My view on the epidemiology of *Listeria* infections. In M. L. Gray (ed.), Second Symposium on Listeric Infection, Montana State College, Bozeman, MT, pp. 133–139.
50. Donnelly, C. E. 1988. *Listeria* and U.S. dairy products: The issues in perspective. *Dairy Food Sanitat. 8*:297–299.
51. Donnelly, C. W., and E. H. Briggs. 1986. Psychrotrophic growth and thermal inactivation of *Listeria monocytogenes* as a function of milk composition. *J. Food Prot. 49*:994–998.
52. Donnelly, C. W., E. H. Briggs, and L. S. Donnelly. 1987. Comparison of heat resistance of *Listeria monocytogenes* by neutrophils and macrophages of bovine origin. Ann. Mtg. Amer. Soc. Microbiol., Atlanta, GA, March 1–6, Abstr. P-27.
53. Donnelly, C. W., E. H. Briggs, C. M. Beliveau, and W. L. Beeken. 1987. In vitro phagocytosis of *Listeria monocytogenes* by neutrophils and macrophages of bovine origin. Ann. Mtg. Amer. Soc. Microbiol, Atlanta, GA, March 1–6. Abstr. P- 27.
54. Doyle, M. P., K. A. Glass, J. T. Beery, G. A. Garcia, D. J. Pollard, and R. D. Schultz. 1987. Survival of *Listeria monocytogenes* in milk during high-temperature, short-time pasteurization. *Appl. Environ. Microbiol. 53*:1433–1438.
55. Durst, J. 1975. The role of temperature factors in the epidemiology of listeriosis. *Zbl. Bakteriol. Hyg., I. Abt. Orig. A 233*:72–74.
56. Durst, J., and A. Sawinsky. 1972. Beiträge zur Untersuchung der Ausbreitungsmöglichkeit der *Listeria monocytogenes. Z. Gesamte Hyg. Grenzgeb. 18*:117–118.
57. Earnshaw, R. G., and J. G. Banks. 1989. A note on the inhibition of *Listeria monocytogenes* NCTC 11994 in milk by an activated lactoperoxidase system. *Lett. Appl. Microbiol. 8*:203–205.
58. El-Gazzar, F. E., and E. H. Marth. 1991. An apparent benzoate-resistant strain of *Listeria monocytogenes* recovered from a milk clotting agent of animal origin. *Milchwissenschaft* (accepted).
59. El-Kest, S. E., and E. H. Marth. 1988. Inactivation of *Listeria monocytogenes* by chlorine. *J. Food Prot. 51*:520–524.
60. El-Kest, S. E., and E. H. Marth. 1988. *Listeria monocytogenes* and its inactivation by chlorine: A review. *Lebensm. Wiss. Technol. 21*:346–351.
61. El-Kest, S. E., and E. H. Marth. 1988. Temperature, pH and strain of pathogen as factors affecting inactivation of *Listeria monocytogenes* by chlorine. *J. Food Prot. 51*:622–625.
62. El-Kest, S. E., and E. H. Marth. 1989. Lethal and sublethal effects caused by freezing *Listeria monocytogenes*. Ann. Mtg. Inst. Food Technol., Chicago, IL, June 25–29, Abstr. 357.
63. El-Kest, S. E., and E. H. Marth. 1989. Unpublished data.
64. El-Shenawy, M. A., and E. H. Marth. 1988. Sodium benzoate inhibits growth of or inactivates *Listeria monocytogenes. J. Food Prot. 51*:525–530.
65. El-Shenawy, M. A., and E. H. Marth, 1988. Inhibition and inactivation of *Listeria monocytogenes* by sorbic acid. *J. Food Prot. 51*:842–847
66. El-Shenawy, M. A., and E. H. Marth, 1989. Inhibition or inactivation of *Listeria monocytogenes* by sodium benzoate together with some organic acids. *J. Food Prot. 52*:771–776.
67. El-Shenawy, M. A., and E. H. Marth. 1989. Behavior of *Listeria monocytogenes* in the presence of sodium propionate. *Intern. J. Food Microbiol. 8*:85–94.
68. El-Shenawy, M. A., and E. H. Marth. 1990. Behavior of *Listeria monocytogenes* in the presence of gluconic acid and during preparation of cottage cheese curd using gluconic acid. *J. Dairy Sci. 73*:1429–1438.

69. El-Shenawy, M. A., H. S. Garcia, and E. H. Marth. 1990. Inhibition and inactivation of *Listeria monocytogenes* by the lactoperoxidase system in raw milk buffer or a semisynthetic medium. *Milchwissenschaft 45*:638–641.

70. El-Shenawy, M. A., A. E. Yousef, and E. H. Marth. 1989. Heat injury and inactivation of *Listeria monocytogenes* in reconstituted nonfat dry milk. *Milchwissenschaft 44*:741–745.

71. El-Shenawy, M. A., A. E. Yousef, and E. H. Marth. 1989. Inactivation and injury of *Listeria monocytogenes* in tryptic soy broth or ground beef treated with gamma irradiation. *Lebensm. Wiss. Technol. 22*:387–390.

72. El-Zawahry, Y. A., and D. B. Rowley. 1979. Radiation resistance and injury of *Yesinia enterocolitica. Appl. Environ. Microbiol. 37*:50–54.

73. Emme, A. E., A. E. Yousef, and E. H. Marth. 1989. Unpublished data.

74. Farber, J. M., G. W. Sanders, S. Dunfield, and R. Prescott. 1989. The effect of various acidulants on the growth of *Listeria monocytogenes. Lett. Appl. Microbiol. 9*:181–183.

75. Farber, J. M., G. W. Sanders, J. I. Speirs, J.-Y. D'Aoust, D. B. Emmons, and R. McKellar. 1988. Thermal resistance of *Listeria monocytogenes* in inoculated and naturally contaminated raw milk. *Int. J. Food Microbiol. 7*:277–286.

76. Farrag, S. A., and E. H. Marth. 1989. Behavior of *Listeria monocytogenes* when incubated together with *Pseudomonas* species in tryptose broth at 7 and 13°C. *J. Food Prot. 52*:536–539.

77. Genigeorgis, C. 1989. Personal communication.

78. George, S. M., B. M. Lund, and T. F. Brocklehurst. 1988. The effect of pH and temperature on initiation of growth of *Listeria monocytogenes. Lett. Appl. Microbiol. 6*:153–156.

79. Glass, K. A., and M. P. Doyle. 1989. Fate and thermal inactivation of *Listeria monocytogenes* in beaker sausage and pepperoni. *J. Food Prot. 52*:226–231, 235.

80. Golden, D. A., L. R. Beuchat, and R. E. Brackett. 1988. Inactivation and injury of *Listeria monocytogenes* as affected by heating and freezing. Ann. Mtg. Amer. Soc. Microbiol., Miami Beach, FL, Abstr. P-45.

81. Gonzales, C. F. 1989. Method for inhibiting bacterial spoilage and resulting decomposition. U.S. Patent No. 4,883,673.

82. Gray, M. L., and A. H. Killinger. 1966. *Listeria monocytogenes* and listeric infections. *Bacteriol. Rev. 30*:309–382.

83. Harris, L. J., T. R. Klaenhammer, and H. P. Fleming. 1989. Sensitivity and resistance of *Listeria monocytogenes* to nisin. Ann. Mtg. Inst. Food Technol., Chicago, IL, June 25–29, Abstr. 354.

84. Harris, L. J., M. A. Daeschel, M. E. Stiles, and T. R. Klaenhammer. 1989. Antimicrobial activity of lactic acid bacteria against *Listeria monocytogenes. J. Food Prot. 52*:784–787.

85. Herald, P. J., and E. A. Zottola. 1988. Attachment of *Listeria monocytogenes* to stainless steel surfaces at various temperatures and pH values. *J. Food Sci. 53*:1549–1552, 1562.

86. Hof, H., H. P. R. Seeliger, A. Schrettenbrunner, and S. Chatzipanagiotou. 1986. The role of *Listeria monocytogenes* and other *Listeria* spp. in foodborne infections. In *Proc. 2nd World Congress, Foodborne Infections and Intoxications*, Berlin, West Germany, pp. 220–223.

87. Hoover, D. G. 1989. Personal communication.

88. Hoover, D. G., P. M. Walsh, K. M. Kolaetis, and M. M. Daly. 1988. A bacteriocin produced by *Pediococcus* species associated with a 5.5-megadalton plasmid. *J. Food Prot. 51*:29–31.

89. Hoover, D. G., C. Metrick, A. M. Papineau, D. F. Farkas, and D. Knorr. 1989. Biological effects of high hydrostatic pressure on food microorganisms. *Food Technol. 42*(3):99–107.

90. Hughey, J. L., and E. A. Johnson. 1987. Antimicrobial activity of lysozyme against bacteria involved in food spoilage and food-borne disease. *Appl. Environ. Microbiol. 53*:2165–2170.

91. Hughey, J. L., P. A. Wilger, and E. A. Johnson. 1989. Antibacterial activity of hen egg white lysozyme against *Listeria monocytogenes* Scott A in foods. *Appl. Environ. Microbiol. 55*:631–638.

92. Huhtanen, C. N., R. K. Jenkins, and D. W. Thayer. 1989. Gamma radiation sensitivity of *Listeria monocytogenes. J. Food Prot. 52*:610–613.

93. Ikonomov, L., and D. Todorov. 1967. Microbiological studies on the pasteurization of ewe's milk. III. Resistance of some pathogenic bacteria. *Vet. Med. Nauki, Sof. 4*:99–108.

94. Joerger, M. C., and T. R. Klaenhammer. 1986. Characterization and purification of helveticin J and evidence for a chromosomally determined bacteriocin produced by *Lactobacillus helveticus* 481. *J. Bacteriol. 167*:439–446.

95. Johnson, E. A. 1988. Personal communication.

96. Johnson, J. L., M. P. Doyle, R. G. Cassens, and J. L. Schoeni. 1988. Fate of *Listeria monocytogenes* in tissues of experimentally infected cattle and in hard salami. *Appl. Environ. Microbiol. 54*:497–501.

97. Junttila, J. R., S. I. Niemelä, and J. Hirn. 1988. Minimum growth temperatures of *Listeria monocytogenes* and non-haemolytic *Listeria. J. Appl. Bacteriol. 65*:321–327.

98. Kamau, D. N., S. Doores, and K. M. Pruitt. 1989. Effect of growth phase, temperature and the level of activation of the lactoperoxidase-thiocyanate-hydrogen peroxide system on growth of *Listeria monocytogenes*. Ann. Mtg. Amer. Soc. Microbiol., New Orleans, LA, May 14–18, Abstr. P-49.

99. Kamau, D. N., S. Doores, and K. M. Pruitt. 1989. The effect of the lactoperoxidase-thiocyanate-hydrogen peroxide system on thermal resistance of *Listeria monocytogenes*. Ann. Mtg. Amer. Soc. Microbiol., New Orleans, LA, May 14–18, Abstr. P-50.

100. Knabel, S. J., H. W. Walker, P. A. Hartman, and A. F. Mendonca. 1990. Effects of growth temperature and strictly anaerobic recovery on survival of *Listeria monocytogenes* during pasteurization. *Appl. Env. Microbiol. 56*:370–376.

101. Kostenbader, K. D., and D. O. Cliver. 1989. Unpublished data.

102. Kovincic, I., I. F. Vujicic, M. Svabic-Vlahovic, M. Mrdjen, M. Vuluc, V. Komnenov-Pupavac, and J. T. Tierney. 1988. Heat resistance of *Listeria monocytogenes* in naturally infected and inoculated cow's milk. *Proc. Intern. Symp. Listeriosis*, Pecs, Hungary, Aug. 22–26, Abstr. 53.

103. Kukharkova, L. L., P. K. Boyarshinov, V. A. Adutskevich, and P. B. Perova. 1960. Data on the hygienic judgement of meat in case of listeriosis. *Veterinariya 37*:74–79.

104. Lang, D. M., E. T. Ryser, and E. H. Marth. 1987. Unpublished data.

105. Larsen, H. E. 1969. *Listeria monocytogenes*. Studies on Isolation Techniques and Epidemiology, Carl Fr. Mortensen, Copenhagen.

106. Larsen, H. E., and A. Gundstrup. 1965. The inhibitory action of various strains of *Bacillus* on *Listeria monocytogenes. Nord. Vet.-Med. 17*:336–341.

107. Lemaire, V., O. Cerf, and A. Audurier. 1988. Heat resistance of *Listeria monocytogenes. Proc. Intern. Symposium on Listeriosis*, Pecs, Hungary, Aug. 22–26, Abstr. 54.

108. Lopes, J. A. 1986. Evaluation of dairy and food plant sanitizers against *Salmonella typhimurium* and *Listeria monocytogenes. J. Dairy Sci. 69*:2791–2796.

109. Marcos, A., and M. A. Esteban. 1982. Nomograph for predicting water activity of soft cheese. *J. Dairy Sci. 64*:1795–1797.

110. Méro, E., and B. Ralovich. 1972. Present situation of human listeriosis in Hungary. *Acta Microbiol. Acad. Sci. Hung. 19*:301–310.

111. Messina, M. C., H. A. Ahamad, J. A. Marchello, C. P. Gerba, and M. W. Paquette. 1988. The effect of liquid smoke on *Listeria monocytogenes. J. Food Prot. 51*:629–631, 638.

112. Mohamed, G. E. E., A. Seaman, and A. Woodbine. 1980. Food antibiotic nisin: Comparative effects on *Erysipelothrix* and *Listeria*. In M. Woodbine (ed.), *Antimicrobials and Agriculture*, Butterworths, London, pp. 435–442.

113. Muriana, P. M., and T. R. Klaenhammer. 1987. Conjugal transfer of plasmid-encoded determinants for bacteriocin production and immunity in *Lactobacillus acidophilus* 88. *Appl. Environ. Microbiol. 53*:553–560.

114. Mustapha, A., and M. B. Liewen. 1989. Destruction of *Listeria monocytogenes* by sodium hypochlorite and quaternary ammonium sanitizers. *J. Food Prot. 52*:306–311.

115. Nichols, J. G. 1989. Personal communication.

116. Ozgen, H. 1952. *Z. Tropenm. u. Paras. 4*:40.

117. Palumbo, S., and A. C. Williams. 1989. Freezing and freeze-injury in *Listeria monocytogenes*. Ann. Mtg. Amer. Soc. Microbiol., New Orleans, LA, May 14–18, Abstr. P-1.

118. Parish, M. E., and D. P. Higgins. 1989. Survival of *Listeria monocytogenes* in low pH model broth systems. *J. Food Prot. 52*:144–147.

119. Patterson, M. 1989. Sensitivity of *Listeria monocytogenes* to irradiation on poultry meat and in phosphate-buffered saline. *Lett. Appl. Microbiol.* 8:181–184.

120. Payne, K. D., E. Rico-Munoz, and P. M. Davidson. 1989. The antimicrobial activity of phenolic compounds against *Listeria monocytogenes* and their effectiveness in a model milk system. *J. Food Prot.* 52:151–153.

121. Petran, R. L., and E. A. Zottola. 1989. A study of factors affecting growth and recovery of *Listeria monocytogenes* Scott A. *J. Food Sci.* 54:458–460.

122. Pfeiffer, J., E. T. Ryser, and E. H. Marth. 1988. Unpublished data.

123. Polyakov, A. A., and M. A. Baranenkov. 1973. Enzymic activity of listeriae under normal conditions and after the action of chemical disinfectants. *Tr. Vses. Nauchno-Issled. Inst. Vet. Sanit.* 45:235–251.

124. Polyakov, A. A., M. A. Baranenkov, and V. P. Andreev. 1972. Structural changes in *Listeria monocytogenes* after the action of disinfecting solutions on them. *Dokl. Veses. Akad. Sel'skokhoz. Nauk.* 3:32–34.

125. Pomanskaya, L. A. 1961. Polymorphism of *Listeria. Zh. Microbiol. Epidemiol. Immunobiol.* 38:124–128.

126. Potel, J. 1951. The morphology, culture and pathogenicity of *C. infantisepticum. Zbl. Bakteriol. Parasitol.* 156:490–496.

127. Pucci, M. J., E. R. Vedamuthu, B. S. Kunka, and P. A. Vandebergh. 1988. Inhibition of *Listeria monocytogenes* by using bacteriocin PA-1 produced by *Pediococcus acidilactici* PAC 1.0. *Appl. Environ. Microbiol.* 54:2349–2353.

128. Raccach, M., R. McGrath, and H. Daftarian. 1989. Antibiosis of some lactic acid bacteria including *Lactobacillus acidophilus* toward *Listeria monocytogenes. Intern. J. Food Microbiol.* 9:25–32.

129. Reimer, L., S. Mottice, and D. Andrews. 1988. The effect of pH on survival of *Listeria monocytogenes.* Annual Mtg. Amer. Soc. Microbiol., Miami Beach, FL, May 8–13, Abstr. C-175.

130. Rosales, J., M. Verder-Elepano, C. E. Franti, and C. Genigeorgis. 1988. Antimicrobial activity of selected food plant sanitizers, cleaners and soaps on *Listeria* species, *Salmonella typhimurium, Escherichia coli* and *Pseudomonas aeruginosa* in the presence or absence of organic matter. *Vet. Med. Res. Rep.*, University of California, Davis, CA.

131. Rosenow, E. M., and E. H. Marth. 1987. Growth of *Listeria monocytogenes* in skim, whole and chocolate milk, and in whipping cream during incubation at 4, 8, 13, 21 and 35°C. *J. Food Prot.* 50:452–459.

132. Rossmoore, K. 1988. The microbial activity of glutaraldehyde in chain conveyor lubricant formulations. In D. R. Houghton, R. N. Smith, and H. O. W. Eggins (eds.), *Proc. 7th Intern. Biodeterioration Symposium*, Cambridge, Elsevier Appl. Sci. Publ. Ltd., England, pp. 242–247.

133. Rossmoore, K., and C. Drenzek. 1989. Unpublished data.

134. Ryser, E. T., and E. H. Marth. 1985. Survival of *Listeria monocytogenes* during manufacture and storage of cottage cheese. *J. Food Prot.* 48:746–750.

135. Ryser, E. T., and E. H. Marth. 1987. Behavior of *Listeria monocytogenes* during the manufacture and ripening of Cheddar cheese. *J. Food Prot.* 50:7–13.

136. Ryser, E. T., and E. H. Marth. 1987. Fate of *Listeria monocytogenes* during manufacture and ripening of Camembert cheese. *J. Food Prot.* 50:372–378.

137. Ryser, E. T., and E. H. Marth. 1988. Survival of *Listeria monocytogenes* in cold-pack cheese food during refrigerated storage. *J. Food Prot.* 51:615–621, 625.

138. Ryser, E. T., and E. H. Marth. 1988. Growth of *Listeria monocytogenes* at different pH values in uncultured whey or whey cultured with *Penicillium camemberti. Can. J. Microbiol.* 34:730–735.

139. Ryser, E. T., and E. H. Marth. 1989. Behavior of *Listeria monocytogenes* during manufacture and ripening of brick cheese. *J. Dairy Sci.* 72:838–853.

140. Schlech, W. F., P. M. Lavigne, R. A. Bortolussi, A. C. Allen, E. V. Haldane, A. J. Wort, A. W.

Hightower, S. E. Johnson, S. H. King, E. S. Nicholls, and C. V. Broome. 1985. Epidemic listeriosis—evidence for transmission by food. *N. Engl. J. Med. 303*:203–206.

141. Seeliger, H. P. R. 1961. *Listeriosis*, Hafner Publishing Co., New York.
142. Seeliger, H. P. R., and D. Jones. 1987. *Listeria*. In *Bergey's Manual of Systematic Bacteriology*, 9th ed., Williams and Wilkins, Baltimore, pp. 1235–1245.
143. Shahamat, M., A. Seaman, and M. Woodbine. 1980. Influence of sodium chloride, pH and temperature on the inhibitory activity of sodium nitrite on *Listeria monocytogenes*. In Technical Series No. 14, Soc. Appl. Bacteriol., Academic Press, London, pp. 227–237.
144. Shahamat, M., A. Seaman, and M. Woodbine. 1980. Survival of *Listeria monocytogenes* in high salt concentrations. *Zbl. Bakteriol. Hyg., I. Abt. Orig. A 246*:506–511.
145. Sielaff, H. von. 1968. Die lebensmittelhygienische Bedeutung der Listeriose. *Monatsh. Veterinärmed. 21*:750–758.
146. Siragusa, G. R., and M. G. Johnson. 1987. Inhibition of *Listeria monocytogenes* by the lactoperoxidase-thiocyanate-hydrogen peroxide antibacterial system. Ann. Mtg. Amer. Soc. Microbiol., Atlanta, GA, March 1–6, Abstr. P-22.
147. Skovgaard, N. 1987. *Listeria*: Major sources and routes of human infection-environment and plants. In A. Schönberg (ed.), Listeriosis-Joint WHO/ROI Consultation on Prevention and Control, West Berlin, December 10–12, 1986, pp. 86–97. Institut für Veterinarmedizin des Bundesgesundheitsamtes, Berlin.
148. Sorrells, K. M., D. C. Enigl, and J. R. Hatfield. 1989. Effect of pH, acidulant, time and temperature on the growth and survival of *Listeria monocytogenes*. *J. Food Prot. 52*:571–573.
149. Spelhaug, S. R., and S. K. Harlander. 1989. Inhibition of foodborne bacterial pathogens by bacteriocins from *Lactococcus lactis* and *Pediococcus pentosaceus*. *J. Food Prot. 52*:856–862.
150. Sperber, W. 1987. Personal communication.
151. Stajner, B., S. Zakula, I. Kovincic, and M. Galic. 1979. Heat resistance of *Listeria monocytogenes* and its survival in raw milk products. *Veterinarski Glasnik 33*:109–112.
152. Stanfield, J. T., C. R. Wilson, W. H. Andrews, and G. J. Jackson. 1987. Potential role of refrigerated milk packaging in the transmission of listeriosis and salmonellosis. *J. Food Prot. 50*:730–732.
153. Stenberg, H., and T. Hammainen. 1955. On determination *in vitro* of the resistance of *Listeria monocytogenes* to sodium chloride and heat and on experimental monocytosis in albino mice. *Nord. Vet. Med. 7*:853–868.
154. Styles, M. F., D. G. Hoover, and D. F. Farkas. 1989. Effects of high hydrostatic pressure on *Listeria monocytogenes* and *Vibrio parahaemolyticus*. Ann. Mtg. Inst. Food Technol., Chicago, IL, June 25–29, Abstr. 356.
155. Sumner, S. S., T. M. Sandros, M. Harmon, V. N. Scott, and D. T. Bernard. 1989. Effect of water activity on the heat resistance of *Salmonella* and *Listeria*. Ann. Mtg. Inst. Food Technol., Chicago, IL, June 25–29, Abstr. 465.
156. Tarjan, V. 1988. The sensitivity of *Listeria monocytogenes* to gamma radiation. *Proc. 10th Intern. Symp. Listeriosis*, Pecs. Hungary, Aug. 22–26, Abstr. P57.
157. Tatini, S. R. 1990. Personal communication.
158. Taylor, S. L. 1986. Unpublished data.
159. Ting, W. T. E., ad K. E. Deibel. 1989. Sensitivity of *Listeria monocytogenes* to spices at two temperatures. Ann. Mtg. Inst. Food Technol., Chicago, IL, June 25–29, Abstr. 474.
160. Urbach, H., and G. Schabinski. 1955. Zur Listeriose des Menschen. *Z. Hyg. Infektionskr. 141*:239–248.
161. Urbain, W. M. 1986. *Food Irradiation*, Academic Press, New York.
162. Vranchen, Z. E., O. N. Shuvaeva, and Y. I. Andryunin. 1974. Soil decontamination in some infectious diseases of animals. *Tr. Vses. Nauchno-Issled. Inst. Vet. Sanit. 49*:226–229.
163. Walker, S. J., P. Archer, and J. G. Banks. 1990. Growth of *Listeria monocytogenes* at refrigeration temperatures. *J. Appl. Bacteriol. 68*:157–162.
164. Welshimer, H. J. 1960. Survival of *Listeria monocytogenes* in soil. *J. Bacteriol. 80*:316–320.
165. Wendorf, W. L. 1989. Effect of smoke flavorings on *Listeria monocytogenes* in skinless franks.

Seminar presentation, Department of Food Science, University of Wisconsin-Madison, Jan. 13.

166. WHO Working Group. 1988. Foodborne listeriosis. *Bull. WHO 66*:421–428.
167. Wilkins, P. O., R. Bourgeois, and R. G. E. Murray. 1972. Psychrotrophic properties of *Listeria monocytogenes. Can. J. Microbiol. 18*:543–551.
168. Wood, L. V., and M. Woodbine. 1979. Low temperature virulence of *Listeria monocytogenes* in the avian embryo. *Zbl. Bakteriol. Hyg., I. Abt. Orig. A 243*:74–81.
169. Yousef, A. E., and E. H. Marth. 1988. Behavior of *Listeria monocytogenes* during manufacture and storage of Colby cheese. *J. Food Prot. 51*:12–15.
170. Yousef, A. E., and E. H. Marth. 1988. Inactivation of *Listeria monocytogenes* by ultraviolet energy. *J. Food Sci. 52*:571–573.
171. Yousef, A. E., and E. H. Marth. 1989. *Bacillus* sp. isolated from spices inactivates *Listeria monocytogenes*. Ann. Mtg. Inst. Food Technol., Chicago, IL, June 25–29, Abstr. 358.
172. Yousef, A. E., M. A. El-Shenawy, and E. H. Marth. 1989. Inactivation and injury of *Listeria monocytogenes* in a minimal medium as affected by benzoic acid and incubation temperature. *J. Food Sci. 54*:650–652.
173. Yousef, A. E., R. J. Gajewski II, and E. H. Marth. 1990. Kinetics of growth and inhibition of *Listeria monocytogenes* in the presence of antioxidant food additives. *J. Food Sci. 55*: (in press).

6

Conventional Methods to Detect and Isolate *Listeria monocytogenes*

INTRODUCTION

Listeria monocytogenes is a nonfastidious organism that can be subcultured on most common bacteriological media (i.e., Tryptose Agar, Nutrient Agar, and Blood Agar); however, attempted isolation or reisolation of listeriae from inoculated or naturally contaminated food and clinical specimens is often unsuccessful. Difficulties encountered in isolating *L. monocytogenes* date back to initial characterization of this pathogen in 1926 when Murray and his co-workers (134) stated, "The isolation of the infecting organism is not easy and we found this to remain true even after we had established the cause of the disease." Although efforts to isolate *L. monocytogenes* from blood and CSF of infected patients have met with considerable success, mainly because of the presence of *Listeria* in pure culture, obvious difficulties arise when food and clinical specimens (tissue biopsies and autopsy specimens) contain small numbers of *L. monocytogenes* in combination with large numbers of other microorganisms.

As shown in Fig. 6.1, direct plating, cold enrichment, warm enrichment and several rapid methods can be used in various combinations to detect *L. monocytogenes* in food, clinical, and environmental samples. Early attempts to isolate small numbers of listeriae from samples containing large populations of indigenous microflora relied on direct plating and often ended in failure. In 1948, Gray et al. (82) introduced the cold enrichment procedure as an alternative method to isolate *L. monocytogenes* from highly contaminated samples. Although this method has contributed much to our present-day knowledge concerning the epidemiology of listeriosis, the prolonged incubation period necessary to obtain positive results is a serious disadvantage. In the years that followed, major strides were made in development of selective enrichment and plating media which ultimately decreased the time needed for analysis from several months to less than 1 week. Recent outbreaks of foodborne listeriosis have underscored the need for faster and more efficient methods to detect small numbers of listeriae in a wide range of food products.

We will now trace development of various cold and warm enrichment broths as well as plating media and methods used to isolate *Listeria* spp., including *L. monocytogenes*, from clinical, environmental, and food samples. Such a task is particularly formidable when one considers that well over 60 different enrichment broths and 60 different plating media have been used during the past 40 years for selective cultivation of *Listeria*. Detection and isolation of listeriae also are complicated by the inability of researchers

120

to identify a single procedure that is sufficiently sensitive to detect *L. monocytogenes* in all types of foods within a reasonable time. Furthermore, many selective enrichment broths and plating media that have been developed fail to allow repair and/or growth of sublethally injured listeriae frequently present in processed foods. Despite these inherent problems, recent research efforts in response to identifiable cases of foodborne listeriosis have led to development of the FDA and USDA procedures. They have been unofficially adopted in the United States as "standard methods" to isolate *L. monocytogenes* from fermented/nonfermented dairy products, seafood and vegetables, and meat/poultry products, respectively. However, in an effort to more rapidly detect both healthy and sublethally injured listeriae in the variety of foods currently being examined, these methods and others that are less widely accepted will undoubtedly undergo further changes as the selective enrichment broths and plating media used in these procedures continue to be improved. While the previously mentioned number of *Listeria* enrichment broths and plating media may at first appear overwhelming, further experimentation with some of the more obscure media formulations outlined in Tables 6.1, 6.2, and 6.3 could prove helpful to individuals involved in improving current *Listeria* detection and isolation procedures.

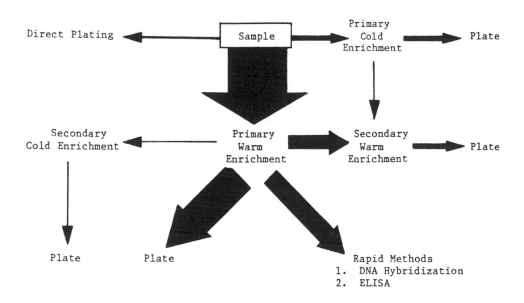

Figure 6.1 Schema for isolation and/or detection of *L. monocytogenes* from food and other biological and environmental samples. Size of arrows denotes current trends in relative numbers of samples analyzed by various methods.

Table 6.1 Fluid Media for Cold Enrichment of *L. monocytogenes* at 4°C

Media (composition/liter)	Samples analyzed	Ref.
*Tryptose Broth (TB)	milk, cheese, brine, whey, meat, tissue, feces, environmental samples	12, 49, 52, 65, 80, 82, 112, 113, 140, 146, 166–168, 170, 180, 195
TB + trisodium citrate (20 g)	cheese	147, 148, 170, 195
*TB + trypaflavine HCl (10 mg) + nalidixic acid (40 mg) + cycloheximide (50 mg)[a]	milk, cheese	11, 14
*Oxoid Nutrient Broth no. 2 (ONB2)	milk, cheese, cabbage, silage, feces, sewage, sludge, water	1, 42, 63, 88, 111, 152, 179, 190
ONB2 + KSCN[a] (3.75 g)	feces	174
ONB2 + KSCN (3.75 g) + Tween 80[a] (1 g)	milk, water, silage, soil, feces	193
Tryptose Phosphate Broth (TPB)	feces, water, sewage, chicken, cheese	72, 100, 151, 195
TPB + thallous acetate[a] (0.2 g)	feces	120
TPB + nalidixic acid[a] (50 mg)	feces	120
TPB + thallous acetate (0.2 g) + nalidixic acid[a] (40 mg)	silage, biological specimens	102
TPB + polymyxin[a] (3120 IU)	tissue, feces, swabs	21
Brain Heart Infusion Broth	cabbage, vegetation, soil	85, 191, 192
Holman Medium[b]	feces, throat swabs	156, 158, 159, 160
Trypticase Soy Broth + Yeast Extract (6 g) (TSB-YE)	snails, frogs, feces, water, milk	22, 37
FDA Enrichment Broth: TSB-YE + acriflavine (15 mg) + nalidixic acid (40 mg) + cycloheximide (50 mg)[a]	cheese, dairy environment	11
TSB-YE + potassium tellurite (50 mg)[a]	snails, frogs, feces, water	22
Thioglycolate Broth (TGB)	feces, throat swabs, meconium	144, 145, 159
TGB + polymyxin B (5000 IU) + bacitracin (5000 IU)[a]	feces	144
Rodriguez Collection Medium A[b]	feces	163
Rodriguez Collection Medium B[b]	feces	163
Rodriguez Collection Medium C[b]	feces	163

*Cold enrichment broths of some importance in food analysis.
[a]Medium also suitable for warm enrichment at 30–37°C.
[b]Formula given in appendix.

Table 6.2 Fluid Media for Warm Enrichment of L. monocytogenes at 30–37°C

Media (composition/liter)	Samples analyzed	Ref.
*FDA Enrichment Broth: Trypticase Soy Broth + yeast extract (6 g) + acriflavine HCl (15 mg) + nalidixic acid (40 mg) + cycloheximide (50 mg) [Difco, BBL][a]	milk, dairy products, meat, poultry, vegetables, seafood	8, 11, 19, 37, 38, 42, 67, 70, 85, 87, 90, 92, 93, 111, 122, 124, 125, 141, 151, 180, 184
FDA Enrichment Broth + 3-[N-Morpholino] propanesulfonic acid-acid free (8.5 g) + 3-[N-Morpholino] propanesulfonic acid sodium salt (13.7 g)	dairy factory environment	32, 103
*Fraser Broth[b] [Difco]	meat, poultry, ice cream, factory environment	32, 38, 68
*University of Vermont Medium[b] (UVM) [Difco, BBL]	meat, poultry, seafood, milk	7, 8, 37, 46, 141, 157
*USDA Listeria Enrichment Broth I (LEB I): UVM + nalidixic acid (20 mg) [Oxoid]	meat, poultry, seafood, milk	7, 9, 38, 67, 70, 87, 93, 111, 132, 139, 141, 157, 184
*USDA Listeria Enrichment Broth II (LEB II): LEB I + acriflavine (12.5 mg)	meat, poultry, seafood, milk	7, 9, 38, 93, 111, 132, 139, 141, 184
Tryptose Broth (TB) + trypaflavine HCl (10 mg) + nalidixic acid (40 mg) + cycloheximide (50 mg)	cheese, milk, meat	14, 139
Doyle and Schoeni Selective Enrichment Broth: TB + glucose (5 g) + dipotassium phosphate (1.5 g) + defibrinated blood (50 ml) + acriflavine HCl (10 mg) + nalidixic acid (40 mg) + polymyxin B (16,000 IU)	cabbage, milk, feces, liver, brain	49, 85, 184
Oxoid Nutrient Broth no. 2 (ONB2) + KSCN (3.75 g)	feces	119, 174
ONB2 + KSCN (3.75 g) + Tween 90 (1 g)	milk, brain, silage, soil, manure	193
ONB2 + KSCN (3.75 g) + glucose (2 g)	soil, manure, silage, grass, cabbage	85, 106
ONB2 + KSCN (3.75 g) + nalidixic acid (10 mg)	milk, dairy products, cabbage	1, 85, 88, 111, 190
ONB2 + KSCN (3.75 g) + nalidixic acid (100 mg)	milk	179
ONB2 + KSCN (37.5 g) + nalidixic acid (100 mg)	sewage, sludge, water, dairy products, meat, poultry, vegetables	38, 190

(continued)

Table 6.2 Continued

Media (composition/liter)	Samples analyzed	Ref.
ONB2 + KSCN (37.5 g) + nalidixic acid (100 mg) + acriflavine (25 mg)	milk	179, 180
ONB2 + KSCN (37.5 g) + acriflavine (2.5 g) + Tween 80 (1 g)	milk, brain, silage, soil, manure	63, 193
ONB2 + nalidixic acid (50 mg) + horse blood (5%)	milk, brain, silage, soil, manure	193
ONB2 + glucose (2 g) + nalidixic acid (40 mg) + thallous acetate (2 g)	grass, silage, soil, manure	106
Listeria Test Broth	meat	189
Tryptose Phosphate Broth (TPB) + nalidixic acid (40 mg)	laboratory cultures	6
TPB + propolis (15 mg)	laboratory cultures	6
TPB + nalidixic acid (40 mg) + propolis (15 mg)	laboratory cultures	6
TPB + nalidixic acid (40 mg) + thallous acetate (0.2 g)	silage, feces	102
TPB + furacin (10 mg)	laboratory cultures	129
Stuart Transport Medium	milk, cabbage	85, 88
Levinthal Broth + nalidixic acid (40 mg) + trypaflavine (40 mg)[b]	feces	156, 157, 159
Levinthal Broth + nalidixic acid (40 mg) + trypaflavine (12 mg)	milk, sausage	38
Holman Medium[b]	clinical samples	156–158
Holman Medium + nalidixic acid (40 mg) + trypaflavine (40 mg)	feces	156, 157, 159
Todd-Hewitt Broth + potassium dichromate (0.83 g) + chromium tri-oxide (2 g) + thionin (50 mg) + na-lidixic acid (100 mg) + amphotericin B (3000 IU)	feces	128
HPB Enrichment Broth	laboratory cultures	62
Nutrient Broth + potassium tellurite (0.5 g)	straw, feces, nasal swabs	81
Peptone + rhamnose + methylene blue + nalidixic acid + polymyxin B	feces	43, 83
Rodriguez Collection Medium A[b]	feces	163
Rodriguez Collection Medium B[b]	feces	163
Rodriguez Collection Medium C[b]	feces	163
Rodriguez Enrichment Medium I [incubated at 22°C][b]	feces	163
Rodriguez Enrichment Medium II [incubated at 22°C][b]	feces	163
Rodriguez Enrichment Medium III [incubated at 22°C][b]	feces, cheese, cabbage	70, 75, 163

(continued)

Table 6.2 Continued

Media (composition/liter)	Samples analyzed	Ref.
*IDF Pre-Enrichment Broth[b]	milk, dairy products	187
*IDF Enrichment Broth[b]	milk, dairy products	42, 187
L-PALCAMY Broth[b]	dairy products, meat, chicken, vegetables	38, 139
University of Montana Broth[b]	clinical specimens	171

*Warm enrichment media of major importance in food analysis.
[a]Commercially available from Difco Laboratories, Detroit, MI; BBL, Cockeysville, MD; Oxoid Ltd., Basingstoke, Hampshire, England.
[b]Formula given in Appendix I.

Table 6.3 Plating media for isolation of *L. monocytogenes*

Media (composition/liter)	Samples analyzed	Ref.
McBride Listeria Agar (MLA): Phenylethanol Agar (35.5 g) + glycine (10 g) + lithium chloride (0.5 g) + sheep blood (5%) [Difco, BBL][a]	feces, brain, liver, milk, dairy products, vegetables	9, 49, 65, 70, 75, 83, 85, 111, 121, 129, 179
MLA + polymyxin B (3 mg)	clinical specimens	65
MLA + nalidixic acid (40 mg)	clinical specimens	65
MLA2: MLA with glycine anhydride (10 g) substituted for glycine (10 g)	nonfat dry milk, cheese, meat, poultry, seafood	33, 51, 121, 122, 129, 139, 157, 164, 166–168
MLA2 + sheep blood (5%)	clinical specimens, cheese, dairy products	1, 12, 61, 88, 111, 167
MLA2 + LiCl (4.5 g)	cheese, meat	59, 169, 170, 194
*FDA-Modified McBride Listeria Agar (FDA-MMLA)[b]	milk, dairy products, meat, poultry, vegetables, seafood	23, 24, 33, 37, 38, 42, 67, 75, 89, 90, 92, 93, 111, 124, 125, 139, 141, 151, 180
ARS-Modified McBride Listeria Agar[b]	dairy products, meat, poultry, vegetables	27, 29, 34, 139
*LPM Agar: MLA2 + LiCl (4.5 g) + moxalactam (20 mg) [Difco, BBL]	dairy products, meat, poultry, vegetables, seafood	9, 24, 30, 33, 34, 37, 38, 67, 70, 87, 89, 90, 93, 111, 116–118, 121, 124, 139, 157
Modified LPM Agar[b]	cheese, meat, poultry, seafood	108, 110
LPMX Agar: LPM Agar + xylose (5 g) + bromcresol purple (50 mg)	meat factory environment	162
*Modified Vogel-Johnson Agar (MVJ agar)[b]	dairy products, meat, poultry, vegetables, seafood	24, 27, 29, 30, 33, 34, 38, 121, 139
*Oxford Agar[b] [Oxoid, Difco]	clinical specimens, feces, cheese, poultry	38, 39, 40, 135, 139, 149, 153
*Modified Oxford Agar[b]	meat, poultry	32
*Merck Listeria Agar: Basal Medium + acriflavine (10 mg) + nalidixic acid (40 mg) [Merck]	dairy products, meat, food processing environment	25, 86, 87
*Gum Base Nalidixic Acid Medium[b] (GBNA) [BBL]	soil, feces, milk, dairy products, meat, poultry, seafood, vegetables	9, 33, 34, 74, 75, 88, 111, 126
GBNA + lithium chloride (5.0 g) + moxalactam (20 mg)	milk, dairy products, poultry	9, 75
*Trypaflavine Nalidixic Acid Serum Agar[b] (TNSA)	throat swabs, feces, milk, cheese, meat	14, 83, 98, 139, 145, 157, 159, 160, 184
Modified Despierres Agar[b]	milk, dairy products, meat, vegetables, seafood	33, 34, 43, 75
Lithium Chloride-Ceftazidime Agar[b] (LCA)	dairy products, meat, poultry, seafood	110

(continued)

Table 6.3 Continued

Media (composition/liter)	Samples analyzed	Ref.
RAPAMY Agar[b]	milk, meat	138, 157
RAPAMY-S Agar: RAPAMY Agar with bovine serum (50 ml) substituted for egg yolk emulsion (25 ml)	milk, meat	157
ALPAMY[b]	milk, cheese, poultry, vegetables	136
PALCAM[b]	cheese, meat, poultry, vegetables	38, 139
CNPA Agar[b]	laboratory cultures, meat	96, 121
Acriflavine Ceftazidime Agar (AC Agar): Columbia Agar Base + acriflavine HCl (10 mg) + ceftazidime (50 mg)	cheese	11, 38, 87, 121, 139
University of Vermont Agar[b]	milk, dairy products, meat, vegetables, seafood	33, 46, 74
Modified Doyle/Schoeni Selective Agar I (MDSSA I)[b]	vegetables	85
MDSSA II: MDSSA I with cycloheximide (200 mg) substituted for acriflavine	food-processing environments	23
Binds Acriflavine Agar[b]	milk, dairy products, vegetables	74
Brackett/Beuchat Listeria Selective Agar[b]	milk, dairy products, vegetables	74
Farber Agar[b]	laboratory cultures	62
University of Montana Agar[b]	clinical specimens	171
Rodriguez Isolation Medium I[b]	feces	163
Rodriguez Isolation Medium II[b]	feces	163
Rodriguez Isolation Medium III (RIM III)[b]	feces, dairy products, seafood	38, 70, 121, 163–165
RIM III + acriflavine HCl (6 mg)	dairy products	164
Modified RIM III (MRIM III): RIM III with sodium phosphate 7-hydrate substituted for sodium phosphate 2-hydrate	dairy products, meat, vegetables, seafood	33, 34, 74
Tryptose Agar (TA)	feces, brain, soil, manure, silage, milk	82, 120, 121, 144, 179, 180, 183
TA + horse serum (10%)	manure, soil, grass, silage, food	106, 186
TA + gallocyanine + pyronine + nalidixic acid	feces	127

(continued)

Table 6.3 Continued

Media (composition/liter)	Samples analyzed	Ref.
TA + KSCN (3.5 g)	laboratory cultures	120
TA + LiCl (0.5 g)	laboratory cultures	120
TA + nalidixic acid (40 mg)	feces, poultry	72, 144
TA + nalidixic acid (50 mg)	laboratory cultures	120
TA + potassium tellurite (0.5 g)	laboratory cultures	120
TA + propolis (15 mg)	laboratory cultures	6, 84
TA + thallous acetate (0.2 g)	laboratory cultures	120
TA + thallous acetate (0.2 g) + KSCN (3.5 g)	laboratory cultures	120
TA + thallous acetate (0.2 g) + nalidixic acid (50 mg)	laboratory cultures	120
TA + nalidixic acid (40 mg) + thallous acetate (50 mg) + trypaflavine (25 mg)	feces	120
TA + nalidixic acid (40 mg) + acriflavine HCl (10 mg)	milk	179
TA + glucose (2 g) + thallous acetate (2 g) + nalidixic acid (60 mg)	manure, soil, grass, silage	106, 230
TA + glucose (5 g) + dipotassium phosphate (1.5 g) + nalidixic acid (40 mg) + polymyxin B (16,000 IU) + sheep blood (5%) + Fe^{3+} (5 mg)	cabbage	85
Tryptose Blood Agar + glucose (5 g)	meat, seafood	33
Tryptose Serum Agar + propolis (15 mg)	laboratory cultures	6
Tryptose Phosphate Agar + esculin (0.5 g) + ferric citrate (0.5 g)	milk	47, 48
Tryptose Soy Agar (TSA) + nalidixic acid (50 mg)	food, soil, feces	126
TSA + nalidixic acid (40 mg)	clinical specimens	65
TSA + nalidixic acid (40 mg) + acriflavine (25 mg)	clinical specimens	65
TSA + nalidixic acid (0.1 mg) + gallocyanin (50 mg) + pyronin (5 mg)	feces	128
TSA + yeast extract (5 g) + nalidixic acid (40 mg) + acriflavine (10 mg) + polymyxin B (14,400 IU) + esculine (5 g) + bromocresol purple (40 mg)	yogurt	176

(continued)

Table 6.3 Continued

Media (composition/liter)	Samples analyzed	Ref.
Blood Agar (BA)	organs, feces, swabs	97, 158
BA + nalidixic acid (40 mg)	feces, clinical specimens, dairy products	15, 97, 164
BA + nalidixic acid (40 mg) + acriflavine HCl (25 mg)	feces, silage	63
BA + nalidixic acid + Columbia colistin + amphoterin	feces	60
Nutrient Agar (NA) + glucose (2 g) + KSCN (3.75 g)	manure, soil, grass, silage	106
NA + glucose (2 g) + thallous acetate (2 g) + nalidixic acid (40 g)	manure, soil, grass, silage	106
NA + potassium tellurite (2.5 g) + nalidixic acid (40 mg)	feces, silage	102
NA + nalidixic acid (40 mg) + horse blood (5%)	manure, soil, grass, silage	106
NA + nalidixic acid (40 mg) + acriflavine (10 mg) + rabbit blood (5%) + equi factor (7500 Units)	laboratory cultures	177
Basal Medium + antibiotics[b]	feces, sewage	53
Serum Agar + nalidixic acid (50 mg)	organs, feces, swabs	158, 159
Oxoid Nutrient Broth no. 2 + KSCN (37.5 g) + nalidixic acid (100 mg) + agar (15 g)	meat, seafood	33

*Plating media of major importance in food analysis.
[a]Commercially available from Difco Laboratories, Detroit, MI; BBL, Cockeysville, MD; Oxoid Ltd., Basingstoke, Hampshire, England; Merck, Darmstadt, West Germany.
[b]Formula given in appendix.

COLD ENRICHMENT

Difficulties in isolating *L. monocytogenes* typically arise when small numbers of listeriae are present in food, environmental, and clinical samples containing large numbers of indigenous microorganisms. Hence, the number of listeriae must be increased, relative to that of the background flora, before the bacterium can be detected.

Thirteen years after the first description of *L. monocytogenes* by Murray et al. (134), Biester and Schwarte (17) observed that *Listerella* (*Listeria*) could be frequently isolated from naturally infected sheep organs that were held in 50% glycerol and refrigerated for several months. Although initial plating of diluted specimens was only rarely successful in isolating the organism, these authors failed to comment on the significance of cold storage.

Following similar chance observations, a young graduate student, M. L. Gray, recognized the benefits of low-temperature incubation in isolating *L. monocytogenes* from clinical specimens. In 1948, Gray et al. (82) reported that in three of five bovine listeriosis cases, *L. monocytogenes* was only isolated after brain tissue diluted in Tryptose Broth was stored 5–13 weeks at 4°C and then plated on Tryptose Agar. Although a few *Listeria* colonies were observed after directly plating the remaining two brain tissue samples on Tryptose Agar, the bacterium was more readily isolated following cold enrichment. Their results clearly showed the ability of *L. monocytogenes* to multiply to detectable levels in the presence of other microbial contaminants during extended storage at 4°C.

Gray's cold enrichment method, in which samples homogenized in Tryptose Broth are incubated at 4°C and plated weekly or biweekly on Tryptose Agar during 3 months of storage, was soon adopted as the "standard procedure" for detecting *L. monocytogenes*. Normally only a few weeks of cold enrichment are required before listeriae can be detected; however, in once instance (79), 6 months of refrigerated storage was necessary before *L. monocytogenes* could be isolated from calf brains. While the cold enrichment procedure admittedly is slow and laborious, this method greatly enhances the likelihood of isolating listeriae from a variety of specimens, including food.

In 13 studies summarized by Bojsen-Møller (21), *Listeria* was identified in 995 tissue and organ specimens from naturally and experimentally infected domestic animals. Using both direct plating and cold enrichment procedures, listeriae were isolated from 684 of 995 (68.7%) specimens, whereas 307 of 995 (30.8%) specimens required cold enrichment before the bacterium could be detected. Furthermore, cold enrichment failed to detect *Listeria* in only 4 of 684 (0.6%) samples that were previously positive by direct plating. A study by Ryser et al. (166) stressed the importance of cold enrichment for recovery of *L. monocytogenes* from cottage cheese manufactured from milk inoculated with the pathogen. Using direct plating, *L. monocytogenes* was recovered from 43 of 112 (38.4%) cottage cheese samples stored at 3°C for up to 28 days, whereas cold enrichment of the same samples in Tryptose Broth for up to 8 weeks led to recovery of listeriae from 59 of 112 (52.7%) samples. Thus, cold enrichment was necessary to detect the pathogen in 16 of 112 (14.3%) cheese samples. Ryser and Marth also found the cold enrichment procedure to be of great value for detecting low levels of *L. monocytogenes* in Cheddar (167), Camembert (168), and brick cheese (170) manufactured from pasteurized milk inoculated with the bacterium.

Despite proven success of the cold enrichment procedure for nearly 40 years, the mechanism by which numbers of *L. monocytogenes* are enhanced during prolonged incubation at 4°C is not fully understood. While cold enrichment exploits the psychrotrophic nature of *L. monocytogenes* and simultaneously suppresses growth of indigenous nonpsychrotrophic organisms, Gray and Killinger (79) indicated that, at times, growth of *Listeria* was too rapid to attribute enhanced isolation of the pathogen to mere multiplication. When this procedure was first described in 1948, Gray et al. (82) suggested possible involvement of an inhibitory factor in bovine brain tissue that suppressed growth of competing organisms. However, this theory has been dispelled by subsequent studies in which enhancement of *Listeria* populations occurred during cold enrichment of such diverse samples as mouse liver (179), oat silage (78), feces (149), sewage (63), cabbage (85), raw milk (179), and cheese (166–168). A more plausible explanation is that degradation of somatic cells during cold enrichment leads to release of intracellular listeriae, which subsequently grow at 4°C. Experimental evidence indicates that sublethally injured listeria may be present in cottage cheese manufactured from skim milk inoculated with the pathogen (166). Thus repair of large numbers of injured cells during cold enrichment in nonselective media (i.e., Tryptose Broth, Nutrient Broth) followed by modest growth also could lead to higher than expected *Listeria* populations.

Over 20 different media formulations have been used successfully for cold-enriching various samples that were either naturally or artificially contaminated with *L. monocytogenes* (Table 6.1). Since incubation at 4°C is in itself partially selective for growth of *L. monocytogenes*, nonselective broths such as Tryptose Broth and Oxoid Nutrient Broth No. 2 (ONB2) rapidly emerged as media of choice, with Tryptose Broth generally recognized as being superior. In earlier studies, cold enrichment was used as the sole enrichment procedure and was followed by plating a portion of the enriched sample on Tryptose Agar at intervals during 2–12 months (172). Following incubation, plates were examined under oblique lighting for typical bluish-green, *Listeria*-like colonies.

Although growth of *L. monocytogenes* is favored at 4°C, other organisms including *Proteus*, *Hafnia*, *Pseudomonas*, enterococci, and certain lactic acid bacteria also can multiply in nonselective media at refrigeration temperatures (2), thus making detection of *Listeria* more difficult. To prevent non-*Listeria* organisms from overgrowing *L. monocytogenes*, investigators began adding inhibitory agents to various nonselective cold enrichment broths (Table 6.1). In 1972 Bojsen-Møller (21) recognized that addition of polymyxin B to Tryptose Phosphate Broth substantially reduced populations of gram-negative rods (i.e., *Escherichia coli*, *Pseudomonas aeruginosa*, and *Proteus* spp.) and enterococci, while at the same time allowing rapid growth of *L. monocytogenes*. Unfortunately, certain species of lactic acid bacteria resistant to polymyxin B can ferment lactose to lactic acid and reduce the pH to the point where *L. monocytogenes* fails to grow (pH < 5.0) at 4°C. Recent attempts at maintaining a pH of 7.2 by adding 0.1 M MOPS [3-(N-morpholino) propane sulfonic acid] to cold-enriched raw milk samples were unsuccessful (88). Hence, occasional neutralization of acid with sodium hydroxide may be necessary to increase recovery of *L. monocytogenes* from highly contaminated samples.

Recovery of *L. monocytogenes* also is enhanced when cold enrichment is used as a secondary enrichment, preceded by a selective primary warm enrichment, as shown in Fig. 6.1. Bannerman and Billie (11) cold-enriched numerous cheese and cheese factory environmental samples in FDA Enrichment Broth (secondary cold enrichment) that were previously incubated at 30°C for 48 h (primary warm enrichment). Their results for 96 *L. monocytogenes* isolates obtained by plating enrichments on two selective agars indicate that 34 and 62 of the isolates were obtained after warm and cold enrichment, respectively. Thus cold enrichment for 28 days resulted in a 64.6% (21/96) increase in recovery of *L. monocytogenes* from cheese and cheese factory samples. Despite substantial increases in environmental recovery of *L. monocytogenes*, the lengthy incubation period involved in cold enrichment makes this procedure impractical for use in routine regulatory analysis of food products.

SELECTIVE AGENTS

Modest, nonspecific nutritional requirements of *L. monocytogenes* have led to difficulties in formulating media that enhance growth of this pathogen. Consequently, efforts

Table 6.4 Ability of Two Enrichment Broths and Four Selective Plating Media
to Recover *L. monocytogenes* from 45 Artificially Contaminated Soft Cheeses
Manufactured in England

Selective plating media	Enrichment broths[a]	
	FDA Enrichment Broth[b]	UVM Broth[b]
FDA-MMLA	0/45	0/45
MMLA (Difco)	0/45	0/45
Merck Agar	3/45	5/45
Oxford Agar	36/45	38/45

[a]Both enrichment broths incubated at 30°C and sampled after 2 and 7 days with/without
KOH and after 1 day of secondary enrichment in the same broth.
[b]Number of samples in which *L. monocytogenes* was detected/number of samples analyzed.
Source: Adapted from Ref. 153.

have primarily focused on inhibition of the indigenous bacterial flora by taking advantage of the resistance of *L. monocytogenes* to various selective agents and antibiotics. While many inhibitory agents have proven to be at least somewhat useful for selective isolation of *L. monocytogenes* from naturally and artificially contaminated biological specimens (Table 6.4), others have demonstrated very little value when added to basal media (Table 6.5). Throughout the following discussion of selective agents, one must keep in mind that formulating media selective for *L. monocytogenes* is not a straightforward process, as many selective agents can partially inhibit growth of the pathogen, particularly when the organism is sublethally injured.

In 1950, Gray et al. (81) examined the potential of potassium tellurite and sodium azide as inhibitory agents in *Listeria*-selective media. Sodium azide prevented growth of *L. monocytogenes* in Tryptose Broth, whereas potassium tellurite was quite selective for the pathogen. However, shortly after these findings were published, Olson et al. (143) observed that potassium tellurite prevented growth of numerous *L. monocytogenes* strains. Substantiation of these findings by other investigators (102,106,120,129,155) has discouraged use of potassium tellurite as a *Listeria*-selective agent.

An outbreak of ovine listeriosis in Japan prompted Shimizu et al. (175) to investigate use of guanofuracin as a *Listeria*-selective agent. Uninhibited growth of *L. monocytogenes* was observed in 1% glucose nutrient broth and 5% sheep blood agar containing 0.01 and 0.0083% guanofuracin, respectively, whereas at the same time, growth of gram-negative rods, spore formers, β-hemolytic streptococci, and staphylococci was completely inhibited. However, α-hemolytic streptococci and enterococci grew in this medium. Although the selective and differential characteristics of this medium were reportedly enhanced by adding 0.01% potassium tellurite, the inhibitory effects of this compound against *L. monocytogenes*, combined with continued difficulties in distinguishing colonies of *Listeria* from other microbial contaminants, have generally led to abandonment of this medium by most investigators (172).

Using the combination of phenylethanol and lithium chloride (Table 6.6), McBride and Girard (129) succeeded in amplifying numbers of *L. monocytogenes* in the presence of gram-negative bacteria. The usefulness of phenylethanol and lithium chloride as *Listeria*-

selective agents has since been confirmed by other investigators to the point where McBride Listeria Agar, which contains these agents, became a widely accepted plating medium for *L. monocytogenes* (49,65,83,85,88,118,122,129,167,168,179). A modification of McBride Listeria Agar (omission of sheep blood and addition of cycloheximide as an antifungal agent) is currently recommended by the FDA for analyzing food samples suspected of harboring listeriae (122,123). Through personal experience, it was found that increasing the lithium chloride concentration to 0.5% [0.05% lithium chloride in the original formulation (129)] increased selectivity of the medium without appreciably decreasing recovery of healthy listeriae (169,170,194).

Several early studies found that addition of potassium thiocyanate to nonselective media enhanced recovery of *L. monocytogenes* by inhibiting a portion of the background microflora. However, more recently researchers (106,120,155) demonstrated partial inhibition of *L. monocytogenes* by potassium thiocyanate. Kramer and Jones (106)

Table 6.5 Selective Agents Unsatisfactory for Recovery of
Listeria when Added to Basal Media

Agent	Concentration (%)
Acetic acid	0.1
Bile	0.1
Boric acid	0.1
Potassium cyanide	0.1
Sodium azide	0.01
Sodium chloride	5
2-3-5 Triphenyltetrazolium chloride	0.005
Acid fuchsin	0.001
Aniline blue	0.001
Bismarck brown	0.001
Brilliant green	0.001
Crystal violet	0.000005
Malachite green	0.001
Methyl green	0.001
Neutral red	0.001
Soluble blue	0.001
Aminoguanidine	NG[a]
Benzyl chloride	NG
Ethyl alcohol	NG
Guanidine hydrochloride	NG
Lysozyme	NG
Sodium phenobarbital	NG
Sodium thiosulfate	NG
Rhamnose + phenyl red	NG

[a]Not given.
Source: Refs. 106, 129.

Table 6.6 Partial List of Inhibitory Agents used in *Listeria*-Selective Media

Agent	Concentration/L	Microorganisms inhibited	Ref.
Acriflavine	10 mg	gram-positives including *Lactobacillus bulgaricus* and *Streptococcus thermophilus*	176
Bacitracin	5000 IU	gram-positives	144
Cefotetan	4–8 mg	*Staphylococcus aureus*	39
Ceftazidime	50 mg	broad spectrum	39, 123
Colistin	20 mg	gram-negatives	184
Cycloheximide	50 mg	fungi	14,122
Fosfomycin	64-512 mg	broad spectrum including *Staphylococcus aureus*	39, 184
Furacin	10 mg	*Escherichia coli, Micrococcus* spp.	129
Laxamoxef	4 mg	*Staphylococcus aureus*	39
Lithium chloride	0.5 g	gram-negatives, except *Pseudomonas* spp.	106,129
Moxalactam	20 mg	broad spectrum	114,118
Nalidixic acid	40 mg	gram-negatives except *Pseudomonas* and *Proteus* spp.	184
Oxolinic acid	15–20 mg	broad spectrum	184
Phenylethanol	2.5 ml	gram-negatives and *Proteus* spp.	106, 129
Polymyxin B	16,000 IU	gram-negatives, including *Pseudomonas* spp., some gram-positives	21, 176
Potassium tellurite	0.5 g	gram-negatives	228, 257
Potassium thiocyanate	3.75 g	most gram-negatives; also *Bacillus* spp. and coryneforms	241
Propolis	15 mg	gram-positives including *Staphylococcus* and *Streptococcus*	261, 236
Rivanol	25 mg	*Staphylococcus, Streptococcus,* and *Pseudomonas* spp.	265
Thallous acetate	0.2 g	gram-negatives	230
Trypaflavine	40 mg	gram-positive cocci	184, 246, 255

postulated that the thiocyanate ion interferes with *Listeria* growth by binding to iron-containing proteins of the cytochrome system. Controversy surrounding effects of potassium thiocyanate also has served to decrease use of this compound in *Listeria*-selective media.

Beerens and Tahon-Castel (15) were first to report the usefulness of nalidixic acid in isolating *L. monocytogenes* from heavily contaminated pathological specimens. Increased numbers of *Listeria* isolations using media containing nalidixic acid primarily resulted from inhibition of indigenous gram-negative bacteria (77). Benefits of adding nalidixic acid to otherwise noninhibitory media were soon confirmed in many laboratories (97,102,145,158,174). Nalidixic acid has since been recognized as one of the most important selective agents and is now used alone or more commonly in combination with other selective agents (i.e., trypaflavine) for isolating *L. monocytogenes* from food and clinical specimens.

Despite successful use of nalidixic acid, Ralovich et al. (159,160) found that certain gram-positive cocci and gram-negative rods grew in the presence of the chemical and created difficulties during attempted isolation of *L. monocytogenes*. Such difficulties led to inclusion of trypaflavine, a known inhibitor of gram-positive cocci, to media containing nalidixic acid. The end result was the selective inhibition of virtually all other bacteria, while growth of *L. monocytogenes* was only slightly decreased (19,143). Additional work revealed that contaminating organisms, predominantly streptococci, grew infrequently on clear media containing both antibiotics and were generally discernible from *L. monocytogenes* with the naked eye. Confirmation of these findings in other European laboratories (20,55,83,99,145,173) has led to widespread use of trypaflavine/nalidixic acid as *Listeria*-selective agents.

In 1972 Seeliger (173) reported that the combined use of acriflavine and nalidixic acid greatly suppressed gram-negative organisms and fecal streptococci without apparently affecting recovery of *L. monocytogenes*. These findings were subsequently confirmed by Bockemühl et al. (20) and others (3,64). In 1984, Rodriguez et al. (163) reported developing a blood agar medium supplemented with acriflavine and nalidixic acid (Rodriguez Isolation Medium—Table 6.3) that was far superior to the earlier formulations of Ralovich et al. (158,160). During the past several years, numerous media containing acriflavine and nalidixic acid with or without other antibiotics have been proposed for selective isolation/enrichment of listeriae from food and environmental samples, including Merck Listeria Agar (25,86,87), which is commercially available in Europe. Additionally, Fraser Broth (68) is a newly developed enrichment medium.

During the early 1950s, thallous acetate was employed as a selective agent for lactic acid bacteria; however, it was not until 1969 that Kramer and Jones (106) recommended the combined use of thallous acetate and nalidixic acid in *Listeria*-selective media. Three years later, Khan et al. (102) found that unlike potassium tellurite, thallous acetate used alone or together with nalidixic acid did not adversely affect recovery of *L. monocytogenes* from biological specimens and silage samples. In 1979, Leighton (120) demonstrated that the combined use of thallous acetate and nalidixic acid completely suppressed growth of *Escherichia coli* strains that were previously resistant to nalidixic acid. Greater inhibition of gram-positive bacteria also occurred when both selective agents were used together rather than separately. Although Leighton (120) recommended a medium composed of Tryptose Phosphate Broth, thallous acetate, and nalidixic acid for recovery of *L. monocytogenes* from mixed bacterial populations, thallous acetate (as well as potassium thiocyanate, potassium tellurite, and lithium chloride) altered the colonial morphology of *L. monocytogenes* from the smooth to the rough form. In view of this experience, most new formulations of *Listeria*-selective media omit thallous acetate.

In 1971, Despierres (43) reported that the combination of polymyxin B and nalidixic acid was useful to recover *L. monocytogenes* from feces, with these antibiotics preventing growth of many background organisms including *Streptococcus faecalis*. During the same year, Ortel (144) proposed another medium containing polymyxin B and bacitracin to isolate *L. monocytogenes* from stool samples. According to Bojsen-Møller (21), gram-negative rods and enterococci failed to grow in Tryptose Phosphate Broth containing polymyxin B, whereas growth of *L. monocytogenes* was relatively unaffected. After examining six different enrichment and isolation media, Rodriguez et al. (163) concluded that little if any benefit was gained by adding polymyxin B to media already containing nalidixic acid and acriflavine. More recently, Doyle and Schoeni (49) successfully isolated *L. monocytogenes* from milk, clinical, and fecal samples following enrichment in a selective broth containing polymyxin B, acriflavine, and nalidixic acid that was somewhat similar to Isolation Medium II developed by Rodriguez et al. (163). While the selective enrichment broth developed by Doyle and Schoeni has gained some attention (122), the necessity for polymyxin B in this medium remains somewhat questionable. Nevertheless, Siragusa and Johnson (176) isolated *L. monocytogenes* from yogurt using a medium containing polymyxin B, nalidixic acid and acriflavine. Their medium reportedly prevented growth of *Streptococcus thermophilus* and *Lactobacillus bulgaricus* and may therefore be particularly suitable for isolating *L. monocytogenes* from fermented dairy products.

Several additional inhibitory agents, including acridine, cycloheximide, propolis, ceftazidime, rivanol, and moxalactam, have enhanced recovery of *L. monocytogenes* from samples containing a mixed microbial flora. Bockemühl et al. (20) reported easy recovery of *L. monocytogenes* from enriched fecal samples using an agar medium that contained nalidixic acid and acridine dye. According to Gregorio et al. (83), use of nalidixic acid together with either acriflavine or trypaflavine gave rise to media that were equally inhibitory to background microflora, suggesting that similar results can be obtained by substituting acriflavine for trypaflavine. The FDA recommends inclusion of cycloheximide in Modified McBride Listeria Agar and FDA Enrichment Broth (123); the latter also contains nalidixic acid and trypaflavine as selective agents. Thus far both media have been successful in recovering *L. monocytogenes* from milk, dairy products, meat, poultry, vegetables, and seafood (226). Aspøy (6) discovered that *L. monocytogenes* was highly resistant to a rather curious substance known as propolis (the sticky secretion of honeybees used to cover the walls and crevices of their hives) as compared to other gram-positive bacteria, i.e., *Streptococcus viridans*, *Staphylococcus aureus*, and *Streptococcus agalactiae*. When propolis was combined with nalidixic acid, virtually all non-*Listeria* organisms were inhibited except *Pseudomonas aeruginosa* and a few fecal streptococci. Thus propolis eventually may prove to be a valuable additive to media for selective isolation of *L. monocytogenes*.

In 1976, Durst and Berencsi (53) found the combination of trypaflavine and nalidixic acid inhibitory to some strains of *L. monocytogenes* and suggested a new medium containing rivanol and nalidixic acid as selective agents. Growth of staphylococci and streptococci was virtually eliminated in media containing rivanol; however, Grønstøl and Aspøy (84) demonstrated that the combined use of rivanol and nalidixic acid failed to adequately inhibit growth of fecal streptococci in heavily contaminated samples containing *L. monocytogenes*. Addition of propolis and polymyxin B to the medium of Durst and Berencsi (53) substantially reduced growth of fecal streptococci and *Corynebacterium* spp. without appreciably affecting growth of *L. monocytogenes*.

Results from recent antibiotic susceptibility tests (144) led Lee and McClain (118) to add moxalactam (a broad-spectrum antibiotic that inhibits many gram-positive and gram-negative bacteria including *Staphylococcus*, *Proteus*, and *Pseudomonas*) to McBride Listeria Agar containing 0.25% phenylethanol and 0.5% lithium chloride. The result was a highly selective medium able to recover *L. monocytogenes* from inoculated samples of raw beef and many other foods. This medium, currently known as LPM Agar, is recommended by the USDA to isolate *L. monocytogenes* from raw meat and poultry (133) and also has been incorporated into the 1989 FDA procedure as a second selective plating medium.

A newly developed broth containing both acriflavine and nalidixic acid has recently replaced USDA Listeria Enrichment Broth II as the secondary enrichment broth of choice in the USDA procedure which is the method most widely used to recover *L. monocytogenes* from meat and poultry products (32).

Resistance of *L. monocytogenes* to cycloheximide prompted development of an enrichment broth that contains acriflavine and nalidixic acid in addition to cycloheximide. The FDA is now recommending this medium, known as FDA Enrichment Broth, for primary enrichment of milk, dairy, seafood, and vegetable products.

Bannerman and Billie (11) used Columbia Agar Base in combination with acriflavine and ceftazidime (AC Agar), a broad-spectrum cephalosporin antibiotic, to isolate *L. monocytogenes* from cheese samples. Their results indicated that AC Agar recovered approximately 50% more *L. monocytogenes* isolates than did the FDA-Modified McBride Listeria Agar. Except for a few enterococci, the combination of acriflavine and ceftazidime inhibited all organisms (i.e., *Enterobacteriaceae*, yeasts, and molds) other than *Listeria* spp. While these results appear promising, van Netten et al. (139) found that PALCAM agar, which contains polymyxin B and lithium chloride along with half or less the concentration of acriflavine and ceftazidime found in AC agar, was superior to the latter medium. After comparing 13 different plating media, these authors also concluded that media containing the combination of ceftazidime and 1.5% lithium chloride afforded more selectivity than did phenylethanol alone. However, increased selectivity will likely result in decreased recovery of stressed/sublethally injured cells that are frequently present in foods.

WARM ENRICHMENT

The principle of warm enrichment is based on selective inhibition of indigenous microflora through addition of inhibitory agents, while at the same time allowing unhindered growth of *Listeria*. Given the many months of incubation required for the cold enrichment procedure, the scientific community soon recognized the need to shorten the length of analysis. In 1950, Gray et al. (81) isolated *L. monocytogenes* from contaminated material that was inoculated into Nutrient Broth containing 0.5% potassium tellurite and incubated at 37°C for 6 to 8 hours before being plated on solid media. Even though subsequent studies showed that this broth is partially inhibitory to listeriae (102,120,143), Gray and his colleagues can still be credited with introducing both the first cold enrichment procedure and the first warm enrichment medium for selective isolation of *L. monocytogenes*. Since 1950, various combinations of the previously described selective agents (Table 6.6) have been added to basal media, i.e., Tryptose Broth, Oxoid Nutrient Broth No. 2, and Tryptose Phosphate Broth, to obtain media suitable for selective enrichment of *Listeria* at 30–37°C. Mavrothalassitis (128) reported an optimum incubation temperature of 30°C for enrichment of *L. monocytogenes* from heavily contaminated samples. Results from at least two additional studies (39,139) also showed that laboratory cultures of *L. monocytogenes*, *L. seeligeri*, and/or *L. ivanovii* were more susceptible to commonly used *Listeria* selective agents (i.e., ceftazidime, cefotetan, laxamoxef, and fosfomycin) when incubated at 37 rather than 30°C. Hence, most warm enrichments are now done at 30°C. As shown in Table 6.2, over 40 different formulations of warm enrichment media have been developed to isolate *L. monocytogenes* from naturally and artificially contaminated food, environmental, and clinical specimens. No doubt, additional formulations could be gathered from the literature and included in Table 6.2; however, such efforts would only add to the confusion already present.

As you will recall from our earlier discussion of selective agents, many warm enrichment broths, including the early formulation by Gray et al. (81), contain inhibitory substances now of questionable value. In 1961, Fuzi and Pillis (69) proposed a medium containing 0.35% potassium thiocyanate for selective enrichment of *L. monocytogenes*. Although some researchers have found potassium thiocyanate useful (55,119,174), others claim that this selective agent is at least somewhat inhibitory to *L. monocytogenes* (106,120,159). The importance of nalidixic acid as a *Listeria*-selective agent was first reported by Beerens and Tahon-Castel (15) in 1966 and was later confirmed by many investigators (20,55,97,102,144,158,174). Despite previous reports indicating partial inhibition of *L. monocytogenes* by potassium thiocyanate (106,120,159), other studies demonstrated that an enrichment broth containing this selective agent in combination with nalidixic acid was useful in isolating *L. monocytogenes* from cabbage (85), milk (88,179), and other dairy products (111). In 1972, Ralovich et al. (159) endorsed Levinthal's Broth and Holman's Medium, both of which contain nalidixic acid and trypaflavine, for selective enrichment of listeriae. Results obtained by Slade and Collins-Thompson (179) indicate that growth of *L. monocytogenes* in Oxoid Nutrient Broth No. 2 containing both nalidixic acid and potassium thiocyanate can be improved by adding acriflavine. Current selective media recommended by the FDA (123,125) and USDA (132,133) for enrichment of food samples containing *L. monocytogenes* are modifications of media proposed by Ralovich et al. (160) and Rodriguez et al. (163) as modified by Donnelly and Baigent (University of Vermont Medium) (46), respectively. Fraser Broth, which is a modification of USDA Listeria Enrichment Broth II (Table 6.2), was found to be advantageous in detecting *Listeria* sp. in enriched food samples. Since Fraser Broth turns black as a result of esculin hydrolysis after 48 hours of incubation when listeriae are present (26), this broth has now replaced USDA Listeria Enrichment Broth II as the preferred medium for secondary enrichment of meat and poultry samples handled according to the USDA procedure (32).

Studies have demonstrated that successful warm enrichment for listeriae is dependent upon both the type and level of indigenous microflora inherent in the sample. Hence, a given selective broth might not provide adequate enrichment of *L. monocytogenes* from samples of raw meat and cheese.

Despite recent efforts toward developing an effective enrichment medium for recovery of *L. monocytogenes* from food, none of the selective enrichment broths listed in Table 6.2 has proven to be totally reliable for analysis of food products containing *Listeria*. Nevertheless, several enrichment broths have moved to the forefront and include FDA Enrichment Broth as well as Fraser Broth and USDA Listeria Enrichment

Broths I and II, most of which are commercially available from BBL or Difco Laboratories in the United States. Truscott and McNab (189) developed a selective enrichment medium called Listeria Test Broth (LTB) (Table 6.2) as an alternative to the University of Vermont Medium [UVM (Table 62) formerly used in the USDA procedure] for detecting *L. monocytogenes* in meat products. After primary and/or secondary enrichment of 50 frozen ground beef samples in both enrichment broths, *L. monocytogenes* was detected in 19 of 50 (38%) and 16 of 50 (32%) samples using UVM and LTB, respectively. Although *Listeria* recovery rates for these two broths are not appreciably different, neither medium alone was able to detect the pathogen in all 29 of 50 (58%) samples that were positive. Finally, L-PALCAMY Broth (Table 6.2) which was developed by van Netten et al. (139) also appears promising for selective enrichment of noninjured listeriae with limited test results already showing that this medium is superior to USDA Listeria Enrichment Broths I and II as well as the Tryptose Broth–based antibiotic medium of Beckers et al. (14) (Table 6.2) for recovery of *L. monocytogenes* from naturally contaminated cheese, minced meat, fermented sausage, raw chicken, and mushrooms. However, given the wide variations in both the type and number of naturally occurring microbial contaminants present in our food supply, it appears unlikely that a single enrichment broth can ever be developed for truly optimal recovery of listeriae from all types of food.

Warm enrichment also can be used in various sequences, as illustrated in Fig. 6.1. As with cold enrichment, protocols have been developed in which warm enrichment precedes—primary enrichment (11)—or follows—secondary enrichment—cold enrichment (1,85,88,179). However, a single primary warm enrichment followed by plating a portion of the sample on one or more selective agar media is presently the most common method to analyze food samples. Currently, the FDA and USDA methods use a single primary warm enrichment and a primary followed by a secondary warm enrichment, respectively. The latter method, which currently includes secondary enrichment in Fraser Broth, provides a certain degree of pH control and may therefore be particularly suited for recovery of sublethally injured listeriae. A detailed description of these procedures will follow our discussion of selective plating media.

PLATING MEDIA

Isolation of *L. monocytogenes* from blood and CSF is a relatively simple procedure since such specimens are normally obtained under aseptic conditions. Provided that the pathogen is present in sufficient numbers, satisfactory results are typically obtained by directly plating a portion of the centrifuged sample on conventional noninhibitory media such as Tryptose Agar, Blood Agar, or Brain Heart Infusion Agar (2). Despite the relative ease with which *L. monocytogenes* can be isolated in pure culture from such specimens, early investigators were frustrated by their inability to recover the pathogen from clinical and pathological specimens containing a mixed microbial flora. Thus a need arose for a selective plating medium on which *L. monocytogenes* could be distinguished from normal background microorganisms.

Experimentation with the previously described selective agents has resulted in well over 70 different formulations for selective plating media to isolate *L. monocytogenes* from food, environmental, and clinical samples. Composition of these plating media and their intended use are given in Table 6.3. Although additional media formulations probably could be retrieved from the early literature, including such additional information in Table 6.3 would only add confusion to an area of *Listeria* research that has yet to be fully understood.

Efforts toward developing a satisfactory solid selective medium to isolate *L. monocytogenes* date back to 1950, just 2 years after introduction of the cold enrichment procedure. In that year, Gray et al. (81) recommended plating samples that were previously warm-enriched in Nutrient Broth containing 0.05% potassium tellurite on either Tryptose Agar or Tryptose Agar containing 0.05% potassium tellurite. Initially, this selective agar medium appeared to yield satisfactory results; however, further studies indicated that use of this medium was not always successful (102,120,143,155).

After discovering the benefits of adding nalidixic acid to enrichment broth (15), Ralovich et al. (158) effectively used serum agar containing nalidixic acid to isolate *L. monocytogenes* from feces, organs, and other clinical specimens. Although the background microbial flora was largely inhibited on this medium, occasionally streptococci and other nalidixic acid–resistant organisms persisted. Ralovich et al. (160) subsequently improved this medium by adding trypaflavine, which led to inhibition of virtually all non-*Listeria* organisms. This medium soon became known as Trypaflavine Nalidixic Acid Serum Agar (TNSA). Following successful use of this medium in many European studies (19,98,144,145,159), Ralovich et al. (155) endorsed TNSA as the plating medium of choice for isolating *L. monocytogenes* from contaminated materials. In 1974, Hofer (94) proposed using a medium prepared from Tryptose Agar containing nalidixic acid, trypaflavine, and thallous acetate. Trypaflavine can be replaced by other acridine dyes including xanthacridine, acriflavine, or proflavinehemisulfate (156). Based on results from European laboratories (44,54,98,156), a Serum or Blood Agar–based medium containing trypaflavine, acriflavine, and nalidixic acid appeared to be satisfactory for selective isolation of *L. monocytogenes* from samples containing a mixed microbial flora.

Despite the successful use of TNSA in many European studies, another selective medium, namely McBride Listeria Agar (MLA), has proven to be more suitable for isolating *L. monocytogenes* from mixed cultures. This medium, introduced by McBride and Girard (129) in 1960, was prepared from Phenylethanol Agar to which lithium chloride, glycine, and sheep blood were added. At least seven subsequent changes in the original formulation of MLA have led to considerable confusion as to the exact composition of this medium. Ironically, the first reported modification of MLA by Bearns and Girard (12) dates back to 1959, nearly 1 year before the original formulation appeared in the literature (129). This medium, named Modified McBride Medium (MLA2, Table 6.3) by the authors and known today as one of several Modified McBride Listeria Agars, is similar to the original formulation except that sheep blood is omitted and glycine anhydride is substituted for glycine; the anhydride reportedly is less inhibitory to *L. monocytogenes* than is glycine (118). With one exception (83), MLA2 has proven to be more *Listeria*-selective than Nalidixic Acid Agar (65,144), Acriflavine Nalidixic Acid Agar (179), or Acridine Nalidixic Acid Agar (65).

The previously mentioned 1986 report in which glycine was found to partially inhibit *L. monocytogenes* (118) prompted many individuals to prepare the various forms of McBride Listeria Agar with glycine anhydride, which is far less inhibitory to listeriae. Nevertheless, two widely used formulations of the original McBride Listeria Agar containing glycine have been commercially available since 1985 in the United States from Difco Laboratories and BBL. Although addition of blood provides a ready means of identifying possible *L. monocytogenes* colonies (virtually all are at least somewhat β-hemolytic) and enhances growth of the pathogen in certain B vitamin– and/or amino acid–deficient media, many individuals prefer to omit blood from the various formulations of McBride Listeria Agar and examine the plates under oblique illumination for blue to bluish-green *Listeria*-like colonies.

In 1987, Lovett et al. (125) added cycloheximide to blood-free MLA2 and named this particularly useful medium FDA-Modified McBride Listeria Agar (FDA-MMLA, Table 6.3). Although one earlier study claimed that TNSA was superior to MLA2, present data indicate that FDA-MMLA (123–125) and MLA2 (1,75,85,88,125,160,179), which contains glycine anhydride, are the McBride Listeria Agar formulations of choice for isolating *Listeria* spp. from food samples—particularly dairy, vegetable, and seafood products—with the FDA formulation serving as one of two plating media (the other being LPM Agar) in the widely used FDA procedure. However, late in 1990 the FDA modified its procedure by replacing FDA-MMLA with Oxford Agar.

The selectivity of MLA2 can be further improved, without affecting recovery of listeriae, by increasing the lithium chloride content to 0.5%. When used with sheep blood, this medium was more inhibitory to background microflora, and hence better suited than MLA2 for recovering *L. monocytogenes* from brick (170), feta (147), and blue cheese (148), as well as cold-pack cheese food (169). In 1986, Lee and McClain (118) added 4.5 g of lithium chloride and 20 mg of moxalactam to MLA2 and named their new medium LPM (Lithium Chloride-*P*henylethanol-*M*oxalactam) Agar. While this selective medium (commercially available in the United States from BBL and Difco Laboratories) is particularly well suited for isolating listeriae from raw meat and poultry as evidenced by its inclusion as the medium of choice in an earlier version of the USDA procedure, LPM Agar has since been replaced by Modified Oxford Listeria Agar (32) (Table 6.3), which produces black *L. monocytogenes* colonies, each with a black halo following 24 hours of incubation. However, as you will recall, LPM Agar was being used along with FDA-MMLA in the FDA procedure to isolate listeriae from dairy products, vegetables, and seafood. According to preliminary data obtained by Rico-Munoz (162), a modified version of LPM Agar called LPMX Agar, which is equally selective and also able to distinguish between xylose-fermenting (i.e., *L. ivanovii*, *L. welshimeri*, and *L. seeligeri*) and non–xylose-fermenting *Listeria* spp. (i.e., *L. monocytogenes*, *L. innocua*, *L. grayi*, and *L. murrayi*), will likely be more helpful to food microbiologists than the earlier nondifferential form of LPM Agar. Hence, it follows that LPMX Agar may eventually replace standard LPM Agar as the second medium of choice in the FDA procedure.

Interest in foodborne listeriosis during the 1980s has led to development of many additional *Listeria*-selective media for examination of milk and dairy products. In 1984, Martin et al. (126) developed Gum Base Nalidixic Acid Medium (GBNA)—a synthetic agar-free solid medium (Table 6.3) superior to the Modified McBride Listeria Agar of Bearns and Girard (12) for isolation of *L. monocytogenes* from raw milk (88). Bailey et al. (9) also found that a modified version of this medium containing lithium chloride and moxalactam (Table 6.3) was suitable for isolating *L. monocytogenes* from raw chicken. According to a 1988 report by Bannerman and Billie (11), a Trypticase Soy Agar–based medium containing acriflavine and ceftazidime (known as AC Agar) was superior to FDA-MMLA (123,125) for recovery of *L. monocytogenes* from soft cheese and cheese factory environments. The following year Siragusa and Johnson (176) described a medium containing nalidixic acid, acriflavine, and polymyxin B that inhibited lactic acid bacteria commonly found in yogurt, and at the same time permitted excellent growth of *L. monocytogenes*. A selective agar medium (85) based on the enrichment broth of Doyle and Schoeni (49), from which acriflavine was omitted and Fe^{3+} was added, compared favorably to the original formulation of McBride Listeria Agar (129). Supplementation of selective (85) and nonselective media (35) with Fe^{3+} enhances growth of *L. monocytogenes* and may be beneficial for isolating sublethally injured cells from food samples containing a mixed microbial flora.

Attempts to isolate *L. monocytogenes* from food products have focused on enhancing the selectivity of currently available blood-free plating media which are normally viewed under oblique illumination, as well as development of alternative media that incorporate differential agents other than blood to aid microbiologists in identifying *Listeria* colonies in mixed cultures. In 1987, Buchanan et al. (27) found the combination of moxalactam, nalidixic acid, and bacitracin effective in allowing growth of *Listeria* spp. while preventing growth of most other foodborne organisms, including micrococci and streptococci. These selective agents were used to formulate Modified Vogel Johnson Agar (MVJ) (Table 6.3) on which *L. monocytogenes* colonies appear entirely black (reduction of tellurite) on a red background (unable to use mannitol). Thus suspected *Listeria* colonies could be readily identified on MVJ without using oblique illumination. Addition of the same three selective agents to the Modified McBride Listeria Agar of Bearns and Girard (12) resulted in Agricultural Research Service Modified McBride Listeria Agar (ARS-MMLA, Table 6.3) which could be used in conjunction with oblique lighting to quantitate *Listeria* in a wide range of milk, dairy, and meat samples. In a subsequent study, Buchanan et al. (29) found MVJ was slightly superior to ARS-MMLA for recovery of *L. monocytogenes* from inoculated samples of milk, dairy products, meat, and coleslaw. Although ARS-MMLA was more selective than MVJ, the black *Listeria*-like colonies that appeared on MVJ were more readily discernible. Initial comparisons of ARS-MMLA and MVJ with LPM Agar indicated that both new media functioned well. In a follow-up study, Buchanan et al. (28) assessed the ability of MVJ and LPM Agar to detect listeriae in retail samples of raw meat, fish, and shellfish. *Listeria* populations were generally too low to be detected by direct plating on either medium. However, using a three-tube/24-hour MPN method employing USDA Listeria Enrichment Broth I (Table 6.2), comparable isolation rates were obtained using both MVJ and LPM Agar. Once again, the differential nature of MVJ proved to be extremely useful for selecting colonies though to be *Listeria* spp.

In 1988, van Netten et al. (43) reported that RAPAMY Agar, a modification of TNSA developed by Ralovich et al. (160) (*R*) that includes acriflavine (*A*), phenylethanol (*P*), aesculin (*A*), mannitol (*M*), and egg yolk emulsion (*Y*) (Table 6.3), was suitable for enumeration of *Listeria* spp. Virtually identical populations were observed when overnight broth cultures of *L. monocytogenes*, *L. seeligeri*, and *L. ivanovii* were surface-plated on RAPAMY and a nonselective agar, with growth of all non-*Listeria* organisms tested, except *Streptococcus faecalis* and *Streptococcus faecium*, completely inhibited on the selective medium. Like Oxford Listeria Agar (40) and nearly 10 other plating media listed in Table 6.3, RAPAMY Agar also gave rise to distinctive black *Listeria* colonies that were surrounded by a dense black halo from esculin hydrolysis. While such characteristic colonies were present against a deep red background (nonuse of mannitol) on RAPAMY Agar, *S. faecalis* and *S. faecium* generally produced colonies with blue-green halos. Although attempts to completely eliminate growth of these two species of enterococci by adding cefoxitin (moxalactam) to this medium failed, preliminary results indicate that RAPAMY Agar can be used to detect and quantify *Listeria* spp. in thermally processed and dried foods that have a total aerobic plate count of $\leq 10^6$ CFU/g and an enterococcus count of $\leq 10^2$ CFU/g. However, as might be expected, high populations of enterococci severely hampered detection of *Listeria* spp. in chicken parts, minced meat, and mold-ripened cheese.

Further attempts by van Netten et al. (136) to eliminate growth of enterococci by adding fosfomycin (20 mg/L) to RAPAMY Agar met with only limited success. Addition of lithium chloride (1.5%) to RAPAMY Agar inhibited many *Listeria* spp.; however, an improved selective and differential medium was obtained when lithium chloride was added to RAPAMY Agar and nalidixic acid was omitted. The resultant medium was named ALPAMY Agar (Table 6.3)—*A*criflavine–*L*ithium chloride–*P*henylethanol–*A*esculin–*M*annitol–Egg *Y*olk emulsion agar. In a study with pure cultures, ALPAMY Agar allowed uninhibited growth of all 10 *L. monocytogenes* strains tested but completely prevented growth of single strains of *L. seeligeri* and *L. ivanovii*. Selectivity tests indicated that ALPAMY Agar supported growth of only 2 of 41 non-*Listeria* organisms—one strain each of *Staphylococcus aureus* and *Micrococcus* sp., both of which could be readily differentiated from *Listeria* colonies. Subsequent studies indicate that ALPAMY Agar is far superior to RAPAMY Agar for detecting listeriae in raw milk and soft cheeses manufactured from raw milk, as well as raw vegetables and chicken.

Farber et al. (62) developed an improved *Listeria*-selective plating medium by combining the positive attributes of McBride Listeria Agar and LPM Agar. In their preliminary formula for "Farber Listeria Agar" (Table 6.3), oxolinic acid was substituted for nalidixic acid. Both agents function by interfering with the activity of DNA gyrase, an enzyme needed to maintain proper DNA structure and resealing of chromosomal nicks (77). Current attempts at improving this formulation are centering around addition of carbohydrates (i.e., glucose and cellobiose) and low levels of acriflavine, along with adjustment of the levels of other selective agents.

As shown in Fig. 6.1, most plating media discussed thus far can be used to isolate listeriae directly from a sample as well as after one or more warm and/or cold enrichments in an appropriate broth. Following inoculation, all plates are normally incubated aerobically at 30–37°C. Plates containing popular selective media such as FDA-MMLA, LPM Agar, and Modified Oxford Agar normally are incubated for 48 hours, whereas plates containing pure or near-pure cultures of *Listeria* on nonselective media can generally be examined after 24 hours. Since growth of *L. monocytogenes* is reportedly enhanced under conditions of reduced oxygen (172), inoculated plates (49,136,138,166–168,170) as well as warm enrichment broths (49) have been incubated under microaerobic conditions (5% O_2:10% CO_2:85% N_2). Although microaerobic incubation may favor recovery of injured and/or stressed cells from food, such incubation conditions are not

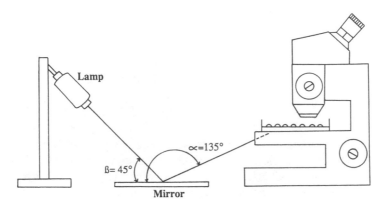

Figure 6.2 Oblique illumination technique developed by Henry (91). Angles of reflected light (β) and transillumination (α) equal 45°and 135°, respectively.

routinely available in many laboratories. Therefore, all but one current protocol for *Listeria*-testing allows samples to be incubated aerobically.

Except for a few recently developed plating media that contain esculin, xylose, mannitol, or other differential agents, most remaining formulations of *Listeria*-selective plating media can be classified into one of two categories based on presence or absence of blood. Recognition of *Listeria*-like colonies on blood-free media such as MMLA, TNSA, and GBNA is greatly facilitated when colonies are observed under oblique illumination with a binocular scanning microscope. Using the Henry technique (91) in which plates are examined under white light transmitted obliquely through the medium at an angle of 45° (Fig. 6.2), listeriae colonies appear as small, round, finely textured, bluish green to bluish gray with an entire margin. In 1984, Martin et al. (126) compared the appearance of *L. monocytogenes* on Nalidixic Acid Agar and Tryptone Soya Gum Base Nalidixic Acid Medium and found that the uniformly transparent nature of the gum-based medium greatly enhanced the bluish-green color of *Listeria* colonies when observed with oblique illumination as described by Henry (91). After observing that the angle of transillumination in the Henry method was 135° (Fig. 6.2), Lachica (109) found that the bluish-green hue of *Listeria* colonies was more easily observed if plates were viewed from the backside at an angle of 45° with a 5× magnification hand lens while colonies were directly illuminated with a high intensity beam of light that traveled perpendicular to the bench surface(β = 135°, Fig. 6.3). This latter method appears to have eliminated many of the problems (i.e., reproducibility and convenience) that have been associated with the traditional technique developed by Henry (91) nearly 60 years ago. However, with enough experience, either of these two procedures can readily differentiate probable *Listeria* colonies from background organisms on even heavily contaminated plates.

As you will recall, *Listeria* spp.including *L. monocytogenes* can hydrolyze esculin. However, while black *Listeria* colonies can be obtained by adding esculin and ferric citrate to suitable selective media (46,48), esculin hydrolysis is by no means unique to listeriae and is therefore of only limited value. Incorporation of potassium tellurite into selective media also results in black colonies of *L. monocytogenes*. Unlike the typical black-yellowish and gray colonies produced by gram-positive cocci, the marginal zone of *Listeria* colonies appears green when the organism is grown on media containing potassium tellurite and viewed with oblique illumination (172).

As you will recall, addition of blood to solid media also can be used to differentiate listeriae, including *L. monocytogenes*, from other microorganisms. When grown on media containing blood, such as McBride Listeria Agar, *L. monocytogenes* colonies are typically surrounded by a narrow zone of β-hemolysis. In some instances, β-hemolytic activity is so weak that the clearing zone cannot be observed until the colony is gently wiped from the agar surface. In 1989, Blanco et al. (18) proposed overlaying previously inoculated plates of blood-free *Listeria* selective agar with a thin layer of blood agar so that the β-hemolytic activity associated with pathogenic listeriae could be directly observed after reincubation of the plates. According to these authors, hemolysis was more readily observed using this procedure than when blood was incorporated into plating media before incubation. However, further work using highly contaminated samples such as raw milk showed that the success of this procedure was primarily dependent upon the selectivity of the initial plating medium with highly selective media yielding the best results. Recognizing the usefulness of this blood overlay technique, USDA officials (32) are currently (early 1990) recommending that this procedure be used with blood-free nonselective agar (i.e., Columbia Blood Agar Base) to determine hemolytic activity of purified *Listeria* strains isolated from meat and poultry products.

Through personal experience, we have found that colonies of *L. monocytogenes* can be easily recognized when plates of blood-containing media are examined from the reverse side, as shown in Fig. 6.4. In this method, light from a 60-watt bulb strikes a concave mirror at an angle of 45° and is reflected up into the culture plate. When the back side of the plate is viewed with the unaided eye, *L. monocytogenes* colonies characteristically have a small opaque or darkened center with a bright area of β-hemolysis

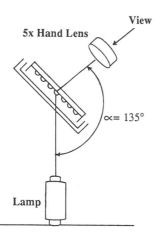

Figure 6.3   Modified Henry technique developed by Lachica (109). Angle of transillumination (β) equals 135°.

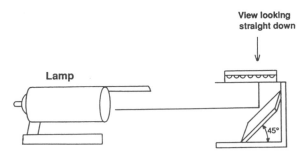

Figure 6.4 Examination of *Listeria* colonies on media containing blood.

underneath the colony which may or may not extend just beyond the margin. All such colonies appear to "light up" when viewed in this manner. In contrast, colonies formed by gram-positive cocci and other contaminants generally lack the light area underneath the colony and appear uniformly opaque. In addition, non-*Listeria* contaminants from cheese samples often show pronounced β- or α-hemolysis on McBride Listeria Agar, which can aid in differentiating these colonies from those formed by *L. monocytogenes*. With practice, a single colony of *L. monocytogenes* can be easily recognized on a plate containing several hundred or more non-*Listeria* contaminants; however, it is imperative that the plates be poured thin (~10–12 ml medium/plate) to allow sufficient illumination.

When confronted with the list of selective plating media in Table 6.3, it is easy to understand why many food microbiologists are confused as to the best medium to use for isolating *Listeria* from a particular food product. In an attempt to ease this confusion, Golden et al. (74), Hao et al. (85), and Cassiday et al. (33) collectively compared 20 selective plating media for their ability to recover uninjured cells of *L. monocytogenes* from samples of pasteurized milk, Brie cheese, ice cream mix, raw cabbage, dry-cured/country-cured ham, and/or raw oysters inoculated to contain approximately 10^2, 10^4, and 10^6 *L. monocytogenes* CFU/g or ml. The combined results of their efforts are in Table 6.7. GBNTSM, MLA2, FDA-MMLA, and MDA were consistently superior to nine other media used by Golden et al. (74) for enumeration of all three inoculum levels of listeriae in samples of pasteurized milk and ice cream mix by direct plating. Ability to recover low levels of listeriae from both products was facilitated by the lack of significant levels of non-*Listeria* contaminants. Five of the 14 plating media used in this study failed to recover *L. monocytogenes* from inoculated samples of pasteurized milk as well as Brie cheese and were therefore omitted for analysis of ice cream and raw cabbage. Examination of Brie cheese containing approximately 10^2 and 10^4 *L. monocytogenes* CFU/g indicated that none of the nine remaining direct plating media were sufficiently selective to prevent overgrowth of listeriae by molds, yeasts, and gram-positive cocci. Despite these inherent difficulties in detecting small numbers of *Listeria*, MRIM III, MLA2, FDA-MLA, and MDA were judged to be satisfactory when Brie cheese contained ≥10^6 listeriae CFU/g. However, subsequent results from the same laboratory (34) indicate that LPM Agar was superior to these four media for recovery of *L. monocytogenes* from Brie cheese. With raw cabbage, enumeration of *Listeria* was a problem only at the lowest inoculum level where large populations of microbial contaminants (i.e., gram-positive and gram-negative rods as well as gram-positive cocci)

Table 6.7 Comparison of Plating Media for Enumeration of *L. monocytogenes* in Inoculated Food Samples

Media	Pasteurized milk	Brie cheese	Ice cream mix	Raw cabbage	Dry-cured ham	Country-cured ham	Raw oysters
Bind's Acriflavine Agar	NG^a	NG	NT^b	NT	NT	NT	NT
Brackett and Beuchat Selective Enrichment Agar	V^c	V	V	V	NT	NT	NT
Modified Rodriguez Isolation Medium III (MRIM III)	V	+^{e}	V	V	–^{d}	+	+
University of Vermont Agar (UVA)	V	V	V	+	–	+	–
Doyle & Schoeni Selective Enrichment Agar (DSSEA)	NG	NG	NT	+/NT	NT	NT	NT
DSSEA + ferric citrate (0.219 g)	NG	NG	NT	+/NT	NT	NT	NT
DSSEA + acriflavine + ferric citrate (0.219 g)	NT	NT	NT	+	NT	NT	NT
DSSEA + acriflavine + sheep blood	NT	NT	NT	V	NT	NT	NT
FDA Enrichment Broth + agar (15 g)	NT$_f$	NT	++	+	–	–	V
Gum Base Nalidixic Acid Tryptose Soya Medium (GBNTSM)	++$_f$	+	+	+	NT	NT	NT
Gum Base Nalidixic Acid Medium (GBNA)	NT	NT$_f$	+	V	NT	NT	–
LPM Agar (LPM)	+	++$_f$	+	++	++	++	–
Modified Listeria Transport Enrichment Broth (MLTEB)	NG	NG	NT	NT	NT	NT	NT
Modified McBride Listeria Agar II (MLA2)	+	+$_f$	+	+	–	NT	V
MLA2 + sheep blood	NT	NT	NT	V	NT	NT	NT
ARS-Modified McBride Listeria Agar (ARS-MMLA)	–	–	–	–	NT	NT	NT
FDA-Modified McBride Listeria Agar (FDA-MMLA)	+	+	+	+	+	V	V
Modified Despierres Agar (MDA)	+	+	+	+	+	V	–
Modified Vogel-Johnson Agar (MVJ)	–	–	–	–	V	+	+
Thiocyanate Nalidixic Acid Agar (TNAA)	V	V	V	V	–	–	–
TNAA + glucose (10 g) + ferric citrate (0.219 g)	NT	NT	NT	+	NT	NT	NT
Trypaflavine Nalidixic Acid Serum Agar (TNSA)	NG	NG	NT	NT	NT	NT	NT
Tryptose Blood Agar + glucose (5 g) (TBAG)	V	V	V	V	–	–	–

^{a}No growth.
^{b}Not tested.
^{c}Variable results.
^{d}Not recommended.
^{e}Growth.
^{f}Strongly recommended.
See Table 6.3 for composition of plating media.
Source: Adapted from Refs. 33, 34, 74, 85.

typically interfered with recovery. At the two higher inoculum levels, *L. monocytogenes* could be readily quantitated by directly plating cabbage samples on MDA, GBNTSM, and MLA2. However, this same investigative team (34) later obtained even better results using LPM Agar.

One year earlier, Hao et al. (85) successfully recovered *L. monocytogenes* from inoculated samples of cabbage using GBNA, DSSEA, DSSEA + ferric citrate, DSSEA + acriflavine + ferric citrate, TNAA + glucose + ferric citrate, and MLA2, but concluded that DSSEA + acriflavine + ferric citrate and MLA2 outperformed the other media tested (Table 6.7). When results from the previous three studies are combined, LPM Agar, GBNTSM, MLA2, FDA-MMLA, and MDA generally emerged as the plating media of choice for detecting uninjured listeriae in dairy and vegetable products. Overall, these findings agree with those of at least four other studies (70,90,111,121) in which LPM Agar outperformed other popular plating media including FDA-MMLA, RIM III, and/or MVJA for recovery of *L. monocytogenes* from raw milk, ice cream, yogurt, soft cheese, and/or vegetables inoculated with the pathogen. In addition, Rodriguez et al. (164) found that RIM III containing 6 rather than 12 g of acriflavine hydrochloride (Table 6.3) did better than the original formulation of McBride Listeria Agar for isolating *L. monocytogenes* in artificially contaminated raw milk and hard cheese. While the best media for recovering listeriae from dairy products and vegetables remain to be defined, FDA-MMLA and LPM Agar appear to be the present plating media of choice in the United States for selective isolation of listeriae from such products as evidenced by their inclusion in an FDA procedure (89,124). Since late 1990, Oxford Agar has replaced FDA-MMLA in the FDA procedure.

Since there are inherent differences between the natural microflora found in various types of food, one can easily surmise that *Listeria*-selective plating media best suited for dairy products and vegetables might be somewhat less than ideal for analysis of meat, poultry, and seafood. Consequently, Cassiday et al. (33) went on to evaluate 10 selective plating media for their ability to enumerate *L. monocytogenes* in artificially contaminated dry- and country-cured ham as well as raw oysters. According to their results (Table 6.7), MDA, FDA-MMLA, and LPM Agar generally recovered approximately equal numbers of uninjured listeriae from dry-cured ham. However, ease in differentiating *L. monocytogenes* colonies from those formed by background contaminants led these authors to recommend LPM Agar for analysis of dry-cured ham. Not surprisingly, LPM Agar also was equal or superior to three other plating media (i.e., MRIM III, MVJA, and UVA) that were deemed acceptable for isolating listeriae from country-cured ham. Unlike both types of ham, high populations of indigenous microflora in raw oysters made detection of listeriae on virtually all 10 plating media extremely difficult. While MRIM III and MVJA supported less growth of listeriae than other marginally acceptable plating media including MLA2, FDA-MMLA, and GBNTSM, MRIM III and MVJA were somewhat more reliable for differentiating *L. monocytogenes* from background contaminants. Therefore, these authors hesitantly recommended MRIM III and MVJA for examination of raw oysters.

Several less extensive studies also have dealt with the ability of various plating media to recover listeriae from meat, poultry, and seafood. According to a 1988 report by Loessner et al. (121), recognition of *L. monocytogenes* in inoculated samples of raw ground beef and scallops was only possible using LPM Agar. Among the three other plating media tested, RIM III and the original formulation of McBride Listeria Agar proved to be insufficiently selective, whereas MVJA was inhibitory to the *L. monocytogenes* strain tested. Unlike these findings, results of Garayzabal and Genigeorgis (70) indicated that LPM Agar and RIM III were acceptable for detecting listeriae in raw meat with both media superior to FDA-MMLA. Working at the USDA, Buchanan et al. (30) also found that LPM Agar and MVJA generally gave comparable recovery of listeriae from naturally contaminated samples of fresh meat, cured meat, poultry, fish, and shellfish. However, presence of both tellurite and mannitol as differential agents in MVJA greatly aided in differentiating *Listeria* colonies from those formed by naturally occurring contaminants including various species of enterococci and staphylococci. In the only other comparative study of *Listeria*-selective media thus far reported, Bailey et al. (9) found that LPM Agar and GBNA fortified with lithium chloride and moxalactam were both superior to unfortified GBNA and McBride Listeria Agar for recovering *L. monocytogenes* as well as other *Listeria* spp. from naturally contaminated raw poultry.

Throughout the previous discussion, we indicated that most investigators found LPM Agar to be among the most useful plating media for selective isolation of listeriae from meat and poultry products. Since this medium was originally developed by USDA officials for such purposes, it is not surprising that LPM Agar was soon recognized as the plating medium of choice in the USDA procedure which has since become the unofficial "standard method" for detecting listeriae in meat and poultry products. However, in May of 1989 USDA officials changed the plating medium in the USDA procedure to Modified Oxford agar, a medium of similar selectivity on which *Listeria* colonies appear black from esculin hydrolysis, thus eliminating the need for Henry's technique to differentiate blue to bluish-green *Listeria* colonies from those formed by other organisms.

While the FDA procedure, employing both FDA-MMLA and LPM Agar, has been used by many persons to isolate listeriae from fish and shellfish, the suitability of these *Listeria*-selective agars in relation to other frequently used plating media has not yet been determined. However, with the current (1990) interest in *Listeria*-contaminated seafood, it appears likely that results from studies designed to address this question will soon be reported. Future studies in which recovery of *L. monocytogenes* from different types of food is compared using a variety of selective plating media will no doubt serve a critical role in establishing suitable plating media to detect and enumerate listeriae in particular foods. However, since it is unlikely that any one selective medium can optimally recover uninjured (or injured) cells of *L. monocytogenes* from all types of food, various isolation media may well have to be tailor-made to detect *Listeria* in particular foods or food groups. Once this has been done, these selective plating media can be used to determine the ability of uninjured *Listeria* cells to grow in different selective broths during warm enrichment of various food samples. Results from such studies may lead to development of various detection and isolation schemes which could then be accurately reviewed and adopted as a series of true "standard methods" for enumeration of uninjured listeriae in different foods or food groups. Despite these rather optimistic projections, it should be remembered that many *Listeria* cells present in food are likely to be sublethally injured, and probably would be unable to grow on or in selective media. The suitability of various selective plating media to detect and enumerate sublethally injured cells of *L. monocytogenes* will be discussed shortly.

PROPOSED METHODS FOR ISOLATING *L. MONOCYTOGENES* FROM FOOD

Despite the usefulness of Gray's time-honored cold enrichment procedure (82), several food-related listeriosis outbreaks during the 1980s emphasized the need for more rapid detection of *L. monocytogenes* in food. The logical approach was to use some of the previously described enrichment broths containing selective agents and to incubate samples at an elevated temperature, generally 30°C. In response to numerous requests from the food industry, several one- and two-stage enrichment schemes have been developed that include both primary warm or cold enrichment followed by secondary warm or cold enrichment.

An outbreak of listeriosis supposedly linked to consumption of pasteurized milk (66) led Hayes et al. (88) to develop the multiple two-stage enrichment procedure outlined in Fig. 6.5 for isolating *L. monocytogenes* from raw milk. Primary cold enrichment in Oxoid Nutrient Broth No. 2 (ONB2) followed by secondary warm enrichment in ONB2 containing KSCN and nalidixic acid and plating on GBNA yielded the highest number of positive milk samples. No statistically significant difference in recovery of listeriae was observed using either Stuart Transport Medium or selective enrichment broth containing potassium thiocyanate and nalidixic acid. Although 15 milk samples were

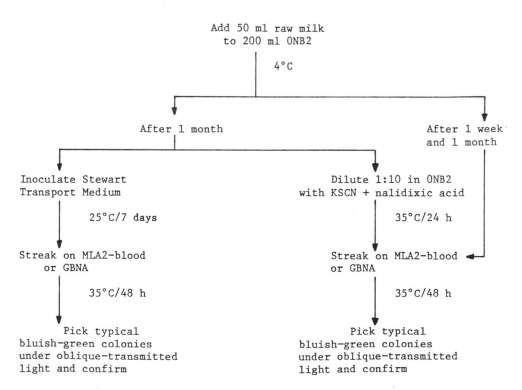

Figure 6.5 Multiple two-stage enrichment procedure for isolating *L. monocytogenes* from raw milk (88).

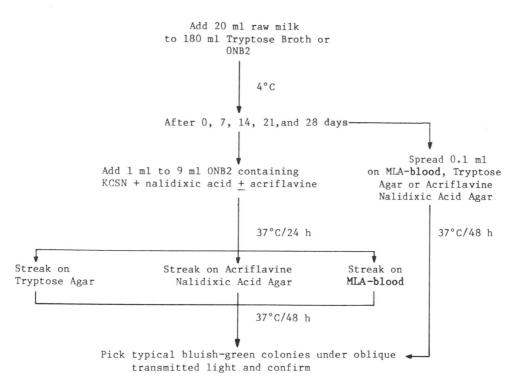

Figure 6.6 Two-stage enrichmnet procedure for isolating *L. monocytogenes* from raw milk (240).

positive when plated on GBNA medium as compared to 11 on MLA2 without blood, the difference was not statistically significant. The authors concluded that primary cold enrichment in ONB2 followed by secondary warm enrichment in selective broth and plating on GBNA medium were most favorable for recovery of *L. monocytogenes* from raw milk.

Slade and Collins-Thompson (179) developed a somewhat shorter two-stage enrichment procedure (Fig. 6.6) to isolate listeriae from foods. Their method was tested using raw milk inoculated to contain approximately 100 *L. monocytogenes* CFU/ml. Results showed that Tryptose Broth was superior to Oxoid Nutrient Broth No. 2 (ONB2) as a primary cold enrichment medium. In addition, diluting milk samples 1:10, rather than 1:5, increased the number of *Listeria* isolations on selective media. The more dilute samples probably maintained a higher pH (≥ 6.0) during cold enrichment as a result of fewer lactic acid bacteria and less lactose being present, which in turn led to faster growth and increased detection of listeriae on solid media.

Original McBride Listeria Agar without blood was the only medium tested that proved useful for plating primary cold enrichments since Tryptose Agar and Trypaflavine Nalidixic Acid Agar were typically overgrown by competing microflora. Favorable results were, however, obtained using Tryptose Agar after secondary warm enrichment. Addition of acriflavine to Thiocyanate Nalidixic Acid Broth proved beneficial for recovery of *L. monocytogenes*. Thus following 7–14 days of cold enrichment in Tryptose

Broth, *L. monocytogenes* was most frequently isolated after plating samples enriched in Thiocyanate Nalidixic Acid Broth on either MLA-B or Tryptose Agar.

A "shortened" enrichment procedure and a two-stage cold/warm enrichment procedure were developed in Canada by Farber et al. (61) for isolating *Listeria* spp. from raw milk. In the "shortened" enrichment procedure (Fig. 6.7), milk samples underwent primary and secondary warm enrichment as well as primary cold enrichment in two selective media. Although no single step within the procedure was completely satisfactory for isolating listeriae from raw milk, the two steps that were most helpful involved surface-plating the primary FDA Enrichment Broth culture on MLA2 + blood after 1 day of incubation at 30°C and surface-plating the 30-day-old cold enriched FDA Enrichment Broth culture (initially incubated 7 days at 30°C) on MLA2 + blood. Collectively, these two steps led to detection of *Listeria* spp. in 31 of 51 (60.8%) positive raw milk samples. Although 11 isolations were made after 1 but not 7 days of primary warm enrichment, 6 isolations were only possible after 7 days of primary warm

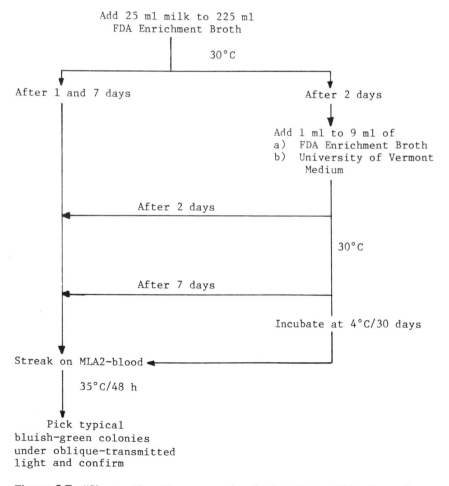

Figure 6.7 "Shortened" enrichment procedure for the isolation of *Listeria* spp. from raw milk (61).

enrichment. Thus incubation of the primary warm enrichment for 7 days before plating on MLA2-blood markedly enhanced recovery of listeriae from raw milk.

The two-stage cold/warm enrichment method, which was the second of two procedures developed by Farber et al. (61), also detected *Listeria* spp. in raw milk samples. Using this procedure (Fig. 6.8), listeriae were isolated from 12 samples that were negative using the "shortened" enrichment procedure. Similarly, 10 samples that were positive for *Listeria* spp. using the "shortened" enrichment procedure were negative with the two-stage cold/warm enrichment method. Thus, when used alone, neither procedure detected listeriae in all positive samples. Following cold enrichment, similar numbers of samples were positive for *Listeria* spp. after warm enrichment in FDA Enrichment Broth and University of Vermont Medium. However, eight raw milk samples were only positive after 2 weeks of cold enrichment as compared to three samples in which listeriae were only detected after 4 weeks of cold enrichment. These results are similar to those of Doyle and Schoeni (49), who also observed that *Listeria* spp. could be more readily isolated from raw milk and from soft, surface-ripened cheese (50) during the first 2 weeks of cold enrichment.

Food-associated outbreaks of listeriosis along with the discovery of *L. monocytogenes* in many European varieties of soft-ripened and smear-ripened cheese prompted two Swiss investigators, Bannerman and Billie (11), to develop a two-stage warm/cold enrichment procedure to detect *Listeria* spp. on cheese and dairy factory surfaces

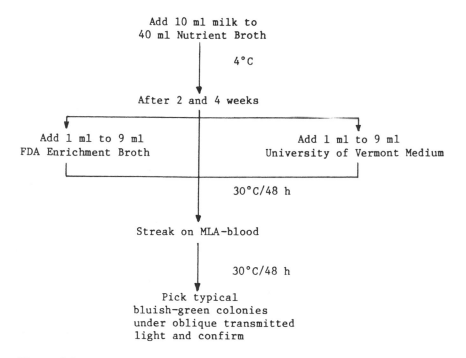

Figure 6.8 Two-stage cold/warm enrichment procedure for the isolation of *Listeria* spp. from raw milk (61).

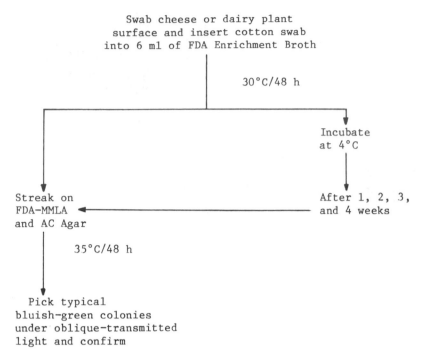

Figure 6.9 Two-stage warm/cold enrichment method for detection of *Listeria* spp. on cheese and dairy factory surfaces (11).

(Fig. 6.9). Their isolation method is similar to the "shortened" enrichment procedure just described (61), with the exception that the secondary warm enrichment step has been eliminated and Acriflavine Ceftazidine Agar (AC Agar) has been included as an additional selective plating medium. Using this method, *Listeria* spp. were isolated from 157 of 1099 (14.3%) cheese and environmental samples. A total of 99 samples were positive for listeriae using both plating media. Following warm enrichment, 56 of 99 (57%) and 35 of 99 (35%) samples were positive after surface-plating enrichment cultures on AC Agar and FDA-MMLA, respectively, whereas 70 of 99 (71%) and 53 of 99 (54%) samples were positive after plating 7-day-old cold enrichment cultures on AC Agar and FDA-MMLA, respectively. Increased selectivity of AC Agar was presumably responsible for detection of approximately 50% more isolates of *Listeria* spp. as compared to FDA-MMLA. According to Kaufmann (101), the Swiss Federal Public Health Office has included this method in its official manual of approved methods for detecting *Listeria* spp. on cheese and dairy factory surfaces.

Important information concerning presence of *Listeria* spp. in food and environmental samples can be gained using the three procedures just described as well as procedures developed by Hayes et al. (88) and Slade and Collins-Thompson (179); however, the need for cold enrichment in these procedures increased the length of analysis to 30–40 days. Hence, while cold enrichment will likely remain an important research tool, the time-consuming nature of this method negates its use in any isolation procedure that is to be adopted by the food industry as a "standard" method.

Rodriguez et al. (165) developed a complicated scheme to examine raw milk that included three noninhibitory collection (primary enrichment) media, three selective (secondary) enrichment media, and one selective plating medium, Rodriguez Isolation Medium III (RIM III), all of which were previously described by Rodriguez et al. (163). The three selective enrichment media used in this protocol (Table 6.2) contained nalidixic acid and trypan blue with or without polymyxin B, whereas nalidixic acid and acriflavine were used as selective agents in the plating medium (Table 6.3). As shown in Fig. 6.10, milk was added to all three collection media (Table 6.1) with Collection Medium B streaked onto RIM III after 7 and 15 days of storage at 4°C. Collection Medium A was incubated at 4°C for 24 hours, subcultured in all three secondary enrichment media, which were incubated at 22°C until a color change occurred, and then samples were streaked on RIM II. A portion of Collection Medium A was also diluted in Collection Medium C, which was streaked on RIM III following 7 and 15 days at 4°C. According to these authors, 11 *L. monocytogenes* isolates were obtained after primary cold enrichment, with Collection Medium C accounting for nine of 11 isolations. Although results for Collection Medium C appear impressive, the increased number of isolations using this medium may have resulted from a more dilute sample, approximately 1:40 as compared to approximately 1:8 in Collection Media A and B. Under these conditions, Collection Medium C would be expected to maintain a higher pH during cold enrichment since fewer lactic acid bacteria and less lactose likely were present, thus providing an improved environment for growth of *L. monocytogenes*. In contrast to cold enrichment, 49 *L. monocytogenes* isolates were obtained following secondary enrichment at 22°C with 16, 32, and one colony originating from Enrichment Media 1, 2, and 3, respectively. Recovery of only one *Listeria* isolate using Enrichment Medium 3 is not surprising, considering that Collection Medium A was diluted approximate 1:68 in Collection Medium C after only 24 hours of enrichment at 4°C. Since transfer of the culture after 24 hours of cold enrichment provides little opportunity for appreciable growth of *L. monocytogenes*, the organism was likely diluted out of the sample. Overall, primary cold enrichment of milk samples diluted approximately 1:8, followed by secondary enrichment in Rodriguez Enrichment Media 1 and 2 incubated at 22°C and plating on an isolation medium containing nalidixic acid and acriflavine, provided the best opportunity for detecting *L. monocytogenes* in raw milk.

In 1986, Doyle and Schoeni (49) used the microaerophilic nature of *L. monocytogenes* in developing a single-stage shortened enrichment procedure to isolate the organism from milk, as well as fecal and biological specimens (Fig. 6.11). In their procedure, the sample was added to an Erlenmeyer flask equipped with a side-arm and then diluted 1:5 in Doyle and Schoeni Selective Enrichment Broth (DSSEB, Table 6.2). Following 24 hours of incubation at 37°C in an atmosphere of 5% O_2:10% CO_2:85% N_2, a portion of the sample was streaked on plates of McBride Listeria Agar (MLA, original formulation with blood), which also were incubated at 37°C for 24 hours under microaerobic conditions. Using DSSEB, *L. monocytogenes* was consistently isolated from raw milk samples inoculated to contain 10 *L. monocytogenes* CFU/ml. In addition, about two and five times as many *L. monocytogenes* isolates were recovered from fecal and biological specimens using DSSEB rather than cold enrichment and direct plating, respectively.

Another enrichment procedure, which is partially based on microaerobic incubation, was developed by Skovgaard and Morgen (178) to isolate *Listeria* spp. from feces, silage,

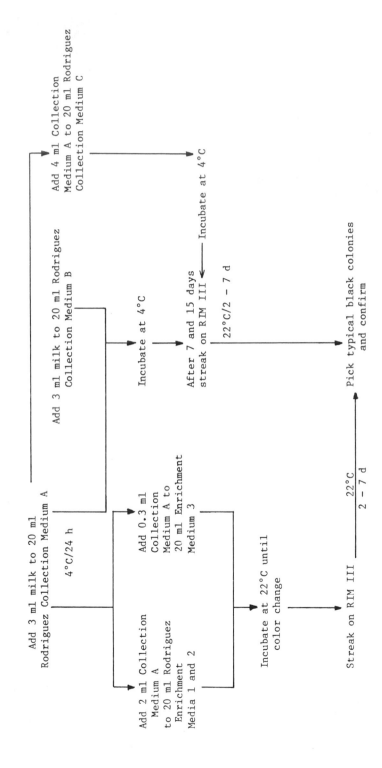

Fig. 6.10 Multistage enrichment procedure for isolating *L. monocytogenes* from milk (165).

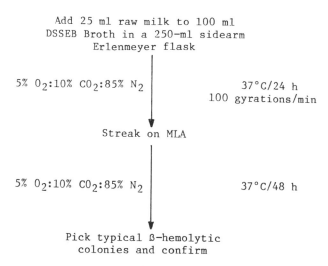

Figure 6.11   Single-stage Doyle and Schoeni shortened enrichment procedure for isolating *L. monocytogenes* from raw milk (49).

minced meat, and poultry. In this two-stage procedure (Fig. 6.12), microaerobic incubation (24 h/30°C/95% air:5% CO_2) of the sample in USDA Listeria Enrichment Broth I (LEB I) is followed by a single aerobic secondary warm enrichment in USDA Listeria Enrichment Broth II (LEB II), after which untreated and KOH-treated samples are

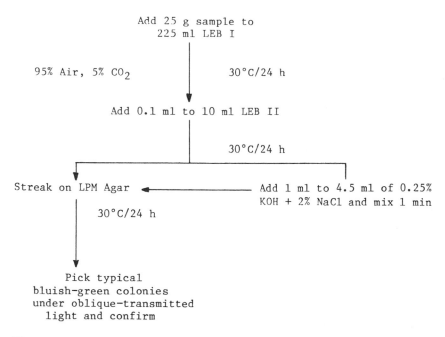

Figure 6.12   Shortened two-stage enrichment procedure to isolate *Listeria* spp. from feces, silage, minced beef, and poultry (178).

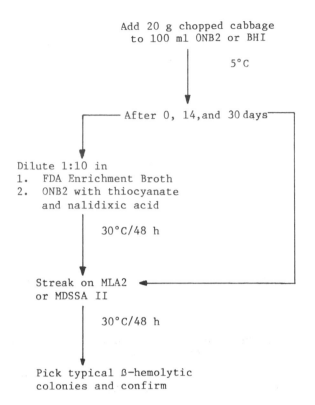

Figure 6.13 Two-stage enrichment procedure for isolating *L. monocytogenes* from cabbage. (Adapted from Ref. 85.)

surface-plated on LPM Agar. Using this isolation scheme, which, with the exception of microaerobic incubation, closely resembles the original USDA procedure (see Fig. 16.19), numerous fecal, silage, minced beef, and poultry samples were positive for *Listeria* spp., including *L. monocytogenes*. Based on these results, the authors concluded that their method was suitable to detect listeriae in heavily contaminated materials, as well as in samples of raw beef and poultry that contained relatively low bacterial populations. Although both procedures just described decrease the *Listeria* detection time to approximately 3 days, incubation of enrichment cultures under microaerobic conditions is particularly awkward and is therefore not feasible for use in large-scale testing programs.

A large listeriosis outbreak in which coleslaw was implicated as the vehicle of infection prompted Hao et al. (85) to compare various media and methods to detect *L. monocytogenes* in cabbage. Preliminary results clearly demonstrated a need for some type of enrichment procedure before *L. monocytogenes* could be isolated from cabbage inoculated with the pathogen. After comparing results from various plating and cold enrichment media, as well as secondary selective enrichment broths, these investigators proposed the two-stage enrichment procedure shown in Fig. 6.13 for isolating *L. monocytogenes* from cabbage. A cold enrichment period of 14 or 30 days at 5°C in Oxoid Nutrient Broth No. 2 (ONB2) or Brain Heart Infusion Broth (BHI) led to increased recovery of listeriae from cabbage following secondary warm enrichment (30°C/48 h) in FDA Enrichment Broth or ONB2 containing potassium thiocyanate and nalidixic acid (Table 6.2). Although Tryptose Broth is generally regarded as one of the best available media for cold enrichment, this medium was not among those chosen for cold-enriching cabbage samples. A comparison of nine selective plating media, both with and without an additional 5 mg of Fe^{3+}/L, led to the recommendation of Modified Doyle/Schoeni Selective Agar II (MDSSA II, Table 6.3) and McBride Listeria Agar with glycine anhydride rather than glycine (MLA2) for isolating *L. monocytogenes* from cabbage. Both media contained 5% sheep blood, which was deemed beneficial for picking *Listeria*-like colonies. As was true for the cold enrichment broths, several popular plating media, including FDA-MMLA and LPM Agar, were not examined in this study. Although there has been widespread success with these two plating media, it would be prudent to determine their efficacy in isolating *L. monocytogenes* from cabbage and other vegetables before recommending this procedure for routine analysis of such products.

RECOMMENDED METHODS FOR ISOLATING *L. MONOCYTOGENES* FROM FOOD

Heightened interest in foodborne listeriosis has led to intense efforts toward devising one or more optimal methods that can be used commercially for screening of food products for listeriae. Although some facets of the previously described isolation methods appear promising, two frequently revised methods developed in the United States by the FDA and USDA have risen to the rank of unofficial "standard methods" to isolate *L. monocytogenes* from nonmeat and meat products, respectively. Despite widespread use of these methods in the United States, Canada, and Western Europe, both procedures are still plagued with difficulties that include the inability to isolate listeriae from all positive samples as well as difficulties in recovering injured cells. In response to these concerns, European scientists working in cooperation with the International Dairy Federation (IDF) have developed a somewhat similar procedure which is partially based on current FDA methodology. In certain situations, the IDF procedure and a modification of this procedure developed in France by COBAC Laboratories were found superior to both of the original FDA and USDA methods. In this section, we will examine some of the positive and negative aspects of these four protocols and then attempt to identify some of the most critical steps involved in isolating *L. monocytogenes* from different foods.

FDA Method

The FDA method, originally developed by Lovett et al. (123,125), is the most frequently used procedure in the United States and Canada to isolate *L. monocytogenes* from milk, milk products (particularly ice cream and cheese), seafood, vegetables, and factory environmental samples. During a series of experiments by the FDA in 1986, the inadvertent isolation of *L. monocytogenes* from an uninoculated sample of French Brie cheese led to exportation of the FDA method to Europe with subsequent testing of French Brie cheese destined for the United States. The original FDA procedure and the revised version, which will be discussed later, were adopted as unofficial "standard methods."

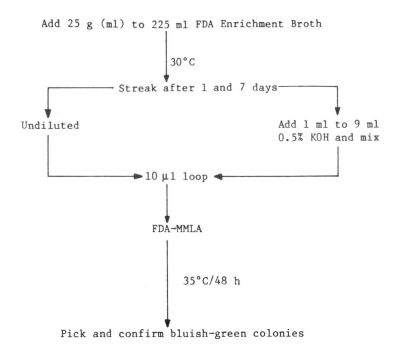

Add 25 g (ml) to 225 ml FDA Enrichment Broth

30°C

Streak after 1 and 7 days

Undiluted

Add 1 ml to 9 ml
0.5% KOH and mix

10 μl loop

FDA-MMLA

35°C/48 h

Pick and confirm bluish-green colonies

Figure 6.14 Original FDA procedure for isolating *L. monocytogenes* from foods, June 1985 to October 1988 (123).

According to the original FDA procedure outlined in Fig. 6.14, a 25-g or 25-ml sample was diluted 1:10 in FDA Enrichment Broth. After 1 and 7 days of aerobic incubation at 30°C, samples of undiluted culture and culture diluted 1:10 in 0.5% KOH were streaked on plates of FDA-MMLA, which were then incubated at 35°C for 48 hours. Following incubation, plates were examined with oblique illumination for bluish-green, *Listeria*-like colonies, which then were picked for confirmation according to results from a series of standard biochemical tests. Because such tests normally take about 2 days to complete, a total of 10–11 days is required to isolate and confirm the presence of *L. monocytogenes* in any food sample.

The FDA procedure has greatly shortened and simplified isolation of *Listeria* spp. from many types of food as compared to earlier methods that were developed to detect the pathogen in clinical specimens. However, intense scrutiny of the original FDA protocol revealed that it was far from perfect for recovering *L. monocytogenes* from all types of dairy products.

In 1987, Doyle and Schoeni (50) compared the original FDA, classical cold enrichment and shortened enrichment procedures (Fig. 6.11) for their ability to recover *L. monocytogenes* from 90 samples of commercially produced, soft, surface-ripened cheese that were previously identified as probably containing *Listeria* spp. Although *L. monocytogenes* was isolated from 41 of 90 (46%) cheese samples, no single procedure detected the pathogen in all positive samples. A total of 21 samples were positive after cold enrichment as compared to only 16 and 13 samples that were positive using FDA and shortened enrichment procedures, respectively. Thus the FDA and shortened enrichment procedure failed to recover *L. monocytogenes* from 5 of 21 (23.8%) and 8 of 21 (38.1%) samples that were positive following cold enrichment. Furthermore, since listeriae were never isolated from the same positive sample by all three enrichment procedures, it appears that the original FDA method was inferior to cold enrichment. Similar results were obtained by Doyle et al. (52) when these same three enrichment procedures were used to isolate *L. monocytogenes* from raw milk samples that had undergone HTST pasteurization. In a 1988 European study, Kaufmann (101) detected *Listeria* spp. in 142 of 207 (68.9%) milk, dairy, and environmental samples using the FDA procedure (Table 6.8). However, the remaining 65 samples were positive following up to 8 weeks of cold enrichment, with listeriae being detected in 45 of 65 (69.2%) samples after 2 weeks of refrigerated storage. Although researchers in Canada (62) and England (151) found negligible differences in numbers of *Listeria* spp. recovered from naturally contaminated samples of raw milk and soft cheese analyzed by the FDA and cold enrichment procedures, once again, both methods failed to detect listeriae in all positive samples.

Some individuals attribute these differences between the FDA and cold enrichment procedures to nonuniform distribution of listeriae within samples such as cheese. However, Doyle and Schoeni (50,52) found cold enrichment superior to the FDA method for analysis of soft, surface-ripened cheese (nonuniform distribution of listeriae expected) as well as pasteurized milk (uniform distribution of listeriae expected). Hence, variations in the ability of the FDA and cold enrichment procedures to detect listeriae in dairy products probably result from inherent differences between the two methods (i.e., media, incubation conditions) and/or presence of microbial competitors rather than nonuniform distribution of listeriae within the product. Although these results indicate that cold enrichment was generally superior to the FDA method, the time-consuming nature of cold enrichment makes this procedure unacceptable as a means to screen

Table 6.8 Comparison of FDA and Cold Enrichment Methods for Recovery of *Listeria* spp. from 207 Positive Milk, Dairy, and Environmental Samples Collected in Switzerland

		Number of positive samples			
	FDA Method[a]	Cold Enrichment Method (weeks)			
Listeria spp.		2	4	6	8
L. monocytogenes	96	35	7	5	3
L. innocua	45	9	4	0	1
L. seeligeri	0	1	0	0	0
L. ivanovii	1	0	0	0	0
Cumulative total	142	187	198	203	207
% Recovery	68.6	90.3	95.7	98.1	100.0

[a]Sampled only after 2 days of enrichment.
Source: Adapted from Ref. 101.

commercial foods for *L. monocytogenes*. Thus the FDA procedure needs to be modified as warranted to detect listeriae faster and more accurately in a variety of foods.

To improve the FDA method outlined in Fig. 6.14, researchers in the United States and Europe reexamined the ability of FDA Enrichment Broth and FDA-MMLA to support growth of healthy listeriae. At the United States Centers for Disease Control, Swaminathan et al. (185) estimated populations of *L. monocytogenes* in commercial Brie cheese by directly plating homogenized cheese samples on FDA-MMLA and testing the homogenates with a three-tube MPN technique in which FDA Enrichment Broth was used as the growth medium. The direct plating and MPN techniques yielded *Listeria* populations of 5×10^5 CFU/g and 2.4×10^5 CFU/g, respectively, indicating that both media and procedures were equally acceptable or unacceptable. According to some European scientists, as also was recently observed for raw seafood (141), recovery of *L. monocytogenes* from Brie cheese was significantly better using FDA rather than USDA Listeria Enrichment Broth, the reasons for which will be discussed in conjunction with the USDA method.

Adoption by French officials of the FDA method for examination of Brie cheese destined for the international market led to a series of European studies which examined the ability of several enrichment broths and plating media, including those in the FDA method, to recover *Listeria* spp. from food products.

One European report by Cox et al. (36) indicates that growth of *L. monocytogenes* in FDA Enrichment Broth at 30°C was somewhat enhanced when pasteurized cheese was added to the medium. However, these researchers observed similar growth curves for group D streptococci and *L. monocytogenes* in FDA Enrichment Broth during incubation at 30°C, indicating that the formulation for this medium may require further refining to optimize recovery of listeriae from soft cheeses.

In another such study conducted in England, Prentice (153) examined two enrichment broths (FDA Enrichment Broth and UVM Broth) and four selective plating media (FDA-MMLA, MMLA, Merck Agar, and Oxford Agar) for their ability to recover *L. monocytogenes* from 45 artificially contaminated samples of English soft cheese manufactured in England. As shown in Table 6.4, comparable results were obtained by enriching cheese samples in either FDA Enrichment Broth or University of Vermont Medium (UVM) and then surface-plating each of the enrichment cultures on the same selective agar. Although FDA Enrichment Broth and UVM appeared to be equally acceptable for enriching soft cheese, with several other researchers in the United States reaching a similar conclusion (7,70), vast differences were seen in the ability of *L. monocytogenes* to grow on the four selective plating media after enrichment. In this particular study, Oxford Agar (Table 6.3) clearly emerged as a best plating medium with *L. monocytogenes* being detected in 36 of 45 (80.0%) cheese samples following enrichment in FDA Enrichment Broth. The three remaining media, including FDA-MMLA, which appears in the FDA protocol, proved to be unacceptable. As previously noted by Golden et al. (74), high levels of non-*Listeria* contaminants present in samples of soft cheese may have contributed to difficulties in isolating listeriae on FDA-MMLA, MLA, and Merck Agar.

In a third European study, Hartmann (86) attempted to recover *Listeria* spp. from routine food samples by surface-plating FDA Enrichment Broth cultures on FDA-MMLA as well as on LPM, AC, and Merck Agar (Table 6.3). In contrast to results of the previous study (153), all four plating media did reasonably well. *Listeria* spp. were detected in 43.7% of the food products using Merck Agar as compared to 43.0, 35.2, and 23.9% of the food products using LPM Agar, FDA-MMLA, and AC agar, respectively (Table 6.9)). More important, the apparent superiority of LPM Agar over FDA-MMLA as a plating medium in the FDA procedure is supported by results from at least four other investigations (70,89,90,111). Findings from one of these studies (70) indicate that enhanced recovery of *Listeria* spp. on LPM Agar was independent of the type of medium (i.e., FDA Enrichment Broth, UVM, Rodriguez Enrichment Medium III) in which naturally contaminated samples of soft cheese and raw meat were enriched. Two factors, namely, (a) examination of samples for all *Listeria* spp. and (b) presence of relatively low levels of non-*Listeria* contaminants in these "routine" food products, may have contributed to increased recovery of listeriae on FDA-MMLA (as well as on the other media) as compared to the previous study by Prentice (153) in which only soft cheeses containing relatively high levels of contaminating microorganisms were examined for *L. monocytogenes*. Thus the natural microflora of individual food products appears to play an important role in recovery of listeriae by the FDA method. In addition, recovery of listeriae from cheese and other foods is influenced by variations in pH that result from growth of the competitive microflora during enrichment. Hence, we must reiterate that it may not be possible to develop a single selective plating medium that is suitable for detection of listeriae in all types of food.

While many researchers have reassessed the suitability of FDA Enrichment Broth and FDA-MMLA to recover *Listeria* from various foods, others have scrutinized the different procedural steps within the original FDA protocol (Fig. 6.14) with primary attention given to (a) length of incubation in FDA Enrichment Broth and (b) presumed benefits derived from diluting a portion of the enrichment culture in 0.5% KOH before plating on FDA-MMLA. According to results from at least four independent investigations in the United States and Canada, primary enrichment at 30°C for more than 48 hours failed to enhance numbers of listeriae isolated from naturally contaminated raw milk (111,180) and inoculated samples of brick (111), Brie (7), Camembert (111), and Colby cheese (111) as well as cold pack cheese food (111), yogurt (111), ice cream

Table 6.9 Recovery of *Listeria* spp. from Routine Food Samples using FDA Enrichment Broth in Combination with Four Solid Selective Plating Media

Sampling times	Number of samples	Solid selective media			
		FDA-MMLA	LPM Agar	AC Agar	Merck Agar
2 days, se[a]	33	12	15	11	18
2 days, se, 7 days	32	10	8	3	12
7 days	77	28	28	20	32
Total	142	50	61	34	62
% Positive	—	35.2	43.0	23.9	43.7

[a]Secondary enrichment in FDA Enrichment Broth followed by 24 hours of incubation at 30°C.
Source: Adapted from Ref. 86.

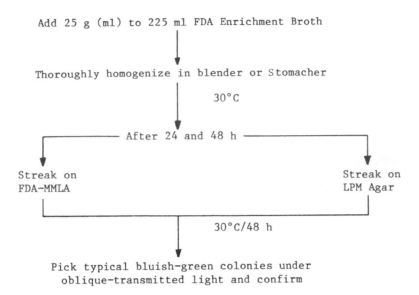

```
        Add 25 g (ml) to 225 ml FDA Enrichment Broth
                              │
                              ▼
    Thoroughly homogenize in blender or Stomacher
                              │
                            30°C
                              │
                              ▼
        ┌───────────── After 24 and 48 h ─────────────┐
        │                                             │
        ▼                                             ▼
    Streak on                                     Streak on
    FDA-MMLA                                      LPM Agar
        │                                             │
        └──────────────────────┬──────────────────────┘
                               │
                            30°C/48 h
                               │
                               ▼
        Pick typical bluish-green colonies under
           oblique-transmitted light and confirm
```

Figure 6.15 Revised FDA procedure for isolating *L. monocytogenes* from food, October 1988 to Fall 1990 when FDA-MMLA was replaced with Oxford Agar (124).

(93,111), and chicken (7). These findings are in direct conflict with earlier laboratory data supplied to the FDA which indicated that recovery of listeriae from cheese could be increased approximately 20% by incubating enrichments for 7 rather than 1 day. Originally Lovett et al. (125) and several other investigators (50, 123,151) reported that pretreatment of the FDA enrichment culture in 0.5% KOH enhanced recovery (i.e., detection) of listeriae from dairy products and other foods by decreasing the numbers of background contaminants. However, numerous other studies (24,71,73,93,107,133,178,180) have shown little if any increase between numbers of listeriae isolated from KOH-diluted and nondiluted FDA Enrichment Broth cultures that were surface-plated on FDA-MMLA.

Based on all of the aforementioned findings, Lovett and Hitchins (124) revised the original FDA procedure in October of 1988 (Fig. 6.15) by (a) reducing the enrichment culture incubation time from 7 to 2 days with sampling after both 1 and 2 days of incubation, (b) eliminating the 0.5% KOH pretreatment, and (c) adding LPM Agar as a second *Listeria*-selective plating medium. This revised FDA procedure is reportedly as sensitive (or more sensitive) as the original FDA procedure and also saves analysis time by allowing laboratory workers to isolate and confirm the presence of *L. monocytogenes* in any food within 5–6 days instead of up to 11 days with the original procedure. Given the newness of the revised FDA method, it is not surprising that as of January 1990, only one report of its use in food surveys or other research endeavors has surfaced in the scientific literature (89). Nonetheless, if current trends continue, the revised FDA procedure, or future revisions of this procedure brought about by the normal evolution of scientific progress, will likely remain among the most popular conventional "standard" methods for isolation of foodborne listeriae.

International Dairy Federation (IDF) Method

Some European scientists also have claimed that the original FDA procedure is sometimes less than ideal for isolating *L. monocytogenes* from dairy products; however, many researchers agree that the FDA method can be revised as was just demonstrated to more accurately detect listeriae in cheese and other materials that are of importance to the dairy industry. Using the original FDA method as a starting point, the IDF recently began to develop a "reference" method to detect *L. monocytogenes* in milk and milk products. Although its protocol, known as the IDF method, has been tested collaboratively in several laboratories using samples of artificially contaminated cheese (Ring Trials), results indicate that this procedure is not yet completely reliable and thus can only be considered as a provisionally recommended method.

As seen in Fig. 6.16, the IDF method (186,187) essentially follows the original procedure developed by the FDA (Fig. 6.14) with the following exceptions: (a) dairy products expected to contain sublethally injured listeriae (i.e., pasteurized milk, fermented milks, yogurt, custards, desserts, and certain cheeses having a pH <5.8 as well as dried milk, whey, butter, and caseinate products) undergo preenrichment in IDF Pre-Enrichment Broth (Table 6.2) followed by primary enrichment in IDF Enrichment Broth (Table 6.2), (b) additional sampling of all products except raw milk following 2 days of primary enrichment, (c) elimination of the KOH treatment before plating primary enrichment cultures on FDA-MMLA (142,153,186), (d) use of IDF Enrichment Broth

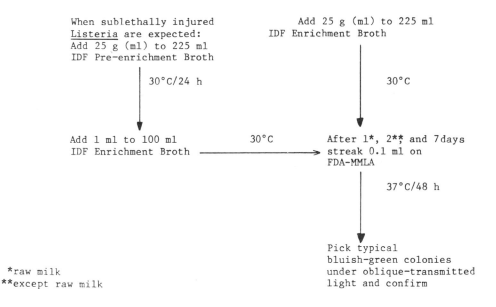

Figure 6.16 Provisional International Dairy Federation (IDF) procedure for isolating *L. monocytogenes* from milk and milk products (186, 187).

[i.e., FDA Enrichment Broth modified to contain 10 instead of 15 mg of acriflavine/L (11,13,186)], and (e) a focus on identification and confirmation of *L. monocytogenes* only rather than all seven *Listeria* spp. (4,186).

The original draft of the IDF procedure also included subenrichment (secondary enrichment) of all 1-day-old primary enrichment cultures at 30°C for 24 hours before surface-plating on FDA-MMLA. Although this step has been eliminated from the protocol adopted in June of 1988 (Fig. 6.16), many scientists involved in developing the IDF method (73,86,142,186) contend that subenriching the 1-day-old primary enrichment culture enhances recovery of listeriae from dairy products, including all varieties of cheese. Some proponents of subenrichment (73,86) recommend that this step be done more than once during the 7-day primary enrichment period. Gledel (73) recently confirmed the importance of subenriching 24-hour-old primary enrichment cultures, but claimed that such a step might be better suited for 7-day-old cultures. However, since *L. monocytogenes* may disappear from the primary enrichment culture anytime during the 7-day incubation period, Gledel (73) also stressed that better results could be obtained by subenriching the primary enrichment culture after 1, 2, and 7 days of incubation at 30°C.

Subenrichment appears to be particularly useful for recovering listeriae from whey as well as from soft, smear-ripened, and processed varieties of cheese (86,142). Although reasons for enhanced recovery of *L. monocytogenes* from such samples following subenrichment remain obscure, the pH of the culture during enrichment is likely to be one of the most important factors affecting growth of *Listeria*. As was true during cold enrichment (21), contaminating microorganisms also can grow during primary warm enrichment and reduce the pH of IDF Enrichment Broth to ≤5.2 (73), which in turn may either partially or completely inhibit growth of listeriae. From this perspective, it appears that the most important benefit obtained from subenrichment (diluting the primary enrichment culture 1:10 in IDF Enrichment Broth) is the resultant increase in pH of the culture medium to a value near neutrality, which will in turn foster growth of listeriae.

Recovery of *Listeria* also is markedly influenced by pH of the enrichment broth during primary warm enrichment. Researchers in Switzerland recovered *L. monocytogenes* from nearly twice as many naturally contaminated samples of Vacherin Mont d'Or soft-ripened cheese when 25-g cheese samples were diluted 1:100 rather than 1:10 in IDF Enrichment Broth. These results are supported by those of another study in which *L. monocytogenes* was isolated from 50 of 100 and 8 of 100 raw meat samples that were diluted 1:100 and 1:10, respectively, in another selective enrichment broth. In both of these studies, samples diluted 1:100 had higher pH values than those diluted 1:10. These results indicate the added benefit of maintaining enrichment cultures at pH values near neutrality.

Success or failure of any detection/isolation procedure is largely dependent on the ability of enrichment and plating media to support rapid growth of *L. monocytogenes* and at the same time prevent growth of non-*Listeria* contaminants. Data compiled by Prentice (153) indicate that the present IDF Enrichment Broth (containing 10 mg of acriflavine/L) is better suited than either FDA Enrichment Broth or UVM Broth for recovery of *L. monocytogenes* from artificially contaminated samples of soft cheese. Since reasonably good results also were obtained using IDF Enrichment Broth in recent interlaboratory studies (Ring Trials), proposals to improve the IDF method have focused on evaluating currently available plating media rather than enrichment broths.

Preliminary results from the 1988 IDF Ring Trials indicate that *L. monocytogenes* was recovered from none of 90 (0%), 8 of 90 (8.8%), and 74 of 90 (82.2%) inoculated samples of soft cheese after plating enrichment cultures on FDA-MMLA, Merck Agar, and Oxford Agar, respectively. As you will recall from data in Table 6.4, similar numbers of inoculated soft cheese samples were positive for *L. monocytogenes* after incubation in both FDA Enrichment Broth and UVM. However, since large variations in numbers of positive cheese samples were observed using different selective plating media, it appears that the plating medium may be more important than the enrichment broth in procedures to detect listeriae in soft cheese and other fermented dairy products. As a result of these observations, the IDF is initiating a new interlaboratory study in which FDA-MMLA, LPM Agar, Oxford Agar, and TNSA will be examined in an attempt to find an optimal plating medium to isolate *L. monocytogenes* from soft cheese. Results from this study and others yet to come may help eliminate a few of the shortcomings of the IDF method, including some of the difficulties encountered in isolating *L. monocytogenes* from certain smear-ripened and raw milk cheeses (142), as well as cheese containing fecal streptococci at levels of $\geq 10^3$ CFU/g (73). Although proposed modifications may give the IDF method a bright future, we need to again emphasize that as of January 1990, the IDF procedure was only provisionally recommended for detection of *L. monocytogenes* in dairy products.

COBAC Method

The Central Laboratory of Food Hygiene in France has recommended a nine-step procedure to detect listeriae in food and environmental samples. This procedure (Fig. 6.17), which has been named the COBAC method by COBAC Laboratories in France (71), is a modified version of the IDF procedure (Fig. 6.16) just discussed in which (a) preenrichment of all samples has been eliminated, (b) KOH treatments for 1-, 2-, and 7-day-old primary enrichment cultures have been added before surface plating on FDA-MMLA, and (c) subenrichment of 7-day-old primary enrichment cultures at 37°C for 24 hours has been added along with direct plating of the subenrichment culture (without KOH treatment) on FDA-MMLA. Girard et al. (71) compared the COBAC method, the original FDA method (Fig. 6.14), and a modified version of the IDF method (Fig. 6.16) in which (a) samples were analyzed after only 1 and 7 days of primary enrichment, (b) KOH treatment was included for 1- and 7-day-old primary enrichments, and (c) subenrichment of the 1-day-old primary enrichment at 37°C for 24 hours was followed by direct plating of the untreated subenrichment culture. Some of the most important steps in optimizing recovery of listeriae from naturally contaminated dairy, meat, and environmental samples were identified. Results of this study showed that *Listeria* spp. were isolated from 62 of 1741 (3.56%), 92 of 1741 (5.28%), and 114 of 1741 (6.55%) samples after 10 days using the FDA, modified IDF, and COBAC methods, respectively. Moreover, the FDA and modified IDF methods failed to detect listeriae in 52 of 114 (45.6%) and 22 of 114 (19.3%) samples, respectively, that were positive using the COBAC method.

Since the COBAC procedure calls for nine platings of enrichment cultures (includ-

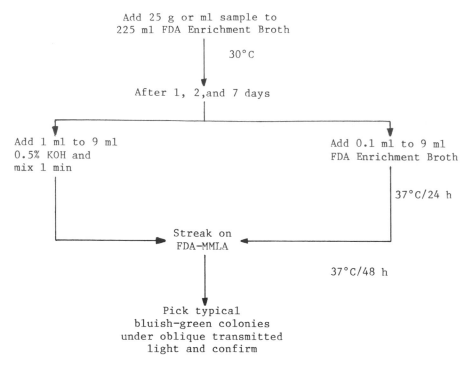

Figure 6.17 COBAC Laboratory method for the isolation of *Listeria* spp. from dairy, meat, and environmental samples (71).

ing subenrichments) as compared to only four and five platings in the FDA and modified IDF methods, respectively, the increased success of the COBAC method over the other two procedures is to be expected. Closer examination of results obtained from the nine-step COBAC method showed that 52.6 and 57.0% of all positive samples were detected after plating untreated and KOH-treated primary enrichment cultures, respectively, on FDA-MMLA. Since diluting enrichment cultures in 0.5% KOH before plating increased the number of positive samples by only 4.4%, simplification of the COBAC procedure by eliminating the three KOH treatments is unlikely to have any appreciable negative effect on recovery of listeriae from food and environmental samples as has already been established in the revised FDA procedure (Fig. 6.15). However, plating of untreated primary enrichment cultures remains an integral step in this and virtually all other conventional isolation methods.

Particularly favorable results were obtained by surface-plating subenrichments of 1-, 2-, and 7-day-old primary enrichment cultures on FDA-MMLA. In the COBAC method, the three subenrichment steps detected listeriae in 90.4% of all positive dairy, meat, and environmental samples. The importance of subculturing the primary enrichment culture is readily apparent when the COBAC and modified IDF methods are compared to the revised FDA procedure, in which subculturing has not yet been included (Fig. 6.18). Within 4 days, *Listeria* spp. were detected in 62.2% of all positive samples using the COBAC and modified IDF methods as compared to only 17.5% of the positive samples using the original FDA procedure. Even more striking is the fact that after analyzing subenriched 2-day-old primary enrichment cultures by the COBAC method, listeriae were isolated from 78% of the positive samples. In contrast, using the original FDA method the level of *Listeria*-positive samples remained at 17.5% for 5 days. Analysis of subenriched 7-day-old primary enrichment cultures in the COBAC method also was beneficial in that this step allowed detection of 20% more positive samples than did the modified IDF method. However, the major advantage of the COBAC method is that 78% of the positive samples were detected after only 5 days as compared to the IDF method, in which 9 days were required to detect 80.7% of the positive samples.

According to results shown in Fig. 6.18, direct plating and particularly subenrichment of both 1- and 2-day-old primary enrichment cultures offer the best possibility for detecting listeriae in dairy, meat, and environmental samples within 5 days. Subenrichment of 7-day-old primary enrichment cultures led to detection of relatively few additional positive samples and at the same time increased the total length of the COBAC method to 10 days. Thus it appears that benefits of subenriching 7-day-old primary enrichment cultures are too small to warrant inclusion of such a step into conventional protocols, many of which are already too lengthy. Although food manufacturers have accepted the FDA method for analysis of food and environmental samples, virtually everyone in the industry is hoping for a "standard method" that will isolate and identify *L. monocytogenes* in less than the current 5–6 days required by the revised FDA procedure. One possibility for increasing the *Listeria* recovery rate of the COBAC

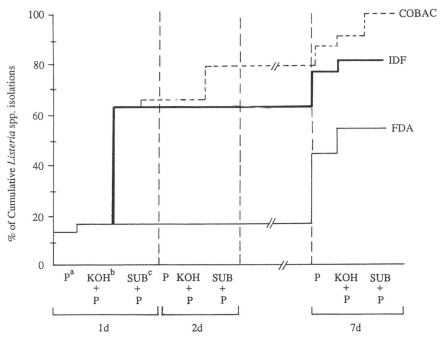

Figure 6.18 Importance of successive steps in recovery of *Listeria* spp. from dairy, meat, and environmental samples. (a) Plate on FDA-MMLA; (b) dilute primary enrichment 1:10 in 0.5% KOH; (c) subenrichment for 24 hours at 30°C. (Adapted from Ref. 71).

method would be to subenrich and plate the primary enrichment broth on FDA-MMLA after 4 instead of 7 days of incubation. Depending on the type of sample being analyzed, better results also might be obtained by plating enrichment cultures on Oxford or LPM Agar instead of FDA-MMLA. Although these changes would allow completion of the COBAC method within 7 days with an additional 2 days required to biochemically confirm *L. monocytogenes* isolates, this protocol would still remain nearly twice as long as the revised FDA procedure. Hence, any potential benefits gained from the aforementioned procedural modifications must be weighed against the increase in time needed for analysis before possible action regarding acceptability of the COBAC method for less perishable food products can be taken.

USDA Method

In the United States, two federal agencies, namely the FDA and the USDA, are responsible for overseeing the microbiological safety of nonmeat (i.e., milk, dairy products, fruits, vegetables, etc.) and meat (including poultry) products, respectively. Two major listeriosis outbreaks linked to consumption of pasteurized milk and Mexican-style cheese prompted the FDA to develop both of the methods described earlier in this chapter for detecting listeriae in foods falling under its jurisdiction. Likewise, continued public concern over presence of listeriae in our nation's food supply prompted the USDA to devise a procedure that could detect naturally occurring *L. monocytogenes* in meat and poultry products.

Since McClain (131) introduced the original USDA procedure in 1986, the method has undergone several significant changes and was revised in May of 1989. The appearance of several procedural modifications in the literature (45,132) has created some confusion as to which enrichment broth was originally recommended by the USDA for analysis of meat and poultry products (45). Several investigators (62,189) used University of Vermont Medium (UVM), developed by Donnelly and Baigent (46), which contained 40 mg of nalidixic acid/L (Table 6.2) instead of the modified version of UVM recommended by McClain and Lee (132) and known as USDA Listeria Enrichment Broth I (LEB I), which contains only 20 mg of nalidixic acid/L (Table 6.2). While the latter medium was originally only used by the USDA for primary enrichment of meat and poultry samples with subsequent secondary enrichments were incubated in USDA Listeria Enrichment Broth II (LEB II), a modified version of LEB I that contained twice as much acriflavine (Table 6.2).

A second major point of confusion is that of sample size. For regulatory testing, the USDA originally enriched 1 g (10 ml of a 25-g sample diluted in 225 ml of LEB I) samples of cooked meat products at 30°C (116). While analysis of 1 g instead of the 25-g sample used in both the original and revised FDA procedures is admittedly far less sensitive, *Listeria* spp. have been detected in numerous samples of vacuum-packaged cooked meat using this procedure. According to Lee (116,117), *Listeria* populations of >100 CFU/g have been readily demonstrated on the surface of retail vacuum-packaged, cooked meats by directly swabbing the surface and then inoculating plates of LPM Agar using a swab/streak technique. Alternatively, *L. monocytogenes* can be quantitated by inserting the same swab into phosphate-buffered saline solution and preparing 10-fold dilutions which can be surface-plated on LPM Agar. Whereas high *Listeria* populations observed on the surface of vacuum-packaged cooked meats may help explain why the organism has been detected in numerous 1-g samples using the original USDA regulatory testing procedure, USDA officials clearly recognize the increased sensitivity gained by analyzing 25-g samples of cooked and raw meat as evidenced by their revised procedure which will be discussed shortly. Hence. to obtain the most accurate results, a 25-g sample should be analyzed whenever possible.

The original USDA method (Fig. 6.19) developed by Lee and McClain in 1986 (118,133) differs markedly from both FDA methods (Figs. 6.14 and 6.15) in that the USDA procedure includes both primary and secondary enrichment for detecting listeriae. Using the original USDA procedure, presumptive *Listeria* colonies can be detected within 3 rather than the 9–11 or 5–6 days using the original and revised FDA methods,

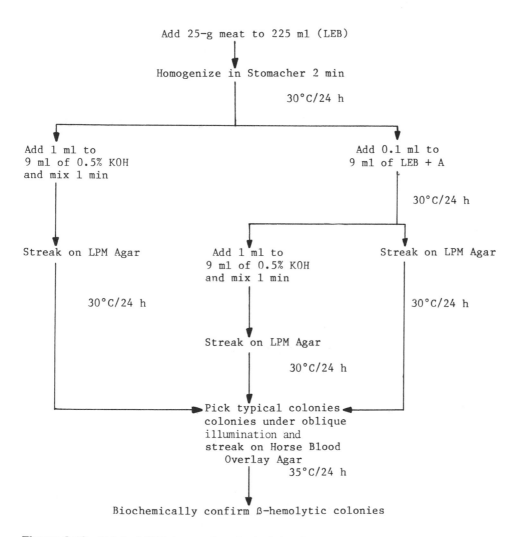

Figure 6.19 Original USDA procedure for isolating *L. monocytogenes* from meat and poultry products, 1986 to April 1989. (Adapted from Refs. 118, 133.)

respectively. Additional variations between these three methods, as well as the previously discussed IDF and COBAC procedures, include use of different primary and/or secondary enrichment broths and LPM Agar instead of FDA-MMLA (now Oxford Agar) as the plating medium.

According to McClain and Lee (133), LEB I (12 mg acriflavine/L) supported excellent growth of pure *L. monocytogenes* cultures. Unfortunately, enriching meat samples in the same medium led to prolific growth of non-*Listeria* organisms, which, in turn, made detection of *L. monocytogenes* colonies on LPM Agar extremely difficult. However, addition of a secondary enrichment step in LEB II (25 mg acriflavine/L) led to detection of approximately 42% more positive samples than with primary enrichment alone.

When the USDA procedure was followed by plating suspected *Listeria* isolates on thin-layer horse blood agar (10 ml of blood-free Columbia Agar Base overlayed with 5 ml of Columbia Agar Base containing 5% horse blood, per plate), *L. monocytogenes* was recovered from 20 of 41 (48.8%), 12 of 23 (52.2%), and 7 of 22 (31.8%) naturally contaminated samples of frozen ground beef, pork sausage, and poultry, respectively. Furthermore, modifying the original USDA procedure to include plating 4-hour primary enrichment, 24-hour primary enrichment, and 24-hour secondary enrichment cultures with and without KOH treatment on LPM Agar led to recovery of *L. monocytogenes* from 34 of 39 (87.2%), 24 of 39 (61.5%), and 5 of 39 (12.8%) positive samples, respectively. These results emphasize the potential benefits gained from sampling primary enrichment cultures early in the USDA protocol. However, as expected, virtually identical numbers of untreated and KOH-treated primary and secondary enrichment cultures were positive for *L. monocytogenes*, which again suggests that the KOH step can be eliminated without adversely affecting results.

Slightly modified versions of the USDA procedure have been used in several studies conducted outside of the United States to analyze various meat and poultry products for listeriae. In Canada, Farber et al. (62) modified the original USDA protocol developed by McClain and Lee (131,132) to include sampling of the primary enrichment culture with and without 24 hours of secondary enrichment after 7 days of incubation. Results showed that 7 or 8 days of enrichment was necessary to detect listeriae in 6 of 13 (46.2%) samples of fermented sausage. In contrast, *L. monocytogenes* was isolated from 24 of 26 (92.3%) samples of minced beef and pork after ≤48 h of primary enrichment in HPB Enrichment Broth (Table 6.2). These findings suggest that listeriae which are presumably less stressed can be recovered more easily from ground meats than sausage in which organisms are more likely to be sublethally injured.

In a second Canadian study, Truscott and McNab (189) compared the ability of UVM (USDA Enrichment Broth I containing 40 mg of nalidixic acid/L) and Listeria Test Broth (Table 6.2) to recover *L. monocytogenes* from ground beef. Eight different protocols were used in which samples underwent primary and/or secondary enrichment in UVM or Listeria Test Broth. Untreated and KOH-treated samples were then surface-plated on LPM Agar only after 24 hours of secondary enrichment. With this procedure, *L. monocytogenes* was isolated from 19 of 50 (38%) samples that underwent primary and secondary enrichment in UVM as compared to 16 of 50 (32%) samples that were positive for listeriae after enrichment in Listeria Test Broth only. Whether primary enrichment in UVM was followed by secondary enrichment in Listeria Test Broth or vice versa, both led to recovery of *L. monocytogenes* from 16 of 50 (32%) samples of ground beef. However, proportions of *Listeria* isolates tested that were later found to be β-hemolytic increased from 13.9% using UVM as the primary and secondary enrichment medium to 23.3% when Listeria Test Broth was used for both enrichments. Despite these encouraging results, none of the eight protocols detected *L. monocytogenes* in more than 65% of the positive samples. These findings are in agreement with those of Doyle and Schoeni (50), who found that no single method could detect *L. monocytogenes* in all positive samples of cheese, beef, and poultry neck skin. Although some samples were positive with or without the KOH treatment, the percentage of positive samples detected using KOH-treated and untreated enrichment cultures was approximately equal. Thus, as previously observed by McClain and Lee (133), the KOH step is of minimal benefit in enhancing recovery of listeriae from meat and poultry products.

Working in Denmark, Skovgaard and Morgen (178) examined samples of minced beef and poultry neck skin using the original USDA procedure (133), which was modified to include incubation in an atmosphere containing 95% air and 5% CO_2. With this method, listeriae were isolated from 45 of 67 (67%) and 16 of 17 (94%) samples of minced beef and poultry neck skin, respectively. Similarly, *L. monocytogenes* was found in 19 of 67 (28%) and 8 of 17 (47%) samples of minced beef and poultry neck skin, respectively.

While the USDA and FDA procedures have not yet been directly compared for their ability to recover *L. monocytogenes* from most products, Swaminathan et al. (185) did examine the suitability of the enrichment and plating media used in both procedures to detect naturally occurring *L. monocytogenes* in Brie cheese. Using a three-tube MPN technique, the estimated population of *L. monocytogenes* was more than 10-fold lower when samples of Brie cheese were enriched in LEB I (9.3×10^3 CFU/g) than in the FDA Enrichment Broth (2.4×10^5 CFU/g). Variations in the ability of both media to support growth of listeriae were traced to differences in the levels of fermentable carbohydrate and protein. Addition of 0.25% D-glucose to LEB I greatly enhanced the growth rate of *L. monocytogenes*. Although addition of 0.3% phytone (papaic digest of soy protein) to this glucose-enriched medium further increased growth of listeriae, highest populations were achieved in FDA Enrichment Broth following 24 hours of incubation at 30°C. A comparison of four selective plating media—TSA, GBNA, LPM Agar, and AC Agar— showed that the latter two media yielded significantly fewer colonies formed by two of three *L. monocytogenes* strains than did the others, whereas the remaining strain formed colonies on LPM Agar only after 96 hours of incubation at 35°C.

As just noted, Swaminathan et al. (185) recovered fewer listeriae from naturally contaminated Brie cheese using USDA- rather than FDA-recommended enrichment media; however, most other comparative studies have yielded markedly different results. In 1989 Lammerding and Doyle (111) found that more listeriae could be detected in inoculated samples of brick, Camembert, and Colby cheese as well as cold pack cheese food, ice cream, and yogurt using the original USDA rather than FDA method. Hitchins (93) also found that the original USDA and FDA methods were at least equally suitable for detecting *L. monocytogenes* in inoculated samples of ice cream. In at least three additional comparative studies, the USDA procedure was judged superior to the FDA method for isolating *L. monocytogenes* from raw ground beef (62), raw chicken (7), and whole and liquid egg. These findings appear to largely result from the greater selectivity of enrichment and plating media used in the FDA protocol. Although difficulties have been encountered using the USDA method with raw seafood (141), the other findings just discussed suggest that the USDA procedure is also reasonably well suited for detecting listeriae in many other foods beside meat and poultry products for which this procedure was originally intended.

Given increased interest regarding presence of *L. monocytogenes* in foods, the USDA's role in food safety and several confirmed cases of listeriosis associated with consumption of meat and poultry products in the United States and elsewhere, it is not surprising that the original USDA procedure was revised in May of 1989 (32). This method, which we shall call the revised USDA procedure (Fig. 6.20), differs from the

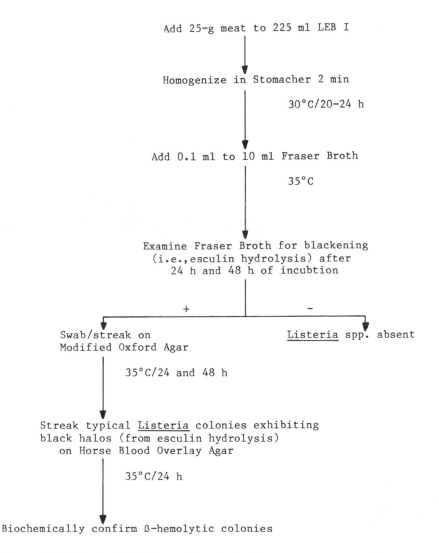

Figure 6.20 Revised USDA procedure for isolating *L. monocytogenes* from meat and poultry products, May 1989 to December 1990 (32).

original protocol in that (a) LEB II has been replaced by Fraser broth (68) [i.e., LEB I to which lithium chloride and ferric ammonium citrate have been added (Table 6.2)] as the secondary enrichment medium, (b) LPM Agar has been replaced by Modified Oxford Agar [i.e., Oxford Agar (40) from which acriflavine, cycloheximide, cefotetan, fosfomycin, and half of the colistin sulfate have been omitted and moxalactam has been added (Table 6.3)] as the only plating medium, and (c) the regulatory sample size has been increased to 25 g. Unlike the original USDA procedure, the revised protocol does not rely on the somewhat questionable ability of many laboratory technicians to identify blue to bluish-green presumptive *Listeria* colonies on clear media using the oblique illumination technique developed by Henry (9). Instead, Fraser Broth and Modified Oxford Agar will both blacken during incubation from the ability of *Listeria* spp. and other possible contaminants (i.e., diphtheroids, aerobic spore-forming bacilli) to hydrolyze esculin with colonies of such organisms exhibiting black halos on Modified Oxford Agar following 24–48 hours of incubation. While LEB I and Fraser Broth allow similar growth of listeriae, the darkening of Fraser broth during incubation is clearly advantageous in that *Listeria*-free samples can be identified with minimal effort after 3 days, thus conserving precious laboratory time and materials. In addition to producing presumptive *Listeria* colonies that are more readily identifiable, Modified Oxford Agar also is somewhat more selective than LPM Agar or the original formulation of Oxford Agar (40), with staphylococci and streptococci both generally unable to grow on Modified Oxford Agar. Since the revised USDA procedure is quite new, no additional information regarding comparison of this method to the FDA procedure or other protocols is currently available. However, USDA officials have acknowledged that their new procedure will be revised as warranted to keep pace with upcoming improvements in *Listeria* isolation/detection methodology.

RECOVERY OF INJURED CELLS

When listeriae are subjected to physical/environmental stresses such as heat (16,33,37,70,75, 76,111,130), multiple freeze/thaw cycles (33,56,57,75,76,111,115), high hydrostatic pressure (95), sanitizing agents (105), food preservatives (33), and gamma irradiation (59,149) as well as acid and drying, many cells became metabolically injured, which results in their inability to grow on selective media. In general, manifestations of sublethal injury acquired by exposing bacterial cells to such physical/environmental stresses typically include (a) leakage of cellular material, (b) increased sensitivity to selective agents, (c) inactivation of certain enzymes such as catalase, superoxide dismutase, aldolase, and lactate dehydrogenase, and (d) structural damage to the cell wall, cell membrane, and ribosomes, as well as DNA and RNA (161,188). However, when incubated in a nonselective, nutritionally rich medium, most sublethally injured bacteria undergo self-repair, which after completion allows the organism to again grow on selective media. Resynthesis of RNA, which is one of the most crucial steps for resuscitation of injured cells, begins during the early stages of the healing process. During this period, protease enzymes help restore normal cell function by degrading damaged cell proteins produced during exposure to environmental stress. Rapid synthesis of lipid material soon reestablishes the integrity of the cell membrane which in turn leads to reconstruction of other cellular lesions, including breaks in double-stranded DNA. Most important, pathogenic bacteria normally retain their pathogenicity after repair of cellular damage (137). Although not yet conclusively proven, *L. monocytogenes* is likely to respond as do most other foodborne pathogens that have been exposed to environmental stress. After pondering the possibility that sublethally injured cells of *L. monocytogenes* might be able to undergo repair in refrigerated foods and then grow to potentially hazardous levels during extended storage, one realizes the importance of being able to detect sublethally injured listeriae in ready-to-eat foods.

As is evident from our previous discussion, few if any *Listeria*-selective agents currently used to inhibit background microorganisms have proven to be completely harmless to *Listeria* spp. One early study demonstrated that potassium dichromate may delay growth of certain *L. monocytogenes* strains belonging to serotypes 3a and 1/2c (128). While results from other experiments indicated that potassium thiocyanate and thallous acetate were less inhibitory to *L. monocytogenes* than potassium tellurite, it also was noted that *Listeria* colonies changed from the smooth to the rough morphological form when grown on media containing potassium thiocyanate or thallous acetate (128). Such a morphological change is a likely indication that selective agents produce an environment that is metabolically stressful to listeriae. While the extent to which potassium tellurite inhibits growth of healthy listeriae was somewhat controversial (27,128), several studies have demonstrated that the presence of as little as 0.001% potassium tellurite, 0.25% phenylethanol, 0.0012% acriflavine, 0.01% polymyxin B sulfate, 5% NaCl, or a combination of these selective agents prevented resuscitation of heat- and acid-injured cells of *L. monocytogenes* (159,182). In 1988, McClain and Lee (133) also reported that healthy *L. monocytogenes* cells had an extended lag phase and slower growth rate in USDA Enrichment Broth I containing 12 mg of acriflavine/L than in the same medium prepared without acriflavine, which further supports the notion that selective agents can produce metabolically stressful conditions.

In 1988, Smith and Archer (182) evaluated 33 different *Listeria*-selective media and found that most, including those recommended by the FDA and USDA, contained inhibitory agents that interfered with detection of heat-injured *L. monocytogenes* cells. Presence of phenylethanol in media currently used by the FDA and USDA was particularly detrimental to repair and subsequent recovery of injured listeriae. Moreover, nearly 10 years earlier Leighton (120) reported that lithium chloride markedly inhibited growth of listeriae. Assuming this is true, present use of lithium chloride in FDA and USDA *Listeria*-selective plating media would be expected to hinder detection of heat-injured listeriae. Of even greater importance are the as yet unknown synergistic effects that various combinations of inhibitory agents might have on repair and growth of *L. monocytogenes* during selective enrichment. Thus it appears that current reliance on numerous combinations of selective agents in enrichment and plating media has made detection of sublethally injured listeriae difficult with the likelihood that *L. monocytogenes* in processed foods may be frequently undetected or underreported.

To assess the ability of selective plating media to quantitate injured listeriae, methods must first be developed to differentiate normal from injured cells. Numerous researchers (16,29,41,56,58,59,182,196) have observed that healthy and sublethally injured listeriae can be differentiated on the basis of the organism's tolerance to various concentrations of NaCl. Buchanan et al. (29) found that unheated *L. monocytogenes* cells grew rapidly on Tryptose Phosphate Agar containing either 0 (TPAT) or 5% NaCl (TPAS), whereas growth of mildly heated cultures was significantly reduced on the same medium containing 5% NaCl. Further refinements of the method indicated that *L. monocytogenes* cultures held at 52°C for 60 minutes readily grew on Tryptose Phosphate Agar containing 1% sodium pyruvate (TPAP); however, plating identical heat-treated cultures on TPAS resulted in a decrease in the number of colonies which was directly proportional to the length of the heat treatment (Fig. 6.21). Thus the TPAP count represents the number of injured plus noninjured cells, whereas the TPAS count represents only the number of noninjured cells. Hence, the number of injured *L. monocytogenes* cells represents the difference between counts on TPAP and TPAS. Using the method just described, these researchers examined 10 different selective plating media for their ability to recover healthy and heat-injured listeriae (Table 6.10). Although similar growth rates for uninjured *L. monocytogenes* cells were observed for all 10 plating media, results concerning the ability of these media to recover thermally injured listeriae were somewhat surprising in that FDA Enrichment Broth + 2% agar completely inhibited growth of injured listeriae and FDA-MMLA failed to detect approximately 39% of the injured cells. UVM containing 2% agar (i.e., a medium similar to USDA LEB I with the exception that the former contains agar and twice as much nalidixic acid) was very similar to FDA-MMLA for recovery of thermally injured listeriae. However, LPM Agar (i.e., the former plating medium of choice in the original USDA procedure), which is now used along with FDA-MMLA in the revised FDA procedure, prevented repair and subsequent growth of all injured cells. In support of these observations, Crawford et al.

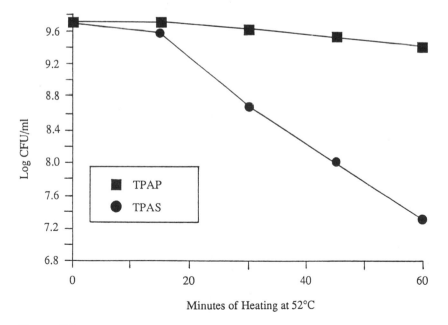

Figure 6.21 Colony formation by injured cells of *Listeria monocytogenes* obtained by heating pure cultures at 52°C. Adapted from Ref. 29.

Table 6.10 Recovery of Thermally Injured *L. monocytogenes* Cells Using Various Selective Plating Media

Media	Recovery of injured cells (%)	T[a] (mg)	NA[b] (mg)	A[c] (mg)	LC[d] (g)	GA[e] (g)	C[f] (mg)	P[g] (ml)	M[h] (mg)
		Concentration of selected inhibitory agents/L of media							
GBNA	102	—	50	—	—	—	—	—	—
TPAT (positive control)	100	—	—	—	—	—	—	—	—
Vogel-Johnson Agar – tellurite	89	—	—	—	5	10[i]	—	—	—
CNP Agar	88	—	45	—	—	—	—	1	—
Phenylethanol Agar	74	—	—	—	—	—	—	2.5	—
UVM + 2% agar	64	—	40	12	—	—	—	—	—
FDA-MMLA	61	—	—	—	0.5	10	200	2.5	—
Vogel-Johnson Agar + tellurite	45	0.2	—	—	5	10[i]	—	—	—
Baird-Parker Agar	30	—	—	—	5	—	—	—	—
TPAS (negative control)	0	—	—	—	—	—	—	—	—
LPM Agar	–21	—	—	—	5	10	200	2.5	20
FDA Enrichment Broth + 2% agar	–25	—	40	15	—	—	50	—	—

[a]Tellurite.
[b]Nalidixic acid.
[c]Acriflavine.
[d]Lithium chloride.
[e]Glycine anhydride.
[f]Cycloheximide.
[g]Phenylethanol.
[h]Moxalactam.
[i]Glycine instead of glycine anhydride.
Source: Adapted from Ref. 29.

(37) also found that FDA-MMLA was superior to LPM Agar (but far inferior to nonselective plating media) for recovery of *L. monocytogenes* cells that were thermally injured during heating in raw and sterile milk. However, early in 1990, Lachica (110) reported that Modified LPM Agar (Table 6.3) in which ceftazidime was substituted for moxalactam recovered 70–95% more thermally injured *L. monocytogenes* cells from laboratory media than did LPM Agar. Most important, Modified LPM Agar compared favorably with nonselective Brain Heart Infusion Agar for detecting injured listeriae. With the exception of GBNA, somewhat different results were obtained when these experiments were repeated using acid-injured *L. monocytogenes* cells. Growth of acid-injured listeriae was partially inhibited on Vogel-Johnson Agar + tellurite and Phenylethanol Agar, whereas CNP Agar, FDA-MMLA, LPM, and UVM + 2% agar generally prevented repair and subsequent growth of injured cells. According to the authors, inhibition of thermally injured listeriae correlated with inclusion of phenylethanol, acriflavine, potassium tellurite, polymyxin B sulfate, sodium thiosulfate, oxgall, and sodium chloride in the various media formulations. While further examination of their data suggests that nalidixic acid has little if any inhibitory effect on growth of thermally injured listeriae, it appears that moxalactam and cycloheximide also may be involved in preventing repair and subsequent growth of this organism.

As previously mentioned, combinations of selective agents within the same medium also might act synergistically to prevent repair and growth of injured cells. For example, fewer injured cells of *L. monocytogenes* were recently recovered from irradiated poultry using Oxford Agar—a highly selective medium containing lithium chloride, cycloheximide, colistin sulfate, acriflavine, cefotetan, and fosfomycin, rather than an earlier formulation of McBride Listeria Agar which contained only phenylethanol and lithium chloride as selective agents (149). While a modified version of Oxford Agar containing only lithium chloride, colistin sulfate, and moxalactam as selective agents is the current plating medium of choice in the revised USDA procedure, future investigations may show that this medium also is somewhat less than optimal for recovery of injured listeriae from meat and poultry products. Although the studies just described provide much needed information concerning the ability of selective media to recover pure cultures of heat- and acid-injured *L. monocytogenes*, overgrowth of both injured and healthy *Listeria* by the natural microflora present in foods has greatly complicated detection of the pathogen. Consequently, Golden et al. (75) and Cassiday et al. (33) evaluated various selective plating media for their ability to quantitate uninjured, heat-injured, and freeze-injured cells of *L. monocytogenes* in artificially contaminated samples of pasteurized whole milk, chocolate ice cream mix, Brie cheese, raw cabbage, dry/country-cured ham, and raw oysters. These seven foods were inoculated to contain 10^2–10^3, 10^4–10^5, or 10^5–10^6 uninjured, heat-injured, or freeze-injured *L. monocytogenes* CFU/g or ml and then plated on up to 10 selective media. The complex design of these two studies (four *L. monocytogenes* strains tested separately × three different inoculum levels × uninjured × heat-injured × freeze-injured × up to 10 different plating media) led to considerable variability within the data in that generally no single plating medium could optimally recover uninjured, heat-injured, and freeze-injured cells of all four *L. monocytogenes* strains from the same food product at all three inoculum levels. Despite the risk of oversimplifying their results, we made some generalizations concerning the acceptability of these plating media to detect uninjured, heat-injured, and freeze-injured listeriae in

Table 6.11   Ability of Various Selective Direct Plating Media to Recover Uninjured, Heat-Injured, and Freeze-Injured Cells of *L. monocytogenes* from Various Foods

Produce	Recovery media	Uninjured	Type of injury Heat-injured	Freeze-injured
Pasteurized whole milk	MLA2	+[a]	+	V[b]
	GBNATSM	++[c]	V[d]	+
	MDA	+	−	V
	FDA-MMLA	+	−	V
Chocolate ice cream mix	MLA2	+	+	V
	GBNATSM	++	+	+
	MDA	+	−	V
	FDA-MMLA	+	−	V
Brie cheese	MLA2	+	+	+
	MDA	+	V	V
	FDA-MMLA	+	V	V
	MRIM III	+	+	V
Raw cabbage	GBNATSM	+	V	+
	MDA	+	+	V
	FDA-MMLA	+	V	V
	UVA	+	+	V
Dry-cured ham	MDA	+	V	V
	FDA-MMLA	+	V	V
	LPMA	++	+	+
	MVJA	V	−	−
Country-cured ham	MRIM III	+	V	V
	UVA	+	V	V
	LPMA	++	V	+
	MVJA	+	−	−
Raw oysters	MLA2	V	−	−
	GBNATSM	V	−	−
	MRIM III	+	V	V
	FDA-MMLA	V	−	−

[a]Recommended.
[b]Variable results.
[c]Strongly recommended.
[d]Not recommended.
Source: Adapted from Refs. 33, 75.

the four products tested. Our generalizations appear in Table 6.11. While all media tested could quantitatively recover uninjured listeriae from pasteurized whole milk and chocolate ice cream mix, Gum Base Nalidixic Acid Trypticase Soy Medium (GBNATSM) and to a lesser extent MLA2 were most useful for detecting both heat- and freeze-injured cells. Relatively low numbers of non-*Listeria* contaminants in these pasteurized dairy products greatly facilitated recovery of *L. monocytogenes* on these less inhibitory plating media. As in the earlier study by Smith and Archer (182), FDA-MMLA was again ill-suited for detecting heat-injured listeriae in pasteurized milk and ice cream mix; however, this same medium proved to be somewhat useful in isolating freeze-injured listeriae from these products. In contrast to the analysis of milk and ice cream mix, detection of uninjured as well as injured listeriae in Brie cheese and raw cabbage required use of selective media with more inhibitory potential to prevent subsequent overgrowth of *L. monocytogenes* by natural microflora. While MRIM III and UVA generally allowed less repair of heat- and freeze-injured listeriae, those cells that overcame the effects of the inhibitory agents were more easily detected as a result of fewer background contaminants. In general, heat- and freeze-injured listeriae were far more difficult to detect in cured ham and raw oysters with virtually none of the media tested being able to suppress background contaminants while simultaneously allowing repair of injured cells. Thus food microbiologists are presently faced with a choice between (a) lower repair rates for injured cells on highly selective media, which would be followed by decreased recovery of survivors, and (b) higher repair rates for injured cells on less selective media, which in turn may lead to complete overgrowth of listeriae by competing microflora. From these results, it appears unlikely that any single plating medium will be found satisfactory for quantitating healthy as well as injured *L. monocytogenes* cells in all types of foods.

To determine the true incidence of *L. monocytogenes* in processed foods, it is clear that most currently available selective plating and enrichment media need to be modified to increase the repair rate for injured cells. Dallmier and Martin (41) found that *L. monocytogenes* cultures lost 50% of their catalase and superoxide dismutase enzyme activity after being heated in phosphate buffer for 19 min at 57.5–59°C and 52–56°C, respectively. However, more important, simultaneous increases in the intracellular levels of hydrogen peroxide (degraded by catalase) and superoxide anion (degraded by superoxide dismutase) paralleled the organism's decreased ability to grow on a nonselective medium containing 5.5% NaCl. Exposing thermally injured listeriae to free hydrogen peroxide also resulted in decreased survival of low rather than high catalase-producing strains. Thus extreme sensitivity of heat- and possibly acid-injured (137) *L. monocytogenes* cells to physiological stress from increased levels of intracellular peroxides may be partly responsible for underestimation of *L. monocytogenes* populations in processed foods.

One possible means of increasing the repair rate for injured cells on selective media is addition of catalase, superoxide dismutase and other oxygen scavenging agents such as sodium pyruvate that prevent formation of hydrogen peroxide and other free radicals. An attempt by Dallmier and Martin (41) to increase the repair rate of thermally injured *L. monocytogenes* cells through anaerobic incubation or through addition of sodium pyruvate and catalase to Tryptic Soy Agar and Tryptic Soy Agar + 5% NaCl was unsuccessful, as was a similar attempt by Smith and Archer (182) to resuscitate thermally injured *L. monocytogenes* cells on McBride Listeria Agar containing 1–3% sodium

Table 6.12 Effect of Different Hydrogen Peroxide
Levels on Survival of *L. monocytogenes* Plated on Nutrient
Agar (NA) Containing Sodium Pyruvate (NaP)

Media	Hydrogen peroxide (%)[a]		
	0.1	1.0	3.0
NA	14[b]	42	52
NA + 0.1% NaP	12	32	43
NA + 1.0% NaP	0	16	29
NA + 5.0% NaP	0	0	13
NA + 10.0% NaP	0	0	0

[a]Sterile 13-mm disks were saturated with aqueous solutions of 0.1,
1.0, and 3.0% hydrogen peroxide and placed in the center of plates
inoculated with a lawn of *L. monocytogenes*.
[b]Inhibition zone (mm).
Source: Adapted from Ref. 62.

pyruvate. However, as shown in Table 6.12, Canadian researchers (62) demonstrated
that sodium pyruvate could be used to protect healthy *L. monocytogenes* cells from the
lethal effects of hydrogen peroxide. Unlike the previous results described by Dallmier
and Martin (41), Farber et al. (62) reported that inclusion of sodium pyruvate in McBride
Listeria Agar as prepared by McBride and Girard (129) enhanced recovery of injured
cells. However, these researchers noted that at least 3 and preferably 7 days of incubation
at 22–25°C was required before most stressed cells could be detected. Since Dallmier
and Martin (41) examined their plates after only 48 hours of incubation at 35°C,
differences observed between the effectiveness of sodium pyruvate in these two studies
may be at least partly the result of changes in incubation times and temperatures. Further
work is needed to determine if recovery of heat-, freeze-, and acid-injured listeriae from
processed foods can be improved by addition of sodium pyruvate and other growth-stim-
ulating agents (i.e., glucose, phytone, vitamins) to FDA-MMLA, LPM Agar, and the
remaining selective plating media shown in Table 6.5. Those involved in such work
should recall that Petran and Zottola (150) reported that 10% fewer healthy *L. monocytogenes*
cells produced colonies on FDA-MMLA than on Plate Count Agar. Hence, a conscious
effort should be made to minimize the number and concentration of inhibitory agents
used in selective media to increase recovery of injured as well as healthy listeriae.

While decreasing the highly selective nature of *Listeria* enrichment and plating
media will enhance recovery of injured cells from food products containing low levels
of microbial contaminants, preenrichment in a less selective medium appears to be
another means of optimizing resuscitation and recovery of heat- and acid-injured listeriae
(37,111,130,171). In support of this argument, van Netten et al. (136) maintained that
ALPAMY Agar alone was not suited for examination of foods suspected of harboring
sublethally injured listeriae. However, stressed cells could be resuscitated on Tryptone
Soya Peptone Yeast Extract Agar containing catalase (15,000 IU/ml) and then formed
colonies made visible by overlaying the plates with ALPAMY Agar.

To enhance repair and recovery of injured listeriae, consideration also must be given to optimization of incubation conditions. While the ideal incubation temperature for recovery of healthy listeriae from contaminated materials is generally assumed to be 30°C, the best incubation temperature for repair of injured cells is widely disputed. In experiments by Bunning et al. (31), *L. monocytogenes* cells were thermally injured by heating freely suspended cells in sterile skim milk at temperatures between 52.2 and 68.9°C, and then quantitated by directly plating samples on Trypticase Soy Yeast Extract Agar. According to these authors, *Listeria* counts were approximately 3- to 10-fold higher when plates were incubated at 25°C for 7 days than at 37°C for 2 days. However, in a similar study (181), thermally injured listeriae were completely or nearly completely resuscitated on Tryptose Phosphate Agar following only 6–9 hours of incubation at 20–40°C. In support of these studies, Lovett (123) also found that the optimum incubation temperature for repair of sublethal injury of listeriae was between 25 and 30°C.

Repair rates at refrigeration temperatures are likely to be less than optimal, as evidenced by one recent report (181) in which thermally injured listeriae failed to resuscitate on Tryptose Phosphate Agar following 9 hours of incubation at 5 or 12°C. However, several reports indicate that heat- and acid-stressed *L. monocytogenes* cells can be resuscitated in laboratory media during extended refrigerated storage. After heat-treating freely suspended *L. monocytogenes* cells in sterile cabbage juice (pH 4.0–5.6) at 50–58°C for up to 10 minutes, Beuchat et al. (16) surface-plated appropriate dilutions on Tryptic Soy Agar and incubated the plates at 30°C. All plates were counted after 24 hours of incubation, and then the plates were held at 5°C for 21 days, transferred to a 30°C incubator for 48 hours and then finally recounted. Using this procedure, *Listeria* counts were up to 10-fold higher on refrigerated than on nonrefrigerated plates. In addition, the effect of prolonged cold storage on subsequent colony formation at 30°C was most evident for cells that had been exposed to the most severe acid and heat treatments during processing. Ryser et al. (166) also found low-temperature incubation useful for recovering *L. monocytogenes* cells that presumably were heat- and acid-injured during manufacture of cottage cheese. Cold enrichment in Tryptose Broth for up to 8 weeks, combined with surface plating enrichments on MLA2 (Table 6.3) at 2-week intervals, led to detection of *L. monocytogenes* in four of eight curd samples (pH 4.7) that had been cooked at 57.2°C for 30 minutes. Cells presumably injured also were recovered from cold-enriched samples of whey, wash water, and washed curd. While these results suggest that cold enrichment in a nonselective medium is a viable means of recovering injured listeriae, five of nine positive samples required 2 weeks of cold enrichment before the pathogen could be detected on MLA2. Nordholt (142) also proposed resuscitation of injured listeriae at 4 to 7°C followed by incubation at 30°C for growth. Nevertheless while the apparent success of cold enrichment was demonstrated in the aforementioned studies, the repair rate for heat- and acid-injured listeriae during refrigerated storage is probably too slow to be of any practical benefit to the food industry.

Given the unofficial "standard" status of the FDA and USDA procedures for detecting healthy listeriae in foods, it is not surprising that these methods have been recently reevaluated for their ability to recover injured listeriae. One report issued in 1987 (5) claimed that the FDA and USDA procedures were unable to detect thermally injured cells of *L. monocytogenes*. However, several more recent studies demonstrated that both procedures can detect limited numbers of sublethally injured listeriae, particularly in foods with relatively low populations of non-*Listeria* contaminants. In one such study, Bradshaw et al. (24) reported that neither the original FDA nor the USDA procedure could detect heat- and cold-stressed *L. monocytogenes* cells in ice cream mix following 24 hours of enrichment at 30°C. However, both procedures were able to recover some injured cells if the samples were enriched for 7 days, with the FDA method reportedly superior. While subsequent experiments also showed that the FDA and USDA procedures were equivalent for detecting heat- and cold-stressed listeriae in inoculated samples of nonfat dry milk, neither procedure recovered all injured cells from ice cream mix or nonfat dry milk. After closer examination of the enrichment broths used in the original FDA and USDA procedures, Bailey et al. (10) concluded that USDA Listeria Enrichment Broth I (LEB I) was superior to FDA Enrichment Broth for recovering thermally injured cells of *L. monocytogenes* from Tryptose Phosphate Broth. Additional experiments which examined the behavior of thermally injured listeriae in the presence of natural contaminants from Brie cheese and chicken indicated that increased recovery of injured listeriae with LEB I was closely related to absence of fermentable carbohydrates and presence of a more efficient phosphate buffering system, both of which helped to maintain a near-neutral pH for optimum resuscitation and growth of the pathogen.

In addition to the previous findings, Crawford et al. (37) also examined the ability of the original FDA, USDA, and cold enrichment procedures, as well as a nonselective method [i.e., Tryptic Soy Yeast Extract Agar and broth substituted for the selective media in the original FDA protocol] to recover nonstressed and heat-stressed *L. monocytogenes* cells from pasteurized milk. Despite comparable results for recovery of nonstressed cells using all four procedures, marked differences were noted for detection of injured cells. Recovery of heat-stressed listeriae led to a $D_{71.7°C}$ of 2.7–3.8 seconds using the nonselective procedure rather than 0.9–1.6 seconds for both the FDA and USDA procedures. While these findings indicate the importance of proper media formulations to detect thermally injured cells, the revised FDA and USDA protocols as well as future changes in these procedures also might lead to enhanced recovery of stressed listeriae.

Throughout this chapter we have stressed the importance of being able to detect sublethally injured cells of *L. monocytogenes* in food. However, given (a) the current lack of evidence indicating that thermally or otherwise injured *L. monocytogenes* cells can undergo self-repair and subsequently grow to as yet unknown hazardous levels in actual foods during extended storage and (b) results from at least one study (37) showing the inability of *L. monocytogenes* cells injured during high-temperature, short-time pasteurization of milk to multiply in the product during cold storage, some persons maintain that the presence of sublethally injured cells in food does not pose a significant public health risk. While their view might eventually prove to be correct, two factors, namely (a) the largely unknown behavior of sublethally injured listeriae in food during extended storage and (b) a recent report (183) indicating that heat-stressed *L. monocytogenes* cells still can produce listeriolysin, an essential virulence factor, compel us to take a more cautious approach. Furthermore, since the oral infective dose for *L. monocytogenes* also is largely unknown, the public health consequences associated with possible repair of injured cells that have escaped detection in food products cannot presently be ignored.

REFERENCES

1. Ajello, G. W. 1986. Personal communication.
2. Albritton, W. L., G. L. Wiggins, W. E. DeWitt, and J. C. Feeley. 1980. *Listeria monocytogenes.* In E. H. Lennette, A. Balows, W. J. Hausler, Jr., and J. P. Truant (eds.), *Manual of Clinical Microbiology*, 3rd ed., American Society for Microbiology, Washington, DC, pp. 139–142.
3. Al-Ghazali, M. R., and S. K. Al-Azawi. 1988. Effects of sewage treatment on the removal of *Listeria monocytogenes. J. Appl. Bacteriol. 65*:203–208.
4. Anonymous. 1988. Determination and detection of *Listeria monocytogenes* in milk and milk products. *Int. Dairy Fed. News 105*:5.
5. Anonymous. 1988. FDA, USDA *Listeria* methods fail to detect injured cells, paper says. *Food Chem. News 29* (36):5–6.
6. Aspøy, E. 1977. Selective effect of propolis in the isolation of *Listeria monocytogenes. Nord. Vet. Med. 29*:440–445.
7. Bailey, J. S., D. L. Fletcher, and N. A. Cox. 1990. Effect of enrichment media and sampling protocol on recovery of *Listeria monocytogenes. J. Food Prot. 53*:505–507.
8. Bailey, J. S., D. L. Fletcher, and N. A. Cox. 1989. Growth of *Listeria monocytogenes* and suppression of microflora from broiler chickens in UVM (University of Vermont) and LEB (*Listeria* enrichment broth). Ann. Mtg., Amer. Soc. Microbiol., New Orleans, LA, May 14–18, Abstr. P-12.
9. Bailey, J. S., D. L. Fletcher, and N. A. Cox. 1989. Recovery and serotype distribution off *Listeria monocytogenes* from broiler chickens in the southeastern United States. *J. Food Prot. 52*:148–150.
10. Bailey, J. S., D. L. Fletcher, and N. A. Cox. 1990. Efficacy of enrichment media for recovery of heat-injured *Listeria monocytogenes. J. Food Prot. 53*:473–477.
11. Bannerman, E. S., and J. Billie. 1988. A selective medium for isolating *Listeria* spp. from heavily contaminated material. *Appl. Environ. Microbiol. 54*:65–167.
12. Beams, R. E., and K. F. Girard. 1959. On the isolation of *Listeria monocytogenes* from biological specimens. *Amer. J. Med. Technol. 25*:120–126.
13. Beckers, H. J. 1988. Personal communication.
14. Beckers, H. J., P. S. S. Soentoro, and E. H. M. Delfgou-van Asch. 1987. The occurrence of *Listeria monocytogenes* in soft cheeses and raw milk and its resistance to heat. *Int. J. Food Microbiol. 4*:249–256.
15. Beerens, H., and M. M. Tahon-Castel. 1966. Milieu a l'acide nalidixique pour l'isolement des *Streptocoques, D. pneumoniae, Listeria, Erysipelothrix. Ann. Inst. Pasteur. 111*:90–93.
16. Beuchat, L. R., R. E. Brackett, D. Y.-Y. Hao, and D. E. Conner. 1986. Growth and thermal inactivation of *Listeria monocytogenes* in cabbage and cabbage juice. *Can. J. Microbiol. 32*:791–795.
17. Biester, H. E., and L. H. Schwarte. 1939. Studies on *Listerella* infection in sheep. *J. Infect. Dis. 64*:135–144.
18. Blanco, M., J. F. Fernandez-Garayzabal, L. Dominguez, V. Briones, J. A. Vazquez-Boland, J. L. Blanco, J. A. Garcia, and G. Suarez. 1989. A technique for the identification of haemolytic-pathogenic *Listeria* on selective plating media. *Lett. Appl. Microbiol. 9*:125–128.
19. Bockemühl, J., H. P. R. Seeliger, and R. Kathke. 1971. Acridinfarbstoffe in Selektivnährböden zur Isolierung von *L. monocytogenes. Med. Microbiol. Immunol. 157*:84–95.
20. Bockemühl, J., E. Feindt, K. Höhne, and H. P. R. Seeliger. 1974. Acridinfarbstoffe in Selectivnährböden zur Isolierung von *L. monocytogenes*. II. Modifiziertes Stuart-Medium: Ein neues *Listeria*-Transport-Anreicherungsmedium. *Med. Microbiol. Immunol. 59*:289–299.
21. Bojsen-Møller, J. 1972. Human listeriosis—diagnostic, epidemiological and clinical studies. *Acta Pathol. Microbiol. Scand.* Section B, Suppl. *229*:1–157.
22. Botzler, R. G. 1973. *Listeria* in aquatic animals. *J. Wildl. Dis. 9*:163–170.
23. Boyle, D. L., and J. N. Sofos. 1989. Development of a culture medium for enumeration of

Listeria monocytogenes in foods. Ann. Mtg., Inst. Food Technol., Chicago, IL, June 25–29, Abstr. 462.

24. Bradshaw, J. G., J. Lovett, and J. T. Peeler. 1989. Parallel comparison of the FDA and USDA procedures for recovery of heat and cold injured *Listeria monocytogenes* from ice cream and nonfat dry milk. Ann. Mtg., Inst. Food Technol., Chicago, IL, June 25–29, Abstr. 530.

25. Breuer, J., and O. Prändl. 1988. Nachweis von Listerien und deren Vorkommen in Hackfleisch und Mettwürsten in Österreich. *Arch. Lebensmittelhyg. 39*:28–30.

26. Buchanan, R. L. 1988. Advances in cultural methods for the detection of *Listeria monocytogenes*. Soc. Ind. Microbiol.—Comprehensive Conference on *Listeria monocytogenes*, Rohnert Park, CA, Oct. 2–5, Abstr. I-14.

27. Buchanan, R. L., H. G. Stahl, and D. L. Archer. 1987. Improved plating media for simplified, quantitative detection of *Listeria monocytogenes* in foods. *Food Microbiol. 4*:269–275.

28. Buchanan, R. L., H. G. Stahl, and M. M. Bencivengo. 1988. Recovery of *Listeria* from fresh retail-level foods of animal origin. Ann. Mtg., Amer. Soc. Microbiol., Miami Beach, FL, May 8–13, Abstr. P-46.

29. Buchanan, R. L., J. L. Smith, H. G. Stahl, and D. L. Archer. 1988. *Listeria* methods development research at the Eastern Regional Research Center, U.S. Department of Agriculture. *J. Assoc. Off. Anal. Chem. 71*:651–654.

30. Buchanan, R. L., H. G. Stahl, M. M. Bencivengo, and F. del Corral. 1989. Comparison of lithium chloride-phenylethanol-moxalactam and modified Vogel-Johnson agars for detection of *Listeria* spp. in retail-level meats, poultry and seafood. *Appl. Environ. Microbiol. 55*:599–603.

31. Bunning, V. K., C. W. Donnelly, J. T. Peeler, E. H. Briggs, J. G. Bradshaw, R. G. Crawford, C. M. Beliveau, and J. T. Tierney. 1988. Thermal inactivation of *Listeria monocytogenes* within bovine milk phagocytes. *Appl. Environ. Microbiol. 54*:364–370.

32. Carnevale, R. A., and R. W. Johnston. 1989. Method for the isolation and identification of *Listeria monocytogenes* from meat and poultry products. United States Department of Agriculture Food Safety and Inspection Service, Laboratory Communication No. 57, Revised May 24. USDA, Washington DC.

33. Cassiday, P. K., R. E. Brackett, and L. R. Beuchat. 1989. Evaluation of ten selective direct plating media for enumeration of *Listeria monocytogenes* in ham and oysters. *Food Microbiol. 55*:113–125.

34. Cassiday, P. K., R. E. Brackett, and L. R. Beuchat. 1989. Evaluation of three newly developed direct plating media to enumerate *Listeria monocytogenes* in foods. *Appl. Environ. Microbiol. 55*:1645–1648.

35. Cowart, R. E., and B. G. Foster. 1985. Differential effects of iron on the growth of *Listeria monocytogenes*: Minimum requirements and mechanism of acquisition. *J. Infect. Dis. 151*:721–730.

36. Cox, L. J., A. Renaud, and M. van Schothorst. 1988. Some studies on methodology for recuperation of *Listeria monocytogenes* from foods with special reference to soft cheeses. *J. Assoc. Off. Anal. Chem. 71*:449. Abstr.

37. Crawford, R. G., C. M. Beliveau, J. T. Peeler, C. W. Donnelly, and V. K. Bunning. 1989. Comparative recovery of uninjured and heat-injured *Listeria monocytogenes* cells from bovine milk. *Appl. Environ. Microbiol. 55*:1490–1494.

38. Curtis, G. D. W. 1989. Pharmacopoeia of culture media in food microbiology—Additional monographs. *Int. J. Food Microbiol. 9*:85–145.

39. Curtis, G. D. W., W. W. Nichols, and T. J. Falla. 1989. Selective agents for *Listeria* can inhibit their growth. *Lett. Appl. Microbiol. 8*:169–172.

40. Curtis, G. D. W., R. G. Mitchell, A. F. King, and E. J. Griffin. 1989. A selective differential medium for the isolation of *Listeria monocytogenes*. *Lett. Appl. Microbiol. 8*:95–98.

41. Dallmier, A. W., and S. E. Martin. 1988. Catalase and superoxide dismutase activities after heat injury of *Listeria monocytogenes*. *Appl. Environ. Microbiol. 54*:581–582.

42. Davidson, R. J., D. W. Sprung, C. E. Park, and M. K. Rayman. 1989. Occurrence of *Listeria*

monocytogenes, Campylobacter spp., and *Yersinia enterocolitica* in Manitoba raw milk. *Can. Inst. Food Sci. Technol. J. 22*:70–74.

43. Despierres, M. 1971. Isolement de *Listeria monocytogenes* dans un milieu défavorable a *Streptococcus faecalis. Ann. Inst. Pasteur 121*:493–501.
44. Dijkstra, R. G. 1976. *Listeria*-encephalitis in cows through litter from a broiler-farm. *Zentralbl. Bakteriol. Hyg. I Abt. Orig. B 161*:383–385.
45. Donnelly, C. W. 1988. Historical perspectives on methodology to detect *Listeria monocytogenes. J. Assoc. Off. Anal. Chem. 71*:644–646.
46. Donnelly, C. W., and G. J. Baigent. 1986. Method for flow cytometric detection of *Listeria monocytogenes* in milk. *Appl. Environ. Microbiol. 52*:689–695.
47. Donnelly, C. W., and E. H. Briggs. 1986. Psychrotrophic growth and thermal inactivation of *Listeria monocytogenes* as a function of milk composition. *J. Food Prot. 49*:994–998.
48. Donnelly, C. W., E. H. Briggs, and L. S. Donnelly. 1987. Comparison of heat resistance of *Listeria monocytogenes* in milk as determined by two methods. *J. Food Prot. 50*:14–17, 20.
49. Doyle, M. P., and J. L. Schoeni. 1986. Selective-enrichment procedure for isolation of *Listeria monocytogenes* from fecal and biologic specimens. *Appl. Environ. Microbiol. 51*:1127–1129.
50. Doyle, M. P., and J. L. Schoeni. 1987. Comparison of procedures for isolating *Listeria monocytogenes* in soft, surface-ripened cheese. *J. Food Prot. 50*:4–6.
51. Doyle, M. P., L. M. Meske, and E. H. Marth. 1985. Survival of *Listeria monocytogenes* during the manufacture and storage of nonfat dry milk. *J. Food Prot. 48*:740–742.
52. Doyle, M. P., K. A. Glass, J. T. Beery, G. A. Garcia, D. J. Pollard, and R. D. Schultz. 1987. Survival of *Listeria monocytogenes* in milk during high-temperature, short-time pasteurization. *Appl. Environ. Microbiol. 53*:1433–1438.
53. Durst, J., and G. Berencsi. 1975. New selective media of rivanol content for *Listeria monocytogenes. Zentralbl. Bakteriol. Hyg. I Abt. Orig. A 232*:410–411.
54. Durst, J., and G. Berencsi. 1976. Contributions to further serovariants of *L. monocytogenes. Zentralbl. Bakteriol. Hyg. I Abt. Orig. A 236*:531–532.
55. Elischerova, K., and S. Stupalova. 1972. Listeriosis in professionally exposed persons. *Acta Microbiol. Hung. 19*:379–384.
56. El-Kest, S. E., and E. H. Marth. 1989. Lethal and sublethal effects caused by freezing *Listeria monocytogenes.* Ann. Mtg., Inst. Food Technol., Chicago, IL, June 25–29, Abstr. 357.
57. El-Kest, S. E., and E. H. Marth. 1989. Unpublished data.
58. El-Shenawy, M. A., A. E. Yousef, and E. H. Marth. 1989. Heat injury and inactivation of *Listeria monocytogenes* in reconstituted nonfat dry milk. *Milchwissenschaft 44*:741–745.
59. El-Shenawy, M. A., A. E. Yousef, and E. H. Marth. 1989. Inactivation and injury of *Listeria monocytogenes* in tryptic soy broth or ground beef treated with gamma irradiation. *Lebensm. Wiss. Technol. 22*:387–390.
60. Fallon, R. J. 1985. Listeriosis. *Lancet ii*:728.
61. Farber, J. M., G. W. Sanders, and S. A. Malcom. 1988. The presence of *Listeria* spp. in raw milk in Ontario. *Can. J. Microbiol. 34*:95–100.
62. Farber, J. M., G. W. Sanders, and J. I. Speirs. 1988. Methodology for isolation of *Listeria* from foods—a Canadian perspective. *J. Assoc. Off. Anal. Chem. 71*:675–678.
63. Fenlon, D. R. 1985. Wild birds and silage as reservoirs of *Listeria* in the agricultural environment. *J. Appl. Bacteriol. 59*:537–543.
64. Fenlon, D. R. 1986. Rapid quantitative assessment of the distribution of *Listeria* in silage implicated in a suspected outbreak of listeriosis in calves. *Vet. Rec. 118*:240–242.
65. Filice, G. A., H. F. Cantrell, A. B. Smith, P. S. Hayes, J. C. Feeley, and D. W. Fraser. 1978. *Listeria monocytogenes* infection in neonates: Investigation of an epidemic. *J. Infect. Dis. 138*:17–23.
66. Fleming, D. W., S. L. Cochi, K. L. MacDonald, J. Brondum, P. S. Hayes, B. D. Plikaytis, M. B. Holmes, A. Audurier, C. V. Broome, and A. L. Reingold. 1985. Pasteurized milk as a vehicle of infection in an outbreak of listeriosis. *N. Engl. J. Med. 312*:404–407.
67. Francis, D. W., and J. Lovett. 1989. Comparison of FDA and USDA methods for isolating

Listeria monocytogenes. Ann. Mtg., Amer. Soc. Microbiol., New Orleans, LA, May 14–18, Abstr. P-39.

68. Fraser, J. A., and W. H. Sperber. 1988. Rapid detection of *Listeria* spp. in food and environmental samples by esculin hydrolysis. *J. Food Prot. 51*:762–765.
69. Fuzi, M., and I. Pillis. 1961. Selektive Züchtung von *L. monocytogenes.* Vortrag 3, Kongress d. ung. Mikrobiol. Gesellsch., Budapest.
70. Garayzabal, J. F., and C. Genigeorgis. 1990. Quantitative evaluation of three selective enrichment broths and agars used in recovering *Listeria* microorganisms. *J. Food Prot. 53*:105–110.
71. Girard, N. 1988. Personal communication.
72. Gitter, M. 1976. *Listeria monocytogenes* in "oven-ready" poultry. *Vet. Rec. 99*:336.
73. Gledel, J. 1988. Personal communication.
74. Golden, D. A., L. R. Beuchat, and R. E. Brackett. 1988. Direct plating technique for enumeration of *Listeria monocytogenes* in foods. *J. Assoc. Off. Anal. Chem. 71*: 647–650.
75. Golden, D. A., L. R. Beuchat, and R. E. Brackett. 1988. Evaluation of selective direct plating media for their suitability to recover uninjured, heat-injured, and freeze-injured *Listeria monocytogenes* from foods. *Appl. Environ. Microbiol. 54*:1451–1456.
76. Golden, D. A., L. R. Beuchat, and R. E. Brackett. 1988. Inactivation and injury of *Listeria monocytogenes* as affected by heating and freezing. Abstr. Ann. Mtg., Amer. Soc. Microbiol., Miami Beach, FL, Abstr. P-45.
77. Goldstein, E. J. C. 1988. Structure of the fluoroquinolone group of antibacterials—introduction. *Suppl. Urol. 32*:4–8.
78. Gray, M. L. 1960. Isolation of *Listeria monocytogenes* from oat silage. *Science 132*:1767–1768.
79. Gray, M. L., and A. H. Killinger. 1966. *Listeria monocytogenes* and listeric infections. *Bacteriol. Rev. 30*:309–382.
80. Gray, M. L., C. Singh, and F. Thorp, Jr. 1956. Abortion and pre- or postnatal death of young due to *Listeria monocytogenes*. III. Studies in ruminants. *Amer. J. Vet. Res. 17*:510–516.
81. Gray, M. L., H. J. Stafseth, and F. Thorp, Jr. 1950. The use of potassium tellurite, sodium azide, and acetic acid in a selective medium for the isolation of *Listeria monocytogenes*. *J. Bacteriol. 59*:443–444.
82. Gray, M. L., H. J. Stafseth, F. Thorp, Jr., L. B. Sholl, and W. F. Riley, Jr. 1948. A new technique for isolating listerellae from the bovine brain. *J. Bacteriol. 55*:471–476.
83. Gregorio, S. B., W. C. Eveland, and H. F. Maassab. 1986. Efficiency of various solid media for the isolation of *Listeria monocytogenes*. Abstr. Ann. Mtg., Amer. Soc. Microbiol., p. 27.
84. Grønstøl, H., and E. Aspøy. 1977. A new selective medium for the isolation of *Listeria monocytogenes*. *Nord. Vet. Med. 29*:446–451.
85. Hao, D.Y.-Y., L. R. Beuchat, and R. E. Brackett. 1989. Comparison of media and methods for detecting and enumerating *Listeria monocytogenes* in refrigerated cabbage. *Appl. Environ. Microbiol. 53*:955–957.
86. Hartmann, V. 1988. Personal communication.
87. Hartmann, V., K. Friedrich, F. Beyer, and G. Terplan. 1988. Verbesserung des Listeriennachweises durch einen Moxalactam-enthaltenden Nährboden. *Deutsche Molkerei-Zeitung 38*:1164–1166.
88. Hayes, P. S., J. C. Feeley, L. M. Graves, G. W. Ajello, and D. W. Fleming. 1986. Isolation of *Listeria monocytogenes* from raw milk. *Appl. Environ. Microbiol. 51*:438–440.
89. Heisick, J. E., D. E. Wagner, M. L. Nierman, and J. T. Peeler. 1989. *Listeria* spp. found on fresh market produce. *Appl. Environ. Microbiol. 55*:1925–1927.
90. Heisick, J. E., F. M. Harrell, E. H. Peterson, S. McLaughlin, D. E. Wagner, I. V. Wesley, and J. Bryner. 1989. Comparison of four procedures to detect *Listeria* spp. in foods. *J. Food Prot. 52*:154–157.
91. Henry, B. S. 1933. Dissociation in the genus *Brucella*. *J. Infect. Dis. 52*:374–402.
92. Hitchins, A. D. 1989. Effect of food microflora concentration on the detectability of *Listeria monocytogenes* in foods. Ann. Mtg., Amer. Soc. Microbiol., New Orleans, LA, May 14–18, Abstr. P–7.

93. Hitchins, A. D. 1989. Quantitative comparison of two enrichment methods for isolating *Listeria monocytogenes* from inoculated ice cream. *J. Food Prot.* 52:898–900.
94. Hofer, E. 1974. Study of occurrence of *L. monocytogenes* in human feces. *Rev. Soc. Bras. Med. Trop.* 8:109–116.
95. Hoover, D. G. 1989. Personal communication.
96. Jay. J. M. 1987. A new selective medium for the recovery of *Listeria* spp. from food. Ann. Mtg., Amer. Soc. Microbiol., Atlanta, GA, March 1–6, Abstr. P-24.
97. Kampelmacher, E. H., and L. M. van Noorle Jansen. 1969. Isolation of *Listeria monocytogenes* from feces of clinically healthy humans and animals. *Zentralbl. Bakteriol. I Abt. Orig. A* 211:353–359.
98. Kampelmacher, E. H., and L. M. van Noorle Jansen. 1972. Further studies on the isolation of *Listeria monocytogenes* in clinically healthy individuals. *Zentralbl. Bakteriol. I Abt. Orig. A* 221:70–77.
99. Kampelmacher, E. H., and L. M. van Noorle Jansen. 1972. Isolierung von *L. monocytogenes* mittels Nalidixinsäuretrypaflavin. *Zentralbl. Bakteriol. Parasit. Abt. I Orig. A* 221:139–140.
100. Kampelmacher, E. H., D. E. Maas, and L. M. van Noorle Jansen. 1976. Occurrence of *Listeria monocytogenes* in feces of pregnant women with and without direct animal contact. *Zentralbl. Bakteriol. Hyg. I. Abt. Orig. A* 234:238–242.
101. Kaufmann, V. 1988. Personal communication.
102. Khan, M. A., A. Seaman, and M. Woodbine. 1972. Differential media for the isolation of *Listeria monocytogenes*. *Acta Microbiol. Acad. Sci. Hung.* 19:371–372.
103. Klausner, R., and C. W. Donnelly. 1989. Personal communication.
104. Klinger, J. D., A. Johnson, D. Croan, P. Flynn, K. Whippie, M. Kimball, J. Lawrie, and M. Curiale. 1988. Comparative studies of nucleic acid hybridization assay for *Listeria* in foods. *J. Assoc. Off. Anal. Chem.* 71:669–673.
105. Knight, M. T., J. F. Black, and D. W. Wood. 1988. Industry perspectives on *Listeria monocytogenes*. *J. Assoc. Off. Anal. Chem.* 71:682–683.
106. Kramer, P. A., and D. Jones. 1969. Media selective for *Listeria monocytogenes*. *J. Appl. Bacteriol.* 32:381–394.
107. Kvendberg, J. E. 1988. Personal communication.
108. Lachica, R. V. 1988. Selective direct plating medium for enhanced recovery of *Listeria monocytogenes* (LM) from foods. Soc. Ind. Microbiol., Comprehensive Conference on *Listeria monocytogenes*, Rohnert Park, CA, Oct. 2–5, Abstr. P-5.
109. Lachica, R. V. 1989. Modified Henry technique for the initial recognition of *Listeria* colonies. Ann. Mtg., Soc. Indust. Microbiol., Seattle, WA, August 13–18, Abstr. P-44.
110. Lachica, R. V. 1990. Selective plating medium for quantitative recovery of food-borne *Listeria monocytogenes*. *Appl. Environ. Microbiol.* 56:167–169.
111. Lammerding, A. M., and M. P. Doyle. 1989. Evaluation of enrichment procedures for recovery of *Listeria monocytogenes* from dairy products. Ann. Mtg., Inst. Food Technol., Chicago, IL, June 25–29, Abstr. 460.
112. Larsen, H. E. 1964. Investigations on the epidemiology of listeriosis—the distribution of *Listeria monocytogenes* in environments in which clinical outbreaks have not been diagnosticated. *Nord. Vet. Med.* 16:890–909.
113. Larsen, H. E., and A. Gundstrup. 1965. The inhibitory action of various strains of *Bacillus* on *Listeria monocytogenes*. *Nord Vet. Med.* 17:336–341.
114. Larsson, S., M. H. Walder, S. N. Cronberg, A. B. Forsgren, and T. Moestrup. 1985. Antimicrobial susceptibilities of *Listeria monocytogenes* strains isolated from 1958 to 1982 in Sweden. *Antimicrob. Agents Chemother.* 28:12–14.
115. Leasor, S. B., and P. M. Foegeding. 1990. *Listeria* species in commercially broken raw liquid whole egg. *J. Food Prot.* 52:777–780.
116. Lee, W. H. 1988. Personal communication.
117. Lee, W. H. 1989. Screening test to detect *Listeria* (<100/g) in food. Ann. Mtg., Amer. Soc. Microbiol., New Orleans, LA, May 14–18, Abstr. P-38.

118. Lee, W. H., and D. McClain. 1986. Improved *Listeria monocytogenes* selective agar. *Appl. Environ. Microbiol. 52*:1215–1217.
119. Lehnert, C. 1964. Bakteriologische, serologische und tierexperimentelle Untersuchungen zur Pathogenese, Epizootologie und Prophylaxe der Listeriose. *Arch. exp. Vet. Med. 18*:981–1027, 1247–1301.
120. Leighton, I. 1979. Use of selective agents for the isolation of *Listeria monocytogenes*. *Med. Lab. Sci. 36*:283–288.
121. Loessner, M. J., R. H. Bell, J. M. Jay, and L. A. Shelef. 1988. Comparison of seven plating media for enumeration of *Listeria* spp. *Appl. Environ. Microbiol. 54*:3003–3007.
122. Lovett, J. 1988. Isolation and enumeration of *Listeria monocytogenes*. *Food Technol. 42*(4):172–175.
123. Lovett, J. 1988. Isolation and identification of *Listeria monocytogenes* in dairy products. *J. Assoc. Off. Anal. Chem. 71*:658–660.
124. Lovett, J., and A. D. Hitchins. 1988. *Listeria* isolation; Revised method of analysis. *Fed. Register 53*:44148–44153.
125. Lovett, J., D. W. Francis, and J. M. Hunt. 1987. *Listeria monocytogenes* in raw milk: detection, incidence, and pathogenicity. *J. Food Prot. 50*:188–192.
126. Martin, R. S., R. K. Sumarah, and M. A. MacDonald. 1984. A synthetic based medium for the isolation of *Listeria monocytogenes*. *Clin. Invest. Med. 7*:233–237.
127. Mavrothalassitis, P. 1975. Etud d'un milieu différentiel pour l'isolement de *Listeria monocytogenes*. *Pathol. Microbiol. 42*:238.
128. Mavrothalassitis, P. 1977. A method for rapid isolation of *Listeria monocytogenes* from infected material. *J. Appl. Bacteriol. 43*:47–52.
129. McBride, M. E., and K. F. Girard. 1960. A selective method for the isolation of *Listeria monocytogenes* from mixed bacterial populations. *J. Lab. Clin. Med. 55*:153–157.
130. McCarthy, S. A., M. L. Motes, and R. M. McPhearson. 1989. Recovery of heat-stressed *Listeria monocytogenes* from laboratory-infected and naturally-contaminated shrimp. Ann. Mtg., Amer. Soc. Microbiol., New Orleans, LA, May 14–18, Abstr. P-10.
131. McClain, D. 1986. Personal communication.
132. McClain, D., and W. H. Lee. 1987. A method to recover *Listeria monocytogenes* from meats. Ann. Mtg., Amer. Soc. Microbiol., Atlanta, GA, May 1–6, Abstr. P-23.
133. McClain, D., and W. H. Lee. 1988. Development of USDA-FSIS method for isolation of *Listeria monocytogenes* from raw meat and poultry. *J. Assoc. Off. Anal. Chem. 71*:660–664.
134. Murray, E. G. D., R. A. Webb, and M. B. R. Swann. 1926. A disease of rabbits characterized by a large mononuclear leucocytosis, caused by a hitherto undescribed bacillus *Bacterium monocytogenes* (n.sp.). *J. Pathol. Bacteriol. 29*:407–439.
135. Neaves, P. 1988. Personal communication.
136. Netten, P. van, I. Perales, and D. A. A. Mossel. 1988. An improved selective and diagnostic medium for isolation and counting of *Listeria* spp. in heavily contaminated foods. *Lett. Appl. Microbiol. 7*:17–21.
137. Netten, P. van, H. Van der Zee, and D. A. A. Mossel. 1984. A note on catalase enhanced recovery of acid injured cells of gram negative bacteria and its consequences for the assessment of the lethality of L-lactic acid decontamination of raw meat surfaces. *J. Appl. Bacteriol. 57*:169–173.
138. Netten, P. van, A. van de Ven, I. Perales, and D. A. A. Mossel. 1988. A selective and diagnostic medium for use in the enumeration of *Listeria* spp. in foods. *Int. J. Food Microbiol. 6*:187–198.
139. Netten, P. van, I. Perales, A. Van de Moosdijk, G. D. W. Curtis, and D. A. A. Mossel. 1989. Liquid and solid selective differential media for the detection and enumeration of *L. monocytogenes* and other *Listeria* spp. *Int. J. Food Microbiol. 8*:299–316.
140. Nieman, R. E., and B. Lorber. 1980. Listeriosis in adults: A changing pattern. Report of eight cases and review of the literature, 1968–1978. *Rev. Infect. Dis. 2*:207–227.
141. Noah, C. W., and N. C. Ramos. 1989. Detecting *Listeria* spp. in naturally contaminated

seafoods: Comparing four enrichment procedures to a modified standard FDA method. *J. Food Prot.* 52:751. Abstr.

142. Nordholt, M. 1988. Personal communication.

143. Olson, C., Jr., L. A. Dunn, and C. L. Rollins. 1953. Methods for isolation of *Listeria monocytogenes* from sheep. *Amer. J. Vet. Res.* 14:82–85.

144. Ortel, S. 1971. Ausscheidung von *Listeria monocytogenes* im Stuhl gesunder Personen. *Zentralbl. Bakteriol. I. Abt. Orig.* 217:41–46.

145. Ortel, S. 1972. Experience with nalidixic acid-trypaflavine agar. *Acta Microbiol. Acad. Sci. Hung.* 19:363–365.

146. Osebold, J. W., J. W. Kendrick, and A. Njoku-Obi. 1960. Abortion in cattle-experimentally infected with *Listeria monocytogenes*. *J. Amer. Vet. Med. Assoc.* 137:227–233.

147. Papageorgiou, D. K., and E. H. Marth. 1989. Fate of *Listeria monocytogenes* during the manufacture, ripening and storage of Feta cheese. *J. Food Prot.* 52:82–87.

148. Papageorgiou, D. K., and E. H. Marth. 1989. Fate of *Listeria monocytogenes* during the manufacture and ripening of blue cheese. *J. Food Prot.* 52:459–465.

149. Patterson, M. 1989. Sensitivity of *Listeria monocytogenes* to irradiation on poultry meat and in phosphate-buffered saline. *Lett. Appl. Microbiol.* 8:181–184.

150. Petran, R. K. L., and E. A. Zottola. 1988. A study of factors affecting the growth and recovery of *L. monocytogenes* strain Scott A. Ann. Mtg., Inst. Food Technol., New Orleans, LA, June 19–22, Abstr. 313.

151. Pini, P. N., and R. J. Gilbert. 1988. A comparison of two procedures for the isolation of *Listeria monocytogenes* from raw chickens and soft cheeses. *Int. J. Food Microbiol.* 7:331–337.

152. Pomanskaya, L. A. 1961. Polymorphism of *Listeria*. *Ah. Mikrobiol. Epidemiol. Immunobiol.* 38:124–128.

153. Prentice, G. A. 1988. Personal communication.

154. Pusch, D. J. 1989. A review of current methods used in the United States for isolating *Listeria* from food. *Int. J. Food Microbiol.* 8:197–204.

155. Ralovich, B. S. 1975. Selective and enrichment media to isolate *Listeria*. In M. Woodbine (ed.), *Problems of Listeriosis, Proceedings of the Sixth International Symposium*, Leicester University Press, Leicester, pp. 286–294.

156. Ralovich, B. 1984. *Listeriosis Research—Present Situation and Perspective*, Akademiai Kiado, Budapest.

157. Ralovich, B. 1989. Data on the enrichment and selective cultivation of listeriae. *Int. J. Food Microbiol.* 8:205–217.

158. Ralovich, B., A. Forray, E. Mero, and H. Malovics. 1970. Additional data on diagnosis and epidemiology of *Listeria* infections. *Zentralbl. Bakteriol. I Abt. Orig.* 214:231–235.

159. Ralovich, B., L. Emody, I. Malovics, E. Mero, and A. Forray. 1972. Methods to isolate *Listeria monocytogenes* from different materials. *Acta Microbiol. Acad. Sci. Hung.* 19:367–369.

160. Ralovich, B., A. Forray, E. Mero, H. Malovics, and I. Szazados. 1971. New selective medium for isolation of *L. monocytogenes*. *Zentralbl. Bakteriol. I Abt. Orig.* 216:88–91.

161. Ray, B. 1986. Impact of bacterial injury and repair in food microbiology: Its past, present and future. *J. Food Prot.* 49:651–655.

162. Rico-Munoz, E. 1989. Modified LPM agar for the isolation of *Listeria monocytogenes* from meat products. Ann. Mtg., Inst. Food Technol., Chicago, IL, June 25–29, Abstr. 461.

163. Rodriguez, D. L., G. S. Fernandez, J. F. F. Garayzabal, and E. R. Ferri. 1984. New methodology for the isolation of *Listeria* microorganisms from heavily contaminated environments. *Appl. Environ. Microbiol.* 47:1188–1190.

164. Rodriguez, D. L., J. F. Fernandez, V. Briones, J. L. Blanco, and G. Suarez. 1988. Assessment of different selective agar media for enumeration and isolation of *Listeria* from dairy products. *J. Dairy Res.* 55:579–583.

165. Rodriguez, D. L., J. F. F. Garayzabal, J. A. V. Boland, E. R. Ferri, and G. S. Fernandez. 1985. Isolation de microorganisms de listeria a partir de lait cru destine a le consommation humaine. *Can. J. Microbiol.* 31:938–941.

166. Ryser, E. T., E. H. Marth, and M. P. Doyle. 1985. Survival of *Listeria monocytogenes* during manufacture and storage of cottage cheese. *J. Food Prot. 48*:746–750, 753.
167. Ryser, E. T., and E. H. Marth. 1987. Behavior of *Listeria monocytogenes* during the manufacture and ripening of Cheddar cheese. *J. Food Prot. 50*:7–13.
168. Ryser, E. T., and E. H. Marth. 1987. Fate of *Listeria monocytogenes* during manufacture and ripening of Camembert cheese. *J. Food Prot. 50*:372–378.
169. Ryser, E. T., and E. H. Marth. 1988. Survival of *Listeria monocytogenes* in cold-pack cheese food during refrigerated storage. *J. Food Prot. 51*:615–621, 625.
170. Ryser, E. T., and E. H. Marth. 1989. Behavior of *Listeria monocytogenes* during manufacture and ripening of brick cheese. *J. Dairy Sci. 72*:838–853.
171. Schiemann, D., S. Shope, and M. Brown. 1989. Development of new isolation media for hemolytic species of *Listeria*. Ann. Mtg., Amer. Soc. Microbiol., New Orleans, LA, May 14–18, Abstr. P-34.
172. Seeliger, H. P. R. 1961. *Listeriosis*, Hafner Publishing Co., New York.
173. Seeliger, H. P. R. 1972. Reviews—A new outlook on the epidemiology and epizoology of listeriosis. *Acta Microbiol. Hung. 19*:273–286.
174. Seeliger, H. P. R., F. Sander, and J. Bockemühl. 1970. Zum kulturellen Nachweis von *Listeria monocytogenes. Z. Med. Mikrobiol. Immunol. 155*:352–368.
175. Shimizu, K., G. Otsuka, and M. Oka. 1954. Guanofuracin media for isolation of *Listeria monocytogenes* and its practical application. *Jap. J. Vet. Res. 2*:1–10.
176. Siragusa, G. R., and M. G. Johnson. 1989. Persistence of *Listeria monocytogenes* in yogurt as determined by direct plating and cold enrichment methods. *Int. J. Food Microbiol. 7*:147–160.
177. Skalka, B., and J. Smola. 1983. Selective diagnostic medium for pathogenic *Listeria* spp. *J. Clin. Microbiol. 18*:1432–1433.
178. Skovgaard, N., and C.-A. Morgen. 1988. Detection of *Listeria* spp. in faeces from animals, in feeds, and in raw foods of animal origin. *Int. J. Food Microbiol. 6*:229–242.
179. Slade, P. J., and D. L. Collins-Thompson. 1987. Two-stage enrichment procedures for isolating *Listeria monocytogenes* from raw milk. *J. Food Prot. 50*:904–908.
180. Slade, P. J., and D. L. Collins-Thompson. 1988. Comparison of two-stage and direct selective enrichment techniques for isolating *Listeria* spp. from raw milk. *J. Food Sci. 53*:1694–1696.
181. Smith, J. L. 1988. Stress-induced injury in *Listeria monocytogenes*. Soc. Ind. Microbiol., Comprehensive Conference on *Listeria monocytogenes*, Rohnert Park, CA, Oct. 2–5, Abstr. I-29.
182. Smith, J. L., and D. L. Archer. 1988. Heat-induced injury in *Listeria monocytogenes. J. Ind. Microbiol. 3*:105–110.
183. Sokolovic, A., and W. Goebel. 1989. Synthesis of listeriolysin in *Listeria monocytogenes* under heat shock conditions. *Infect. Immun. 57*:295–298.
184. Spoloor, D., M. L. Dal Santo, and F. Zilio. 1989. Rassegna delle tecniche di ricerca ed isolamento per via colturale delle listerie. *Indust. Aliment. 28*:577–583.
185. Swaminathan, B., P. S. Hayes, and V. A. Przybyszewski. 1988. Evaluation of enrichment and plating media for isolating *Listeria monocytogenes. J. Assoc. Off. Anal. Chem. 71*:664–668.
186. Terplan, G. 1988. Personal communication.
187. Terplan, G. 1988. Provisional IDF-recommended method: Milk and milk products—detection of *Listeria monocytogenes*. Int. Dairy Federation, Brussels.
188. Tomlins, R. I., and Z. J. Ordal. 1976. Thermal injury and inactivation in vegetative bacteria. In F. A. Skinner and W. B. Hugo (eds.), *Inhibition and Inactivation of Vegetative Microbes*. Academic Press, NY, pp. 153–190.
189. Truscott, R. B., and W. B. McNab. 1988. Comparison of media and procedures for the isolation of *Listeria monocytogenes* from ground beef. *J. Food Prot. 51*:626–628, 638.
190. Watkins, J., and K. P. Sleath. 1981. Isolation and enumeration of *Listeria monocytogenes* from sewage, sewage sludge and river water. *J. Appl. Bacteriol. 50*:1–9.
191. Welshimer, H. J. 1968. Isolation of *Listeria monocytogenes* from vegetation. *J. Bacteriol. 95*:300–303.

192. Welshimer, H. J., and J. Donker-Voet. 1971. *Listeria monocytogenes* in nature. *Appl. Microbiol. 21*:516–519.

193. Wood, D. 1969. Isolation of *Listeria monocytogenes*. In D. A. Shapton and G. W. Gould (eds.), *Soc. Appl. Bacteriol. Technical Series*, No. 3, Academic Press, London, pp. 63–69.

194. Yousef, A. E., and E. H. Marth. 1988. Behavior of *Listeria monocytogenes* during manufacture and storage of Colby cheese. *J. Food Prot. 51*:12–15.

195. Yousef, A. E., E. T. Ryser, and E. H. Marth. 1988. Methods for improved recovery of *Listeria monocytogenes* from cheese. *Appl. Environ. Microbiol. 54*:2643–2649.

196. Yousef, A. E., M. A. El-Shenawy, and E. H. Marth. 1989. Inactivation and injury of *Listeria monocytogenes* in a minimal medium as affected by benzoic acid and incubation temperature. *J. Food Sci. 54*:650–652.

7

Rapid Methods to Detect
Listeria monocytogenes in
Food and Environmental Samples

INTRODUCTION

For nearly 100 years food microbiologists have relied on various agar media to isolate and quantify the myriad of microorganisms present in food. Hence, this science of "agarology" was logically adopted by investigators to enumerate *Listeria* spp. in clinical, environmental, and food samples, as discussed in the preceding chapter. Several outbreaks of foodborne listeriosis during the 1980s led to development of the current (1990) FDA and USDA enrichment/plating procedures to detect *L. monocytogenes* in dairy and meat products, respectively. Although these two "standard methods" have drastically shortened the time of analysis as compared to the traditional cold enrichment procedure, the 3- to 6-day period needed to determine that a particular food sample is free of *L. monocytogenes* is unacceptable to large segments of the food industry which deal with highly perishable products such as fluid milk, raw meat, poultry, and seafood. Thus a need exists for faster methods to detect *L. monocytogenes* and other foodborne pathogens in foods with a short shelf life.

Using traditional agar methodology, detection of microorganisms including *L. monocytogenes* is contingent upon formation of visible colonies from which isolates can be obtained and then purified and confirmed using the previously described battery of biochemical and serological tests, all of which are costly, labor intensive, and time consuming. Provided that sufficient numbers of samples are processed, several rapid test strip methods and automated systems can be economically used to decrease the time needed for biochemical confirmation from 5–7 days to less than 24 hours. Recent advances in allied fields of immunology and microbial genetics also have led to development of fluorescent antibody assays, enzyme-linked immunosorbent assays, and DNA hybridization (DNA probe) assays, which can be used to detect *L. monocytogenes* in foods within several hours following primary and/or secondary warm enrichment. Several of these assays are available commercially and can be used effectively to screen large numbers of food samples for presence of *Listeria* spp. Progress toward rapid identification of listeriae in food has surpassed earlier expectations expressed in a survey conducted by the FDA (1). However, before any of these rapid methods can be adopted as "standard," scientists first must agree on a standard enrichment/plating procedure that can be used to measure the sensitivity and selectivity of these newly developed assays. Once this is done, various rapid methods can be compared to a true "standard method" for possible approval by the Association of Official Analytical Chemists. Following approval, newly developed rapid assays will likely revolutionize detection of *L. monocytogenes* and other foodborne pathogens and, at the same time, propel food microbiology from a science of "agarology" into a new era of enzyme assays, DNA probes, and other similar forms of "high technology."

ACCELERATED STANDARD BIOCHEMICAL TESTS

As you will recall from Chapter 1, a minimum of 1–2 days is required to complete most standard biochemical tests commonly used to speciate listeriae. However, during the last few years several "shortcuts" have been proposed to accelerate biochemical confirmation of presumptive *Listeria* isolates. According to a 1989 report by Lachica (4,64), *L. monocytogenes* colonies were much larger on Lithium Chloride–Ceftazidime Agar (LC Agar) (see Table 6.3) than on other selective plating media following 20 hours of incubation at 35°C and an additional 20 hours of incubation at 30°C. More important, the resulting *Listeria* colonies that appeared blue to bluish-green under oblique illumination were large enough to permit multiple tests on individual colonies. The "RAP-ID" identification procedure which the author employed is actually an accelerated version of the traditional protocol which is based on results from the following six tests: (a) a rapid CAMP test using discs impregnated with staphylococcal β-hemolysin, (b) rhamnose fermentation, (c) xylose fermentation, (d) catalase production, (e) KOH viscosity, an indirect means of determining the gram reaction, and (f) tumbling motility as observed microscopically. When plating media for the first three tests were heavily inoculated over a very small surface area, results for the entire battery of tests allowed positive identification of *L. monocytogenes*, *L. seeligeri*, *L. welshimeri*, *L. ivanovii*, and *L. innocua/L. grayi/L. murrayi* after only 8 hours. Overall, combined use of LC Agar and the "RAP-ID" method permitted quantitative detection and identification of *L. monocytogenes* and most other *Listeria* spp. in naturally contaminated, ready-to-cat foods within 48 hours. Since this procedure requires no extensive training, special equipment, or reagents, the cost-effective nature of this rapid identification scheme should be of particular benefit to small, less sophisticated testing laboratories.

   In addition to the isolation/identification scheme just described, several individual biochemical tests have been modified to more rapidly identify *Listeria* isolates. In 1989, Hunt and Sado (49) described a combined CAMP/xylose fermentation agar stab test that successfully speciated pure culture of *L. monocytogenes*, *L. ivanovii*, *L. seeligeri*, *L. innocua/L. grayi/L. murrayi*, and *L. welshimeri/L. denitrificans* within 24 hours. When heavily inoculated, a buffered broth containing 0.2% esculin and 5% sodium chloride also was able to identify organisms belonging to the genus *Listeria* after only 2 hours of incubation (50). However, since *Listeria* spp. and enterococci will both darken this medium after 2 hours of incubation, additional biochemical tests are required to eliminate false-positive reactions.

   While not generally regarded as a biochemical means of identification, changes that occur in laboratory media from microbial metabolic activity can be closely monitored by electrical impedance, i.e., a method in which resistance to flow of an alternating electrical current through a growth medium is quantified. Using such an approach, Phillips and Griffiths (82) found that *Listeria* spp. produced a uniformly strong capacitance signal during growth in Acriflavine–Ceftazidime Broth (AC Agar) (see Table 6.3). More important, this signal was distinctly different from those produced by other potential contaminants able to grow in AC broth, including *Enterobacter agglomerans*, *Pseudomonas aeruginosa*, and various *Bacillus* spp. Although these findings suggest that electrical impedance measurements can be used for early detection of *Listeria* spp. in mixed cultures, the apparent inability of this method to differentiate between *L. monocytogenes* and other *Listeria* spp. lessens the value of impedance monitoring for food samples that frequently contain only nonpathogenic listeriae.

MINIATURIZED BIOCHEMICAL TESTS

Use of miniaturized techniques for rapid biochemical identification of microorganisms began in the late 1940s when Weaver and his students (104) heavily inoculated small tubes of bacteriological media with pure cultures of unknown organisms. This concept has steadily grown in popularity so that today various kits are commercially available for rapid biochemical identification of medically important microorganisms. Several of these kits have been adapted for rapid identification of *Listeria* spp. These miniaturized systems can provide biochemical identification of *L. monocytogenes* isolates within 4 to 24 hours; however, all of these test kits require that the organism first be isolated in pure culture. As mentioned in the previous chapter, obtaining listeriae in pure culture from food and environmental samples is not always an easy task. Using the revised FDA procedure, 3–4 days normally elapse before a colony thought to be *Listeria* spp. appears on solid media. Thus, although the following test kits will allow rapid and economical biochemical confirmation of *L. monocytogenes*, the recently developed enzyme-linked immunosorbent assays and DNA hybridization assays appear to be much more beneficial in that both techniques bypass the need for a pure culture or isolated colony and can quickly detect organisms belonging to the genus *Listeria* in enrichment broth cultures containing a diverse microbial flora.

After the groundwork was laid during the late 1960s, Analytab Products Inc. (API) was among the first firms to commercially introduce miniaturized biochemical tests kits for identification of enteric pathogens. In the years that followed, additional API test kits were developed to identify anaerobic organisms of medical importance as well as streptococci, lactobacilli, and yeasts. All of these kits consist of a series of microtubules that contain various dehydrated substrates. After reconstituting the substrates by adding a suspension of the test organism, the kits are incubated according to the manufacturer's instructions. Depending on the type of kit being used, results are typically available after 4–24 hours of incubation.

One of these kits, the API 20 STREP system, which was originally developed to speciate streptococci, has proven useful for identifying *Listeria* spp. According to Mac Gowan et al. (68), the API 20 STREP system successfully identified 147 known clinical and environmental isolates of *Listeria* spp. to genus level after only 4 hours of incubation. While this system could not distinguish *L. monocytogenes* from *L. seeligeri*, hemolytic listeriae (i.e., *L. monocytogenes*, *L. seeligeri*, and *L. ivanovii*) could be readily differentiated from nonhemolytic species (i.e., *L. innocua*, *L. welshimeri*, *L. grayi*, *L. murrayi*). Furthermore, inclusion of mannitol and ribose in this test kit allowed the authors to distinguish *L. ivanovii* from other hemolytic listeriae and *L. grayi/L. murrayi* from the two remaining nonhemolytic species. Not surprising, the API-ZYM system (i.e., an enzyme-based kit developed to differentiate streptococci) also has proven useful for rapid confirmation and characterization of listeriae to the genus level (17,87). However, neither of these two API kits is presently able to confirm *Listeria* isolates as *L. monocytogenes*.

Like the API system, the MICRO-ID system, which was introduced by Organon Teknika in 1976, was originally intended for rapid (4 hours) identification of the *Enterobacteriaceae*. This test kit contains filter paper discs impregnated with reagents that detect specific enzymes and/or metabolic products from unknown bacterial isolates. Each of 15 separate wells in the test kit contains a particular substrate to be acted on by a bacterial enzyme as well as a detection system which reacts with the metabolic end-product to produce a readily identifiable color change.

In 1988, the MICRO-ID system was adapted by Robison et al. (86) to identify nonenteric bacteria, including *Listeria* spp. A total of 108 *L. monocytogenes* cultures, two cultures of *L. ivanovii*, and one culture each of *L. innocua*, *L. grayi*, *L. murrayi*, *L. welshimeri*, and *L. seeligeri* were examined using the MICRO-ID system. Following 4 hours of incubation, the test kit identified all *Listeria* cultures as belonging to octal codes 44041 (97 *L. monocytogenes* and six other *Listeria* spp.), 44040 (one *L. monocytogenes* and one *L. ivanovii*), or 44071 (10 *L. monocytogenes*). In addition, nine different bacterial species in the genera *Streptococcus*, *Staphylococcus*, *Micrococcus*, *Bacillus*, and *Lactobacillus* were correctly identified as non-*Listeria* spp. Subsequently, 105 presumptive *Listeria* strains isolated from dairy and environmental samples by the FDA procedure and 135 presumptive *Listeria* strains isolated from meat and meat-processing facilities by the USDA procedure were biochemically confirmed as *Listeria* spp. using traditional bacteriological media and the MICRO-ID system (Table 7.1). Overall, 159 and 162 strains were identified as belonging to the genus *Listeria* using the MICRO-ID system and conventional bacteriological media, respectively, thus indicating a false-negative rate of only 1.85% (3/162) for the rapid method. Although neither method could identify

Table 7.1 Use of the MICRO-ID System and Selected Conventional Biochemical Tests to Identify Presumptive *Listeria* Strains Isolated from Food and Food-Processing Factories

Sample	Number of strains	Isolation procedure	Conventional		MICRO-ID	
			Listeria spp.	non-*Listeria* spp.	*Listeria* spp.	non-*Listeria* spp.
Dairy products/ dairy factories	105	FDA	75	30	73	32
Meat products/ meat factories	135	USDA	87	48	86	49
Total	240		162	78	159	81

Source: Adapted from Ref. 85.

L. monocytogenes with absolute certainty (serological testing also is necessary), virtually identical results were available within 4 hours using the MICRO-ID system as compared to approximately 5–7 days using conventional media, thus indicating the usefulness of the rapid test kit.

Two additional rapid methods, the Minitek System and the Vitek Automicrobic System (AMS), also have been used to identify *Listeria* spp. The Minitek and MICRO-ID systems are somewhat similar in that both test kits use discs impregnated with appropriate substrates and reagents so a color change occurs after incubation. However, unlike the MICRO-ID system, substantial growth of the test organism must occur in the Minitek system before a color change can be observed. Therefore, this test requires approximately 18–24 hours to complete as compared to only 4 hours for the MICRO-ID system. Unlike the previous two test kits, the Vitek-AMS is a fully automated and computerized method for rapid biochemical identification of microorganisms. This system automatically does a series of 30 tests per sample in which biochemical reactions are monitored hourly during incubation by passing a light beam through each of 30 wells in a single "test card" containing the sample. Data concerning changes in light transmission that result from biochemical tests done on the sample are fed into a microcomputer which maintains a library of biochemical test results for all organisms able to be identified by the system. Using this method, positive results are normally available in 4–24 hours.

Several recent studies have evaluated the Vitek-AMS as an alternative to doing the more traditional, time-consuming biochemical tests for identification of *Listeria* spp. isolated from food and environmental samples. Knight et al. (62) found that the Vitek-AMS successfully identified 229 of 236 (97.0%) *Listeria* strains isolated from food-processing facilities. Using this rapid method, 95% of all positive isolates were confirmed after only 6–8 hours of incubation. The seven remaining isolates that were unidentified by the Vitek-AMS were subsequently confirmed as *Listeria* spp. using conventional biochemical tests. Thus the Vitek-AMS yielded a fairly acceptable false-negative rate of 2.97%. However, results obtained during a later FDA survey of raw vegetables (43) were even more impressive with each of 105 *Listeria* isolates yielding identical biochemical test results when examined by both the Vitek-AMS and traditional methods.

In another study, Doores et al. (26) compared the FDA identification procedure which uses conventional bacteriological media to the Minitek System and the Vitek-AMS for identification of *Listeria* spp. A total of 79 isolates from raw milk were presumptively identified as listeriae and confirmed to genus level using the FDA identification method (conventional bacteriological media), a modified Minitek procedure, and the Vitek-AMS for gram-positive bacteria. The FDA, Minitek, and Vitek-AMS methods yielded positive results within 5–7 days, 24 hours, and 5–13 hours, respectively, with excellent correlation being observed between the latter two rapid methods when compared to the FDA identification procedure. The Vitek-AMS also could speciate the organisms, provided that tests for hemolysis and rhamnose fermentation were included in the system. Despite impressive preliminary results obtained with the Vitek-AMS, only large research and industrial laboratories are likely to be able to justify the costs involved in owning, operating, and maintaining such a system. In contrast to the Vitek-AMS, the low cost of analysis and the nearly identical results obtained with the Minitek and MICRO-ID systems make them suitable for use in virtually any laboratory situation.

GAS CHROMATOGRAPHY

Quantitation of various biochemical components of bacterial cell extracts, particularly volatile and nonvolatile fatty acids, by gas-liquid chromatography is used routinely in large clinical laboratories to identify anaerobic bacteria of medical importance. Gas-liquid chromatography is based on the partition of volatile solutes between a flowing carrier gas phase and a liquid phase coated on inert particles. In theory, any compound that is volatile or becomes volatile at a temperature up to ~375°C can be detected and quantitated using this method.

Widespread use of gas-liquid chromatography as a tool to identify unknown bacterial isolates led to a recent investigation in which capillary column gas chromatography was employed to rapidly identify *Listeria* spp. and related bacteria. Using this method to quantitate cellular fatty acids, Sasser and Roy (90) speciated isolates of *L. monocytogenes*, *L. innocua*, *L. ivanovii*, and *L. grayi/L. denitrificans* 24 hours after obtaining pure cultures. Following growth at 28°C, the ratio of the free fatty acid 14:0/ISO 14:0 was >6 for *L. monocytogenes* and *L. innocua* but <6 for *L. ivanovii*. *L. monocytogenes* and *L. innocua* could be distinguished according to different ratios for the free fatty acids ANTEISO 15:0 and ANTEISO 17:0. Similarly, *L. grayi/L. denitrificans* contained the free fatty acids 16:0 and ISO 16:0 at a ratio >4, which is in direct contrast to levels in the other *Listeria* spp. examined. Using free fatty acid ratios, all *Listeria* spp. tested also were readily differentiated from organisms belonging to the related genera of *Brochothrix*, *Erysipelothrix*, *Kurthia*, and *Lactobacillus*. These results are similar to those of a subsequent study (40) in which *L. monocytogenes*, *Erysipelothrix rhusiopathiae*, *Rhodococcus equi*, *Actinomyces pyogenes*, *Arcanobacterium haemolyticum*, *Oerskovia xanthineolytica*, *Corynebacterium*, and other related groups could be differentiated from each other according to fatty acid composition. Identification of *Listeria* spp. using free fatty acid analysis yields rapid and precise results. However, as was true for miniaturized biochemical tests, this method also requires a pure culture which, as previously stated, easily may take 4 days to obtain. Thus, when combined with relatively high costs of equipment and the need for a skilled technician, use of gas chromatography to identify listeriae in food samples appears to be of little practical benefit to the food industry as compared to the enzyme-linked immunosorbent assays and DNA hybridization assays, which will be discussed shortly.

FLUORESCENT ANTIBODY TECHNIQUES

One of the procedures which meets the criterion of speed is the fluorescent antibody (FA) technique. Since its inception in 1942, this method has been used extensively in clinical microbiology laboratories to detect such pathogens as *Salmonella* spp., *Escherichia coli*, *Clostridium botulinum*, *Clostridium perfringens*, and *Treponema pallidum*, the causative agent of syphilis. However, the FA technique was not used successfully to identify pathogens in food until 1962 when several Russian scientists adopted this procedure for detecting salmonellae in milk (7). As a consequence of their work, widespread application of FA methodology to detect other foodborne pathogens, including *L. monocytogenes*, followed.

The FA technique is based on selective fluorescence which results from specific binding of a fluorescently labeled antibody to antigens on the bacterial cell surface. When properly treated, the bacterial cell surface is completely coated with the antigen–antibody complex and emits fluorescence which can be observed with a fluorescence-detecting microscope. Antibodies can be labeled with one of several fluorescent markers including rhodamine B, fluorescein isocyanate, and fluorescein isothiocyanate, the last of which is most common.

Bacterial cells can be labeled fluorescently in one of two ways using either a direct or an indirect FA technique with both techniques normally applied to bacterial cells that have been fixed to glass microscope slides. In the direct method, fluorescently labeled antibody binds directly to surface antigens, thus coating the entire surface of the bacterial cell (Fig. 7.1). In contrast, the indirect method is a two-step procedure in which binding of an unlabeled antibody (homologous antibody) to the bacterial cell surface is followed by binding of a fluorescently labeled antibody to the homologous antibody (Fig. 7.2). Thus in the indirect method, the labeled antibody detects presence of the homologous antibody which is bound to the surface antigen, whereas in the direct method, the labeled antibody binds directly to the surface antigen. Although both FA techniques eliminate the need for a pure bacterial culture, the indirect method offers a second advantage in that one need not prepare labeled antibody that is specific for each organism of interest.

Difficulties and delays in isolating *L. monocytogenes* from some types of clinical specimens, coupled with the often life-threatening conditions of listeric infection in newborn infants, make the FA technique particularly attractive as a rapid diagnostic tool. In 1962, Smith et al. (96) were first to accurately identify *L. monocytogenes* using the direct FA technique. In their study, all of 30 *L. monocytogenes* isolates obtained from human and animal sources were brilliantly fluorescent following treatment with a specific polyvalent somatic antiserum labeled with fluorescein isothiocyanate. In contrast, the labeled antiserum failed to react with 180 gram-positive and gram-negative

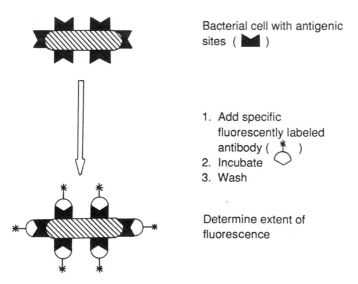

Bacterial cell with antigenic sites (   )

1. Add specific fluorescently labeled antibody (   )
2. Incubate
3. Wash

Determine extent of fluorescence

Figure 7.1   Direct fluorescent antibody technique.

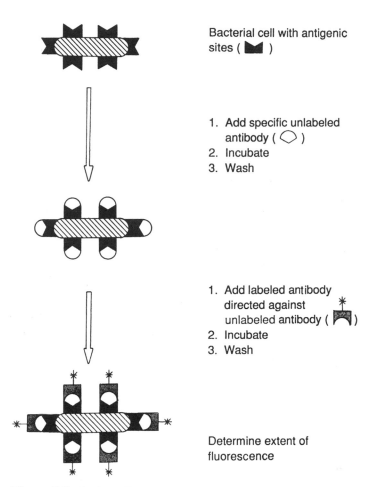

Bacterial cell with antigenic
sites ( )

1. Add specific unlabeled
   antibody ( )
2. Incubate
3. Wash

1. Add labeled antibody
   directed against
   unlabeled antibody ( )
2. Incubate
3. Wash

Determine extent of
fluorescence

Figure 7.2   Indirect fluorescent antibody technique.

non-*Listeria* organisms. Eveland (31) later used a similar direct FA technique to identify *L. monocytogenes* in cerebrospinal fluid of a patient, thus attesting to the usefulness of this procedure.

Preliminary results from the earlier study by Smith et al. (96) also suggested that the FA technique could be used successfully to detect *L. monocytogenes* in formalin-fixed tissues. Their observations were soon substantiated by Biegeleisen (12) and Villella et al. (101); both confirmed previous cases of human listeriosis by direct FA examination of formalin-fixed, deparaffinized tissue sections made from specimens taken during autopsy. These findings indicate that retrospective analysis of autopsy specimens taken from likely victims of listeriosis can provide valuable epidemiological information concerning prevalence of this illness.

In addition to identifying *L. monocytogenes* in mixed culture, the FA technique also can provide information concerning the serotype of the organism. In 1963, Nelson and Shelton (75) found that fluorescein isothiocyanate–labeled antisera to *L. monocytogenes* serotypes 1 and 3 led to specific fluorescent staining of organisms of serotypes 1, 2, and 3, whereas no fluorescence was observed for organisms of serotypes 4a and 4b. In contrast, *L. monocytogenes* strains of serotypes 4a and 4b were brilliantly fluorescent with labeled type 4b antisera, whereas organisms of serotypes 1, 2, and 3 were not fluorescent in the presence of the same antisera. Antigenic analysis of *L. monocytogenes* has shown that organisms of serotypes 1, 2, and 3 share a common heat-stable somatic antigen-factor III, whereas factor V is common to serotypes 4a, 4b, 4c, and 4e. Thus results of this study can be explained by the specific binding of labeled antisera to factor III (serotypes 1, 2, and 3) or factor V (serotypes 4a and 4b). With the exception of *Staphylococcus aureus*, specificity tests of both labeled antisera failed to demonstrate cross-staining or nonspecific staining with other bacterial species.

Fluorescein isothiocyanate–labeled antisera specific for *L. monocytogenes* serotypes 1 and 4, as well as a polyvalent antiserum able to detect serotypes 1, 2, 3, and 4, have been available commercially (Difco Laboratories) since 1975. These antisera can be used for direct FA analysis of cerebrospinal fluid, meconium, tissue impression smears, or isolated cultures and reportedly will detect approximately 98% of all known strains of *L. monocytogenes*. Although this commercial test kit provides a means for rapid presumptive identification of *L. monocytogenes*, results obtained from direct FA analysis must be confirmed by biochemical characterization of the organism in pure culture.

Direct FA analysis also has been applied to detect *L. monocytogenes* in various foods. As early as 1977, Khan et al. (53) inoculated samples of sterile lamb, minced beef, and sausage meat to contain approximately 1×10^4 *L. monocytogenes* CFU/g and analyzed the products with FA using the previously described commercial types 1, 4, and polyvalent antisera. Although *L. monocytogenes* was observed in smears of crude meat homogenates after counterstaining with Eriochrome Black to decrease background fluorescence, preenrichment of meat homogenates in a selective broth for 6–24 hours before FA analysis greatly facilitated detection of listeriae. Under these conditions, *L. monocytogenes* was brightly fluorescent while background fluorescence and cross-reactions with natural meat microflora (i.e., staphylococci and streptococci) were eliminated. Furthermore, when samples were preenriched, counterstaining was deemed unnecessary. These researchers also evaluated the ability of the direct FA technique to detect *L. monocytogenes* in pasteurized milk inoculated with the pathogen. After proper fluorescent staining of undiluted milk smears, listeriae appeared as bright yellowish-green cells against a black background. However, as in previous studies (16,47,91), labeled *L. monocytogenes* antisera cross-reacted with micrococci/streptococci which led to many highly fluorescent cells, some of which were brighter than *Listeria*. Despite use of proper controls, including FA analysis of *Listeria*-free specimens, this technique had only limited success when applied to milk.

In response to public health concerns regarding *Listeria*-contaminated dairy products, researchers in Yugoslavia (102) reexamined the possibility of using the direct FA technique to identify *L. monocytogenes* in naturally contaminated cow's milk. After treating dried milk smears with acetone to release possible intracellular listeriae, all samples from which the pathogen was originally isolated using conventional microbiological methods were positive with the direct FA technique. Furthermore, several culture-negative samples also were positive for *L. monocytogenes* by direct FA analysis, thus proving the sensitivity of such a test.

Working in England, McLauchlin and Pini (71) also developed a rapid (i.e., <2 hours) direct immunofluorescence test to detect *L. monocytogenes* in soft cheese. According to the authors, previously characterized *L. monocytogenes*-specific monoclonal antibodies (72) were conjugated to fluorescein isothiocyanate and applied to dried, acetone-fixed smears of soft cheese. Using this technique, *L. monocytogenes* was identified in seven soft cheeses which generally contained >10^4 listeriae CFU/g by direct plating. While the direct immunofluorescence test failed to detect the pathogen in 18 other *Listeria*-positive cheeses, eight of which contained >10^4 *Listeria* CFU/g by direct plating, the authors noted that the latter eight cheeses had rinds. Hence, lack of recovery may be more closely related to nonhomogeneity of these samples than to the direct immunofluorescence test itself.

Although results from the latter two studies appear far more promising, several serious disadvantages typically encountered during direct FA analysis of meat and dairy products include (a) nonspecific cross-reactivity of labeled *Listeria* antisera with streptococci, micrococci, and staphylococci, (b) poor visual resolution of listeriae from background microflora based on fluorescence intensity, and (c) the time-consuming and subjective nature of visual microscopic examination. To circumvent some of these problems associated with conventional fluorescence microscopy analysis, Donnelly and Baigent (24) attempted to automate the FA procedure by using flow cytometry to detect *L. monocytogenes* in milk. Briefly, flow cytometry provides a means of rapidly characterizing any cell population according to parameters such as morphology, nucleic acid content, and surface antigenicity. After passing a suspension of fluorescently labeled cells individually through a laser beam, the entire cell population can be characterized according to degree of light scattering, fluorescence, and absorbance.

Using an indirect FA technique (Fig. 7.2) (fluorescein isothiocyanate–labeled goat anti-rabbit immunoglobulin bound to commercial anti-*Listeria* antisera types 1 and 4) in combination with quantitation of DNA (fluorescently labeled with propidium iodide) and cell size (determined by the degree of light scattering), Donnelly and Baigent (24) adapted flow cytometry to distinguish *L. monocytogenes* from such common raw milk contaminants as *Streptococcus faecalis*, *Streptococcus agalactiae*, *Streptococcus uberis*, *Staphylococcus epidermidis*, and *Staphylococcus hyicus*. However, as in previous studies (16,91), *L. monocytogenes* and *Staphylococcus aureus* remained indistinguishable because of the high degree of cross-reactivity with *Listeria* antibodies. Resolution between these two organisms was further complicated by their virtually identical DNA profiles. To circumvent this problem, Listeria Enrichment Broth III of Rodriguez et al. (88) was modified to prevent growth of *S. aureus* and other common raw milk contaminants that previously obscured detection of *L. monocytogenes*. This modified enrichment medium, as you will recall from the previous chapter, also is known as University of Vermont Medium, and is very similar to the medium used in the USDA procedure for isolating *L. monocytogenes* from meat products. Flow cytometric analysis of raw milk samples inoculated to contain approximately 9 *L. monocytogenes* CFU/ml resulted in a minimum detection level of approximately 1×10^6 *Listeria* CFU/ml following 24 hours of enrichment at 37°C. Using measurements of DNA content followed by determinations of cell size and immunofluorescence, *L. monocytogenes* could be presumptively identified in 24-hour-old enrichment cultures within 4 hours.

In a subsequent study, Donnelly et al. (25) compared their flow-cytometric/selective enrichment procedure just described to the classical cold enrichment method for detection of *L. monocytogenes* in raw milk. Using the cold enrichment procedure, *L. monocytogenes* was detected in 15 of 939 (1.6%) raw milk samples obtained from over 50 farms. Although 66 of 939 (7.0%) samples were positive for listeriae after flow cytometric analysis, the pathogen could be confirmed in only 10 of these samples. Hence, use of flow cytometry led to false-positive and false-negative rates of 5.96 and 0.53%, respectively, as compared to cold enrichment. Since flow cytometry is a noncultural method, some of these false-positive reactions may have resulted from detection of nonviable or injured cells unable to grow during cold enrichment. More important, however, this rapid method failed to detect *L. monocytogenes* in 5 of 15 samples that were positive after cold enrichment, thus yielding a false-negative rate of 33.3%. Current work toward developing highly specific monoclonal antibodies is likely to decrease the unacceptably high rates for false-positive and false-negative reactions. If these improvements are made, flow cytometry may become a technically acceptable method to rapidly screen milk samples for *L. monocytogenes*; however, the sophisticated nature and excessive cost of the instrumentation is likely to limit use of flow cytometry to only the largest food microbiology and reference laboratories.

ENZYME-LINKED IMMUNOSORBENT ASSAY

A far simpler method to rapidly detect *L. monocytogenes* is the enzyme-linked immunosorbent assay (ELISA). Unlike the FA technique, which is subjective, labor intensive, and difficult to automate, ELISA is relatively objective, far less labor intensive, and can be automated with relative ease. These considerations, along with the simple and inexpensive nature of the test and necessary equipment, have made ELISA feasible in many small laboratories and in developing countries. Consequently, considerable research effort has focused on developing ELISA methods to detect numerous pathogenic microorganisms, including *L. monocytogenes*, in clinical, food, and environmental samples.

The ELISA technique, which is based on the assumption that either an antibody or antigen can be linked to an enzyme with the resulting complex retaining immunological as well as enzymatic activity, is among the most recent developments in labeled reagent assays. As just inferred, ELISA can be used to detect either antibody or antigen. Assays for antibody are most often accomplished using an indirect method (Fig. 7.3) in which an enzyme-labeled anti-immunoglobulin (conjugate) is bound to an unlabeled antibody (antibody being detected) specifically linked to an antigen, which in turn is attached to a polystyrene well of a microtiter plate. Since specificity of the indirect assay is associated with the unlabeled antibody, relatively few types of conjugates are needed to detect antibodies produced during various disease states. After thorough washing to remove unbound conjugate, the appropriate enzyme substrate is added to produce a color change. The amount of bound conjugate, enzymatically labeled with either horseradish peroxidase or alkaline phosphatase, can then be quantitated spectrophotometrically or determined visually.

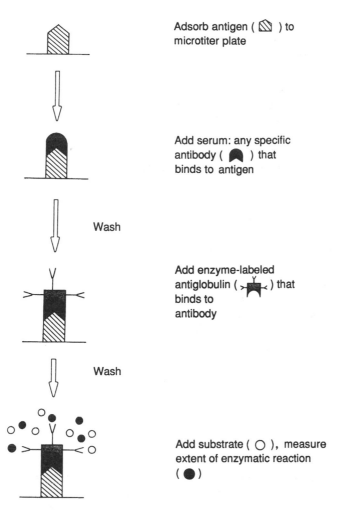

Adsorb antigen (⬙) to microtiter plate

Add serum: any specific antibody (⬤) that binds to antigen

Wash

Add enzyme-labeled antiglobulin (⤳Y⤲) that binds to antibody

Wash

Add substrate (○), measure extent of enzymatic reaction (●)

Figure 7.3 Indirect ELISA for detection and quantitation of antibodies.

Several recently described indirect ELISA techniques are sufficiently sensitive to detect small quantities of antibodies directed against *L. monocytogenes*. One such assay developed by Meyer and Brunner (73) was superior to a tube agglutination method for detecting low levels of antibodies to O (somatic) and H (flagellar) antigens of *L. monocytogenes* serotypes 1 and 4b which predominate. An outbreak of listeriosis in Canada linked to consumption of contaminated coleslaw afforded Hudak et al. (48) an opportunity to compare a newly developed indirect ELISA technique to the conventional complement fixation and microagglutination tests for diagnosing cases of perinatal listeriosis. The ELISA test for IgM (immunoglobulin M) antibodies to *L. monocytogenes* identified 79% of the cases as positive and 78% of the controls as negative, whereas the same test for IgG (immunoglobulin G) antibodies to the pathogen led to 76% of the cases being reported as positive and 90% of the controls being reported as negative. Somewhat similar results for the standard microagglutination and complement fixation tests led the authors to conclude that all three techniques are at best specific and predictive in ruling out infections, but lack the necessary sensitivity to confirm cases of listeriosis.

Although detection of *Listeria* antibodies through indirect ELISA may eventually prove useful to track the spread of foodborne listeriosis, major emphasis has been placed on developing ELISA techniques that will identify antigens from specific *Listeria* spp. in foods. During the past decade, ELISA methods have helped food microbiologists screen a wide range of products for such microbiological hazards as *Staphylococcus aureus* and *Clostridium perfringens* enterotoxins, botulinal toxins, and various myco-toxins, as well as salmonellae, shigellae, *Escherichia coli* O157:H7, and most recently *Listeria* spp.

Enzyme immunoassays to detect antigens can be divided into two major classes: competitive and noncompetitive. Although both types have proven useful to food microbiologists, the competitive assay which requires use of purified antigens poses difficulties for many laboratories. Therefore, recent efforts toward developing an ELISA technique to detect *L. monocytogenes* in food have focused on two types of noncompet-itive assays: the indirect and double antibody sandwich methods. The indirect procedures to detect antigens and antibodies (Fig. 7.3) are identical with the exception that in the indirect procedure for antigen detection, the ELISA is done on a dry nitrocellulose membrane (instead of a polystyrene microtiter plate) to which the organism has been transferred through direct contact with an agar plate or hydrophobic-grid membrane filter (HGMF) containing visible colonies. In the double antibody sandwich ELISA (Fig. 7.4), a highly specific antibody is first bound to the polystyrene surface of a microtiter plate well. A heat or chemically inactivated extract of the food sample containing antigenic material from the organism in question is then added to the microtiter well containing the bound antibody. Following incubation and washing to remove unbound antigen, conjugate enzymatically labeled with either horseradish peroxidase or alkaline phospha-tase is added to the well containing antigen–antibody complex. After incubation and washing, bound conjugate is detected through addition of enzyme substrate and a color development solution. The degree of color change, determined either visually or spec-trophotometrically, is directly proportional to the amount of antigen in the test sample.

The success of any immunological-type assay (i.e., agglutination, complement-fixation, or ELISA test) is largely determined by the specificity of the antibody, along with the number of antigenic sites to which the antibody can selectively bind. Thus it is not surprising that antisera and antibody production methods have undergone several radical changes over the past 25 years.

Before 1975, antibody production techniques bordered on a scientifically practiced form of art in which rabbits or other laboratory animals were injected with increasing quantities of antigen over 3–4 weeks. After bleeding the animals, the serum fraction was separated from blood and clarified by centrifugation. The result was an antiserum that contained a mixture of antibodies (polyclonal antibodies) only some of which would react with the antigen in question. A similar procedure for preparation of O and H *Listeria* antisera was described by Seeliger in 1961 (91). Preparation of control antisera for use in agglutination (66) and precipitation (74) tests followed essentially the same procedure. During 1988 and 1989, several researchers (10,89) reported that highly monospecific antisera to various *Listeria* spp. could be obtained by subjecting crude preparations to

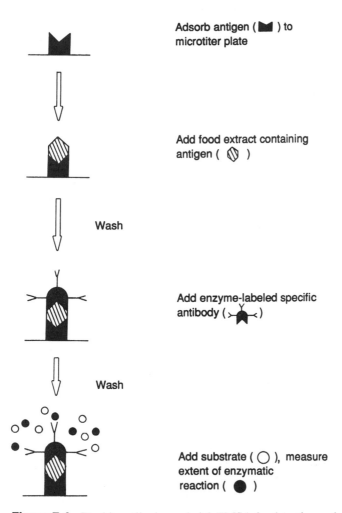

Adsorb antigen (◣) to
microtiter plate

Add food extract containing
antigen (◊)

Wash

Add enzyme-labeled specific
antibody (>─◆─<)

Wash

Add substrate (○), measure
extent of enzymatic
reaction (●)

Figure 7.4   Double antibody sandwich ELISA for detection and quantitation of antigens.

various absorption, concentration and filtration techniques, with one of these preparations proving satisfactory for a sandwich-type ELISA. Although the latter two antisera
are not yet commercially available, laboratories lacking animal facilities can obtain
satisfactory unlabeled as well as fluorescently labeled (fluorescein isothiocyanate, FITC)
types 1, 4, and polyvalent antisera from Difco Laboratories.

Despite their inherent lack of specificity, polyclonal antibodies have been used with
several ELISA techniques to detect *L. monocytogenes* in food samples. In 1988, Siragusa
et al. (92) developed an enzyme immunoassay for *L. monocytogenes* in which washed
antigens from whole cells or cell wall fragments were adsorbed to microtiter plates. An
indirect ELISA technique (Fig. 7.3) was used in which bound antigen was treated with
commercially prepared FITC conjugated polyclonal antibody (Difco) directed against
L. monocytogenes followed by an anti-FITC horseradish peroxidase conjugated anti-

body. After addition of enzyme substrate, highest absorbance values, as determined spectrophotometrically, were obtained from treated cell wall fragments. Three years earlier, Kamisango et al. (52) used a simplified ELISA technique to identify teichoic acids in biotin-labeled cell wall extracts of *L. monocytogenes*. Such an assay should prove useful to screen various antibody preparations for anti-*Listeria* activity.

Needs of the food industry that emerged during the 1980s led to development of a rapid 2-hour polyclonal antibody-based double antibody sandwich ELISA to detect the seven presently recognized *Listeria* spp. in food and environmental samples (8,42). This test, known as the Tecra Listeria Visual Immunoassay, is now commercially available through Bioenterprises Pty. Ltd., Australia, and Minnesota Mining and Manufacturing Co., Inc. (3M). To increase the numbers of listeriae to detectable levels (i.e., $>10^5$ *Listeria* CFU/ml) food and environmental samples to be examined by this assay must first undergo selective enrichment. Food samples (25 g) are diluted 1:10 in FDA Enrichment Broth and incubated for 24 hours at 30°C after which a portion of the primary warm enrichment sample is secondarily enriched in FDA Enrichment Broth an additional 18–24 hours at 30°C. In contrast, environmental samples undergo a single warm enrichment in USDA Enrichment Broth (formula in appendix) for 24 hours at 30°C. A double antibody sandwich ELISA (Fig. 7.4) is then done by adding 0.2 ml of the heat-inactivated enrichment culture to a commercially prepared microtiter plate well containing bound *Listeria*-specific polyclonal antibody. After thorough washing, an enzyme-labeled *Listeria*-specific polyclonal antibody is added. Following additional washing to remove unbound labeled antibody, enzyme substrate is added to produce a color change from clear to green for positive samples.

According to results from one follow-up study (8,9) in which over 1000 food and environmental samples were examined, the Tecra Listeria Visual Immunoassay yielded average false-positive and false-negative rates of 0.84 and 0%, respectively. However, given the need for enrichment and the relatively high cost of this assay (~$7.50/test), the entire protocol can likely be made more attractive and cost-efficient by using Fraser Broth or a similar enrichment medium that changes color in the presence of listeriae. Such a modification would provide a ready means for eliminating negative samples while at the same time not compromising the sensitivity of the test. While this assay is proving to be useful, readers are reminded that all positive results must be confirmed by streaking the original enrichment culture on FDA-Modified McBride Listeria Agar or other suitable plating media. Any suspect colonies that subsequently appear on these plates should be confirmed according to recognized morphological, biochemical, and serological methods.

The discovery of monoclonal antibody technology has led to dramatic changes in methodology for antibody production. In 1975, Köhler and Milstein (63) published their now classic paper which describes manufacture of monoclonal antibodies, predefined highly specific antibodies, by means of permanent tissue culture cell lines. Although various steps in the procedure for monoclonal antibody production have undergone technical improvements, the basic methodology originally described by Köhler and Milstein has remained unchanged for over 10 years.

Briefly, monoclonal antibodies are prepared by first immunizing an appropriate laboratory animal with the antigen of interest to predefine the specificity of hybridoma cells. After several weeks, antibody-producing spleen cells are collected from the immunized animal and fused to a cell line which gives rise to hybridomas that permit production of immunoglobulins. After using an ELISA technique to screen for hybridoma clones that secrete antibodies possessing desired characteristics, selected hybridoma clones are grown in mass culture with the resultant monoclonal antibody being recovered from the supernatant liquid following centrifugation. Alternatively, selected hybridoma cells can be injected into BALB/c mice, which leads to production of solid tumors able to secrete milligram quantities of the desired monoclonal antibody into the serum and ascitic fluid. Production of useful monoclonal antibodies by laboratories of even modest size and means has led to rapid growth of hybridoma technology to treat cancer patients, diagnose diseases, and identify various pathogenic microorganisms including salmonellae and *Listeria* spp.

Monoclonal antibodies directed against *L. monocytogenes* were first produced in 1984 by Ziegler and Orlin (105), who fused tumor cells with spleenic B cells obtained from mice immunized with the pathogen. Using three forms of listerial antigens— (a) heat-killed cells of *L. monocytogenes*, (b) purified soluble listerial proteins, and (c) macrophages that had ingested heat-killed *Listeria* cells, 93 of 600 (15.5%) hybridomas exhibited some antibody reactivity to at least one of the three antigenic forms. Of 31 hybridomas tested, 22 (70%) produced monoclonal antibodies that reacted only with *L. monocytogenes*, 20 (91%) of which exhibited some degree of serotype specificity, whereas two (6%) were specific for the genus *Listeria* (tested against *L. grayi*, *L. murrayi*, and *L. denitrificans*) and seven (23%) reacted with *Listeria* spp., and at the same time cross-reacted with *Bacillus subtilis*, *Staphylococcus aureus*, *Escherichia coli*, and/or *Staphylococcus epidermidis*. Although these researchers recognized the obvious importance of their findings to diagnosticians, no mention was made concerning future efforts to develop a *Listeria*-specific assay using the monoclonal antibodies that they had uncovered.

Using similar hybridoma screening techniques, at least two other research groups have identified one or more monoclonal antibodies that react with organisms belonging to the genus *Listeria* (39) as well as specific species including *L. monocytogenes* (39,94) and *L. innocua* (94). Furthermore, one recently discovered monoclonal antibody (100) reportedly reacted only with β-hemolysin produced by *L. monocytogenes* serotypes 1/2a, 1/2c, and 3a (i.e., not serotypes 1/2b or 4b), thus suggesting that structural differences exist between β-hemolysins produced by different serotypes. Although most of the monoclonal antibodies uncovered during these investigations are still being evaluated for possible use in ELISA-type *Listeria* diagnostic test kits, preliminary results from several of the studies appear promising.

Advances in hybridoma/monoclonal antibody technology, coupled with numerous recalls of *Listeria*-contaminated dairy products and pleas from the food industry for a rapid, easy, and inexpensive method to detect listeriae in foods, have prompted development of an ELISA for detecting *Listeria* spp., including *L. monocytogenes*, in various food and environmental samples. The 2-hour double antibody sandwich ELISA (Fig. 7.5), known as the Listeria-Tek Assay, was commercially introduced by Organon Teknika Corp. in November of 1987 and has attracted much attention. The discussion that follows will focus on development and commercialization of this assay, as well as its many applications for the food industry.

Using the previously described techniques for monoclonal antibody production (63), Butman et al. (13) laid the groundwork for developing the Listeria-Tek Assay by

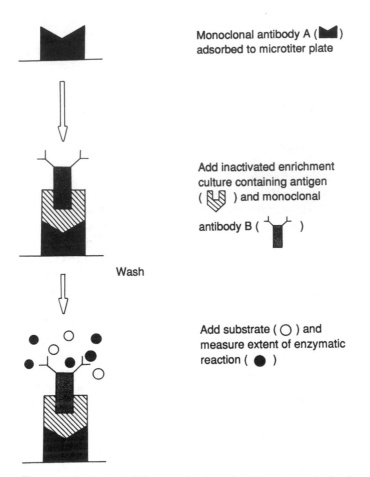

Monoclonal antibody A (⬛) adsorbed to microtiter plate

Add inactivated enrichment culture containing antigen (◹) and monoclonal

antibody B (⊥)

Wash

Add substrate (○) and measure extent of enzymatic reaction (●)

Figure 7.5   Listeria-Tek assay for detecting *Listeria* spp. in food samples.

characterizing 511 hybridomas, 37 (7.2%) of which reacted positively with a heated extract of *L. monocytogenes* in an indirect ELISA. Further characterization of these hybridomas led to discovery of 15 monoclonal antibodies that reacted specifically with a heat-stable antigenic protein (MW 30,000–38,000) common to 26 strains of *L. monocytogenes* (representing serotypes 1, 1a, 1b, 1/2a, 1/2b, 2, 3, 3a, 3b, 4a, 4b, 4c, 4d, and 4e) as well as various strains of *L. ivanovii*, *L. innocua*, *L. grayi*, *L. murrayi*, and *L. seeligeri*. Extensive testing of these 15 monoclonal antibodies by both indirect ELISA and Western blot (immunoblot) techniques failed to uncover any cross-reactivity with heated extracts from *Actinomyces pyogenes*, *Bacillus cereus*, *Citrobacter freundii*, *Enterobacter aerogenes*, *Erysipelothrix rhusiopathiae*, *Escherichia coli*, *Lactobacillus casei*, *Micrococcus varians*, *Salmonella typhi*, and various species of pseudomonads, staphylococci, and streptococci.

Subsequently, researchers at Organon Teknika (6,29,30,69,97) used two of these genus-specific monoclonal antibodies just described to develop a one-step ELISA procedure to detect *Listeria* spp. in dairy and meat products, as well as environmental samples. After enriching food and environmental samples 40–52 hours in a selective medium, a double monoclonal antibody sandwich ELISA procedure (Fig. 7.5), known as the Listeria-Tek Assay, is done on the enrichment culture. Using this technique, presumptive results concerning presence or absence of *Listeria* spp. in dairy, meat, and environmental samples are available an average of 48 hours after initiation of enrichment.

Since the lower detection limit for the Listeria-Tek Assay is between 5×10^4 and 2×10^5 *Listeria* CFU/ml (6), preparation of samples for the test involves several different selective enrichment procedures, depending on the type of material to be analyzed (2). Dairy products (25 g or ml) are diluted 1:10 in FDA Enrichment Broth containing MOPS buffer (FDA Enrichment Broth + MOPS) (see Table 6.2) and incubated at 30°C for 44 ± 4 hours In contrast, environmental samples are collected on a swab or sponge which is placed in 10 or 100 ml of FDA Enrichment Broth + MOPS, respectively, and incubated at 30°C for 44 ± 4 hours. Unlike dairy and environmental samples, meat products (25 g) are diluted 1:10 in phosphate buffer and thoroughly blended, after which 10 ml of the blended sample is added to 10 ml of double strength USDA Listeria Enrichment Broth I (2x formula) (see Table 6.2) and incubated at 30°C. After 24–26 hours of incubation, 0.1 ml of the enriched culture is added to 10 ml of single-strength USDA Listeria Enrichment Broth I containing 37 mg of acriflavine/L and incubated an additional 24–26 hours at 30°C.

The Listeria-Tek Assay (6) is a one-step double antibody sandwich ELISA procedure (Fig. 7.5) in which antigenic material from a heat-inactivated enrichment culture is incubated with a horseradish peroxidase–labeled monoclonal antibody in polystyrene micro-ELISA wells that have been commercially precoated with an unlabeled "capture" monoclonal antibody. Following 60 minutes of incubation at 37°C, the microtiter plate wells are washed six times and an enzyme substrate (tetra-methylbenzidine) is added to produce an intense blue color. After an additional 30 minutes of incubation at ambient temperature, the enzymatic reaction is stopped by addition of acid which turns the reaction mixture yellow. Results are then read using a spectrophotometer, with the entire assay being completed within 2 hours. Since two different monoclonal antibodies are used in this procedure, one for antigen capture and one for antigen detection, this test is extremely sensitive and specific. In addition to providing fast results that are easily interpreted, the Listeria-Tek Assay also is safe to do since only heat-killed organisms are used. Furthermore, this assay reportedly has a very low false-negative rate, indicating that *Listeria*-negative samples require no further testing. While the Listeria-Tek Assay provides an excellent means for screening large numbers of samples for presence or absence of listeriae, preliminary results show that this test can be far more cost effective (present cost ~$15.00/test) if samples are enriched in a selective/differential medium such as Fraser Broth rather than in a medium that is only selective (38). Using this protocol, the Listeria-Tek assay need only be done on presumptive positive cultures that exhibited a color change, i.e., blackening from esculin hydrolysis.

According to the manufacturer, at least 15 major food manufacturers/testing laboratories in the United States and several large food manufacturers in England have adopted this assay for routine analysis of food products (6). However, until this non–*L. monocytogenes* specific *Listeria* assay and others such as the aforementioned Tecra Listeria Visual Assay are approved by the Association of Official Analytical Chemists, all *Listeria*-positive samples must be confirmed using standard cultural, biochemical,

Table 7.2 Comparison of the Listeria-Tek and FDA Cultural Methods for Detection of *L. monocytogenes* in Inoculated Dairy Products

Product	Inoculation level (CFU/g or ml)	Number of samples analyzed	Number of positive samples	
			FDA Method	Listeria-Tek assay
Milk (2% fat)	0	10	0	0
	0.2	20	20	20
	2	20	20	20
Ice cream	0	10	0	0
	0.2	20	20	20
	2	20	20	20

Source: Adapted from Ref. 85.

and serological methods. The necessity for proper confirmation is readily apparent when one recalls that *L. monocytogenes* is the only *Listeria* sp. currently considered to constitute a serious public health hazard if in food.

Several other studies (69,85) compared the Listeria-Tek Assay to conventional culture techniques (FDA and USDA methods) for recovery of *Listeria* spp. from dairy, meat, and environmental samples. Results from Robison (85) (Table 7.2) indicate that the Listeria-Tek Assay and FDA cultural method are equally effective for detecting *Listeria* in samples of milk and ice cream inoculated to contain 0.2–2 *L. monocytogenes* CFU/g or ml. In a similar study, Hitchins et al. (46) inoculated ice cream to contain approximately 0.1–1000 *L. monocytogenes* CFU/g and then analyzed the product for listeriae using the Listeria-Tek, FDA, and USDA procedures. All three methods again yielded comparable results and could easily detect one organism in a 25-g sample. Siragusa et al. (95) compared the USDA and Listeria-Tek methods to detect *Listeria* in samples of sterile chicken homogenate that were inoculated to contain approximately 50–500 *L. monocytogenes* CFU/g in combination with a mixture of taxonomically related, thermoduric non–spore-forming bacteria. As in previous studies, comparable results were obtained using both procedures. In addition, no false-positive reactions were recorded using the Listeria-Tek Assay. In a follow-up study by the same authors (93), the Listeria-Tek Assay again was useful to detect *L. monocytogenes* in chicken samples that were analyzed after 6 days of refrigerated storage.

In 1988, researchers at Organon Teknika (69,85) concluded that the Listeria-Tek Assay generally was superior to the FDA and USDA methods for detecting *Listeria* spp. in naturally contaminated food and environmental samples (Table 7.3). Combining the results from both in-house studies, 98 of 842 (11.6%) and 49 of 842 (5.8%) samples were positive using the Listeria-Tek and recognized cultural methods, respectively. Conventional culture techniques led to confirmation of listeriae in 69 of 98 (70.4%) samples that were positive according to the Listeria-Tek Assay. Thus *Listeria* spp. were detected in 20 additional samples using rapid rather than conventional detection methods. Although the Listeria-Tek Assay produced a high percentage of false-positive results (29.6%), the actual value is likely to be considerably lower since heavy contamination interfered with confirmation of listeriae in 41 dairy factory samples.

Another enzyme immunoassay recently developed in Canada by Farber and Speirs (32) uses monoclonal antibodies directed against flagellar antigens for rapid detection

Table 7.3 Comparison of Listeria-Tek ELISA Assay and FDA/USDA Cultural Methods for Detection of *Listeria* sp. from Naturally Contaminated Dairy, Meat, and Environmental Samples

Type of sample	Number of samples analyzed	Cultural method		Listeria-Tek	Listeria-Tek confirmations
		FDA	USDA		
Dairy products[a]	394	0	NA[b]	2	1
	39	0	NA	7	7
Dairy factory environments	259	34	NA	69	41[c]
	43	3	NA	4	4
Meat products	34	NA	1	2	2
	29	NA	3	3	3
Meat factory environments	19	NA	4	5	5
	25	NA	4	6	6
Total	842	37	12	98	69

[a]Products included ice cream, novelty ice cream, ice milk, sour cream, imitation cheese, low moisture cheese, dried cheese, spices, and gelatin.
[b]Not analyzed.
[c]All 41 samples heavily contaminated with competing microflora.
Source: Adapted from Refs. 69, 85.

of *Listeria* spp. in food. In their study, hybridomas producing antibodies against *Listeria* flagellar antigens were generally prepared according to the original method of Köhler and Milstein (63) and then screened for sensitivity using an indirect ELISA (Fig. 7.3). After further characterization of these monoclonal antibodies by Western blotting and electrophoretic separation followed by immunoblotting, three classes of immunoglobulins were discovered that reacted only with *Listeria* strains containing A, B, and/or C flagellar antigen, i.e., *L. monocytogenes, L. innocua, L. ivanovii, L. seeligeri,* and *L. welshimeri.* These same monoclonal antibodies failed to react with *L. grayi, L. murrayi,* and *L. denitrificans* or cross-react with any of 30 non-*Listeria* spp. from 15 different genera. Using these monoclonal antibodies, a nitrocellulose membrane ELISA (indirect immunodot or immunoblot assay) was developed to examine samples of raw milk and soft-ripened cheese that were naturally contaminated with approximately 10^3–10^4 *L. monocytogenes* CFU/ml or g. Various quantities of milk were filtered through hydro-

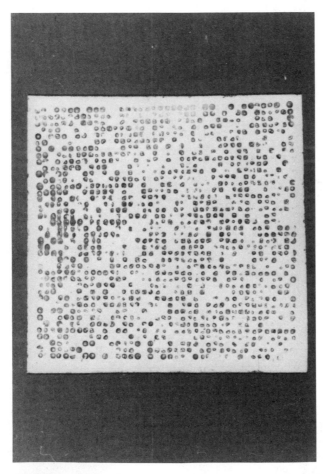

Figure 7.6 Indirect immunoblot assay done on a hydrophobic grid membrane filter showing *Listeria* colonies (black dots) recovered from naturally contaminated raw milk. (Used with permission of J. M. Farber, Health and Welfare, Canada.)

phobic-grid nitrocellulose filter membranes which were placed on Modified McBride Listeria Agar without sheep blood (MLA2-blood) (see Table 6.3) and incubated at 30°C for 48 h. Appropriately diluted samples of soft-ripened cheese were directly plated on MLA2-blood and incubated at 30°C for 48 h. Following incubation, an indirect immunodot assay was done directly on the nitrocellulose membranes through which milk samples were filtered (Fig. 7.6). In contrast, cheese samples were analyzed using an indirect immunoblot assay in which *Listeria* organisms were transferred to a non-hydrophobic-grid nitrocellulose membrane by placing the membrane in direct contact with visible colonies obtained on Modified McBride Listeria Agar without sheep blood (Fig. 7.7). After applying a blocking solution both types of nitrocellulose membranes were treated with an unlabeled monoclonal antibody directed against flagella of *Listeria*, followed by a peroxidase-labeled conjugate (Fig. 7.3). After addition of enzyme substrate and proper color development, *Listeria* colonies isolated from naturally contami-

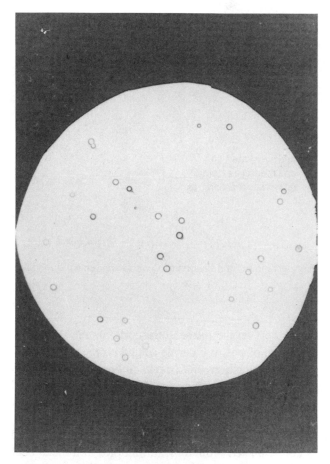

Figure 7.7   Indirect immunodot assay done on a nitrocellulose membrane filter showing *Listeria* colonies (black-ringed circles) recovered from naturally contaminated cheese. (Used with permission of J. M. Farber, Health and Welfare, Canada.)

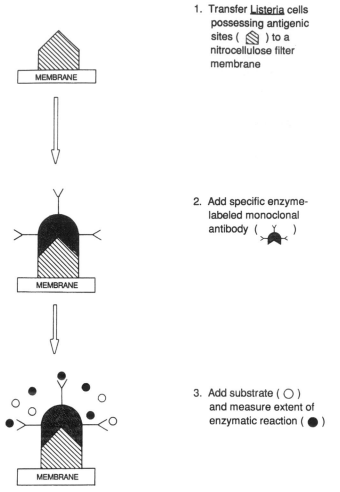

1. Transfer <u>Listeria</u> cells
   possessing antigenic
   sites (   ) to a
   nitrocellulose filter
   membrane

2. Add specific enzyme-
   labeled monoclonal
   antibody (   )

3. Add substrate (○)
   and measure extent of
   enzymatic reaction (●)

Figure 7.8 Immunoblot/Direct ELISA technique for detection of *Listeria* spp. on solid media.

nated raw milk were visible as purple dots on the nitrocellulose membrane (Fig. 7.6).
For cheese samples (Fig. 7.7), the pattern of positive purple ringed circles obtained by
ELISA correlated well with the pattern of bluish-green *Listeria* colonies on agar plates
when observed with oblique illumination. Thus, following the 40-hour incubation period
for colony formation, positive results were obtained within 4 hours by doing the ELISA
directly on the nitrocellulose membrane.

In a later study, Farber et al. (33) examined the potential of their assay just described
to detect *Listeria* spp. in naturally contaminated ground meat. Samples of minced beef
and pork were first enriched according to a modified version of the USDA procedure,
after which colonies thought to be *Listeria* were transferred to a nitrocellulose membrane
and subjected to the previously described indirect immunoblot assay. Using this method,

meat samples containing *Listeria* spp. yielded positive results as evidenced by formation of purple spots on nitrocellulose membranes.

Farber et al. (33) adapted their monoclonal antibodies for use in both an indirect (Fig. 7.3) and double antibody sandwich (Fig. 7.4) ELISA that can be done in microtiter plate wells. Thus far, limited trials indicate that both procedures are satisfactory to detect *Listeria* spp. in minced meat and/or fermented sausage. Although the various ELISA methods developed by Farber et al. (32,33) have not yet reached the commercial stage, their findings may lead to an alternative to the Listeria-Tek Assay. Farber et al. (32) are attempting to produce monoclonal antibodies to the hemolysin protein of *L. monocytogenes*. If successful, a two-stage assay may be on the horizon in which food samples can first be screened for *Listeria* spp. using antiflagellar monoclonal antibodies and then, if necessary, be examined for *L. monocytogenes* using a more specific immunological probe.

In contrast to the two previous studies, Durham and Mattingly (27,28) developed a monoclonal antibody-based, genus-specific, immunoblot/direct ELISA (Fig. 7.8) for rapid detection of *Listeria* spp. on agar plates. As in the previous study, colonies suspected as *Listeria* must first be transferred from an agar plate (or hydrophobic-grid membrane filter) to a nitrocellulose membrane. The membrane is then treated in a protein-blocking solution and incubated with horseradish peroxidase–labeled monoclonal antibody that is specific for the genus *Listeria*. Following addition of enzyme substrate (3-amino-9-ethylcarbazole), areas correlating with *Listeria* colonies on original agar plates turn red within 10 minutes.

The scientific literature also contains a report of a novel enzyme conjugated phage technique, known as the Phage Rapid Identification Assay, to identify *Listeria* as well as *Salmonella*, *Escherichia coli*, *Staphylococcus*, and *Bacillus* (3,65). This non-immunological assay is somewhat similar to an ELISA in that an enzymatically labeled virus (phage) binds to specific receptor sites found on the cell wall of *Listeria* spp. Following removal of unbound labeled phage, an enzyme substrate is added along with a color indicator. A subsequent change from colorless to brown then develops only if enzyme-conjugated phage particles are bound to listeriae. Preliminary results indicate that this assay can detect as few as 250 *Listeria* cells/ml. However, the researchers cautioned that their assay is still in the experimental stage and probably will not be commercially available for some time.

DNA HYBRIDIZATION ASSAYS

Nucleic acid hybridization technology offers an exciting approach for rapid and definitive identification of virtually any organism in clinical, food, and environmental samples. Advances in optimizing hybridization conditions and DNA sequencing technology have resulted in introduction of nucleic acid hybridization assays to detect foodborne pathogens including *Salmonella* (37,80), *Yersinia* (34,51,80), *Campylobacter* (84), and enteropathogenic strains of *Escherichia coli* (45). Difficulties in recovering *Listeria* from food samples using the numerous available cultural procedures, coupled with the lack of a standard identification scheme, have led to development of at least six different labeled DNA probes to detect *L. monocytogenes* or other pathogenic/nonpathogenic listeriae; also developed is an isotopic (58) and colorimetric-based nucleic acid hybridization assay to identify foodborne organisms in the genus *Listeria*. While both of these assays have been introduced commercially by Gene-Trak Systems (Framingham, MA), the isotopic assay has been superseded by a colorimetric version of the same assay with the former no longer commercially available. In addition, a more specific DNA hybridization assay developed by the FDA which only detects *L. monocytogenes* (19) also has undergone extensive testing in the United States, Canada, and England. Results from these tests should be forthcoming.

The principle of the nucleic acid hybridization assay is quite simple (Fig. 7.9) and is based on the fact that any given organism contains sequences of nucleotides (compounds formed from one molecule each of a sugar [deoxyribose in DNA, ribose in RNA], phosphoric acid, and a purine base [adenine (A) or guanine (G) in DNA] or pyrimidine base [cytosin (C) or thymine (T) in DNA and uracil (U) in place of thymine in RNA] within the organism's DNA or RNA genetic makeup that are unique and specific to that particular organism). Once specific nucleotides of a gene coding for a particular trait

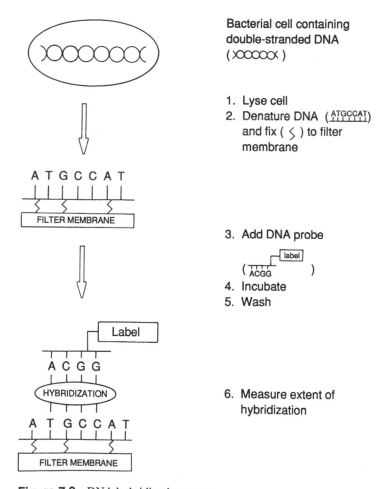

Figure 7.9 DNA hybridization assay.

(i.e., β-hemolysin or other virulence factor) have been identified and sequenced, a radioactive- or enzyme-labeled DNA probe (a homologous DNA fragment) is synthesized to reflect the complementary purine/pyrimidine base-pair sequence in the gene of interest. After the double strand of DNA is denatured to produce two single strands, the DNA probe will reanneal or hybridize with the single strand of target DNA coding for a particular trait only where the base pairs correspond exactly, i.e., adenine binding to thymine (or uracil in RNA) and guanine binding to cytosine.

Hybridization assays follow one of two basic approaches depending on whether double-stranded DNA (genomic or plasmid) or single-stranded RNA is used as the nucleic acid target. In either situation, the organism to be identified must be propagated to sufficient numbers ($>10^4$ cells/ml), collected on a filter membrane by vacuum filtration and then lysed to release target nucleic acids. In the DNA approach (Fig. 7.9), double-stranded target DNA from the organism in question is denatured into complementary single strands of DNA and fixed to the membrane filter. After a short prehybridization step, the filter is immersed and incubated in a hybridization solution that contains a specific DNA probe radioactively labeled with phosphorous (^{32}P) or an enzyme (streptavidin-alkaline phosphatase). The specific nucleotide sequence within the single-stranded DNA molecule then hybridizes with the labeled DNA probe. After washing away unbound or unhybridized probe, the extent of hybridization between labeled probe and target DNA from the organism in question can be detected using a scintillation counter or spectrophotometer, depending on the type of label employed. The degree of radioactive or enzymatic activity emitted above a threshold value (negative control) indicates the presence or absence of the organism in question in the sample. The RNA approach is identical to the DNA approach with the exception that single-stranded ribosomal RNA (rRNA) rather than single-stranded DNA functions as the target nucleic acid. Although less commonly used, the RNA approach offers one major advantage in that rRNA is present in multiple copies (1,000–10,000 copies/cell), which leads to natural amplification of the target nucleic acid as well as the subsequent radioactive or enzymatic signal following hybridization.

While the basis for DNA hybridization dates back to the 1950s, it is only since 1985 that DNA probe–based diagnostic assays have been commercially introduced into food microbiology laboratories. In 1985, Gene-Trak Systems (Framingham, MA) was the first company to commercially introduce a DNA probe-based assay for detecting salmonellae in foods. The success of this assay and a similar assay for *Campylobacter* (84), both of which have since received AOAC approval, led to further research efforts toward developing a DNA probe–based assay to detect *Listeria* spp. in food and environmental samples. Working at Gene-Trak Systems, Klinger et al. (59) synthesized a DNA probe that was specific for the genus *Listeria*. After obtaining nucleotide sequence information from *Listeria* spp. specific regions of 16S rRNA, complementary DNA sequences (DNA probes) were synthesized and purified by chromatography. These DNA probes were then radioactively labeled with ^{32}P and screened for specificity in a dot-blot/DNA hybridization assay against 139 *Listeria* isolates (89 *L. monocytogenes* isolates) representing all seven species as well as 48 gram-positive and 25 gram-negative non-*Listeria* bacterial species representing at least 19 different genera. The end result was a genus-specific DNA probe that reacted with all 139 *Listeria* isolates, but failed to react with any of the non-*Listeria* organisms tested.

Klinger et al. (58,59) subsequently developed and introduced the first DNA probe–based assay, known as the Gene-Trak Isotopic Listeria Assay (Gene-Trak Systems, Framingham, MA), for rapid detection of *Listeria* spp. in dairy and environmental samples. This assay, which was commercially available during 1988 and 1989, has since been replaced by a nonisotopic colorimetric assay which can accurately detect *Listeria* spp. in a much wider range of food and environmental samples.

According to representatives from Gene-Trak Systems (3,70), the genus-specific limitation of both Gene-Trak Listeria Assays was a deliberate policy decision which was made because of the occasional pathogenicity of listeriae other than *L. monocytogenes* (i.e., *L. ivanovii* and *L. seeligeri*). Therefore, this assay was designed to determine the presence or absence of all *Listeria* spp., including *L. monocytogenes*, in food and environmental samples. However, despite knowledge gained from the Gene-Trak Listeria Assay that a particular food sample contains *Listeria* spp., *L. monocytogenes* is currently the only *Listeria* spp. of importance in foodborne illness. Hence, if a ready-to-eat food product is found to contain listeriae by using the Gene-Trak Listeria Assay, the organism must be isolated from the enriched food sample and biochemically identified to determine what corrective measures need to be taken. If the organism proves to be *L. monocytogenes*, the food product must be removed from the marketplace and reprocessed or destroyed; however, at this time (1990) destruction of food products containing *Listeria* spp. other than *L. monocytogenes* appears to be unwarranted. In contrast to positive food samples, the recommended response to environmental samples positive for *Listeria* spp. is somewhat different. In food plant sanitation programs, any environmental sample testing positive for *Listeria* spp. by the Gene-Trak Assay (or any other method) should trigger immediate corrective action (i.e., thorough cleaning and sanitizing of the affected area and a review of the factory's sanitation program to try and pinpoint the source of contamination), regardless of the *Listeria* spp. present, since nonpathogenic listeriae are considered to be potential indicators of *L. monocytogenes*.

The Gene-Trak Isotopic Listeria Assay (58), which is no longer available, generally followed the previously described DNA hybridization procedure (Fig. 7.9), but was based on detection of a unique 16S rRNA rather than DNA sequence by using the aforementioned radioactively labeled DNA probe. As was true for the various ELISA techniques discussed earlier, food and environmental samples also underwent selective enrichment to increase numbers of listeriae to detectable levels, i.e., 10^4–10^5 cells/ml before DNA hybridization. Briefly, food samples (25 g) were homogenized in 225 ml of FDA Enrichment Broth (FDA-EB) (see Table 6.2), whereas swab or environmental samples were added directly to 25 ml of FDA-EB. After 24 hours of incubation at 30°C, all samples were diluted 1:100 in modified FDA-EB buffered to pH 7.2 with MOPS (see Table 6.2) and incubated an additional 24 hours at 35°C (secondary enrichment).

Following incubation, 1 ml of the secondary enrichment culture was added to a vacuum filter membrane and treated with mutanolysin/lysozyme and sodium hydroxide to lyse the cells and denature rRNA, respectively. After washing, the denatured target nucleic acids were fixed to a membrane filter using ethanol. The filters were then immersed in a prehybridization solution and incubated 30 minutes at 65°C, after which the solution was decanted and hybridization solution containing the radioactively labeled genus-specific DNA probe was added. Following 2 hours of incubation at 65°C, filters were washed to remove unbound probe, after which the extent of hybridization was

Table 7.4 Comparison of the Gene-Trak Assay to "Standard" Cultural Methods for Detection of *L. monocytogenes* in Artificially Inoculated Food Samples

Type of food sample	Number of samples tested	Inoculum level (cells/g)	Positive samples (%)		False negatives[a] (%)	
			Gene-Trak assay	Culture method[b]	Gene-Trak assay	Culture method
Milk	4	3–18	100	100	0	0
	4	250	100	100	0	0
Ice cream	14	2–8	100	85.7	0	14.3
	4	174	100	100	0	0
Cheese[c]	8	0.7–74	75	62.5	25	37.5
Dairy products[d]	186	0.4–4	29	18.0	71	82
Meat and seafood[e]	66	0.4–4	70	67.0	30	33

[a] All inoculated samples assumed to be positive.
[b] FDA method—all dairy products; USDA method—meat and seafood.
[c] Imported Brie and Gouda, domestic Brie, and cream cheese.
[d] Vanilla ice cream, milk (2% fat), chocolate milk, cream cheese, and Gouda, Camembert, and Brie cheeses.
[e] Beef and turkey frankfurters, frozen fish, shrimp, and lobster.
Source: Adapted from Refs. 58, 59.

quantitated by counting the amount of radioactivity on each filter membrane in a Gene-Trak beta detector or scintillation counter. Using the Gene-Trak Isotopic Listeria Assay, up to 28 samples could be processed and hybridized at one time. Hybridization results were available within 4 hours, with the entire assay, including enrichments, taking approximately 2.5 days to complete.

To determine the sensitivity and specificity of this hybridization assay, selected food samples were inoculated to contain various levels of each of seven *Listeria* spp. and then simultaneously analyzed using both the Gene-Trak Isotopic Listeria Assay and the original FDA or USDA cultural procedure. According to company representatives, the Gene-Trak Isotopic Listeria Assay presumptively identified *L. monocytogenes* in all milk and ice cream samples regardless of inoculum level (Table 7.4). In contrast, the FDA cultural method proved highly satisfactory for detecting *L. monocytogenes* in milk, but failed to recognize the pathogen in 2 of 14 (14.3%) ice cream samples containing 2 to 8 *Listeria* cells/g. Although neither procedure was completely acceptable for detecting listeriae in cheese and other dairy products as well as meat and seafood, the Gene-Trak Isotopic Listeria Assay outperformed recognized cultural methods by a narrow margin. The hybridization assay and the FDA cultural method were generally equally reliable for detecting *L. innocua*, *L. seeligeri*, and *L. ivanovii* in inoculated samples of ice cream and cheese; however, the rapid procedure proved to be somewhat less effective for detecting these three *Listeria* spp. in inoculated milk samples. With the exception of ice cream inoculated with *L. welshimeri*, both methods generally yielded irregular results for milk and ice cream samples inoculated with *L. welshimeri*, *L. murrayi*, and *L. grayi*. Despite occasional failures of the Gene-Trak Isotopic Listeria Assay to detect nonpathogenic listeriae, this rapid method was generally equal to or superior to both the original FDA and USDA "standard methods" for detecting *L. monocytogenes* in various inoculated foods. Of equal importance was that presumptive results concerning presence or absence of listeriae in food products were obtainable within 2.5 days using the Gene-Trak Isotopic Listeria Assay as compared to 5–6 days using "standard" cultural procedures.

In two later studies (58,59), the Gene-Trak Isotopic Listeria Assay also compared favorably with the FDA cultural procedure to detect listeriae in naturally contaminated dairy, food, and environmental samples (Table 7.5). After testing over 800 food and environmental samples, the Gene-Trak Isotopic Listeria Assay was reported to have a

Table 7.5 Comparison of the Gene-Trak Listeria Assay and FDA "Standard" Cultural Method for Detection of *Listeria* spp. in Naturally Contaminated Dairy Food and Environmental Samples[a]

Type of sample	Number of samples tested	Number of positive samples	
		Gene-Trak assay	FDA cultural method
Dairy foods	468	15 (13)[b]	0
Dairy foods	151	9 (9)	10
Food manufacture and processing environments	200	43	43

[a]Submitted to an independent commercial testing laboratory.
[b]Confirmed by culture.
Source: Adapted from Refs. 58, 59.

false-negative rate of 6.7–12.2% (58,59) as compared to ~22% for the FDA cultural method (60).

Results concerning performance of this previously available hybridization assay were very encouraging. After comparing the FDA "standard" cultural method to the Gene-Trak Isotopic Listeria Assay and the Listeria-Tek ELISA, Knight et al. (61) found both rapid methods were superior to the "standard" plating procedure. Using all three procedures, analysis of 207 environmental and 168 dairy samples resulted in 32 *Listeria*-positive samples with isolation rates of 25, 27, and 30% for the FDA, Gene-Trak, and Listeria-Tek procedures, respectively. Thus reliable results concerning presence or absence of *Listeria* spp. in a particular food product were obtained after only 2.5 days with either of the two rapid methods just discussed, as compared to 5–6 days using "standard" cultural procedures.

Two major obstacles hindering widespread use of this assay included a maximum 10-day shelf life for the radioactive probe (^{32}P half-life $\cong$ 14.3 days) and the need for special licensing to handle the radioactively labeled DNA probe and accompanying waste materials. Recognizing these shortcomings, Gene-Trak Systems introduced an enzymatically labeled nonradioactive DNA probe assay in 1989 known as the Gene-Trak Colorimetric Listeria Assay for qualitative detection of *Listeria* spp. in dairy, meat, and seafood products as well as environmental samples. This highly successful Listeria assay, which is similar to three others developed to identify *Salmonella* spp. (14), pathogenic strains of *Escherichia coli*, and *Yersinia enterocolitica* (80), has now replaced the Isotopic Listeria Assay, which is no longer commercially available.

As was true for the isotopic method, food and environmental samples to be examined by the Gene-Trak Colorimetric Listeria Assay must undergo 24 hours of enrichment in one of several commonly used *Listeria*-selective broths (Fig. 7.10) (55,56). However, unlike the isotopic method, all enrichment cultures to be examined by the Gene-Trak Colorimetric Listeria Assay are swabbed onto LPM Agar plates rather than transferred to a secondary enrichment broth. Following 24 hours of incubation, as much surface growth as possible is collected on a cotton swab and suspended in phosphate-buffered saline solution. The Colorimetric Listeria Assay is then done on 0.3 ml of this bacterial suspension with the remainder reserved for conventional confirmation of listeriae in the event of a positive test result.

The Gene-Trak Colorimetric Assay (Fig. 7.11) can be divided into four main stages: (a) cell lysis, (b) hybridization, (c) capture, and (d) detection. In the first stage, cell lysis is achieved by exposing the bacterial suspension to lysozyme, mutanolysin, and proteinase K for 30 minutes. Following cell lysis, a fluorescein isothiocyanate-labeled *Listeria*-specific DNA "detector" probe (identical to the probe used in the former Gene-Trak Isotopic Assay but labeled with fluorescein rather than ^{32}P) and a *Listeria*-specific DNA "capture" probe containing a tail (i.e., "sticky end") with approximately 100–200 deoxyadenosine monophosphate residues are added to the sample which now contains free single-stranded 16S rRNA (Fig. 7.12). A specially prepared polystyrene "dipstick" coated with deoxythymidine is then inserted into the sample tube (Fig. 7.13). After 1 hour of incubation, the "detector" and "capture" probes will have selectively hybridized with any rRNA from organisms belonging to the genus *Listeria*. Furthermore, the "sticky end" of the capture probe will have hybridized with deoxythymidine on the dipstick. After thorough washing to remove all unbound probe, the dipstick is treated with an

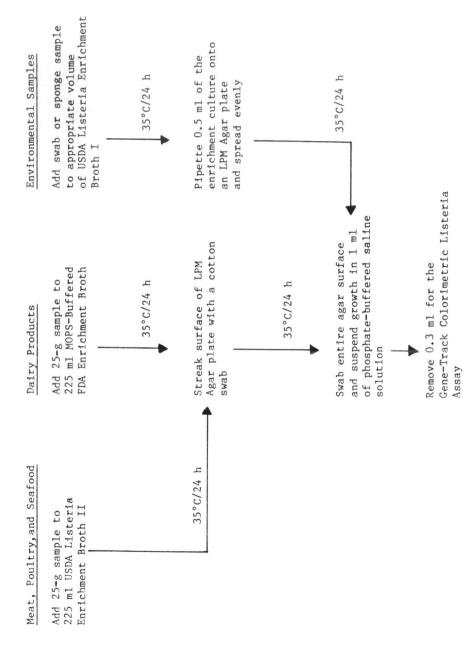

Figure 7.10 Sample enrichment protocols for the Gene-Trak Colorimetric Listeria Assay. (Adapted from Refs. 55–57.)

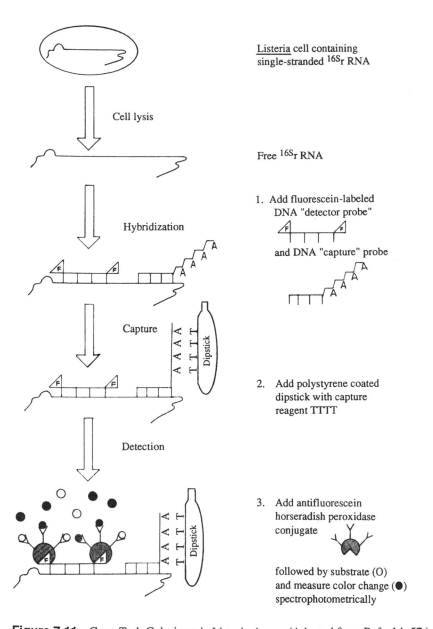

Figure 7.11 Gene-Trak Colorimetric Listeria Assay. (Adapted from Refs. 14, 57.)

antifluorescein antibody conjugated to horseradish peroxidase. The enzyme-labeled antibody selectively binds to the fluorescein-labeled DNA "detector" probe. Following 20 minutes of incubation at ambient temperature, the dipsticks are thoroughly washed, blotted, and immersed in a substrate/chromogen solution containing hydrogen peroxide and tetramethyl benzidene (Fig. 7.14). Finally, after 30 additional minutes of incubation, the color change that develops is arrested by addition of sulfuric acid and then the color is quantitated spectrophotometrically by measuring absorbance at 450 nm. According to the manufacture, readings of >0.10 indicate presence of listeriae in test samples.

When examined for specificity, 195 isolates of *L. monocytogenes* and 96 other *Listeria* strains representing *L. innocua*, *L. ivanovii*, *L. seeligeri*, *L. welshimeri*, *L. murrayi*, and *L. grayi* reacted positively in the Gene-Trak Colorimetric Listeria Assay (41,56,57). Of equal importance is the fact that pure cultures of 65 non-*Listeria* species belonging to 27 different genera [including such closely related organisms as *Jonesia denitrificans* (formerly classified as *L. denitrificans*) and species of *Brochothrix*, *Enterococcus*, *Streptococcus*, and *Staphylococcus*] were not detected by this assay when present at concentrations of 10^8–10^9 CFU/ml.

Further investigations have shown that this nonisotopic assay compares favorably to the original FDA and USDA methods for detecting listeriae in dairy and seafood products (Table 7.6). When various dairy products were inoculated to contain 1–100 *Listeria* CFU/25-g sample, the Gene-Trak and FDA methods yielded false-negative rates of 4.5 and 58.0%, respectively, thus indicating that the nonisotopic assay is far superior to the original FDA procedure for detecting listeriae in fermented and nonfermented dairy products. This was particularly true for raw milk and surface/mold-ripened cheeses from which isolation of listeriae traditionally has been difficult. While the original FDA and USDA procedures yielded false-negative rates of 11.8 and 8.6%, respectively, for detection of *Listeria* spp. in various inoculated seafoods, the Gene-Trak assay again was superior with a false-negative rate of only 5.3%. With the exception of shellfish, identical results were obtained when the Gene-Trak and original USDA procedures were used to detect listeriae in naturally contaminated meat and seafood (Table 7.7). However, the nonisotopic assay was superior to the original USDA method for detecting listeriae in naturally contaminated environmental samples, with a false-negative rate of 4.5 rather than 10.0%. Hence, given (a) the high degree of specificity for *Listeria* spp., (b) favorable comparisons to the original FDA and USDA methods, (c) moderate cost—~$10.00/sample, (d) relative simplicity, and (e) the rapid nature of the Gene-Trak Colorimetric Listeria Assay, such nonisotopic assays eventually may revolutionize detection of listeriae and other pathogens in the food industry.

While the Gene-Trak Colorimetric Listeria Assay just discussed is the only nonisotopic DNA hybridization assay for listeriae that is widely available, an *L. monocytogenes*, rather than a *Listeria* spp.–specific nonisotopic hybridization assay, was recently developed in the Netherlands by Notermans (76). As of February 1990 this assay was reportedly available on a limited basis.

Continued expansion of research in DNA probe technology will likely lead to further commercialization of more nonisotopic DNA hybridization assays that can differentiate between *L. monocytogenes* and other pathogenic as well as nonpathogenic *Listeria* spp. As an example, two Canadian scientists (81) succeeded in preparing a chromogen-labeled DNA probe from the hemolysin gene of *L. monocytogenes* that was previously

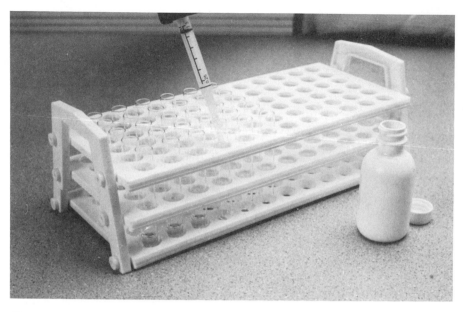

Figure 7.12 Gene-Trak Colorimetric Listeria Assay: Addition of fluorescein-labeled DNA "detector" probe and DNA "capture" probe to suspension of lysed cells. (Used with permission of W. King, Gene-Trak Systems, Framingham, MA.)

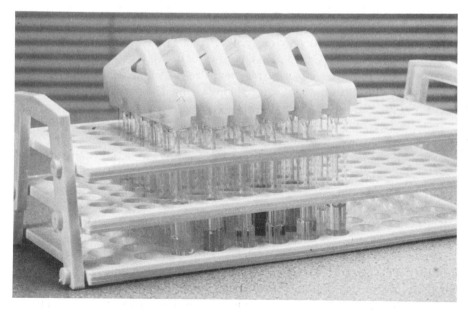

Figure 7.13 Gene-Trak Colorimetric Listeria Assay: Addition of polystyrene-coated dipstick containing capture reagent followed by antifluorescein horseradish peroxidase conjugate and enzyme substrate. (Used with permission of W. King, Gene-Trak Systems, Framingham, MA.)

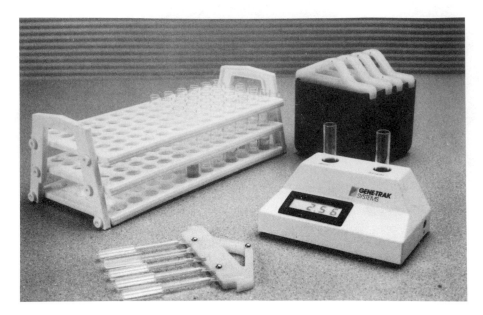

Figure 7.14 Gene-Trak Colorimetric Listeria Assay: Addition of color stop solution followed by a determination of absorbance at 450 nm. (Used with permission of W. King, Gene-Trak Systems, Framingham, MA.)

cloned into *Escherichia coli*. When this probe was used in a colony hybridization assay, *L. monocytogenes* colonies appeared as a series of purple dots on hydrophobic-grid membrane filters, with 21 potentially cross-reactive non-*Listeria* organisms yielding negative results. After labeling a previously developed DNA probe with biotin and digoxigenin, researchers at the Centers for Disease Control in Atlanta (54) also could distinguish between colonies of *L. monocytogenes* and avirulent *Listeria* spp. that were blotted onto nylon membranes from selective plating media. Under stringent conditions, the probe reportedly hybridized with a 13 kilobase DNA fragment from *L. monocytogenes* and a 3.5 kilobase DNA fragment from some strains of *L. seeligeri* while under less stringent conditions, hybridization was observed with a 6–7 kilobase fragment from *L. innocua*, *L. ivanovii*, and *L. seeligeri*. Using this procedure, low numbers of *L. monocytogenes* could be readily distinguished from avirulent listeriae and non-*Listeria* organisms, thus sharply reducing the number of colonies that need to be biochemically confirmed.

Another nonisotopically labeled probe for detection of *Listeria* was recently constructed by Plautz and Liewen (83). This probe was obtained by enzymatically restricting the entire genome of *L. monocytogenes* and then inserting the resulting DNA fragments into a plasmid which was transformed into *Escherichia coli*. Appropriate DNA fragments were then recovered from *E. coli* and enzymatically labeled with streptavidin–alkaline phosphatase to produce DNA probes. Preliminary results indicate that at least one probe hybridized to *Listeria* DNA immobilized on a nylon membrane, but failed to react with DNA from *Salmonella typhi*, *Micrococcus lysodeikticus*, *Streptococcus faecalis*, or *Pseudomonas fluorescens*. Despite these encouraging results, further characterization of

Table 7.6 In-House Comparison of the Gene-Trak Colorimetric Listeria Assay and the Original FDA/USDA Procedures for Detecting *Listeria* spp.[a]

Sample	Number of samples analyzed	Total number of positive samples	Number of positive samples		
			Gene-Trak Assay	FDA	USDA
Dairy products					
Pasteurized milk	13	8	8(8)[b]	6	ND[c]
Raw milk	24	22	22(22)	4	ND
Ice cream	24	16	16(15)	11	ND
Infant formula	12	8	8(8)	8	ND
Hard cheese	33	12	12(12)	2	ND
Semi-soft cheese	9	1	1(1)	0	ND
Surface-ripened cheese	51	23	22(21)	14	ND
Mold-ripened cheese	57	22	22(20)	2	ND
Total	222	112	111(107)	47	ND
Seafood products					
Cooked shrimp	64	55	54(54)	53	50
Raw shrimp	84	70	67(67)	62	69
Crabmeat	24	24	22(22)	18	22
Surimi	24	22	22(22)	20	20
Oysters	20	16	14(12)	12	10
Total	216	187	179(177)	165	171

[a]25-g samples of dairy and seafood products inoculated to contain 1–100 *L. monocytogenes*, *L. innocua*, or *L. ivanovii* CFU/sample.
[b]Number of positive samples subsequently confirmed using standard cultural methods.
[c]Not determined.
Source: Adapted from Refs. 41, 55.

Table 7.7 Comparison of the Gene-Trak Colorimetric Assay to the Original USDA Method for Detecting *Listeria* spp. in Naturally Contaminated Food and Environmental Samples

Sample	Total number of samples	Total positive	Number of positive samples Gene-Trak Assay(C)[a]	USDA
Food				
Raw ground meats	80	67	67(67)	67
Raw sausage	30	10	10(10)	10
Cured meat	10	4	4(4)	4
Shellfish	10	6	3(3)	6
Squid	10	0	0(0)	0
Fish cakes	10	0	0(0)	0
Environment				
Dairy factory	38	19	19(19)	18
Meat factory	62	8	7(7)	6

[a]Number of positive samples subsequently confirmed using standard cultural methods.
Source: Adapted from Refs. 41, 55.

the probe's sensitivity and selectivity for *Listeria* spp. will be necessary to ascertain the full commercial potential of this DNA probe.

In an attempt to identify only pathogenic strains of listeriae, one research team in West Germany (67) identified and isolated the genes encoding for production of hemolysin, listeriolysin O, CAMP factor, and a delayed hypersensitivity-inducing protein (DTH-18) from one *L. monocytogenes* isolate. These genes were subsequently labeled with ^{32}P and used as DNA probes to screen various *Listeria* spp. and other foodborne organisms. Although DNA fragments homologous to hemolysin, listeriolysin O, and the CAMP factor were generally present in all *Listeria* spp. tested except *L. grayi* and *L. murrayi*, the 1.1 kilobase DNA fragment encoding for the DTH factor only hybridized with corresponding DNA from the two major pathogenic *Listeria* spp.—*L. monocytogenes* and *L. ivanovii*. When the latter DNA probe encoding for the DTH factor was subsequently used to screen 284 *Listeria* strains representing all known species, biovars and serovars (77,78), hybridization was observed among all 117 *L. monocytogenes* strains belonging to serogroups 1/2a, 1/2b, 1/2c, 3a, 3b, 3c, 4c, 4d, 4e, 4ab, and 7. While DNA from the single reference strain of *L. ivanovii* and 77 of 78 *L. monocytogenes* serotype 4b isolates also hybridized with the probe, none of the 10 *L. monocytogenes* strains classified as serotype 4a yielded a positive reaction. However, given the rarity of *L. monocytogenes* serotype 4a isolates (i.e., only 10 of >3,000 isolates in the author's culture collection) and the fact that no hybridization was observed with any strains of *L. innocua*, *L. seeligeri*, *L. welshimeri*, *L. grayi*, and *L. murrayi*, this DNA probe encoding for the DTH factor offers promise for identifying virulent listeriae in food, environmental, and clinical samples.

Efforts also have focused on constructing a DNA probe that will only hybridize with nucleic acid from *L. monocytogenes*. The success of such an assay depends on identifying and cloning a DNA fragment which specifically codes for a trait that is unique to *L. monocytogenes*, and preferably only pathogenic strains of the organism. Therefore, researchers also have attempted to construct DNA probes that code for virulence factors specific to *L. monocytogenes*. Stephens et al. (98) recently examined the ability of natural and synthetic DNA probes specific for cholera toxin to hybridize with preparations of purified DNA from *L. monocytogenes*. Using a dot blot assay, DNA from 7 of 11 (63.6%) *L. monocytogenes* strains hybridized with the probe, suggesting that some pathogenic strains of *L. monocytogenes* contain DNA sequences that may code for a toxin related to cholera toxin.

The apparent association of β-hemolytic activity with intracellular survival of *L. monocytogenes* in mice makes the DNA segment encoding for β-hemolysin or listeriolysin (an extracellular thiol-dependent hemolytic protein) a prime candidate for an *L. monocytogenes*-specific DNA probe. In response to this observation, the gene encoding for hemolytic activity was recently sequenced (23) and fragmented by many researchers for use in probes that can distinguish between *L. monocytogenes* and other *Listeria* spp.

Beginning in 1987, FDA officials (19) obtained a 500-base-pair DNA fragment from the *L. monocytogenes* β-hemolysin gene that was cloned into an *Escherichia coli* plasmid by Flamm at Washington State University (35). Following growth of *E. coli* and simultaneous multiplication of the plasmid, cells were lysed to release the plasmid which was harvested by density gradient centrifugation. The original DNA fragment was then reisolated using restriction enzymes and purified by agarose gel electrophoresis and electroelution. Once purified, the 500-base-pair fragment encoding for hemolytic activity was radioactively labeled with ^{32}P using nick translation. Pure cultures of *L. monocytogenes* (18 strains), *Listeria* spp. (34 strains including *L. innocua*, *L. ivanovii*, *L. seeligeri*, *L. grayi*, *L. murrayi*, and nonspeciated *Listeria*), and 10 non-*Listeria* β-hemolytic organisms were used to assess the specificity and selectivity of the DNA probe. After colonies of the aforementioned organisms were obtained on agar media and replicated onto nitrocellulose filter membranes, the cells were lysed using a combination of microwave radiation and sodium hydroxide. The resulting DNA was then fixed to the filter membrane after which the labeled DNA probe was added and allowed to hybridize overnight. Following two 1-hour washes, the extent of hybridization on the filter membrane was determined using autoradiography—a process in which an image is produced by placing the filter membrane in close contact with a photographic emulsion. According to the authors, 10 of 18 (55.5%) *L. monocytogenes* strains that were previously positive for the CAMP test (a test for production of β-hemolysin) hybridized with the DNA probe that was directed against the gene encoding for β-hemolysin. [After conducting further biochemical tests, Datta et al. (21) reported that the eight nonreactive *L. monocytogenes* strains were misidentified and were most likely nonhemolytic strains of *L. innocua*.] Eleven nonspeciated *Listeria* isolates that were positive for the CAMP test also hybridized with the DNA probe and were therefore most likely strains of *L. monocytogenes*. Additionally, *Listeria* spp. that produced a negative CAMP test and β-hemolytic organisms that belonged to other genera failed to hybridize with the probe. Although researchers have long been plagued by immunological cross-reactions between β-hemolysin of *L. monocytogenes* and streptolysin O of streptococci, the DNA probe failed to cross-react with β-hemolytic strains of *Streptococcus pyogenes* and *Streptococcus agalactiae*.

In a follow-up study, Datta et al. (21,22) used the DNA probe just described to identify β-hemolytic strains of *L. monocytogenes* in naturally contaminated samples of raw milk, ricotta cheese, and European semi-soft cheese. Unlike the 48-hour selective enrichment procedure required before doing the Gene-Trak Listeria Assay, these researchers surface-plated appropriate dilutions of homogenized food samples directly on to LPM Agar (see Table 6.3) plates. After 24 hours of incubation, an exact replicate of the colony configuration was prepared by allowing a filter membrane to come in direct contact with the agar surface. The DNA hybridization assay was then done on the filter membrane as described in the preceding paragraph. After analyzing 34 raw milk samples, 12 of which were thought to contain *L. monocytogenes*, the pathogen was detected in only one sample at the level of ≥6000 CFU/ml. Similarly, the DNA probe assay yielded positive results from 1 of 3 samples of semi-soft cheese and 4 of 4 samples of ricotta cheese with populations of approximately 7.7×10^4 and 1.2×10^6 *L. monocytogenes* CFU/g, respectively. All DNA probe-positive colonies also were positive for the CAMP test, thus indicating the specificity of this assay for *L. monocytogenes*. Even though *L. monocytogenes* comprised only 0.1–1.0% of the total number of colonies on nonselective media, colonies of *L. monocytogenes* were easily enumerated using the DNA hybridization assay. Detection of *L. monocytogenes* was further enhanced using LPM Agar with approximately 70–80% of the colonies on this medium reacting positively to the DNA probe.

This probe-based assay developed by the FDA appears to be valuable both as a screening method and a rapid means of estimating *L. monocytogenes* populations in food samples, particularly when relatively high members of listeriae can be expected. Theoretically, the assay has a minimum detection level of 10 *L. monocytogenes* CFU/g of food; however in practice, the organism was never detected at levels less than 6.0×10^3, 7.7×10^4, and 1.2×10^6 CFU/g in samples of milk, semi-soft cheese, and ricotta cheese, respectively. Unlike the Gene-Trak Listeria Assay, which can be done on selectively enriched food samples and completed within 2.5 days, the hybridization assay for *L. monocytogenes* requires 2 days alone and cannot be done until colonies appear on solid media. Although the sensitivity of this assay undoubtedly could be improved by selectively enriching food samples for 1–2 days before streaking the culture on *Listeria*-selective solid media, such a step would increase the total time of analysis to 4–5 days. Furthermore, the quantitative nature of the test would be lost.

Given the proven ability of DNA hybridization to rapidly detect both pathogenic and nonpathogenic listeriae in mixed culture, development of hemolysin-based DNA probes for *Listeria* spp. has received considerable attention in the United States and Western Europe. Working at the FDA, Datta et al. (18,19) found that a listeriolysin O gene fragment from *L. monocytogenes* was useful in a probe-based colony hybridization assay to differentiate *L. monocytogenes* from other hemolytic and nonhemolytic *Listeria* spp. Similarly, researchers in Colorado (11) used a ^{32}P-labeled fragment from the listeriolysin O gene in combination with DNA amplification and agarose gel electrophoresis to detect as few as 10^3 *L. monocytogenes* cells after hybridization. Working at the Pasteur Institute in Paris, Chenevert et al. (15) also isolated a 651-base-pair fragment from the *L. monocytogenes* listeriolysin O gene that was useful as an isotopically labeled probe to differentiate *L. monocytogenes* from *L. innocua*, *L. ivanovii*, *L. seeligeri*, *L. welshimeri*, and *L. murrayi*. Under less stringent hybridization conditions, this probe also reacted with DNA from *L. ivanovii*, thus allowing differentiation between pathogenic and nonpathogenic strains of *Listeria*.

While the hemolysin/listeriolysin gene of *L. monocytogenes* has been the prime focus of most researchers in developing *L. monocytogenes*–specific DNA probes, gene fragments encoding for other virulence factors also may prove useful as potential probes. For example, Flamm et al. (36) cloned another gene (designated *msp*) from *L. monocytogenes* that encoded for a major virulence-associated extracellular polypeptide with a molecular mass of ~60 kilodaltons. When a subsequently constructed 500-base-pair fragment of the *msp* gene was labeled with ^{32}P and used as a probe against DNA from 15 clinical isolates of *L. monocytogenes* and single strains of *L. innocua*, *L. ivanovii*, *L. seeligeri*, *L. murrayi*, *L. grayi*, and *L. denitrificans* (recently reclassified as *Jonesia denitrificans*) as well as six gram-positive non-*Listeria* organisms, hybridization only was observed with DNA from *L. monocytogenes* under stringent conditions. Thus the *msp* gene is highly conserved in *L. monocytogenes*. Furthermore, each of five *L. monocytogenes* strains tested excreted a 60 kilodalton polypeptide that was immunologically related to the *msp* gene product. DNA sequences related to the *msp* gene were, however, observed in *L. innocua*, *L. seeligeri*, and *L. ivanovii* under nonstringent conditions, thus indicating that these three *Listeria* isolates produced an extracellular peptide similar to that in *L. monocytogenes*. While these findings also were consistent with immunological data, it appears that the *msp* gene–based probe can be used under strict hybridization conditions to differentiate *L. monocytogenes* from other *Listeria* spp.

Except for the isotopic and nonisotopic probes developed by Gene-Trak Systems, most remaining DNA probes have been designed to hybridize with DNA rather than rRNA. However, as you will recall, about 10^4 copies of target rRNA are present in each cell rather than just a single copy of target DNA. Thus use of RNA probes offers an opportunity to develop a highly sensitive hybridization assay.

With this in mind, Wallbanks et al. (103) determined the base-pair sequence of the 16S rRNA molecule for all seven *Listeria* spp. Researchers in the United States (99) and Canada (79) also are actively identifying *L. monocytogenes* rRNA fragments that may be useful as probes for rapid detection of the pathogen in various foods. According to Swaminathan et al. (99), electrophoretic separation of *L. monocytogenes* DNA fragments followed by hybridization with a ^{32}P-labeled rRNA probe from *Escherichia coli* and autoradiography revealed distinct patterns for each *L. monocytogenes* strain tested. Given an apparent association between the hybridization pattern and results from isoenzyme and phage typing, these preliminary findings suggest that rRNA:DNA hybridization may be another useful means of typing epidemiologically important *L. monocytogenes* isolates associated with foodborne listeriosis outbreaks.

CONCLUSION

As was true for selective plating and enrichment media discussed in the preceding chapter, development of DNA probes, ELISA assays, and other rapid techniques also has generated some debate over which method is best suited to detect *L. monocytogenes* and other *Listeria* spp. in food and environmental samples. To minimize some of this confusion, Heisick et al. (44) compared the ability of the ELISA Listeria-Tek Assay of Organon Teknika Corp., the Isotopic DNA Hybridization Assay of Gene-Trak Systems (the colorimetric assay was not yet available commercially at the time of the study), an *L. monocytogenes*–specific DNA probe procedure developed by the FDA, and the original FDA culture method to detect listeriae in 309 samples of naturally contaminated raw vegetables and 59 samples of raw milk obtained from cows inoculated with *L. monocytogenes*. While the pathogen was detected in 98 to 100% of the raw milk samples by each of the four methods examined, these assays varied widely in their ability to recover presumably low levels of listeriae from naturally contaminated raw vegetables, with no single assay identifying all positive samples. Overall, the FDA *L. monocytogenes*–specific gene probe correctly identified 38 of 44 (86%) positive samples, with the traditional FDA culture, Organon Teknika ELISA and Gene-Trak genus-specific probe methods identifying listeriae in 33 of 44 (75%), 30 of 44 (68%), and 20 of 44 (45%) samples, respectively. Although the Gene-Trak Isotopic Assay yielded the fewest positive samples along with the most false-positives, this assay (originally designed for only dairy and environmental samples) has since been replaced by the nonisotopic assay which is now widely used in the United States for analyzing many types of food and environmental specimens.

While the USDA (5) and, presumably, many other regulatory agencies in the United States and elsewhere, are actively evaluating the recently developed DNA probes, ELISA assays and other rapid methods to detect listeriae in foods, the way to establish a suitable "approval" system for these methods is still controversial, particularly when one considers that no single method has yet identified all positive samples in any given study. Coupled with this problem is the debate over the use of *L. monocytogenes*–specific or genus-specific assays.

Although some researchers and regulatory authorities may disagree, it appears that the new commercially available nonisotopic Gene-Trak Colorimetric Listeria Assay is among those best suited to rapidly screen large numbers of food and environmental samples for listeriae. However, since *L. monocytogenes* is currently the only *Listeria* spp. of public health concern, all food samples yielding positive results by this method need to be examined using standard cultural and biochemical methods to rule out the presence of *L. monocytogenes*. The greatest benefit of such a rapid method accrues to manufacturers of highly perishable foods so they can readily identify potential problems regarding *Listeria* contamination before their products reach consumers. The Gene-Trak Colorimetric Listeria Assay also provides food manufacturers with a rapid means of assessing the factory environment for listeriae. If food processors are following good sanitary practices, ready-to-eat foods and environmental samples should be free of all pathogenic and nonpathogenic *Listeria* spp. Hence, in such situations the Gene-Trak Colorimetric Listeria Assay can probably be used effectively with few if any samples requiring further testing to confirm presence of *L. monocytogenes*. While in-house *Listeria* testing is strongly discouraged, food manufacturers can conduct such work provided that the laboratory is in a separate building completely removed from all facets of food processing. Nevertheless, given the risks associated with accidental spread and/or introduction of listeriae including *L. monocytogenes* into food-processing facilities and the complexity of analysis, examination of both food and environmental samples for listeriae is probably best left to commercial testing laboratories.

REFERENCES

1. Anonymous. 1988. Food safety diagnosis through biotechnology seen. *Food Chem. News.* *30*(4):9–11.
2. Anonymous. 1988. *Listeria-Tek Instruction Manual for Detection of Listeria in Foods*, Organon Teknika Corp., Durham, NC.
3. Anonymous. 1988. Rapid methods for *Listeria* testing available but unapproved. *Food Chem. News 30*(7):9–10.
4. Anonymous. 1989. Faster method for identifying *Listeria* reported. *Food Chem. News.* *31*(14):27–28.
5. Anonymous. 1989. FSIS rapid test approval rule ignores standard procedures, NFPA says. *Food Chem. News 31*(35):30–31.
6. Anonymous. 1989. Testing for *Listeria. Dairy Ind. Intern. 54*(4):35.
7. Arkhangel'skii, I. I., and V. M. Kartoshova. 1962. Accelerated methods of detecting *Salmonella* in milk. *Veterinariya 9*:74–78.
8. Atrache, V., C. A. Van Huhyn, M. Ash, B. Wreford, A. Geczy, and S. Soldevila. 1989. A rapid immunoassay for detection of *Listeria* in food and environmental samples. *Proc. International Seminar on Modern Microbiological Methods for Dairy Products*, Santander, Spain, May 22–24, Poster 3C.
9. Atrache, V., C. A. Van Huhyn, M. Ash, B. Wreford, A. Geczy, P. Sutherland, and G. Davey. 1988. A rapid enzyme immunoassay for detection of *Listeria* in food and environmental samples. Presented as a poster at Ann. Mtg., Assoc. Off. Anal. Chem., Palm Beach, FL, Aug. 30.
10. Bennett, R. W. 1988. Production of flagellar ("H") and somatic ("O") sub-factor antibodies to *Listeria monocytogenes*. Ann. Mtg., Inst. Food Technol., New Orleans, LA, June 19–22 (Abstr.)
11. Bessesen, M., R. T. Ellison III, Q. Luo, H. A. Rotbart, and M. J. Blaser. 1989. Detection of *Listeria monocytogenes* by DNA. Ann. Mtg., Amer. Soc. Microbiol., New Orleans, LA, May 14–18 (Abstr.)
12. Biegeleisen, J. Z. 1964. Immunofluorescence techniques in retrospective diagnosis of human listeriosis. *J. Bacteriol. 87*:1257–1258.
13. Butman, B. T., M. C. Plank, R. J. Durham, and J. A. Mattingly. 1988. Monoclonal antibodies which identify a genus-specific *Listeria* antigen. *Appl. Environ. Microbiol. 54*:1564–1569.
14. Chan, S. W., S. Wilson, H.-Y. Hsu, W. King, D. H. Halbert, and J. D. Klinger. 1989. Model non-isotopic hybridization systems for detection of foodborne bacteria: Preliminary results and future prospects. In S.-D. Kung, D. D. Bills, and R. Quatrano (eds.), *Biotechnology and Food Technology—Proceedings of the First International Symposium*, Butterworths, Boston, pp. 219–237.
15. Chenevert, J., J. Mengaud, E. Gormley, and P. Cossart. 1989. A DNA probe specific for *L. monocytogenes* in the genus *Listeria. Int. J. Food Microbiol. 8*:317–319.
16. Cherry, W. B., and M. D. Moody. 1965. Fluorescent antibody techniques in diagnostic bacteriology. *Bacteriol. Rev. 29*:222–250.
17. Corrall, F. del, and R. L. Buchanan. 1989. Evaluation of the API-ZYM system for identification of *Listeria*. Ann. Mtg., Amer. Soc. Microbiol., New Orleans, LA, May 14–18, Abstr. P-35.
18. Datta, A. R. 1989. Probes for identifying *Listeria. J. Amer. Med. Assoc. 262*:1629–1630.
19. Datta, A. R., J. Russell, and B. A. Wentz. 1989. Detection of *Listeria monocytogenes* by natural and synthetic listeriolysin O specific gene. Ann. Mtg., Amer. Soc. Microbiol., New Orleans, LA, May 14–18, Abstr. P-31.
20. Datta, A. R., B. A. Wentz, and W. E. Hill. 1987. Detection of hemolytic *Listeria monocytogenes* by using DNA colony hybridization. *Appl. Environ. Microbiol. 53*:2256–2259.
21. Datta, A. R., B. A. Wentz, and W. E. Hill. 1988. Identification and enumeration of beta-hemolytic *Listeria monocytogenes* in naturally contaminated dairy products. *J. Assoc. Off. Anal. Chem. 71*:673–675.
22. Datta, A. R., B. A. Wentz, D. Shook, and M. W. Trucksess. 1988. Synthetic oligodeoxyribonucleotide for detection of *Listeria monocytogenes. Appl. Environ. Microbiol. 54*:2933–2937.

23. Domann, E., and T. Chakraborty. 1989. Nucleotide sequence of the listeriolysin gene from a *Listeria monocytogenes* serotype 1/2a strain. *Nucleic Acids Res. 17*:6406.
24. Donnelly, C. W., and G. J. Baigent. 1986. Methods for flow cytometric detection of *Listeria monocytogenes* in milk. *Appl. Environ. Microbiol. 52*:689–695.
25. Donnelly, C. W., G. J. Baigent, and E. H. Briggs. 1988. Flow cytometry for automated analysis of milk containing *Listeria monocytogenes*. *J. Assoc. Off. Anal. Chem. 71*:655–658.
26. Doores, S., C. Marshall, and J. Amelang. 1988. Comparison of the FDA procedure with Minitek and Vitek AMS for the identification of *Listeria* sp. Ann. Mtg., Amer. Soc., Microbiol., Miami Beach, FL, May 8–13, Abstr. P-7.
27. Durham, R. J., and J. A. Mattingly. 1988. A rapid method for the detection of *Listeria* colonies on agar plates. Ann. Mtg., Inst. Food Technol., New Orleans, LA, June 19–22, Abstr.
28. Durham, R. J., and J. A. Mattingly. 1988. Enzyme immunostaining for *Listeria* colonies on nitrocellulose membranes. Ann. Mtg., Amer. Soc. Microbiol., Miami Beach, FL, May 8–13, Abstr. P-6.
29. Durham, R. J., B. T. Butman, and B. J. Robison. 1989. The use of an ELISA, Listeria-Tek™, for the rapid detection of *Listeria* in food and environmental samples. *J. Food Prot. 52*:748. Abstr.
30. Durham, R. J., B. J. Robinson, and B. T. Butman. 1989. ELISA methods for rapid detection of *Listeria* and *Salmonella*. *Proc. International Seminar on Modern Microbiological Methods for Dairy Products*, Santander, Spain, May 22–24, Poster 3C.
31. Eveland, W. C. 1963. Demonstration of *Listeria monocytogenes* in direct examination of spinal fluid by fluorescent-antibody technique. *J. Bacteriol. 85*:1448–1450.
32. Farber, J. M., and J. I. Speirs. 1987. Monoclonal antibodies directed against the flagellar antigens of *Listeria* species and their potential in EIA-based methods. *J. Food Prot. 50*:479–484.
33. Farber, J. M., G. W. Sanders, and J. I. Speirs. 1988. Methodology for isolation of *Listeria* from foods—a Canadian perspective. *J. Assoc. Off. Anal. Chem. 71*:675–678.
34. Feng, P. 1989. Oligonucleotide probes specific for *Yersinia pseudotuberculosis*. Ann. Mtg., Amer. Soc. Microbiol., New Orleans, LA, May 14–18, Abstr. P-13.
35. Flamm, R. K. 1988. Molecular genetics of *Listeria monocytogenes*: Cloning of a hemolysin gene, demonstration of conjugation, and detection of native plasmids. Doctoral dissertation, Washington State University, Pullman.
36. Flamm, R. K., D. J. Hinrichs, and M. F. Thomashow. 1989. Cloning of a gene encoding a major secreted polypeptide of *Listeria monocytogenes* and its potential use as a species-specific probe. *Appl. Environ. Microbiol. 55*:2251–2256.
37. Flowers, R. S., M. A. Mazola, M. S. Curiale, D. A. Gabis, and J. H. Silliker. 1987. Comparative study of a DNA hybridization method and conventional culture procedure for detection of *Salmonella* in foods. *J. Food Sci. 52*:781–785.
38. Fraser, J. A., and W. H. Sperber. 1988. Rapid detection of *Listeria* spp. in food and environmental samples by esculin hydrolysis. *J. Food Prot. 51*:762–765.
39. Gavalchin, J., M. L. Tortorello, M. Landers, and C. A. Batt. 1988. Monoclonal antibody detection of *Listeria monocytogenes*. Ann. Mtg., Inst. Food Technol., New Orleans, LA, June 19–22, Abstr.
40. Graevenitz, A. von, G. Osterhout, and J. Dick. 1989. Use of cellular fatty acid composition for the identification of aerobic gram-positive non-sporeforming rods. Ann. Mtg., Amer. Soc. Microbiol., New Orleans, LA, May 14–18, Abstr. C-380.
41. Halbert, D. N., W. King, S. M. Raposa, A. R. Johnson, J. E. Warshaw, J. D. Klinger, M. A. Mazola, and J. M. Lawrie. 1989. A colorimetric detection assay for *Listeria* using nucleic acid probes. Ann. Mtg., Inst. Food Technol., Chicago, IL, June 25–29, Abstr. 353.
42. Hapke, B. 1989. Personal communication.
43. Heisick, J. E., D. E. Wagner, M. L. Nierman, and J. T. Peeler. 1989. *Listeria* spp. found on fresh market produce. *Appl. Environ. Microbiol. 55*:1925–1927.
44. Heisick, J. E., F. M. Harrell, E. H. Peterson, S. McLaughlin, D. E. Wagner, I. V. Wesley, and J. Bryner. 1989. Comparison of four procedures to detect *Listeria* spp. in foods. *J. Food Prot. 52*:154–157.

45. Hill, W. F., J. M. Madden, B. A. McCardell, D. B. Shah, J. A. Jagow, W. L. Payne, and B. K. Boutin. 1983. Foodborne enteropathogenic *Escherichia coli*: Detection and enumeration by DNA hybridization. *Appl. Environ. Microbiol. 45*:1324–1330.

46. Hitchins, A. D., R. Durham, B. Butman, and J. A. Mattingly. 1988. Comparison of culture methods and an ELISA for the ability to detect *Listeria* in ice cream. Ann. Mtg., Inst. Food Technol., New Orleans, LA, June 19–22, Abstr.

47. Hopfer, R. L., R. Pinzon, M. Wenglar, and K. V. I. Rolston. 1985. Enzyme release of antigen from *Streptococcus faecalis* and *Listeria monocytogenes* cross-reactive with Lancefield Group G typing reagents. *J. Clin. Microbiol. 22*:677–679.

48. Hudak, A. P., S. H. Lee, A. C. Issekutz, and R. Bortoussi. 1984. Comparison of three serological methods—enzyme-linked immunosorbent assay, complement fixation, and microagglutination—in the diagnosis of human perinatal *Listeria monocytogenes* infection. *Clin. Invest. Med. 7*:349–354.

49. Hunt, J., and P. Sado. 1989. Rapid *Listeria* identification using stab CAMP and stab xylose tests. Ann. Mtg., Amer. Soc. Microbiol., New Orleans, LA, May 14–18, Abstr. P-37.

50. Igo, J. D., and D. P. Murthy. 1989. *Listeria monocytogenes*: A protocol for rapid identification. *Med. J. Austral. 150*:607.

51. Jagow, J. A., and W. E. Hill. 1986. Enumeration by DNA hybridization of virulent *Yersinia enterocolitica* colonies in artificially contaminated food. *Appl. Environ. Microbiol. 51*:441–443.

52. Kamisango, K.-I., M. Nagaoka, H. Fujii, and I. Azuma. 1985. Enzyme assay of teichoic acids from *Listeria monocytogenes*. *J. Clin. Microbiol. 21*:135–137.

53. Khan, M. A., A. Seaman, and M. Woodbine. 1977. Immunofluorescent identification of *Listeria monocytogenes*. *Zbl. Bakteriol. Hyg. I Abt. Orig. A 239*:62–69.

54. Kim, C., L. M. Graves, B. Swaminathan, L. W. Mayer, and B. P. Holloway. 1989. Discrimination of *Listeria monocytogenes* from other *Listeria* species by colony hybridization with non-radioactively labeled probe. Ann. Mtg., Amer. Soc. Microbiol., New Orleans, LA, May 14–18, Abstr. D-231.

55. King, W. 1989. Personal communication.

56. King, W., S. Raposa, J. Warshaw, A. Johnson, D. Halbert, and J. D. Klinger. 1989. A new colorimetric nucleic acid hybridization assay for *Listeria* in foods. *Int. J. Food Microbiol. 8*:225–232.

57. King, W., S. Raposa, J. Warshaw, A. Johnson, K. Whippie, M. Ottaviani, A. Shah, M. Kimball, D. Halbert, J. Lawrie, J. Klinger, and M. Mazola. 1990. A colorimetric assay for the detection of *Listeria* using nucleic acid probes. In A. J. Miller, J. L. Smith, and G. A. Somkuti (eds.), *Foodborne Listeriosis*, Elsevier Scientific Publishing Co., Amsterdam, pp. 117–124.

58. Klinger, J. D., and A. R. Johnson. 1988. A rapid nucleic acid hybridization assay for *Listeria* in foods. *Food Technol. 42*(7):66–70.

59. Klinger, J. D., A. Johnson, D. Croan, P. Flynn, K. Whippie, M. Kimball, J. Lawrie, and M. Curiale. 1988. Comparative studies of nucleic acid hybridization assay for *Listeria* in foods. *J. Assoc. Off. Anal. Chem. 71*:669–673.

60. Klinger, J., D. Croan, P. Flynn, A. Johnson, K. Whippie, M. Ottaviani, G. Mock, N. Curron, M. Kimball, M. Curiale, and J. Lawrie. 1988. DNA probe hybridization assay for identification of *Listeria* species in food and environmental samples. Ann. Mtg., Amer. Soc. Microbiol., Miami Beach, FL, May 8–13, Abstr. P-33.

61. Knight, M. T., J. F. Black, D. W. Wood, and J. A. Mattingly. 1988. Comparison of FDA Lovett, Gene-Trak and ELISA *Listeria* methods. Ann. Mtg., Inst. Food Technol., New Orleans, LA, June 19–22, Abstr.

62. Knight, M. T., J. F. Black, and D. W. Wood. 1988. Industry perspectives on *Listeria monocytogenes*. *J. Assoc. Off. Anal. Chem. 71*:682–683.

63. Köhler, G., and C. Milstein. 1975. Continuous cultures of fused cells secreting antibody of predefined specificity. *Nature 256*:496–497.

64. Lachica, R. V. 1989. Rapid identification scheme for *Listeria monocytogenes*. Ann. Mtg., Amer. Soc. Microbiol., New Orleans, LA, May 14–18, Abstr. P-36.

65. Lane, J. S., J.DeAntoni, R. Johnson, R. O'Bear, M. Lamb, R. V. Eden, W. J. Hubbard, and R. E. Birch. 1987. Detection of food pathogens using the phage rapid identification assay system. Ann. Mtg., Inst. Food Technol., Las Vegas, NV, Abstr.

66. Larsen, S. A., G. L. Wiggins, and W. L. Albritton. 1980. Immune response to *Listeria*. In H. R. Rose and H. Friedman (eds.), *Manual of Clinical Immunology*, 2nd ed., Amer. Soc. Microbiol., Washington, DC.

67. Leimeister-Wächter, M., and T. Chakraborty. 1988. Gene probes for the detection of *Listeria* spp. 10th International Symposium on Listeriosis, Pecs, Hungary, Aug. 22–28, Abstr. 37.

68. Mac Gowan, A. P., R. J. Marshall, and D. S. Reeves. 1989. Evaluation of API 20 STREP system for identifying *Listeria* species. *J. Clin. Pathol. 42*:548–550.

69. Mattingly, J. A., B. T. Butman, M. C. Plank, R. J. Durham, and B. J. Robinson. 1988. Rapid monoclonal antibody-based enzyme-linked immunosorbent assay for detection of *Listeria* in food products. *J. Assoc. Off. Anal. Chem. 71*:679–681.

70. Mazola, M. A. 1988. Personal communication.

71. McLauchlin, J., and P. N. Pini. 1989. The rapid demonstration and presumptive identification of *Listeria monocytogenes* in food using monoclonal antibodies in a direct immunofluorescence test (DIFT). *Letters Appl. Microbiol. 8*:25–27.

72. McLauchlin, J., A. Black, H. T. Green, J. Q. Nash, and A. G. Taylor. 1988. Monoclonal antibodies show *Listeria monocytogenes* in necropsy tissue. *J. Clin. Pathol. 41*:983–988.

73. Meyer, S., and H. Brunner. 1981. Enzyme-immuno-assay in listeriosis: Detection of antibody and antigen. *Zbl. Bakteriol. Hyg., I Abt. Orig. A 248*:469–478.

74. Muraschi, T. F., and V. N. Tompkins. 1963. Somatic precipitinogens in the identification and typing of *Listeria monocytogenes. J. Infect. Dis. 113*:151–154.

75. Nelson, J. D., and S. Shelton. 1963. Immunofluorescent studies of *Listeria monocytogenes* and *Erysipelothrix insidiosa*. Application to clinical diagnosis. *J. Lab. Clin. Med. 62*:935–942.

76. Notermans, S. 1990. Personal communication.

77. Notermans, S., K. Wernars, and T. Chakraborty. 1988. The use of the *Listeria monocytogenes* DTH gene for the detection of pathogenic biovars. 10th International Symposium on Listeriosis, Pecs, Hungary, Aug. 22–26, Abstr. 38.

78. Notermans, S., T. Chakraborty, M. Leimeister-Wächter, J. Dufrenne, K. J. Heuvelman, H. Maas, W. Jansen, K. Wernars, and P. Guinee. 1989. Specific gene probe for detection of biotyped and serotyped *Listeria* strains. *Appl. Environ. Microbiol. 55*:902–906.

79. Pandian, S. 1988. Identification of the rRNA genes of *Listeria monocytogenes*. Society for Industrial Microbiology–Comprehensive Conference on *Listeria monocytogenes*, Rohnert Park, CA, Oct. 20, Abstr. P-14.

80. Parsons, G. 1988. Development of DNA probe-based commercial assays. *J. Clin. Immunoassay 11*:152–160.

81. Peterkin, P. I., and A. N. Sharpe. 1989. Chromogen-labelled DNA probe for the *Listeria monocytogenes* hemolysin gene used in the detection of foodborne *Listeria*. *J. Food Prot. 52*:748. Abstr.

82. Phillips, J. D., and M. W. Griffiths. 1989. An electrical method for detecting *Listeria* spp. *Lett. Appl. Microbiol. 9*:129–132.

83. Plautz, M. W., and M. B. Liewen. 1988. Construction of a DNA probe for detection of *Listeria*. Ann. Mtg., Inst. Food Technol., New Orleans, LA, June 19–22, Abstr.

84. Rashtchian, A., J. Eldredge, M. Ottaviani, M. Abott, G. Mock, D. Lovern, J. Klinger, and G. Parsons. 1987. Immunological capture of nucleic acid hybrids and application to nonradio-active DNA probe assays. *Clin. Chem. 33*:1526–1530.

85. Robison, B. 1988. *Rapid Detection of Listeria and Salmonella by Enzyme Immunoassay*, Organon Teknika, Durham, NC.

86. Robison, B. J., T. Donlevy, S. Keelan, and R. S. Flowers. 1988. Use of MICRO-ID and selected biochemical tests to rapidly identify *Listeria* sp. and *Listeria monocytogenes*. Ann. Mtg., Amer. Soc. Microbiol., Miami Beach, FL, May 8–13, Abstr. P-35.

87. Rocourt, J., and B. Catmel. 1985. Caracterisation biochimique des deux genres *Listeria*. *Zbl. Bakteriol. Hyg. A 260*:221–231.

88. Rodriguez, L. P., G. S. Fernandez, J. F. F. Garayzabal, and E. R. Ferri. 1984. New methodology for the isolation of *Listeria* microorganisms from heavily contaminated environments. *Appl. Environ. Microbiol. 47*:1188–1190.
89. Ruppenthal, T., and S. Wetherell. 1989. Initial characterization of affinity purified antibody specific for *Listeria* spp. using an enzyme immunoassay. Ann. Mtg., Amer. Soc. Microbiol., New Orleans, LA, May 14–18, Abstr. P-32.
90. Sasser, M., and M. Roy. 1988. Fatty acid analysis for rapid identification of the species of *Listeria* and related bacteria. Ann. Mtg., Amer. Soc. Microbiol., Miami Beach, FL, May 8–13, Abstr. P-44.
91. Seeliger, H. P. R. 1961. *Listeriosis*, Hafner Publishing Co., New York.
92. Siragusa, G. R., and M. G. Johnson. 1988. An EIA for *Listeria monocytogenes* cells and cell wall fragments. Ann. Mtg., Poultry Sci. Assoc., Baton Rouge, LA, July 25–28, Abstr.
93. Siragusa, G. R., and M. G. Johnson. 1988. Detection by conventional culture methods and a commercial ELISA test of *Listeria monocytogenes* added to cooked chicken. Ann. Mtg., Poultry Sci. Assoc., Baton Rouge, LA, July 25–28, Abstr.
94. Siragusa, G. R., M. G. Johnson, and L. N. Raymond. 1989. Production of a monoclonal antibody for *Listeria monocytogenes* and *L. innocua* and its use in bacterial assays. Ann. Mtg., Amer. Soc. Microbiol., New Orleans, LA, May 14–18, Abstr. P-16.
95. Siragusa, G. R., K. J. Moore, and M. G. Johnson. 1988. Persistence on and recovery of *Listeria* from refrigerated processed poultry. *J. Food Prot. 51*:831–832. Abstr.
96. Smith, C. W., J. D. Marshall, Jr., and W. C. Eveland. 1960. Identification of *Listeria monocytogenes* by the fluorescent antibody technic. *Proc. Soc. Exp. Biol. Med. 103*:842–845.
97. Sorin, M. L., M. Garnier, M. Bonneau, and R. Robinson. 1989. Test de détection rapide des *Listeria* dans les produits laitiers. *Sci. Aliments 8*:229–234.
98. Stephens, M., B. McCardell, and J. Madden. 1988. DNA:DNA homology between genes for cholera toxin. Ann. Mtg., Amer. Soc. Microbiol., Miami Beach, FL, May 8–13, Abstr. P-42.
99. Swaminathan, B., L. M. Graves, C. M. Carlone, and B. D. Plikaytis. 1988. Molecular epidemiology of *Listeria monocytogenes* by ribosomal RNA typing. Ann. Mtg., Amer. Soc. Microbiol., Miami Beach, FL, May 8–13, Abstr. D-61.
100. Swaminathan, B., W. E. Dewitt, G. M. Carlone, S. E. Johnson, L. Pine, G. Malcolm, C. Kim, and L. Williams. 1989. A monoclonal antibody specific for the beta hemolysin of certain serotypes of *Listeria monocytogenes*. Ann. Mtg., Amer. Soc. Microbiol., New Orleans, LA, May 14–18, Abstr. B-255.
101. Villella, R. L., L. W. Halling, and J. Z. Biegeleisen. 1963. A case of listeriosis in the newborn with fluorescent antibody histologic studies. *Am. J. Clin. Pathol. 40*:151–156.
102. Vlahovic, M. S., I. Kovincic, M. Mrdjan, Lj. Maslovaric, V. Pupavac, S. Bobos, and B. Trbic. 1988. The possibility of identification of *Listeria monocytogenes* in naturally infected cow's milk using fluorescent technic. Tenth International Symposium on Listeriosis, Pecs, Hungary, August 22–26, Abstr. P-71.
103. Wallbanks, S., M. D. Collins, U. M. Rodrigues, and R. G. Kroll. 1989. Nucleic acid probes to the 16S RNA of the genus *Listeria*. Proc. International Seminar on Modern Microbiological Methods for Dairy Products, Santander, Spain, May 22–24, Poster 3b.
104. Weaver, R. H. 1954. Quicker bacteriological results. *Am. J. Med. Technol. 20*:14–26.
105. Ziegler, H. K., and C. A. Orlin, 1984. Analysis of *Listeria monocytogenes* antigens with monoclonal antibodies. *Clin. Invest. Med. 7*:239–242.

8

Foodborne Listeriosis

HISTORICAL OVERVIEW

Discovery of several listeriosis outbreaks during the 1980s that were positively linked to consumption of cheese and raw vegetables has led to inclusion of *L. monocytogenes* in the current "list" of bonafide foodborne pathogens. However, in retrospect the concept of listeriosis as a foodborne illness actually can be traced back to when *L. monocytogenes* was first isolated. Nine years before Murray et al. (130) described *L. monocytogenes* in 1926, Atkinson (36) reported an outbreak of meningitis among five 2- to 9-year-old Australian children, caused by a small gram-positive, diphtheroid-type bacillus that was probably *L. monocytogenes*. Similarly, two additional listeriosis outbreaks (55,159) accounted for 7 of 36 listeriosis cases recorded in the literature between 1917 and 1943 (111). Hence, to explain these three small outbreaks, along with at least 26 other listeriosis outbreaks that have included 1347 documented cases of listeriosis between 1949 and 1987 (Table 8.1), one might reasonably postulate that food-to-human transmission of *L. monocytogenes* occurred in at least some instances.

Early animal feeding studies also support the notion that listeriosis can be acquired through consumption of contaminated food. The first accurate description of *L. monocytogenes* in 1926 by Murray et al. (130) included trials in which three of six 32-day-old rabbits were successfully infected via the oral route. Results from subsequent post-mortem examinations agreed with the previously observed pathological findings for naturally occurring listeriosis in rabbits. Fourteen years later, Julianelle (104) reported that white mice died of generalized listeric infections after consuming drinking water inoculated with *L. monocytogenes*. From these observations, both authors concluded that ingestion of *L. monocytogenes* followed by penetration of the gastrointestinal tract by the bacterium is one means by which listeriosis can be acquired.

As you will recall from our previous discussion of animal listeriosis, lactating cows can shed *L. monocytogenes* in milk for long periods as a consequence of listeric mastitis or abortion. Of greater importance are reports that clinically normal cows can shed listeriae in their milk for at least 12 months (98,164). Although *L. monocytogenes* was not isolated from both the udder and milk of mastitic dairy cattle until 1944 (180), Burn (55) postulated as early as 1936 that milk could serve as a possible vehicle of infection in humans. Two years later, Schmidt and Nyfeldt (159) also suspected a causal relationship between listeriosis in humans and dairy cows during a small listeriosis outbreak in Denmark but were unable to confirm milk as the vehicle of infection.

Given the preceding information, it is not surprising that consumption of raw milk was suspected as the most likely cause of the first documented foodborne outbreak of

Table 8.1 Apparent and Confirmed Common-Source Outbreaks of Listeriosis Involving 10 or More Cases

Location	Year	Number of cases	Possible vehicle of infection	Ref.
Halle, East Germany	1949–1957	~100	Raw milk, sour milk, cream, cottage cheese	36,88,144, 145,150,162
Jena, East Germany	1954	26	Unknown	170
Soviet Union	1956	19	Pork, mouse	91
Bremen, West Germany	1960–1961	81	Unknown	79
Halle, East Germany	1966	279	Unknown	137
Auckland, New Zealand	1969	13	Unknown	42
Anjou, France	1975–1976	162	Unknown	59
Johannesburg, South Africa	1977–1978	14	Unknown	100
Western Australia	1978–1979	12	Raw vegetables	167
Massachusetts, USA	1979	20	Raw vegetables, milk	96
Auckland, New Zealand	1979–1980	10	Unknown	148
Auckland, New Zealand	1980	22	Shellfish, raw fish	117
East Cambria, England	1981	11	Cream	85,126
Slovakia	1981	49	Unknown	148
Maritime Provinces, Canada	1981	41	Coleslaw[a]	158
Christchurch, New Zealand	1981–1982	18	Unknown	74
Houston, Texas, USA	1983	10	Unknown	57
Saxony, West Germany	1983	25	Unknown	131
Massachusetts, USA	1983	49	Pasteurized milk	80
Vaud, Switzerland	1983–1987	122	Vacherin Mont d'Or cheese[a]	47,54
Los Angeles, CA, USA	1985	142[b]	Mexican-style cheese[a]	118
Denmark	1985–1987	35	Unknown	152,156
Linz, Austria	1986	20	Raw milk, vegetables	2,169
Los Angeles, CA, USA	1986–1987	33	Raw eggs	161
Los Angeles, CA, USA	1987	11	Butter	125
England	1987	23	Unknown	127

[a]Vehicle of infection positively identified.
[b]Estimated number of cases as high as 300.

listeriosis. This outbreak, which occurred in Halle, East Germany, between 1949 and 1957 (Table 8.1), was accompanied by additional outbreaks in Jena, East Germany, and Prague, Czechoslovakia, with all three outbreaks prompting numerous investigations dealing with various epidemiological aspects of the disease. In 1955, the scientific literature on *Listeria* that had accumulated over nearly 50 years was admirably reviewed by H. P. R. Seeliger in his monograph entitled simply *Listeriosis* (in German). Interest in this disease was so great that over 150 publications appeared in the literature between 1955 and 1957. Consequently Seeliger extensively revised and updated his monograph in 1957 (in German) and again in 1961 (in English) (162) to the point where his book has to this day remained the leading source of information on the subject.

During this period of keen interest, Seeliger (162) and other European researchers (48,99,113,174) emphasized the likely importance of food in dissemination of listeriosis, which, in turn, resulted in some of the first studies dealing with the organism's suggested ability to survive during pasteurization of milk, as described in Chapter 5. Although a heightened awareness of *L. monocytogenes* led to documentation of at least nine listeriosis outbreaks (613 cases) in the 20-year period from 1960 to 1980 (Table 8.1), a lack of any clear link to food along with continued difficulties in isolating this organism from food and environmental sources are two likely reasons for a "leveling off" of interest in foodborne listeriosis during this period. While *L. monocytogenes* was not yet included in the list of recognized foodborne pathogens published by the World Health Organization in 1976 (3), three years later this pathogen was placed under the heading of "Bacteria Not Conclusively Proved to Be Foodborne" in the second edition of the well-known book *Foodborne Infections and Intoxications*, edited by Riemann and Bryan (151).

In 1981, the status of *L. monocytogenes* began to change when Schlech et al. (158) reported that 17 of 41 (41.5%) people died of listeriosis after consuming coleslaw from which *L. monocytogenes* was later isolated. This outbreak provided the first conclusive evidence that humans can contract listeriosis by consuming contaminated food and also demonstrated that foods other than dairy products can become contaminated with *L. monocytogenes* and thus constitute a health risk to certain segments of the population. Two years later, three additional listeriosis epidemics were documented (Table 8.1), including one widely publicized outbreak in which consumption of pasteurized milk was epidemiologically linked to 49 cases of listeriosis (including 14 deaths) in Massachusetts. However, it must be emphasized that *L. monocytogenes* was never isolated from the incriminated milk.

Any remaining doubt concerning the ability of *L. monocytogenes* to produce foodborne illness completely vanished in June of 1985 when consumption of Jalisco brand Mexican-style cheese was directly linked to at least 142 cases of listeriosis, including 48 deaths, in Los Angeles (118). Thus the two listeriosis outbreaks just mentioned and involving consumption of contaminated coleslaw and Mexican-style cheese, along with another major foodborne listeriosis outbreak in Switzerland that resulted from consumption of contaminated Vacherin Mont d'Or soft-ripened cheese, have generated worldwide concern over presence of *Listeria* in dairy products and many other foods including meat, poultry, eggs, seafood, and vegetables. Consequently, *L. monocytogenes* has now moved to the ranks of a bonafide foodborne pathogen in current food microbiology textbooks (63,103,140).

Since recent concern about foodborne listeriosis has centered around dairy products, it is only fitting to begin this chapter by reviewing the known cases of listeriosis in which nonfermented and fermented dairy products were suspected and/or proven as vehicles of infection. Special attention will be given to the two cheese-related listeriosis epidemics in California and Switzerland as well as the 1983 outbreak in Massachusetts that was supposedly linked to consumption of pasteurized milk. Similar evidence for involvement/possible involvement of other foods, including red meat, poultry, eggs, seafood, fish, vegetables, and fruit products in cases of human listeriosis will be presented in the remaining pages of this chapter.

RAW MILK

Sporadic cases of bovine mastitis and abortion in which *L. monocytogenes* was intermittently shed in milk over several lactation periods have been recorded in the literature for nearly 50 years. Dairy cows that appear healthy also can serve as reservoirs for *L. monocytogenes* and secrete the organism in milk. After it has been obtained from the cow, milk may be further contaminated through inadvertent contact with feces and silage, both of which often contain *Listeria* and are normally present in the dairy farm environment. Considering the present estimate that approximately 4% of raw milk contains a detectable level of *L. monocytogenes*, it is easy to understand why raw milk was suspected as one of the most likely sources of infection in several large European outbreaks of listeriosis.

The first evidence for foodborne transmission of *L. monocytogenes* can be found in a series of anecdotal reports from Germany (88,162). During the reconstruction period that followed the end of World War II, a sharp increase in the number of stillborn infants was observed at an obstetrical clinic in Halle, East Germany, with approximately 100 cases recorded up to 1952. Working in an antiquated laboratory, Potel (143) concluded that these stillbirths were the result of an infection with *Corynebacterium infantiseptica*. However, in 1952 Seeliger suggested and later confirmed that this rash of stillbirths was caused by *L. monocytogenes* (88). Unpasteurized milk as well as sour milk, cream, and cottage cheese were suspected by Seeliger (162) as possible vehicles of infection in several cases observed in Halle. Subsequently, Potel (145) isolated identical serotypes of *L. monocytogenes* from a mastitic cow and from stillborn twins delivered by a woman who had consumed this milk before parturition. On this basis, Potel can be credited with the first description of foodborne listeriosis in humans. During this outbreak, raw milk for pregnant women was generally available only through black markets, which in turn suggests that consumption of raw milk was likely responsible for additional cases of listeriosis (88). After this listeriosis epidemic ended in 1957, two subsequent outbreaks involving 180 and 160 cases were identified in Halle between 1960 and 1961 (79) and in 1966 (137), respectively. Fischer (79) also described a cluster of listeriosis cases that occurred in Bremen, West Germany, between 1960 and 1961. While the mode of transmission and primary reservoir for *L. monocytogenes* was never identified in these outbreaks, involvement of milk appears unlikely since most of these cases were reported during a time in which production and sale of milk were both rigidly controlled.

Since the postwar listeriosis outbreak in Halle in which raw milk was linked to at least one stillbirth, only two additional case studies have been published in which raw bovine milk has been mentioned as a possible cause of listeric infection. In the first of these cases, reported in 1973 (52), a 28-year-old Canadian woman went into premature labor and delivered an infant that died of listeriosis 33 hours after delivery. Shortly before giving birth, the mother recalled purchasing raw milk and cream; however, these products were no longer available for testing. The second case involved a 43-year-old male AIDS patient in California who contracted listeric meningitis in 1987. Following rigorous antibiotic therapy and complete recovery, the patient admitted being a regular consumer of commercially available raw milk. While the investigating team made no attempt to confirm raw milk as the vehicle of infection, the possible role of raw milk in this case suggests that current (1990) efforts by the FDA and Centers for Disease Control to inform AIDS patients about the potential threat of listeriosis, salmonellosis, and other foodborne illnesses associated with consumption of certain high-risk foods (e.g., raw milk, surface-ripened cheese, undercooked poultry) should continue.

The threat of contracting milkborne listeriosis generally appears to be confined to susceptible individuals who routinely consume raw bovine milk, with no listeric infections yet linked to consumption of raw milk from other animals including ewes and goats. Thus, even when given the ability of *L. monocytogenes* to infect humans and produce mastitis in animals, it is still surprising to learn that researchers in Yugoslavia (173) were recently able to link one case of neonatal listeriosis to consumption of contaminated human breast milk. According to their report, a 24-day-old infant girl contracted listeriosis after receiving breast milk from her mother. Thirteen days after onset of symptoms, *L. monocytogenes* serotype 4b was isolated from the infant's cerebrospinal fluid and blood as well as the mother's milk. The infant recovered fully 3 days after cessation of breast feeding. Interestingly, excess breast milk from the mother was given to a newborn litter of three Doberman puppies, and all three dogs became ill with vomiting, diarrhea, and bloody stools. One of the animals died, and the same serotype of *L. monocytogenes* as found in breast milk was detected in a stool specimen from one of the two survivors. While this is currently the only report linking listeriosis to consumption of human breast milk, the medical profession should be aware of the possibility for such transmission, particularly in apparent nosocomial cases of neonatal listeriosis.

PASTEURIZED MILK

Until 1985, the only proven foodborne listeriosis outbreaks associated with dairy products involved consumption of raw milk. However, this changed when Fleming et al. (80) epidemiologically linked consumption of a specific brand of whole and 2% pasteurized milk to 49 cases of listeriosis that occurred in Massachusetts between June and August of 1983. As seen in Table 8.2, 42 (86%) of the cases occurred in adults and seven (14%) in mother-infant pairs. Fourteen of 49 individuals died giving a mortality rate of 29%. Two years later, Todd (168) calculated the total cost of this outbreak at $1.89 million ($1.37 million—deaths, $387,000—hospitalization, $70,000—investigation, $61,000—financial/legal costs) or $38,614 per case excluding legal settlements.

While all adults had underlying conditions that resulted in immunosuppression, symptoms expressed during the course of illness varied, depending on the person's age and degree of immunosuppression. Forty of 49 isolates were available for serotyping, and 32 (80%) of them were of serotype 4b, later defined as the epidemic strain.

Table 8.2 Characteristics of Adult and Perinatal Listeriosis Cases Identified in Massachusetts Between June 30 and August 30, 1983

Case profile	Number of cases (%)	
	Adult	Perinatal
Total cases	42 (86)	7 (14)
Total fatalities	12 (29)	2 (29)
Sex: M/F	27/15	2/5
Clinical syndrome		
Meningitis	13 (31)	3 (42)
Septicemia	29 (62)	2 (29)
Death in utero	—	2 (29)
Underlying condition		
Cancer	20 (48)	—
Cirrhosis/Alcoholism	7 (17)	—
Diabetes	5 (12)	—
Corticosteroid therapy	4 (9)	—
Renal transplant	2 (5)	—
Myelofibrosis	2 (5)	—
Chronic hepatitis	1 (2)	—
Intravenous drug abuse	1 (2)	—

Source: Adapted from Ref. 80.

Two case-control studies, one matched for neighborhood of residence and the other for the patients' underlying condition, indicated that development of listeriosis was strongly associated with drinking a specific brand of pasteurized whole or 2% milk. Further epidemiological investigations showed (a) a correlation between increased consumption of the specific brand of whole or 2% milk and contracting listeriosis, (b) a lower incidence of disease among individuals who drank skim or 1% milk produced by the same dairy, (c) an association between several cases of listeriosis in Connecticut and consumption of the same brand of whole or 2% milk, and (d) an association with a specific phage type of *L. monocytogenes* (phage type 2425A), which was isolated from all 19 listeriosis victims who reportedly drank the specific brand of whole or 2% milk.

While these epidemiological studies strongly suggest that this outbreak resulted from consuming whole or 2% milk, the microbiological findings were far less convincing in that *L. monocytogenes* was never isolated from the incriminated pasteurized milk. The milk implicated in this listeriosis outbreak was processed at a single dairy factory and pasteurized at 77.2°C (171°F)/18 seconds (147), well in excess of the minimum requirement [71.7°C (161°F)/15 sec] specified in the Pasteurized Milk Ordinance. Furthermore, no defect was identified that could have led to improper pasteurization and no source of postpasteurization contamination was ever found within the dairy factory. Shortly after the outbreak ended, a survey conducted by the Centers for Disease Control (80,87,93) indicated that 15 of 124 (12%) raw milk samples collected from the factory milk supply, from individual farms, and a milk cooperative that supplied the factory were positive for

L. monocytogenes. Although several different serotypes were identified, including 1a, 3b, 4a/b, and the epidemic serotype (4b), the phage type that was epidemiologically linked to the outbreak was never isolated from raw milk or the incriminated pasteurized milk.

Although the epidemiological evidence gathered by Fleming et al. (80) suggests this outbreak resulted from drinking a particular brand of pasteurized whole or 2% milk, the means by which *L. monocytogenes* found its way into the milk remains a mystery. Although postpasteurization contamination of the milk cannot be excluded, it seems unlikely since inspections failed to uncover *L. monocytogenes* in the dairy factory environment. Since whole and skim milk were processed each day using the same equipment, it is also difficult to postulate a means by which only whole milk would have been subjected to postpasteurization contamination.

To further support the involvement of pasteurized milk in this outbreak, the authors concluded that "intrinsic contamination of the milk and survival of some organisms despite adequate pasteurization is both consistent with the results of this investigation and biologically plausible;" the latter conclusion was based on the faulty but at the time frequently quoted pasteurization study by Bearns and Girard (41). Consequently, the apparent association of listeriosis with consumption of pasteurized milk raised immediate concerns as to the safety of the product, which in turn led to a series of studies that examined the heat resistance of *L. monocytogenes* (all of which were discussed in Chapter 5). Nearly 2 years after the outbreak was reported in the *New England Journal of Medicine*, Donnelly et al. (63) found that the "open tube" method used by Bearns and Girard (41) was flawed and concluded that freely suspended *L. monocytogenes* cells were unlikely to survive normal HTST pasteurization at 71.7°C (161°F) for 15 seconds. Knowing that this pathogen can exist within milk leukocytes and that the milk in the Massachusetts outbreak was not clarified, but rather passed through a milk sock (coarse filter) that did not remove leukocytes, many researchers postulated that presence of *L. monocytogenes* within these leukocytes enhanced the organism's resistance to pasteurization. Subsequent studies addressing this issue have generally shown insignificant differences in the degree of thermal resistance between free and internalized *L. monocytogenes* cells suspended in milk (66,134). Using milk containing relatively large numbers of intracellular listeriae, several workers demonstrated that *L. monocytogenes* can survive minimum requirements for pasteurization; however, commingling of milk from many farms before pasteurization would result in much lower levels of listeriae (i.e., ≤10 CFU/ml) (33,119,166) with many if not most organisms present only extracellularly as a result of leukocytic breakdown during the first 24–48 hours of cold storage. Hence, on this basis both the scientific community and the World Health Organization contend that *L. monocytogenes* will not survive minimal milk pasteurization at 161°F/ 15 seconds (177). In support of this position, *L. monocytogenes* has not yet been demonstrated to have survived pasteurization in a commercial dairy product that met minimum HTST pasteurization requirements.

While numerous FDA Class I recalls of other pasteurized dairy products including 2%, 1%, and skim milk as well as chocolate milk, ice milk mix, ice milk, ice cream mix, ice cream, ice cream novelties, sherbet, and various cheeses have been well publicized in the United States, in virtually all instances *L. monocytogenes* was present in the immediate manufacturing environment, which strongly suggests postpasteurization contamination. Given this information, the likelihood of *L. monocytogenes* having survived pasteurization at ~77.2°C (171°F)/18 seconds in the Massachusetts outbreak appears remote at best.

Since *L. monocytogenes* was never isolated from the pasteurized milk implicated in the Massachusetts outbreak or the dairy factory environment, some investigators have questioned whether this listeriosis outbreak actually resulted from drinking milk (62). In 1988, several design flaws were discovered in the case-control studies (62) that included missing questions and data on questionnaires, as well as a disproportionate number of follow-up interviews between cases and controls, any of which might have given an unfair bias. Contrary to the view of the authors (80), the cases were generally clustered around the Boston area in a manner that was not consistent with the distribution pattern of the milk. Furthermore, inconsistencies in the data were noted between exposure to the implicated milk and isolation of the *L. monocytogenes* strain supposedly responsible for the epidemic (62). Discovery of these discrepancies in the various case-control studies has since led to a lawsuit which is currently (1990) pending against the Centers for Disease Control; however, it appears unlikely that a definitive answer as to the involvement of milk or some other food product in this outbreak can be reached through the judicial system.

OTHER NONFERMENTED DAIRY PRODUCTS

A search of the early literature has uncovered only a few inconclusive reports suggesting that listeriosis can be contracted by consuming nonfermented dairy products other than raw and possibly pasteurized milk. After the first massive outbreak of listeriosis was reported in Halle, East Germany, between 1949 and 1957, Seeliger (162) indicated that in addition to raw milk, sour milk and cream also were considered as possible sources of infection in several cases. While it is certainly possible for such products to contain *L. monocytogenes*, the exact role of raw milk and cream in these cases was never determined. During the latter half of 1981, an apparent common-source listeriosis outbreak was recorded in East Cambria, England in which identical phage- and serotypes of *L. monocytogenes* were isolated from 11 patients (126). Even though epidemiological evidence indicated a possible association with consumption of pasteurized cream (39,85), the exact mode of transmission was never verified. Similarly, Ralovich (148) learned of a personal account in which *L. monocytogenes* was isolated from cream-based rice soup that was associated with a foodborne illness; however, the etiological role of *Listeria* was never proven.

Following the widely publicized 1985 listeriosis outbreak in California in which numerous deaths were directly linked to consumption of contaminated Mexican-style cheese, Los Angeles County officials instituted an active surveillance program for listeriosis and made the disease reportable (124). These efforts eventually led to discovery of a cluster of 11 perinatal listeriosis cases among Hispanics during November and December of 1987 (123). Seven of 11 *L. monocytogenes* isolates obtained from the victims were of serotype 1/2a. While a subsequent case-control study identified butter as a possible vehicle of infection (odds ratio = 4.0), this first-time association between consumption of butter and listeriosis was not culturally confirmed. Absence of *Listeria* spp. from butter tested by the FDA during the Dairy Initiatives Program (33) and new evidence indicating that large numbers (~92–97%) of *L. monocytogenes* are lost in buttermilk and washings when butter is manufactured from inoculated cream (136) suggest that butter does not appear to be a major vehicle for transmission of listeriae.

Attempts to implicate frozen dairy products as vehicles of infection in listeriosis cases are of relatively recent origin. In 1986, FDA officials investigated an incident in which *L. monocytogenes* was isolated from amniotic fluid following the premature delivery of an infected infant who died 5 days later (9). After learning that the 21-year-old mother consumed ice cream sandwiches 3 days before delivery, all suspect product was withdrawn from store shelves; however, follow-up studies failed to incriminate ice cream as the source of infection.

Beginning in 1985, enhanced surveillance of the dairy industry by the FDA resulted in numerous recalls of *Listeria*-contaminated frozen dairy products including ice cream, ice milk, sherbet, and ice cream novelties as well as ice milk, ice cream, and milk shake mix. Since consumption of such products is thought to constitute a public health risk, preliminary epidemiological results from the U.S. Centers for Disease Control suggesting a possible link between consumption of ice cream and a cluster of 31 listeriosis cases including 14 deaths, in the Philadelphia, Pennsylvania, area appeared to have some merit (15). However, inability to isolate *L. monocytogenes* from ice cream eliminated this product as the vehicle of infection (16, 160). After repeated attempts to (a) identify a common epidemic strain and (b) isolate *Listeria* from cheese and other dairy products as well as meats and vegetables ended in failure, the Centers for Disease Control finally retracted their previous statement and concluded that a common-source outbreak of foodborne listeriosis had not occurred in the Philadelphia area (14,160).

Although well over 3 million gallons of frozen dairy products thought to be contaminated with *Listeria* have thus far been recalled from the market at a cost in excess of $66 million (17), not one case of listeriosis has been directly linked to consumption of such products. Apparent low levels of *L. monocytogenes* in frozen dairy products resulting from postpasteurization contamination combined with the organism's obvious inability to grow during frozen storage (44) are but two reasons why these products appear to constitute a relatively low risk to public health.

FERMENTED DAIRY PRODUCTS

Certain species of lactic acid–producing bacteria can be used to ferment fluid milk into a wide array of dairy products including cultured buttermilk, sour cream, and yogurt as well as hundreds of varieties of cheeses. Thus far no listeriosis outbreaks have been positively linked to consumption of contaminated yogurt, sour cream, or cultured buttermilk; however, the same cannot be said for cheese. As early as the 1950s, cheese was suspected of playing a role in foodborne listeriosis. However, since June of 1985, two major listeriosis outbreaks have been directly linked to consumption of contaminated cheese, thus confirming its role in foodborne listeriosis. The first such outbreak involved consumption of Mexican-style cheese in California and was followed by a second major outbreak in Switzerland, which was traced to contaminated Vacherin Mont d'Or soft-ripened cheese. Both of these outbreaks will now be reviewed in some detail, after which several isolated cases of cheeseborne listeriosis also will be discussed.

As just mentioned, the notion that humans can contract listeriosis by consuming

Listeria-contaminated cheese is not new. Along with raw milk, sour milk, and cream, Seeliger (162) suggested a possible relationship between consumption of cottage cheese and several cases of listeriosis that occurred in Halle, East Germany, mentioned earlier. Nonetheless, it must be stressed that cottage cheese was never confirmed as the vehicle of infection. A search of the scientific literature revealed no additional reports suggesting involvement of cheese in cases of listeriosis during the 30 years that followed the Halle incident.

Mexican-Style Cheese: California, 1985

In June of 1985 the ability of cheese to serve as a vehicle for foodborne listeriosis became evident when consumption of Jalisco brand Mexican-style cheese was linked to a massive listeriosis outbreak in southern California. This outbreak, which later proved to be among the deadliest of all known outbreaks of foodborne disease recorded in the United States, prompted much research activity in the United States, Canada, and Western Europe, most of which is reviewed elsewhere in this book. Before dealing with the facts of this outbreak, it is appropriate to chronologically review the "detective work" conducted by various governmental agencies (Fig. 8.1) that linked this outbreak to Mexican-style cheese, and also led to a nationwide recall of the product on June 17, 1985.

According to information appearing in local newspapers, the first listeriosis case associated with this outbreak was diagnosed in Los Angeles County during the first week of January 1985, with one and three additional cases documented during the second and fourth weeks of January, respectively. Unknown to public health officials, the rate of listeric infections continued to increase with six and nine cases reported in Los Angeles County during February and March, respectively.

Several important chance happenings led to discovery of this outbreak in the weeks that followed. The first hint of a possible problem was uncovered at the Los Angeles County–University of Southern California (USC) Medical Center—a vast medical complex at which about 17,000 infants are delivered each year (101,102). In early April Carol Salminen, a nurse epidemiologist who monitored infection rates at this facility, uncovered five additional cases of listeriosis among Hispanic mother/infant pairs during the previous 2 weeks. Under normal circumstances, only three to five listeric infections would be observed annually at this hospital. After consulting with the medical director of the labor and delivery service, who had developed a personal interest in listeriosis and maintained a log of listeric infections over the previous 10 years, Salminen informed health officials at the Los Angeles County Department of Health Services on May 6 that nine listeriosis victims had been treated at the USC Medical Center since January of 1985. Once notified, health officials at the Los Angeles County Department of Health Services and the Orange County Health Care Agency began surveying area hospitals for additional cases of listeriosis. After the reported number of listeric infections increased from 16 to 67 in just a few days, Los Angeles County health officials contacted the California Department of Health Services and the Centers for Disease Control (CDC) on May 10 for investigative assistance. At the same time, 200 area hospitals in Los Angeles and Orange County were requested to report all listeriosis cases to the health department.

Ten days later, health officials and epidemiologists from CDC began the first of two

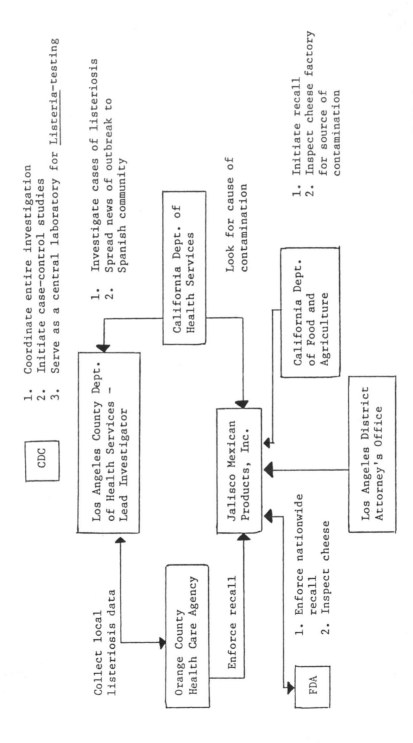

Figure 8.1 Primary roles of local, state, and federal agencies in investigating the 1985 listeriosis outbreak in California.

case-control studies in which listeriosis victims, most of whom were Hispanic, and healthy individuals were interviewed about various environmental factors, behavioral patterns, and consumption of over 60 food items including fresh fruits and vegetables as well as water, milk, and cheese. On May 29, an open package of Jalisco brand Mexican-style cheese was taken from one of the victims' refrigerators and sent to CDC in Atlanta for analysis. After CDC investigators provided preliminary confirmation of *L. monocytogenes* in this opened package of Mexican-style cheese on June 8, 20 packages of Mexican-style cheese of various brands, including two packages of Queso Fresco and Cotija Jalisco brand cheese, were purchased at area markets near the victim's place of residence and sent to CDC for analysis (118). One June 10, results from the case-control study described earlier clearly demonstrated that individuals who had consumed Mexican-style cheeses were at increased risk of contracting listeriosis. Armed with this information, investigators immediately began a second case-control study in which individuals were questioned about the names and brands of Mexican-style cheese consumed. After statistical analysis, on June 12 these data revealed a definite link between consumption of Jalisco brand Mexican-style cheese and development of listeriosis (118), FDA officials were immediately advised of the impending problem with Jalisco cheese. The confirmation of *L. monocytogenes* serotype 4b in two unopened packages each of Jalisco-brand Queso Fresco and Cotija Mexican-style cheese—the last piece of evidence needed to initiate a Class I recall of the product—was provided by the CDC on June 13. (Subsequent studies eventually confirmed the presence of the epidemic *L. monocytogenes* strain in 82% of all Jalisco brand products purchased at area supermarkets.) With this information in hand, the California Department of Food and Agriculture immediately closed the Jalisco cheese factory and announced a statewide recall for these two varieties of Mexican-style cheese, ~80% of which were sold through retail outlets in Los Angeles and Orange County. On June 14, state officials expanded this recall to include the firm's entire line of 44 products (predominantly cheese), consumption of which was already blamed for at least 28 deaths. Hence, in the weeks that followed, health officials were faced with the enormous task of checking ~28,000 Los Angeles-area supermarkets, family-owned grocery stores, and restaurants to ascertain that all Jalisco brand products were removed from shelves. FDA officials also ordered a Class I recall of all Jalisco brand products distributed in California and in 12 other primarily western states (4). Three days later, this recall was expanded to include all 26 states in which the products were sold as well as the United States Protectorates of Guam, American Samoa, and the Marshall Islands (6). When this recall was completed on June 22, nearly 250 tons of Jalisco brand Mexican-style cheese and other dairy products were ready for burial in a landfill site overlooking the San Gabriel Valley.

Although the number of individuals who actually contracted listeriosis after eating the tainted cheese has been a debatable issue for some time, the exact figure will never be known since mild listeric infections in individuals who did not seek medical attention obviously went unreported. Newspaper accounts have placed the total number of listeriosis cases occurring in California between January 1 and August 15 at nearly 300, including 85 fatalities. While about half of these cases were concentrated within the Hispanic communities of Los Angeles and Orange County, a substantial number of listeriosis victims also reportedly resided in the San Diego area, which made the collection of reliable data more difficult. In addition, at least 15 cheese-related listeriosis cases were uncovered outside California (Colorado, Oregon, Texas, and Connecticut) with three fatalities reported in Texas.

While the total number of listeriosis cases reported in Los Angeles County during the 12-month period immediately following the outbreak decreased to 94, the calculated annual crude incidence rate of ~12 cases/million population is still approximately twice the national average (124). However, these findings are not too surprising when one considers that this outbreak certainly made area physicians, hospital personnel, and public health authorities keenly aware of this disease. In all likelihood, these factors in combination with mandatory reporting of this previously obscure illness are largely responsible for the abnormally high incidence of listeriosis in Los Angeles County.

In 1988, Linnan and 14 other members of the investigative team (118) published their findings concerning 142 cases of listeriosis that were linked to consumption of Jalisco brand cheese in Los Angeles County between January 1 and August 15, 1985. Although nearly 160 additional cases occurred elsewhere in California (Orange, San Diego, and Fresno counties) and in other states, logistical concerns limited their studies to Los Angeles County. During the 7.5-month epidemic period, 93 reported listeriosis cases (65.5%) involved pregnant women or their offspring and 49 (34.5%) involved nonpregnant adults (Fig. 8.2, Table 8.3). Forty-eight of the 142 listeriosis victims died, giving an overall mortality rate of 33.8%. Thirty deaths occurred among the 87 early fetal/neonatal cases; however, no late fetal/neonatal or maternal deaths were reported. All but 1 of the 49 nonpregnant adults had a predisposing condition such as cancer (3 patients), steroid dependency (12 patients), chronic illness (23 patients), age > 65 (5

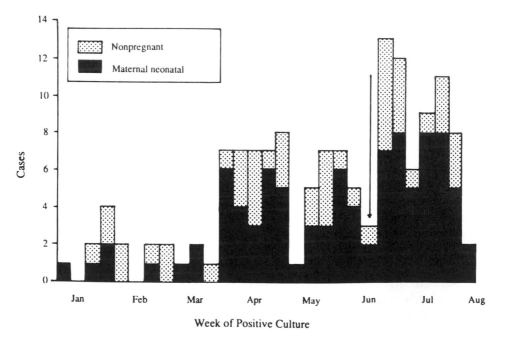

Figure 8.2 Listeriosis cases classified according to risk group in Los Angeles County, January 1 to August 15, 1985. Arrow designates the time of recall (118).

Table 8.3 Clinical and Demographic Data on 142 Listeriosis Cases Occurring in Los Angeles County, California, Between January 1 and August 15, 1985

Variable	Fetal or neonatal		Maternal	Nonpregnant adults
	Early	Late		
No. of patients	87	6	93	49
Mean age	32 weeks gestation	38 weeks gestation	26 yr	58 yr
Race or ethnic group: number (%)				
Hispanic	—	—	81 (87)	14 (29)
White	—	—	10 (11)	26 (53)
Black	—	—	0	7 (14)
Asian	—	—	2 (2)	2 (4)
Fatalities (%)	30 (34)	0	0	18 (37)
Epidemic phage type (%)	—	—	75	27
Mean birth weight (kg)	2.54	3.15	—	—
Septicemia (%)	88	17	52	71
Meningitis (%)	2	67	0	14
Septicemia + meningitis (%)	6	17	0	14
Other positive culture (%)	4	0	48	2

Source: Adapted from Ref. 118.

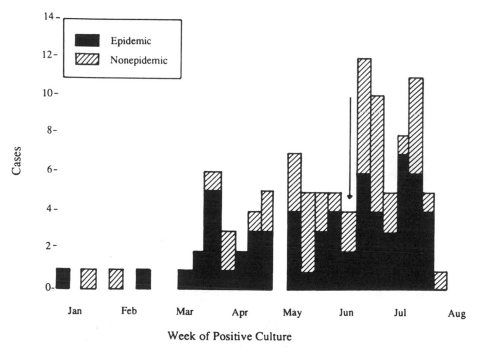

Figure 8.3 Listeriosis cases classified according to epidemic and nonepidemic phage types in Los Angeles County, January 1 to August 15, 1985. Arrow designates the time of recall.

patients), or acquired immunodeficiency syndrome (3 patients), which placed these individuals at greater risk (than the normal population) of developing listeric infections.

After identifying the epidemic *L. monocytogenes* strain as belonging to serotype 4b, all 105 clinical isolates available for study were phage-typed and compared to the strain isolated from Jalisco brand Mexican-style cheese. Results showed that 86 of 105 (82%) clinical isolates were serotype 4b, with the remaining 19 non–serotype 4b isolates originating from listeriosis victims whose illnesses were presumably not related to consumption of contaminated cheese. Of the 86 isolates identified as *L. monocytogenes* serotype 4b, 63 (73%) strains were of the same phage type as strains isolated from the contaminated cheese, thus confirming the involvement of Jalisco brand cheese in this outbreak (Fig. 8.3). The 23 remaining clinical isolates belonging to nonepidemic phage types presumably represented non–cheese-related background cases of listeriosis that occurred throughout the year. Sporadic sale of tainted cheese in a few family-owned grocery stores and restaurants, along with a likely listeriosis incubation period of 3 days to 2 weeks, are both at least partly responsible for those cases which occurred beyond the middle of July.

While these statistics are fairly typical for human listeriosis cases, the most striking feature in Table 8.3 is that 81 of the 93 mother/infant pairs that contracted listeriosis were of Hispanic origin. Furthermore, many of these economically disadvantaged Hispanics sought treatment at the Los Angeles County–USC Medical Center. The clustering of cases at a single medical facility was instrumental in uncovering this outbreak of foodborne listeriosis, since this epidemic would have likely gone unnoticed if the cases had been distributed evenly among the nearly 200 major hospitals in metropolitan Los Angeles.

As previously mentioned, epidemiologists and health officials used data collected from two case-control studies to trace this outbreak first to Mexican-style fresh cheese and then to Jalisco brand Queso Fresco and Cotija cheese. The fact that these strong-flavored cheeses are a common part of the Hispanic diet and not widely consumed by other individuals was another key to determine the exact source of this listeriosis epidemic.

Thus recognition of this outbreak was largely possible because of the use of the Los Angeles County–USC Medical Center by many economically disadvantaged listeriosis victims and the predominance of cases among Hispanics, which in turn precipitated the involvement of Mexican-style cheeses, i.e., products which few other groups of individuals consume on a regular basis. Hence one can easily speculate the cluster of cases would not have been observed if a nonethnic food such as Cheddar cheese, milk, standard fruits or vegetables—all of which are consumed by most individuals—had been contaminated with *L. monocytogenes*. Under such circumstances, an epidemic would probably have gone undetected. Without the increased awareness of foodborne listeriosis that this outbreak brought to the scientific community, additional cases of foodborne listeriosis, including the 1987 listeriosis outbreak linked to consumption of Vacherin Mont d'Or soft-ripened cheese, would likely have gone unnoticed, as the Swiss outbreak previously had for almost 10 years. Hence while Murray et al. (130) can be credited with the first accurate description of *L. monocytogenes*, those individuals who investigated the 1985 listeriosis outbreak in California (and to a lesser extent, outbreaks of listeriosis associated with coleslaw and possibly pasteurized milk in Canada and Massachusetts, respectively) can be credited with fostering the emergence of *L. monocytogenes* as a serious foodborne pathogen of worldwide concern.

Once Jalisco brand cheese was positively identified as the vehicle of infection, local, state, and federal investigators were confronted with the task of determining how the cheese became contaminated (see Fig. 8.1). Additional testing of Jalisco brand cheese indicated that *L. monocytogenes* was present in cheese manufactured from January to mid-June, thus indicating an ongoing problem at the cheese factory. Once this information was obtained, investigators focused their attention on three areas: (a) raw milk supply, (b) adequacy of pasteurization, and (c) possible contamination of the cheese during manufacture, packaging, and/or ripening. However, before interpreting the results from these investigations, it would be prudent to deal with methods used to manufacture those varieties of Mexican-style cheese that were directly linked to cases of listeriosis and also with behavior of *L. monocytogenes* in the finished product.

Queso Fresco or fresh cheese (also known as Ranchero, Estilo Casero, or Quesito) is among the most popular and widely distributed Mexican-style cheeses. Unlike most cheese varieties, Queso Fresco is traditionally prepared without use of a lactic acid bacteria starter culture. Curd is produced by coagulating warm skim milk with rennet or a similar coagulant. The resulting curd-whey is drained through cheese cloth, after which the curd is salted, packed into hoops, and pressed under weights for several days. The final product, which is consumed without additional aging, has a slightly grainy texture and can be sliced or shredded for cooking.

Cotija, also known as Queso Seco (dry cheese) or Queso Anejo (aged cheese), is another white cheese. After the coagulum is cut, recovered curd is pressed in large round hoops and cured at least 3 months to produce a dry, sharp-flavored, odorous cheese, which in some respects resembles Italian Parmesan.

It is important to realize that the cheesemaking procedures used for these Mexican-style cheeses produce favorable conditions for multiplication of *L. monocytogenes* in the final product. The relatively high moisture content of these cheeses, along with the lack of a starter culture which led to pH values in the finished product of ≥5.6, both played crucial roles in allowing *L. monocytogenes* to grow in the cheese during refrigerated storage (95). According to Lee (116), surface and interior samples of frozen Jalisco brand cheese examined some months after the recall contained 1.4×10^4 and 5.0×10^4 *L. monocytogenes* CFU/g, respectively, which supports the hypothesis that the pathogen grew in cheese during refrigerated storage since numbers of listeriae increase approximately 10-fold during cheesemaking as a result of entrapment within curd particles. If one assumes that the pathogen did not grow in cheese during storage, then the milk from which the cheese was prepared would have had to contain unreasonably high levels of listeriae (~1000–5000 CFU/ml) to produce the populations observed by Lee in the finished product. It also is noteworthy that the epidemic strain of *L. monocytogenes* that was designated as strain California (CA) by Ryser and Marth (153) has since proven to be less hardy in Cheddar (153), Camembert (154), brick (155), Colby (183), feta (139), and blue cheese (138) than strains Scott A (clinical isolate from 1983 "milkborne" listeriosis outbreak in Massachusetts), V7 (raw milk isolate from Massachusetts), and/or Ohio (OH) (isolated from Liederkranz cheese manufactured in Ohio).

Comprehensive sanitation inspections of the cheese factory were done immediately after the recall to assess the possibility that the cheese was contaminated during manufacture, packaging, and/or storage. Although the factory received a satisfactory sanitation rating of 85 on a scale of 100, numerous problem areas were cited which included suspended filth on electrical wires near cheese vats, peeling paint above a pasteurizer vat, condensate dripping on cheese in a walk-in refrigerator, and a major ant infestation. Some environmental samples (e.g., vat condensate and floor drains) were positive for the epidemic phage type of *L. monocytogenes* (118). While these environmental sources could have contributed to sporadic contamination of the finished product, the fact that the pathogen was isolated from 22 of 85 lots of cheese produced between January and mid-June indicates that an ongoing problem existed in the factory. Hence, contact between cheese and the factory environment was likely not the major route of contamination in this outbreak.

At the time of the recall, government officials considered faulty pasteurization as one of the most likely means by which the cheese became contaminated. Initial inspections of the cheese factory uncovered various pasteurization problems related to record-keeping and recording charts; however, the time and temperature at which milk was pasteurized exceeded minimum requirements [71.7°C (161°F)/15 sec]. Dye-testing later revealed a number of pin-sized holes in the pasteurization unit's heat transfer plates which separate raw and pasteurized milk. However, since further inspection demonstrated that the booster pumps of the pasteurizer had maintained a higher pressure on the pasteurized rather than raw milk side of the heat exchanger, raw milk would not have passed through the pinholes found in the pasteurizer plates. Hence, pasteurization failure was no longer suspected as the source of contamination (5).

Final reports indicate that *L. monocytogenes* most likely entered the cheese during manufacture through direct addition of raw milk. Toward the end of June 1985 investigators documented that the firm received nearly 700,000 pounds (~10%) more raw milk between April 1 and June 12, 1985, than could have been pasteurized given the capacity of their pasteurizer. Additionally, on several days only 150,000 of 200,000 pounds of milk received was pasteurized. These enormous discrepancies between raw milk received and amount that was pasteurized suggest that unpasteurized milk was deliberately mixed with pasteurized milk for cheesemaking (118). This conclusion also is supported by the fact that cheese supposedly prepared from pasteurized milk contained excessive levels of alkaline phosphatase—a native, heat-labile enzyme normally destroyed during proper pasteurization. However, some caution must be used in interpreting these results since Pratt-Lowe et al. (146) recently demonstrated that California Queso Fresco cheese occasionally contains microorganisms which produce a heat-labile alkaline phosphatase similar to that found in raw milk. Under these conditions, cheese prepared from properly pasteurized milk may falsely appear as having been manufactured from raw milk. Continued preparation of Mexican-style cheese from a mixture of raw and pasteurized milk also is compatible with the pattern of listeriosis cases that occurred over a period of 7 months. Toward the end of July 1985, investigators visited 27 dairy farms that supplied raw milk to the cheese factory (118,122). While no *Listeria* spp. were detected in raw milk or milk filters from dairy farms supplying the Jalisco cheese factory, the same epidemic phage type of *L. monocytogenes* was isolated from jocoque (a sour cream–like product) and cottage cheese byproducts produced by another company that shared the same raw milk source with Jalisco cheese. However, no cases of listeriosis were epidemiologically linked to consumption of either of these two products. According to Hird (95), the epidemic strain of *L. monocytogenes* was uncommon in California during the 11-year period preceding the outbreak, with only 3–5 *L. monocytogenes* serotype 4b isolates belonging to the same epidemic phage type. Even though the epidemic strain of *L. monocytogenes* was never isolated from raw milk, evidence described in the preceding paragraphs strongly suggests that raw milk was the probable source of the pathogen.

Major outbreaks of foodborne disease not only cause great human hardship but also major financial difficulties due to lost product and employee wages as well as medical bills and lawsuits. Jalisco Mexican Products, Inc. was forced to close its doors and declare bankruptcy shortly after its products were recalled because the company could no longer meet expenses. On March 27, 1986, Los Angeles County prosecutors filed 60 misdemeanor charges against the president and vice-president of the company for alleged shortcuts and inadequate safety precautions that routinely occurred in the factory during cheesemaking (13). On May 20, 1986, the vice-president of the firm was sentenced to 60 days in jail, 2 years of probation, and was fined $9,300 in connection with manufacturing and selling *Listeria*-contaminated cheese (12). In addition to investigative costs, which reportedly totaled $617,204, the company also is believed to be facing up to $700 million in lawsuits filed by some of the victims (168). Once the lawsuits are settled, one of the deadliest outbreaks of foodborne illness in United States history will finally come to rest.

After criticism for not recalling the contaminated Jalisco brand cheese sooner, state and federal officials issued a Class I recall for Mexican-style cheese produced by a second firm in the Los Angeles area. Although this *Listeria*-contaminated cheese was supposedly prepared from raw milk as shown by the presence of phosphatase (8), the recall was subsequently downgraded to Class II (i.e., a situation in which use of the product may cause temporary or medically reversible adverse health consequences) after laboratory results confirmed that these cheeses contained *L. innocua*—a nonpathogenic *Listeria* sp.—rather than *L. monocytogenes*. Later investigators also showed that this cheese was prepared from properly pasteurized milk. Hence, one must conclude that false-positive results were obtained with the phosphatase test, as described earlier in this chapter.

Vacherin Mont d'Or Soft-Ripened Cheese: Switzerland, 1983–1987

Human listeriosis has been observed in Switzerland for many years (67), particularly in the Canton of Vaud, which borders France to the west and Lake Geneva to the south. The early scientific literature contains several reports of sporadic listeric infections that occurred in and around Lausanne, the population center of Vaud. Over 20 years ago, Piolino and de Kalbermatten (142) reviewed five cases of adult listeriosis that were diagnosed at the Vaudois University Hospital Medical Center in Lausanne (VUHC) between December 1964 and February 1967. *Listeria monocytogenes* serotype 4b was isolated from four of five patients who exhibited symptoms of meningioencephalitis. While no common source of infection was demonstrated among these individuals, the authors suggested a possible role of domestic livestock in spreading listeriosis.

In 1981, Yersin et al. (182) reviewed 10 cases of listeriosis in adults (ages 35–76 years) that were diagnosed at VUHC between January 1974 and January 1980. (Ten cases of neonatal/infant listeriosis also were reportedly treated at this hospital during the same period.) All 10 adult listeriosis patients suffered from one or more underlying illnesses, which increased their chance of developing listeric infections. During this 6-year period, two cases of septicemia, six of meningitis-encephalitis, and two of encephalitis were recorded, including five deaths (50% mortality rate). As in the previous study, none of the adult cases of listeriosis could be traced to an exact source of infection.

More recently, Malinverni et al. (121) noted that only 20 sporadic listeriosis cases were diagnosed at VUHC between 1974 and 1982 with a mean of three cases per year. Thus these figures reflect an endemic rate of approximately five listeriosis cases/10^6 population in the Canton of Vaud during this 9-year period. In sharp contrast to these findings, a cluster of 25 listeriosis cases (14 adults and 11 maternal/fetal) was observed at the same medical facility between January 1983 and March 1984 (120,121) with 15 additional cases documented in surrounding hospitals (e.g., Geneva and Neuchatel) in Western Switzerland during the same 15-month period (11,120).

This listeriosis epidemic was somewhat atypical in that most adult listeriosis victims had been in good health before the outbreak. In addition, an unusually high incidence of brain-stem encephalitis was observed among patients. Eleven of 14 adults were treated at VUHC for meningitis and/or encephalitis, five of whom eventually died, giving a mortality rate of 45%. Septicemia was observed in the remaining three patients, two of whom were pregnant women.

According to Bille (45) and Malinverni et al. (120), 38 of 40 (95%) L. monocytogenes strains isolated from listeriosis victims during the epidemic period were of serotype 4b, whereas only 9 of 15 (60%) clinical isolates obtained during the previous 6-year epidemic period were serotype 4b. More important, 33 of 36 (92%) L. monocytogenes serotype 4b cultures were of two unique phage type configurations as compared to only 4 of 9 (44%) serotype 4b cultures obtained during the previous 6 years. This, in turn, suggests that a common-source listeriosis outbreak had occurred in western Switzerland between January 1983 and March 1984.

Unlike endemic cases of listeriosis treated between 1974 and 1982, most listeric infections recorded during the epidemic period were diagnosed during the winter months. However, listeriosis cases were uniformly distributed throughout the general population and were apparently unrelated to listeriosis in animals. Despite an in-depth investigation that included interviews with patients and a search for L. monocytogenes in several hundred food items, neither the source nor the mode of Listeria transmission could be found.

Working under the assumption that a similar listeriosis outbreak might occur the following winter, public health officials initiated a case-control study using listeriosis cases that were diagnosed in French-speaking Switzerland between November 1, 1984, and April 30, 1985 (11,45). Overall, 16 cases (7 adults and 9 mother-infant pairs) were analyzed and compared to 49 controls matched for age, sex, and underlying conditions. Fifteen of 16 (94%) patients were infected with L. monocytogenes serotype 4b with 5 of 16 (31%) isolates belonging to the same phage type. While these five cases suggest a possible epidemic focus, data obtained from questionnaires dealing with professional and home exposure as well as types of food consumed (e.g., milk products and raw vegetables) were inconclusive.

Following the 1985 listeriosis outbreak in California linked to consumption of Mexican-style cheese, Swiss officials initiated a series of surveys to determine the incidence of *Listeria* spp. in different dairy products, the results of which are summarized in Chapter 10. During one such survey of soft, semi-hard, and hard cheeses, Breer (53) isolated *L. monocytogenes* from 5 of 25 surface samples of Vacherin Mont d'Or cheese, a soft, smear-ripened cheese that is manufactured only from October to March and consumed primarily in and around the Canton of Vaud. Subsequent test results indicated that all *L. monocytogenes* isolates from Vacherin Mont d'Or cheese were of serotype 4b and also demonstrated that two *L. monocytogenes* phage types isolated from the cheese were identical to most clinical strains isolated during the 1983 to 1986 epidemic period. Investigators in Switzerland (45) then examined over 200 types of domestic and imported soft cheeses, 8–10% of which were contaminated with *L. monocytogenes*. However, these strains as well as other isolates from food and dairy products were of serotypes and/or phage types distinctly different from those of the two strains found on the surface of Vacherin Mont d'Or cheese.

A subsequent review of hospital records indicated that 122 listeriosis cases involving 58 adults (Table 8.4) and 64 mother/infant pairs were diagnosed in the Canton of Vaud between 1983 and 1987 (54) (epidemic rate of ~50 cases/10^6 population/yr) as compared to only 28 cases between 1974 and 1982 (endemic rate of ~5 cases/10^6 population/yr). Interestingly, 84% of the cases that occurred during the epidemic period were diagnosed between October and April. Thirty-four of 122 patients died, giving a mortality rate of 28%.

Overall, 111 of 120 (93%) clinical isolates available from the epidemic period were of serotype 4b with 98 of 111 (85%) serotype 4b strains matching the two epidemic phage types that were isolated from Vacherin Mont d'Or cheese. Several years later, Nocera et al. (133) examined 19 clinical isolates from this epidemic and found that these isolates belonged to the same electrophoretic enzyme type. (However, upon further testing these strains exhibited four distinct restriction endonuclease profiles.) Interestingly, this epidemic strain was identified as being of the same electrophoretic type as strains isolated during the 1985 listeriosis outbreak in California (141). The fact that the

Table 8.4 Description of 58 Adult Listeriosis Cases Diagnosed in Western Switzerland Between 1983 and 1987

Variable	Manifestation		
	Bacteremia	Meningitis	Meningioencephalitis
No. of patients (%)	12 (20)	23 (40)	23 (40)
Median age	72	69	54
Underlying illness[a] (%)	67	39	35
Epidemic strains involved (%)	58	77	86
Mortality (%)	25	30	35

[a]Includes leukemia, lymphoma, cancer, alcoholism, immunosuppressive drug therapy, diabetes, and acquired immunodeficiency syndrome (AIDS).
Source: Adapted from Ref. 54.

dominant phage type associated with the Swiss outbreak was similar to the phage type of the California epidemic strain (141) raises some interesting epidemiological questions as to why these closely related strains were responsible for the two largest outbreaks of cheeseborne listeriosis thus far recorded. However, the exact importance in foodborne listeriosis of this particular electrophoretic enzyme type as compared to others cannot yet be adequately assessed until more information is available regarding the distribution of different electrophoretic enzyme types in nature along with the ability of these various enzyme types to grow and/or survive in dairy products and produce disease in laboratory animals.

While the two previous case-control studies failed to uncover the source of this epidemic, a third case-control study conducted in 1987 demonstrated that 31 of 37 (84%) cases had consumed Vacherin Mont d'Or cheese as compared to only 20 of 51 (39%) controls (47). In addition, investigators were able to isolate the epidemic strain of *L. monocytogenes* from a piece of Vacherin Mont d'Or cheese that had been partially consumed by one of the victims. Armed with this information, Swiss authorities halted production of Vacherin Mont d'Or cheese on November 20, 1987, and recalled the product throughout Switzerland (18,23,47).

Most of the tainted cheese was marketed in Switzerland; however, small quantities were exported to other countries, including England and the United States. Hence, on November 25, 1987, health officials in England warned the general public not to consume Vacherin Mont d'Or cheese, which was reportedly available at a small number of delicatessens and specialty cheese shops in and around London (1,19). Similarly, FDA officials in the United States became concerned after a major newspaper reported that five specialty shops in New York City and a chain of 37 stores in Connecticut had been distributing the cheese since November 1987 (18). These recall efforts were largely successful since all known listeriosis cases linked to consumption of this cheese were confined to Switzerland.

Immediately after the recall, Swiss authorities began investigating possible routes by which Vacherin Mont d'Or cheese could have become contaminated with *L. monocytogenes*. According to Bille (46,47), the cheese implicated in this listeriosis outbreak was produced at 40 different factories located in western Switzerland. All contaminated cheese was reportedly prepared from *Listeria*-free cow's milk. Following coagulation of milk, the resulting curd was dipped into wooden hoops and allowed to drain for 1–2 days. When thoroughly drained, the hooped cheeses were transported to one of 12 cellars (i.e., caves), located throughout western Switzerland and ripened for ~3 weeks on wooden shelves during which time the cheeses were turned daily and brushed with salt water. Once ripened, the cheeses were packaged for sale and the wooden hoops were returned to the cheese factory.

From this description, it is apparent that ample opportunity existed for contamination of Vacherin Mont d'Or cheese, particularly during ripening. In fact, the epidemic strain(s) was detected in 18.5% of surface (rind) samples from Vacherin Mont d'Or cheese at levels of 10^4–10^6 *L. monocytogenes* CFU/g and also on 6.8% of wooden shelves and 19.8% of brushes used in the ripening cellars.

In all likelihood, this outbreak began several years before when *L. monocytogenes* entered one of the 40 dairy factories, possibly through the raw milk supply. While this outbreak was first detected in 1983, the epidemic strain initially was isolated from a listeriosis victim in 1977, which suggests that this outbreak may have been developing for at least 7 years. Investigations showed that nearly half of the 12 ripening cellars were contaminated with one or both epidemic strains of *L. monocytogenes*, thus suggesting that the pathogen was likely spread from one cellar to others through production and distribution practices. This theory is strongly supported by the fact that cheeses produced at any of the 40 factories were normally transferred between different cellars for ripening and/or distribution. The practices of brushing cheeses with salt water, ripening cheese in wooden hoops, and returning these hoops to the cheese factory appear to be important factors in disseminating *L. monocytogenes* to different ripening cellars.

Following the recall, all 40 factories in which Vacherin Mont d'Or cheese was manufactured were thoroughly cleaned and sanitized. More important, all wooden material (i.e., shelves, boxes, hoops, etc.) was removed from ripening cellars and burned. The cellars were then thoroughly cleaned, sanitized, and refitted with metal shelves and easily sanitized equipment. Once this work was completed, experimental batches of Vacherin Mont d'Or cheese were produced during a 2-month period and examined for the epidemic strain of *L. monocytogenes* to assure government officials that the pathogen was eliminated from all ripening cellars. These clean-up efforts proved to be highly successful, with only two cases of listeriosis being reported in western Switzerland between January and September of 1988 (46). Both cases resulted from infections with *L. monocytogenes* strains other than those isolated from Vacherin Mont d'Or cheese.

As a result of this outbreak, several steps have been taken to control and limit the extent of listeriosis in Switzerland (45,46). First, health authorities have begun to systematically screen high-risk foods for presence of *L. monocytogenes* and have adopted a zero tolerance for the pathogen in 10-g samples. Second, physicians and laboratories are now required to notify health officials of every new case (i.e., clinical isolate) of listeriosis occurring throughout Switzerland. Finally, a national *Listeria* Reference Center has been established to collect human, animal, food, and environmental isolates of *Listeria* and to examine these strains in terms of serotype, phage type, enzyme type, and DNA restriction patterns. It is hoped that these efforts will identify the exact endemic rate of human listeriosis in the general population and lead to faster recognition of possible future listeriosis outbreaks as well as the vehicles involved.

Additional Reports of Cheeseborne Listeriosis

Other than listeric infections associated with the aforementioned outbreaks in California and Switzerland, only two additional well-documented cases of nonfatal listeriosis have been directly linked to consumption of contaminated cheese, both of which occurred in England. The first such case involved a healthy, nonpregnant 36-year-old woman who developed meningitis on January 9, 1986, 9 days after consuming a full fat, soft French cheese (10,85). According to Bannister (39), identical phage types of *L. monocytogenes* serotye 4b were isolated from the woman's cerebrospinal fluid and a partially consumed package of cheese. However, the fact that six unopened packages of the same cheese failed to yield viable listeriae suggests that the cheese may have become contaminated in the refrigerator rather than during manufacture.

In response to the 1987 outbreak of listeriosis in Switzerland and the discovery of *L. monocytogenes* in an increasing variety of foods, health officials in England began treating all reported listeriosis cases as possibly foodborne. Follow-up questions about different foods consumed by victims led to discovery of a second cheese-related case of listeriosis in February of 1988 (92). According to official reports (26,38,128), a previously healthy, nonpregnant 40-year-old woman was admitted to a London hospital with meningitis following a 4-day bout with a "flu-like" illness. Identical phage-types of *L. monocytogenes* serotype 4b were eventually isolated from the woman's cerebrospinal fluid, stool, and an open package of Anari raw goat's milk cheese (a Greek-style soft cheese) from which the victim had consumed ~85 g 24 hours before onset of symptoms. Four additional unopened packages of Anari cheese (from the same lot) purchased from a retail store yielded the same *L. monocytogenes* strain at levels of $3.0–5.0 \times 10^7$ CFU/g. Consequently, this cheese was withdrawn from the market in February of 1988 with production not resuming until the summer of 1988.

Following news of this foodborne listeriosis case, McLauchlin et al. (128) examined the extent to which other dairy products produced by this manufacturer were contaminated with listeriae and attempted to identify the exact source of contamination. The Anari goat's milk cheese responsible for the aforementioned case of listeric meningitis came from a one-man, off-farm dairy factory at which Halloumi, Cheddar, feta, soft chive, and Gjestost cheese as well as yogurt also were produced from goat's milk. According to these investigators, 16 of 25 (64%) retail cheeses and 12 of 24 (50%) cheeses obtained directly from the factory over a period of 11 months yielded *L. monocytogenes* serotype 4b with all goat's milk cheese varieties except feta testing positive for the pathogen. Although 22 of 24 (92%) positive cheeses contained <10 *L. monocytogenes* CFU/g, the two remaining cheeses that were purchased from a retailer 10 weeks before their sell date contained $>10^5$ *L. monocytogenes* CFU/g, thus suggesting that the pathogen proliferated in the cheese during retail storage. This hypothesis was subsequently confirmed using naturally contaminated (<10 *L. monocytogenes* CFU/g) 2- to 3-day-old Anari and Halloumi cheeses that were periodically analyzed for numbers of listeriae during 8 weeks of refrigerated storage. While no listeriae were detected in samples of raw goat's milk or yogurt obtained directly from the factory, *L. monocytogenes* serotype 4b was recovered from shelving within the factory, which in turn suggests that the cheese most likely became contaminated during the final stages of manufacture or packaging. Most important, phage typing indicated that 66 of 68 (97%) *L. monocytogenes* isolates recovered from various cheeses and factory shelving were identical to the strain isolated from the patient's cerebrospinal fluid and stool. With the aforementioned evidence, there appears to be little doubt that this case of listeric meningitis resulted from consumption of Anari goat's milk cheese in which *L. monocytogenes* likely grew to high numbers during retail storage.

While the only confirmed cases of cheeseborne listeriosis in the United States have been those associated with consumption of Jalisco brand Mexican-style cheese in 1985, cheese has been suggested as a vehicle of infection in several additional cases of listeriosis. These primarily unconfirmed reports include (a) isolation of *Listeria* from the blood of a 7-day-old infant in California whose mother consumed a raw milk cheese two weeks before delivery (7); (b) three cases of listeriosis in Arizona in which the victims consumed non–Jalisco brand soft Mexican-style cheese; (c) a possible association between listeriosis and consumption of Italian cheese; (d) one case of listeriosis in California in which a woman delivered an aborted fetus after eating Monterey Jack cheese prepared from raw milk; (e) an alleged listeric abortion by a woman in New York who consumed contaminated feta cheese; (f) one case in which *L. monocytogenes* serotype 4b was isolated from a 3-year-old Washington state girl and cheese found in her family's refrigerator (30); (g) isolation of an identical *L. monocytogenes* strain (same phage type and electrophoretic enzyme type) from a listeriosis patient in Philadelphia and from cheese that the victim reportedly consumed (140); and (h) one case involving a healthy woman from New Jersey who supposedly contracted listeriosis after consuming Ricotta cheese containing 10^2–10^6 *L. monocytogenes* CFU/g (116).

Despite the recall of approximately 600 million pounds of French soft-ripened cheese in 1986 (see Chapter 10), no cases of listeriosis were linked to consumption of this cheese in the United States. However, several cases were documented in both Canada and England (39). In one of these Canadian cases, *L. monocytogenes* serotype 1b of the same electrophoretic enzyme type was isolated from the blood of a 66-year-old man and opened packages of imported soft cheese that he consumed (75). The same strain was later identified in unopened packages of cheese produced by the same manufacturer, thus confirming the role of cheese in this isolated case of listeric bacteremia. While the scientific literature contains one additional report of an AIDS patient in England who contracted listeric meningitis after consuming Staffordshire cheese, the two non–phage typable strains of *L. monocytogenes* serotype 1/2a recovered from the patient's cerebrospinal fluid and cheese were subsequently found to exhibit different DNA restriction enzyme patterns, thus negating cheese as the vehicle of infection.

MEAT PRODUCTS

Foods of animal origin have long been recognized as potential vehicles of infection, with meat-associated cases of salmonellosis and botulism recorded in the scientific literature as early as the 1890s. Following confirmation of *L. monocytogenes* as a human and animal pathogen during the 1920s, listeriosis was subsequently identified as a zoonosis, a disease transmissible from animals to humans. Hence, when listeric infections in domestic livestock began to be identified with some regularity during the 1930s and 1940s, some individuals, including Wramby (181), who in 1944 first identified *Listeria* in raw meat, began to speculate that consumption of meat products could play a role in the spread of human listeriosis.

As you will recall from Chapter 2, asymptomatic shedding of *L. monocytogenes* in feces by apparently healthy cattle, sheep, and pigs is not unusual with the pathogen normally present in 2–16% of samples of cattle feces. More recently, Hofer (97) detected *L. monocytogenes* in 11 of 61 (18%) fresh stool samples obtained from apparently healthy beef cattle just before processing in a Rio de Janeiro slaughterhouse. In all fairness, while present laws forbid the sale of meat from diseased animals and also require proper disposal of entire carcasses, it is evident that *Listeria*-laden fecal material from asymptomatically infected domestic livestock can contaminate the slaughterhouse environment. These findings, along with those of earlier studies (77,82,83,165,176,178,179), suggested that certain occupational groups such as veterinarians and slaughterhouse workers may, because of increased contact with *Listeria*-contaminated material from domestic livestock, be at greater risk of becoming infected with *L. monocytogenes* than individuals having little if any contact with domestic animals.

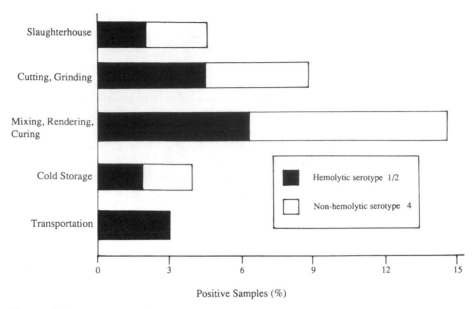

Figure 8.4 Incidence of *L. monocytogenes* in feces collected from employees working in different areas of a smoked meat/sausage factory in Czechoslovakia. (Adapted from Ref. 70.)

Table 8.5 Incidence of *L. monocytogenes* in Fecal Samples Collected from Apparently Healthy Workers in Various Areas of the European Meat Industry

Area within meat industry	Country	Number of workers examined	Number of workers carrying *L. monocytogenes* in feces (%)	Ref.
Meat processing	Czechoslovakia	322	20 (6.2)	70
Butcher shop	Czechoslovakia	294	9 (3.1)	70
Slaughterhouse/ Meat canning	Denmark	1147	55 (4.8)	50
Meat processing	France	53	4 (7.5)	132
Slaughterhouse	Hungary	90	19 (21.1)	149
Slaughterhouse	Hungary	2055	86 (4.2)	129
Meat processing	Hungary	879	22 (2.5)	51
Office/Technical	Hungary	121[a]	0	51
Office	Netherlands	92[a]	11 (11.8)	108
Slaughterhouse	Netherlands	98	13 (13.3)	108
Total		4938	226 (4.6)	

[a]Excluded from total.

Beginning in 1970, studies were conducted to assess the prevalence of *L. monocytogenes* in fecal samples collected from individuals employed in the European meat industry (Table 8.5). According to Elischerová et al. (70), *L. monocytogenes* occurred twice as often in stool samples from individuals in Czechoslovakia involved in the manufacture of smoked meat sausage products rather than in the retail sale of raw meat.

Upon further examination of their data, highest fecal carriage rates in 322 employees working at a smoked meat/sausage factory occurred among individuals involved in cutting/grinding (8.9%) and mixing/rendering/curing of raw meat (14.6%) with a much lower incidence for individuals working in the slaughterhouse (4.5%) or in areas of cold storage and transportation (Fig. 8.4). Except for employees involved in transportation, approximately equal percentages of *L. monocytogenes* serotypes 1/2 and 4 were isolated from the remaining workers. The fact that employees working in both meat-processing areas had an opportunity to consume products during manufacture may help explain the disproportionately high fecal carriage rate of *Listeria* among these two groups.

Results from several earlier Czechoslovakian studies lend further support to oral transmission of *Listeria* via meat products. Beginning in 1972 Elischerová and Stupalová (68) isolated *L. monocytogenes* from the hands and gowns of 1 of 30 and 2 of 30 clinically healthy meat industry workers, respectively, who also exhibited unusually high antibody titers for *L. monocytogenes* compared to most individuals employed in animal breeding and production. Additionally, this organism was detected in six fecal samples from meat production (sausage manufacture)/ice-house employees who had an opportunity to consume crude and semi-crude product during work. These individuals also exhibited elevated O and H serum agglutinin titers against *L. monocytogenes* serotye 1. The potential to become an *L. monocytogenes* carrier via the oral route again was proposed in 1977 when Elischerová et al. (69) detected this pathogen on the hands and gowns of 9 of 46 (19.6%) and 10 of 46 (21.7%) meat production workers, respectively.

Results from six additional surveys (Table 8.5), three of which were conducted in Western Europe, also suggest that *L. monocytogenes* is occasionally present in stool specimens from individuals employed in the meat industry. While the fecal carriage rate for *Listeria* in Hungarian meat industry workers appears to be similar to that observed in other European countries, Ralovich et al. (149) detected *L. monocytogenes* in 19 of 90 (21%) stool samples collected from healthy employees working at a slaughterhouse that processed swine. Interestingly, of the 19 workers that shed listeriae, eight (42%) cleaned and prepared intestines, four (32%) slaughtered swine, one each (5%) dealt with emergency slaughter and transporting manure, and three (16%) individuals were employed as veterinarians. Although the occupational breakdown of *Listeria* shedders was generally similar to that observed by Elischerová et al. (70) (Fig. 8.4), the overall incidence of carriers at this particular slaughterhouse was about three to eight times higher than in other European factories. This unusually high carriage rate among workers appears to be related to a temporary increase in the incidence of *L. monocytogenes* in throats of incoming swine, since fecal carriage rates among these workers decreased to 4–5% the following year (129). While these findings indicate that increased exposure to *L. monocytogenes* in the meat industry can lead to an increased carriage rate among workers, it should be emphasized that all of these presumably healthy individuals were asymptomatic carriers of the pathogen and showed no signs of illness. This is further reinforced by Borbély and Méró (51), who found that while 22 of 879 (2.5%) meat-processing workers at this same facility excreted *L. monocytogenes* in their feces, the pathogen was never isolated from 121 office/technical personnel who were generally not exposed to meat products. However, Kampelmacher et al. (108) reported virtually identical fecal carriage rates for *L. monocytogenes* among office and slaughterhouse workers in The Netherlands, thus casting some doubt on the importance of animal contact in fecal excretion of this pathogen by humans.

Overall, the *L. monocytogenes* fecal carriage rate for employees within the European meat industry reportedly ranged from 2.5 to 21.2% with an average of approximately 4.6%. While these findings appear to indicate a higher-than-normal *L. monocytogenes* fecal carriage rate for workers in the meat industry, this does not appear to be true when one recalls that between 1.8 and 9.0% of the normal healthy human population (differing by age, sex, and occupation) carry *L. monocytogenes* in their feces. While veterinarians and other individuals participating in delivery of newborn livestock are admittedly at increased risk of contracting cutaneous listeric infections (109), healthy workers in other agriculture-related professions, including the meat industry, do not appear to be at any increased risk of harboring *L. monocytogenes* or contracting listeriosis, as has long been maintained by Kampelmacher et al. (108–110) and Seeliger (163). Perhaps the most compelling evidence comes from the fact that in most listeriosis cases, humans have had absolutely no contact with domestic livestock, let alone diseased animals. Thus, as suggested by Seeliger (163), *L. monocytogenes* appears to be a normal transient bacterium of the intestinal tract with potential pathogenic properties.

Healthy individuals working in the meat industry do not appear to be at any increased risk of contracting listeriosis; however, the same is not likely true for pregnant women and individuals in poor health (e.g., immunocompromised individuals, alcoholics, AIDS patients) that may still be in the workforce. This is illustrated by the findings of Elischerová and Stupalová (68), who noted that 11 of 49 (22.4%) pregnancies among 31 Czechoslovakian women working in the meat industry terminated in abortion, stillbirth, or premature delivery of an infected infant with the rate for the latter more than 10 times greater than that of the general population.

Despite the argument presented thus far, a search of the early scientific literature has largely uncovered only circumstantial evidence linking or in some instances only suggesting involvement of meat products in actual clinical cases of human listeriosis (Table 8.6). Beginning in 1955, consumption of contaminated pork (probably undercooked) was suggested as the possible cause of 27 listeriosis cases in the Soviet Union (90,114). The following year, Gudkova et al. (91) isolated *L. monocytogenes* from the viscera of pigs on a Russian farm where several individuals contracted listeric infections presumably after ingesting pork from an infected group of pigs. In 1960, Olding and Philipson (135) investigated one adult and three perinatal cases of listeriosis that occurred within a three-block area of Uppsala, Sweden, during the previous 2 years. Although repeated attempts to isolate *L. monocytogenes* from water, milk, vegetables, and meat ended in failure, the fact that meat was the only food item obtained from the same source by all four individuals suggests the possible involvement of unspecified meat products in this apparently common-source outbreak.

In the only other early recorded incident involving meat products from domesticated animals, ground meat from a dead calf was suspected of transmitting *L. monocytogenes*

Table 8.6 Human Listeriosis Cases in Which Consumption of Meat Products Was Suggested as a Possible Source of Infection

Area	Year	Number of cases	Possible vehicle of infection	Ref.
USSR	1955	27	Pork	90,114
USSR	1956	19	Pork	91
Sweden	1958–59	4	Meat	135
The Netherlands	early 1960s	1	Ground veal/beef	107
Newfoundland/Canada	1963	1	Rabbit	52
United States	1986–87	Unknown	Uncooked hot dogs	161
Philadelphia, PA	1987	Unknown	Salami	27
Italy	1988?	1	Cooked pork	58
Spokane, WA	1989	1	Cooked ground beef	30
San Francisco, CA	1989	1	Cooked Cajun pork sausage	32

to the wife of a Dutch farmer in the early 1960s (107). While involvement of meat in this case of listeriosis appears plausible, the remainder of the suspected meat was sterilized during canning, thus eliminating any hope of confirming the causative agent.

During a review of listeric infections in Canada over a 21-year period, Bowmer et al. (52) uncovered one case in which a pregnant woman in Newfoundland delivered an infant who died 1 month later from listeric meningitis. Ten days before the infant became ill, the mother recalled skinning, cooking, and eating two previously frozen hares that were brought from New Brunswick, thus suggesting rabbit meat as a possible vehicle of infection. While less commonly consumed than meats from domesticated animals, it appears that rabbit meat also may serve as a potential source of *L. monocytogenes*, as evidenced by a long history of listeric infections among rabbits (88,89,162,175). In fact, the first type-strain of *L. monocytogenes* was isolated by Murray et al. (130) in 1924 from the blood of infected rabbits. Several European scientists have expressed some concern about the incidence of *L. monocytogenes* in rabbit meat, along with possible risks of consuming such potentially contaminated products.

Despite such circumstantial evidence suggesting that consumption of contaminated meat products can lead to cases of human listeriosis, the possible involvement of meat products in listeric infections received little if any further attention before 1981, primarily because listeriosis had not yet been associated with any foods other than raw milk. However, this has changed as a result of three major listeriosis outbreaks that were positively linked to consumption of contaminated coleslaw, Mexican-style cheese, and Vacherin Mont d'Or soft-ripened cheese in 1981, 1985, and 1987, respectively. Several factors, namely, (a) the long-time association of *L. monocytogenes* with domestic livestock, (b) the ability of *L. monocytogenes* to grow at refrigeration temperatures, and (c) questions from public health authorities prompted numerous studies on incidence and behavior of this pathogen in raw and processed meat products (see Chapter 11) and also led to increased surveillance and reporting of listeriosis cases. After CDC officials in Atlanta began receiving information about scattered cases of listeriosis occurring throughout the United State, Schwartz et al. (161) initiated a retrospective epidemiological study to identify possible food products that might be associated with sporadic cases of listeriosis.

According to their report, which appeared in 1988 in *Lancet*, an active *L. monocytogenes* surveillance program was established in Missouri, New Jersey, Oklahoma, Tennessee, Washington, and Los Angeles County, California, in January of 1986. During the following 18 months (12 months in Los Angeles County), 154 listeriosis cases were identified in a population of 34 million people with approximately one-third and two-thirds of the patients being classified as newborn infants and elderly or immunocompromised adults, respectively. Overall, 82 of these 154 individuals agreed to participate in a retrospective case-control study in which patients were interviewed and asked to answer a series of questions relating to demographic characteristics, underlying illnesses, medication, exposure to other sick individuals or animals, excavation work, and dietary history. The latter included questions pertaining to consumption of raw fruits and vegetables, poultry, eggs, and dairy products as well as raw, processed, and pickled meats. After comparing their answers to those from 239 controls (individuals without listeriosis) that were matched to the cases in terms of age and underlying illness, listeriosis victims were significantly more likely than controls to have consumed uncooked frankfurters or undercooked chicken. Furthermore, statistical analysis showed that individuals who consumed uncooked frankfurters and undercooked chicken were 6.1 and 3.2 times more likely to contract listeriosis, respectively, than individuals who do not consume these products. Overall, epidemiological evidence from this study suggested that consumption of these foods accounted for 30 of 154 or 20% of all listeriosis cases reported in the surveillance area with 1 in 1200 to 1 in 6000 and 1 in 1500 to 1 in 7500 individuals likely to contract listeriosis after consuming uncooked frankfurters and undercooked chicken, respectively (28). Thus, assuming that 1600 cases of listeriosis occur annually in the United States, these investigators speculated that 255 and 102 of these cases may be attributed to eating uncooked frankfurters and undercooked chicken, respectively.

Although this case-control study identified uncooked frankfurters and undercooked chicken as risk factors in sporadic cases of listeriosis, it is important to stress that such epidemiological investigations cannot establish causality. Furthermore, one must also remember that lack of an association with other foods does not necessarily mean that consumption of such products poses no risk of listeriosis. Nonetheless, despite several shortcomings of this retrospective case-control study that have been echoed by the scientific community (22,51) [i.e., (a) omission of questions concerning cooking methods and consumption of foods such as seafood that have been less commonly associated with listeriosis, (b) limited ability to identify risk factors when exposure was very common or very rare, and (c) difficulty in obtaining accurate diet histories, including the possibility of cases more clearly recalling what they consumed before their illness than controls], recent results from microbiological surveys (see Chapters 11 and 12), along with a 1988 report by the American Meat Institute indicating that 5–10% of prepackaged frankfurters produced in the United States were contaminated with *L. monocytogenes* (20), support the possibility of contracting listeriosis from consuming uncooked frankfurters or undercooked chicken as was suggested in the case-control study by Schwartz et al. (161). During their work, these researchers (27,161) also identified another processed meat product consumed without further cooking, namely salami, as a possible risk factor in a 1987 listeriosis outbreak in Philadelphia that claimed 14 lives. However, CDC officials again lacked the bacteriological data to positively link consumption of the salami to illness.

While results from the study just discussed are by far the most convincing, it must be stressed again that as of July 1990, no raw, cooked, or otherwise processed meat product has been conclusively proven as the vehicle of infection in any case of human listeriosis reported in the United States or elsewhere. While it is important to remember that such a relationship can only be shown conclusively by isolating the identical *L. monocytogenes* serotype and phage or isoenzyme type from the patient and the food consumed as well as unopened packages of the implicated food, numerous North American and European surveys have uncovered low to moderate levels of *L. monocytogenes* in a wide range of commercially available raw, processed, and ready-to-eat meat products (see Chapter 11). Even before Schwartz et al. (27, 161) announced preliminary results from their study, the meat industry (25) maintained that susceptible individuals who consume *Listeria*-contaminated dry sausage, frankfurters, luncheon meats, and other packaged pasteurized products are at low to moderate risk of contracting listeriosis.

Beginning in 1988, researchers on both sides of the Atlantic Ocean uncovered three listeriosis cases in which consumption of meat products was suspected as the most likely cause of infection (Table 8.5). In the first such case, a previously healthy Italian man contracted a nonfatal case of listeric meningitis several days after consuming cooked home-made pork sausage that was later shown to contain $\sim3 \times 10^6$ *L. monocytogenes* CFU/g (58). According to the investigators, the clinical and sausage isolates were both identified as belonging to serotype 4, the most common serotype encountered in clinical cases of listeriosis. Unfortunately, the exact source of contamination was never determined; however, antiquated sausage-making practices in combination with storage of the sausage at ambient rather than refrigeration temperature were cited as playing major roles in this isolated case of listeric meningitis. Nevertheless, while numbers of listeriae present in the sausage were probably more than sufficient to induce illness, some caution still must be used in evaluating the role of sausage in this case since both isolates were never classified further according to phage or enzyme type.

Two unconfirmed cases of apparent meatborne listeriosis also have been recorded in the United States and include (a) a 76-year-old man from Spokane, Washington, who reportedly died from an infection with *L. monocytogenes* serotype 4b after consuming cooked ground beef; however, only serotype 1a was recovered from the ground beef and so it is an unlikely source of the infection (30) and (b) an incident in which *L. monocytogenes* serotype 4b was isolated from cooked Cajun pork sausage that was consumed by an elderly San Francisco man who developed a nonfatal case of listeriosis (32). Approximately 1000 pounds of this sausage was subsequently recalled from the market after investigators recovered *L. monocytogenes* serotype 4b from similar unopened packages of sausage. Even though the two *L. monocytogenes* strains isolated from the patient and the sausage were not further classified according to phage or isoenzyme type, isolation of the same *L. monocytogenes* serotype from unopened packages of sausage and the ability of investigators to presumably trace the source of contamination to natural sausage casings imported from China (65) provides fairly conclusive evidence that consumption of Cajun pork sausage was directly responsible for this case of foodborne listeriosis.

Continued surveillance of listeriosis cases by the CDC officials has uncovered a direct link between consumption of contaminated turkey frankfurters and listeric meningitis in an Oklahoma breast cancer patient (40) (to be discussed shortly) and also led to a nationwide recall of the product (31) along with radical change in the USDA-FSIS policy regarding presence of *L. monocytogenes* in cooked, ready-to-eat, or otherwise processed meat and poultry products. (A detailed discussion of these policy changes regarding meat and poultry products can be found in Chapter 11 and 12, respectively.) In the light of this information, some public health officials are now advising high-risk individuals (i.e., pregnant women, immunocompromised adults, and the elderly) to thoroughly reheat previously cooked and chilled poultry and meat products before they are consumed. Hence, the proven ability of *L. monocytogenes* to grow and/or survive in many refrigerated raw, processed, and ready-to-eat foods, including meat and poultry products, together with extensive food histories now being obtained from many listeriosis victims in the United States and England, make it highly probable that meat products, particularly frankfurters and ready-to-eat meats, will be positively linked to cases of human listeriosis in the future.

POULTRY PRODUCTS

Shedding of *L. monocytogenes* in fecal material from both clinically and subclinically infected domestic fowl (61) appears to place poultry workers at a somewhat higher than normal risk of contracting superficial listeric infections, particularly conjunctivitis. This probable association between handling infected poultry and contracting listeric conjunctivitis is partially based on a 1951 report by Felsenfeld (76), who, 7 years earlier, identified listeric conjunctivitis in two employees who dressed poultry in Illinois. Upon further investigation, *L. monocytogenes* was isolated from the spleens of five birds that were not dressed in the same shop but came from an area in Illinois in which avian listeriosis was previously observed, thus suggesting poultry as the probable source of infection.

While reports of listeric conjunctivitis can be found in the early scientific literature, including several cases in which patients reportedly had contact with birds suffering from undetermined illnesses (86), the 1951 report by Felsenfeld (76) remains one of the few instances where avian listeriosis was linked to listeric conjunctivitis in humans.

A search of the early scientific literature has uncovered only two reports indicating that contact with infected poultry can lead to the internal listeric infections for which *L. monocytogenes* is best known. In 1958, Gray (86) mentioned numerous instances in which Central European women gave birth to *Listeria*-infected infants following contact with sick or dead birds; however, evidence for the link between listeriosis and contact with infected poultry was only circumstantial.

Similarly, Embil et al. (71) identified a woman in Nova Scotia, Canada, who gave birth to an infected infant that died of listeriosis 1 hour after delivery. While it is important to note that the mother reportedly prepared poultry for sale in a family-owned store during the previous 8 months, researchers once again failed to positively link this listeriosis case to contact with raw poultry by not isolating the pathogen from raw chickens sold at the store.

Given the preceding evidence, Kampelmacher (107) suggested as early as 1962 that consumption of contaminated poultry might lead to cases of human listeriosis. While this view also was adopted 10 years later by Méró and Ralovich (129), foodborne transmission of *L. monocytogenes* by consumption of a contaminated poultry product was not documented until November 1988 (112). As was true for meat products, failure to positively link consumption of contaminated poultry to human listeriosis until recently is related to the generally inaccurate methods that were previously available to isolate *L. monocytogenes* from poultry and other foods containing a complex microflora and to a generalized lack of concern about foodborne listeriosis.

Following the two major cheese-associated outbreaks of listeriosis described earlier, public health officials in the United States and England implemented active/semiactive surveillance programs to obtain more accurate data concerning the incidence of listeriosis in the general population. Attempts also were made to trace the source of reported infections to consumption of dairy products and other foods such as poultry which at the time had not yet been linked to listeriosis. As a result of these efforts, three cases of listeriosis have since been positively linked to consumption of poultry products, which, in turn, has led to inclusion of poultry products in the list of foods that may pose a potential threat of listeriosis to susceptible individuals. These three recently recognized cases of poultryborne listeriosis will now be reviewed in some detail.

Working in England, Kerr et al. (29,112) identified the first case of listeriosis clearly linked to consumption of contaminated poultry. According to their November 1988 report, a 31-year-old pregnant woman with a 24-hour history of flu-like symptoms was admitted to a hospital and subsequently delivered a dead 23-week-old fetus. Upon further investigation, it was found that the woman had consumed a heated chicken dish prepared from cooked-and-chilled chicken 5 days before onset of symptoms, with the remaining chicken refrigerated and consumed 3 days later in a salad. Thus the woman had a maximum incubation time before illness of only 4 days as compared to the more typical 7–30 days for listeriosis. Following bacteriological analysis, an identical phage type of *L. monocytogenes* serotype 4 was found in samples of chicken and fetal liver. Other foods in question were tested with no evidence of *Listeria* contamination, thus confirming chicken as the vehicle of infection in this case of listeriosis.

Considerable research and regulatory activity, prompted by reports suggesting that 12–25% of the cook-chill poultry products marketed in England may be contaminated with *L. monocytogenes*, uncovered a second case of poultry-associated listeriosis early in 1989. According to this report (106), *L. monocytogenes* serotype 1/2a was cultured from the blood of a 52-year-old immunocompromised woman who was receiving steroids for systemic lupus erythematosus. Three to 5 days before onset of vomiting and diarrhea, the hospitalized woman and her 29-year-old son shared some ready-cooked chicken nuggets which he had purchased at a carry-out, fast-food restaurant. Detailed questioning later revealed that the son experienced a short-lived illness with diarrhea and vomiting on the same night that his mother became sick. Subsequently, the son's stool sample yielded *L. innocua* as well as *L. monocytogenes* serotypes 1/2a and 1/2c with the DNA homology pattern of the serotype 1/2a isolate being identical to that of the *L. monocytogenes* strain originally isolated from the woman's blood. While *L.*

innocua and an *L. monocytogenes* strain of unreported serotype and DNA homology pattern were recovered from uncooked chicken nuggets, these investigators failed to detect *L. monocytogenes* in a subsequent lot of cooked chicken nuggets obtained from the same source.Nonetheless, the source of infection in both the woman and her son presumably was the commercially cooked chicken nuggets of the "fast-food" variety, which, while served hot, were most likely undercooked, thus allowing *L. monocytogenes* to survive in sufficient numbers to cause illness.

Although this is only the second case of poultryborne listeriosis recorded in England, similar cases have likely gone undetected because of inadequacies in reporting and difficulties encountered in linking these illnesses to consumption of poultry or any other food. These two cases of poultryborne listeriosis and a recent survey of listeriosis cases in Scotland which included identification of possible food-related risk factors associated with the disease have prompted the funding needed to initiate a formal case-control study which will attempt to correlate consumption and/or handling of high-risk foods (i.e., poultry, cheese, prepared salads, delicatessen items) with human listeric infections (56). Such studies in England, the United States, and elsewhere will result in an expanded number of reported cases of foodborne listeriosis and list of foods that already have been associated with this illness.

Despite the controversial nature of many epidemiological studies, such efforts have already played an important role in identifying possible risk factors associated with foodborne listeriosis. As you will recall from our discussion of meatborne listeriosis in the preceding section of this chapter, undercooked chicken was recently identified as a possible vehicle of infection by CDC officials during a large case-control study conducted in conjunction with an active surveillance program in Oklahoma and five other states (161).

During this program, CDC officials discovered a breast cancer patient in Oklahoma who was hospitalized for listeric septicemia and meningitis in December 1988 (31,40). In an attempt to identify the vehicle of infection, CDC officials went to the woman's home, obtained foods from her refrigerator, and isolated *L. monocytogenes* from various foods, including an opened package of turkey frankfurters that contained 1.1×10^3 *L. monocytogenes* CFU/g. A swab applied to the refrigerator's interior also yielded the pathogen. While CDC investigators initially concluded that the woman had contaminated the food herself, public health officials from Oklahoma began examining the same brands of retail products that were in the woman's refrigerator and were positive for *L. monocytogenes*. Interest soon focused on turkey frankfurters after officials learned that the woman consumed one turkey frankfurter daily after warming it for 45–60 seconds in a microwave oven. Although CDC investigators isolated *L. monocytogenes* serotype 1/2a from 2 of 3 unopened retail packages of the same brand of turkey frankfurters, all remaining unopened packages of food other than turkey frankfurters were *Listeria*-free. The *L. monocytogenes* strain isolated from the woman was subsequently identified as of the same serotype (1/2a) and electrophoretic enzyme type as the strain isolated from both opened and unopened packages, thus confirming turkey frankfurters as the vehicle of infection in the first case of poultryborne listeriosis reported in the United States.

Once USDA-FSIS officials were advised of the situation by CDC representatives on April 14, 1989, government officials prompted the Texas manufacturer to issue an immediate Class I recall for approximately 600,000 pounds of turkey frankfurters that were marketed by retail and institutional establishments in 23 states (31). Although the exact source of contamination was never determined, this incident prompted USDA-FSIS to toughen its regulatory policy regarding *Listeria*-contaminated poultry and meat products (see Chapter 11).

EGGS AND EGG PRODUCTS

Acquiring listeriosis through consumption of contaminated eggs and egg products has been considered for nearly 40 years; however, unlike poultry products, no such cases have been firmly documented. Geurden and Devos (84), who in 1952 isolated *L. monocytogenes* from a necrotic lesion in the oviduct of an infected hen, were first to suggest that eggs might serve as a possible vehicle of infection. Nonetheless, these authors also admitted that a 35-year-old man who consumed raw eggs from this infected flock of chickens showed no signs of listeriosis. Three years later, Urbach and Schabinski (170) found that guinea pigs who were fed artificially infected eggs in which *L. monocytogenes* had grown to very high levels soon died of listeric septicemia, thus suggesting that humans also might develop listeriosis by consuming contaminated eggs.

During the same year (1955), Dedié (60) reported an interesting case in which a pregnant woman, who owned nine chickens, gave birth to a *Listeria*-infected infant. Although 26 eggs from these chickens proved to be negative for *L. monocytogenes*, the H and O agglutination titers of the chickens increased dramatically during the 4-week period in which the eggs were collected, thus suggesting that the chickens were recently exposed to this pathogen. Subsequent attempts to isolate *L. monocytogenes* from 200 eggs laid by experimentally infected hens ended in failure. However, the fact that *L. monocytogenes* was detected in feces and nasal secretions from these birds suggests that externally contaminated eggs may constitute a potential source of infection and a potential source for cross-contamination of other foods if the eggs are handled improperly.

As is true for meat and poultry workers, listeric infections among apparently healthy individuals employed in the egg industry are extremely rare. In fact, a search of the literature uncovered only one documented case in which a 39-year-old male egg factory worker became infected with *L. monocytogenes* and subsequently died of meningitis in 1965 (108). Other than the fact that 29.1 and 10.6% of the egg factory workers carried *L. monocytogenes* in their feces 4 and 16 months after the man's death, respectively, no further evidence was reported to incriminate eggs in this fatal case of listeric meningitis. Hence, at this time it appears that healthy egg factory workers need not take any special precautions to guard against listeriosis.

Despite the previous inability to link a single case of listeriosis to consumption of eggs or egg products, the recognized ability of *L. monocytogenes* to grow in egg products along with emergence of this organism as a bonafide foodborne pathogen may well change this picture in the future. This prediction is supported by the fact that CDC officials (160) recently identified a possible cluster of listeriosis cases in Los Angeles County in which 6 of 33 cases and 4 of 101 matched controls consumed raw eggs (odds ratio = 6.4) over a 5-month period spanning 1986–1987.

While epidemiological investigations can never conclusively prove causality, the possible associations discovered in such studies will likely prompt public health authorities to seriously consider eggs and other foods (e.g., seafood, fruits) as potential vehicles of infection, which, in turn, may lead to their implication in future cases of listeriosis.

SEAFOOD PRODUCTS

Despite the recent discovery of *L. monocytogenes* in a variety of raw and processed seafoods including shrimp, crabmeat, lobster tails, surimi, and various finfish (see Chapter 13), most attempts to directly link consumption of such products to cases of human listeriosis have proven unsuccessful. However, as was true for egg products, a few scattered reports attesting to the possible involvement of seafoods in listeric infections have found their way into the scientific literature. Two such reports from New Zealand include (a) a 1971 observation that two pregnant women delivered *Listeria*-infected infants after presumably consuming raw fish sometime during their pregnancies (42), and (b) a cluster of 22 perinatal listeriosis cases between January and November of 1980 in which results of food histories suggested, at best, a weak association between consumption of contaminated shellfish/raw fish and development of listeriosis (117). In 1980, Vilde et al. (171) also published a report suggesting that a 48-year-old immunocompromised French woman had contracted listeriosis after consuming contaminated oysters. However, as already implied, a causal link between consumption of seafood and listeriosis was never clearly proven in any of these reports.

The most convincing case for direct involvement of fish in human listeriosis is that of a 54-year-old Italian woman who in 1988 or 1989 contracted nonfatal meningitis 3–4 days after consuming undercooked fish from which *L. monocytogenes* was subsequently isolated (73). The fact that the two *L. monocytogenes* isolates from the patient's cerebrospinal fluid and a left-over portion of the fish both were of serotype 4 and were identical in terms of phage type and restriction analysis of chromosomal DNA confirms fish as the vehicle of infection in this case of listeric meningitis. According to the investigators, survival and transmission of the pathogen was most likely the result of undercooking since the fish was eaten and refrigerated after steaming. However, the mode by which this fish became contaminated still is a mystery.

The case of listeric meningitis just discussed along with other recently reported cases of foodborne listeriosis that have been positively linked to consumption of dairy as well as ready-to-eat meat and poultry products suggest it would be naive to assume that *L. monocytogenes* poses any less danger to public health when present in cooked and/or ready-to-eat seafood than in other foods. Hence, as you will see in Table 13.1, FDA officials have maintained a policy of "zero tolerance" for *L. monocytogenes* in all ready-to-eat foods and have already (mid 1990) issued 15 Class I recalls involving well over 45,000 pounds of cooked/ready-to-eat seafood. These recalls for presence of the pathogen and the fact that CDC officials now include various shellfish (and presumably finfish) in food history questionnaires given to listeriosis victims in five states as well as Los Angeles County (21,24,161) make it likely that additional cases of listeriosis will be positively linked to consumption of fish and seafood in the future.

FOODS OF PLANT ORIGIN

Evidence for transmission of listeriosis through foods of plant origin probably dates back to 1922 when investigators in Iceland described a "listeriosis-like" illness in silage-fed animals (88). This apparent relationship between consumption of improperly fermented silage and listeriosis in ruminants was clarified in 1960, and now numerous reports of silage-related listeriosis outbreaks in sheep and cows can be found in the scientific literature. While additional cases of animal listeriosis associated with consumption of other types of animal feed have been primarily limited to scattered reports involving cattle that grazed on Ponderosa pine needles in western Canada, one 1977 outbreak of listeriosis in chinchillas was attributed to a batch of meal containing beet pulp (78). However, *L. monocytogenes* was never isolated from the incriminated feed.

Given the evidence linking cases of animal listeriosis to consumption of contaminated plant material, it is reasonable to suspect that raw vegetables (e.g., cabbage, lettuce) and fruits are responsible for a certain percentage of listeriosis cases appearing in the human population, as was first suggested by Blendon and Szatalowicz (49) in 1967. Evidence for involvement of raw fruits in cases of human listeriosis is currently limited to one 1984 unpublished report from Connecticut suggesting a possible link between listeriosis and consumption of unwashed strawberries and/or blueberries. In contrast, the ability of certain segments of the population to succumb to listeriosis after consuming contaminated raw vegetables has been well documented during the last 10 years.

In 1986, Ho et al. (96) published results from an earlier epidemiological investigation in which raw vegetables were suggested as a possible vehicle of infection in an outbreak of listeriosis that occurred among patients in eight Boston-area hospitals during September and October of 1979. However, it is noteworthy that 1 year before these findings were published, Schlech et al. (158) published their landmark report describing the first confirmed North American outbreak of foodborne listeriosis in which 41 Canadians became ill in 1981 after consuming coleslaw contaminated with *L. monocytogenes*. Hence, it seems unlikely that the listeriosis outbreak in Boston would have been reported if Schlech et al. (158) had not published their results first.

In the outbreak described by Ho et al. (96), 23 patients admitted to Boston-area hospitals acquired systemic listeric infections during September and October of 1979, with *L. monocytogenes* isolates from 20 of 23 (87%) patients identified as serotype 4b (Fig. 8.5). In contrast, only 19 listeriosis cases were identified at the same eight hospitals during the 26-month period immediately preceding the outbreak. Unlike the previously described foodborne outbreaks of listeriosis, which included pregnant women, neonates, and adults, all 20 outbreak-related cases of listeriosis from which *L. monocytogenes* serotype 4b was isolated were adults ranging in age from 46 to 89 years; half of them were immunocompromised as a result of cancer, chemotherapy, or steroid treatment. Overall, 18 of 20 (90%) and 8 of 20 (40%) patients suffered from listeric bacteremia and meningitis, respectively. Although 5 of 20 (25%) patients died, two of these deaths were related to underlying illnesses rather than listeriosis.

A series of epidemiological case-control studies revealed that cases were more likely than controls (i.e., listeriosis patients treated at the same eight hospitals during the 26-month period preceding the outbreak) to have (a) become infected with *L.*

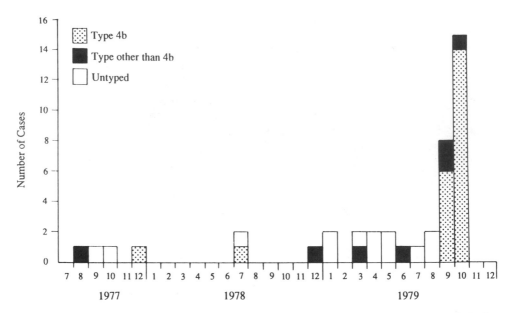

Figure 8.5 Number of listeriosis cases in eight Boston-area hospitals that resulted from infection with serotype 4b, non–serotype 4b, and untypeable strains of *L. monocytogenes* between July 1977 and December 1979. (Adapted from Ref. 96.)

monocytogenes serotype 4b rather than another serotype, (b) acquired listeriosis during hospitalization, (c) exhibited gastrointestinal symptoms, and (d) received antacids or cimetidine before onset of illness. More important, results from food histories revealed that cases were more likely than controls to have consumed tuna, chicken salad, and cottage as well as hard cheese. While it was at first difficult to develop a scenario by which this apparent common-source outbreak could have resulted from consumption of three seemingly unrelated foods obtained from different distributors, hospital kitchen records revealed that all three foods were commonly used in salads containing lettuce, celery, and/or tomatoes. Thus, in the light of the 1981 Canadian listeriosis outbreak involving coleslaw, these researchers postulated that the Boston outbreak was the result of victims having consumed raw lettuce, celery, and/or tomatoes that were contaminated with listeriae. However, since no attempt was made to isolate *L. monocytogenes* from these vegetables at the time of the outbreak, the exact source of infection will always remain in question.

Coleslaw: Canada, 1981

Two years after this presumed vegetableborne outbreak of listeriosis in Boston, Schlech et al. (158) positively identified coleslaw as the vehicle of infection in a major outbreak of listeriosis that occurred in the Maritime Provinces of Canada. According to their report, 34 perinatal and 7 adult cases of *L. monocytogenes* serotype 4b infection were diagnosed between March 1 and September 1 of 1981 in Nova Scotia, New Brunswick, and Prince Edward Island as compared to 22 cases in the 26-month period immediately preceding the outbreak (Fig. 8.6). Perinatal cases were characterized by acute febrile illness in pregnant women followed by spontaneous abortion (five cases), stillbirth (four cases), live birth of a seriously ill infant (23 cases), or live birth of a healthy infant (two cases). [Detailed clinical and laboratory findings concerning 15 of these cases diagnosed at Grace Maternity Hospital in Halifax, Nova Scotia, were subsequently reported by Evans et al. (72).] Additionally, six cases of meningitis and one case of pneumonia/septicemia were diagnosed in seven nonimmunocompromised adults (six men and one nonpregnant woman) who were 21–81 years old. Fifteen of 34 (44%) perinatal and 2 of 7 (29%) adult victims died giving an overall mortality rate of 41% (115).

Two case-control studies were subsequently initiated to assess possible risk factors for acquisition of listeriosis. The first study examined medical, residential, occupational, travel, and educational history as well as exposure to animals and information concerning gardening and outdoor activities, whereas the second case-control study involved a general history of foods consumed during the 3 months before onset of illness. Analysis of results from the first case-control study failed to implicate a common environmental source for this outbreak. While initial data collected from food histories also failed to implicate any particular food, results from a second questionnaire that included names of several food items found in the refrigerator of a man who developed pneumonia and septicemia indicated that cases were more likely than controls to have consumed both coleslaw and radishes. Multivariate analysis later showed that ingestion of radishes was associated with consumption of coleslaw rather than illness. However, repeated interviews with cases and controls who had previously denied eating coleslaw revealed that 100% of the cases but only 40% of the controls remembered consuming the product during the 3-month period before the outbreak.

Armed with this information, investigators visited the home of one of the patients,

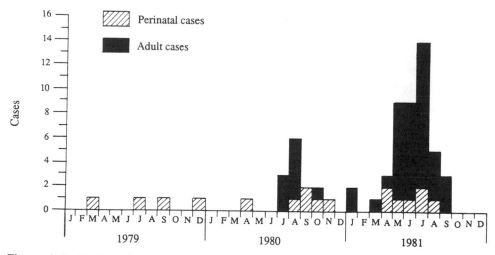

Figure 8.6 Number of perinatal and adult cases of listeriosis recorded in the Maritime Provinces of Canada from January 1979 to December 1981. (Adapted from Ref. 158.)

sampled foods from the refrigerator, and then isolated *L. monocytogenes* from coleslaw but no other foods obtained from the patient's refrigerator. The strain isolated from coleslaw was soon identified as serotype 4b, the same serotype isolated from all 34 victims. To prove that the patient had not inadvertently contaminated the coleslaw, investigators obtained two unopened packages of coleslaw from two different Halifax-area supermarkets and recovered *L. monocytogenes* serotype 4b from each package. Audurier et al. (37) later reported that 28 of 31 (90.3%) *L. monocytogenes* serotype 4b isolates obtained from blood, cerebrospinal fluid, and/or placental material between January and September of 1981 were of the same phage type. Any remaining doubt concerning the role of coleslaw in this outbreak was eliminated by a 1988 report (34,35) indicating that 27 of 29 (93%) clinical and 2 of 2 coleslaw isolates were of the same electrophoretic enzyme type. Additionally, 16 of 18 (89%) isolates of *L. monocytogenes* serotype 4b from sporadic cases of listeriosis were of electrophoretic enzyme types other than that associated with the outbreak. Thus Schlech et al. (158) can be credited with providing the first concrete evidence that consumption of contaminated food, in this instance coleslaw, can cause a listeric infection in humans.

After coleslaw was confirmed as the infectious vehicle in this outbreak, Schlech et al. (158) attempted to determine the route by which the coleslaw became contaminated. Investigators soon traced the tainted coleslaw to a regional manufacturer whose product had been distributed exclusively in the Maritime Provinces of Canada. While repeated microbiological testing of environmental samples from the coleslaw factory failed to uncover the source of contamination, review of factory records along with recent data on animal listeriosis revealed that the manufacturer had received at least 2250 kg of cabbage from a farmer who grew cabbage and raised sheep. Furthermore, the farmer lost two sheep in his flock to listeriosis—one in 1979 and one in 1981. A review of the farmer's agronomic practices indicated that cabbage was routinely fertilized with both raw and composted sheep manure obtained from animals that were presumably fecal carriers of *L. monocytogenes*. Moreover, the final October cabbage crop was held in a large cold-storage shed until early spring. Such storage practices, which somewhat resemble cold enrichment, may have led to an increase in numbers of *L. monocytogenes* in the cabbage. Although none of the implicated cabbage crop (other than that which was previously manufactured into coleslaw and contained the epidemic strain of *L. monocytogenes*) was available for testing, and none of the farm environmental samples, including raw sheep manure, yielded *Listeria*, the aforementioned circumstantial evidence still supports an indirect link between sporadic cases of ovine listeriosis on a cabbage farm and cases of listeriosis in humans consuming a *Listeria*-contaminated product. Several additional observations—(a) crops grown in Canada, the United States, and industrialized European nations are routinely fertilized with material other than raw manure, (b) the recent discovery that 82% of all *L. monocytogenes* strains isolated during one large survey of raw vegetables marketed in the United States were of serotype 1a (94), and (c) most *L. monocytogenes* strains isolated from animal sources, including feces, in North America are of serotype 4 rather than 1—support transmission of *L. monocytogenes* from raw sheep manure to cabbage. Hence, raw manure should not be used to fertilize vegetables that will be consumed without cooking.

Additional Reports of Listeriosis Associated with Products of Plant Origin

Despite the proven link between coleslaw and development of listeriosis in the Canadian outbreak just discussed, consumption of raw vegetables, fruits and other types of produce has not generally been deemed to constitute a major public health threat. This lack of concern has resulted because consumption of raw produce has been infrequently associated with most forms of foodborne disease. However, after consumption of Mexican-style and Vacherin Mont d'Or soft-ripened cheese was directly linked to two separate listeriosis outbreaks (see earlier discussion in this chapter), public health officials on both sides of the Atlantic Ocean became increasingly interested in the possibility that nondairy foods such as meat, poultry, seafood, and raw produce could transmit *L. monocytogenes* to humans.

As of July 1990, the scientific literature contained reports of three additional cases in which consumption of a product of plant (or microbial) origin was directly linked to human listeriosis. In November 1988 Kerr et al. (112) reported that a 29-year-old pregnant woman in England miscarried after a 2-week history of pyrexia and rigors. An identical phage type of *L. monocytogenes* serotype 4b was subsequently isolated from placental swabs and maternal/fetal blood samples as well as a 3-month-old bottle of vegetable rennet (may have been microbial rennet) that was discovered in the woman's refrigerator, thus implicating vegetable rennet which was presumably used to produce a custard-like product.

In the second of these three listeriosis cases, an 80-year-old previously healthy man in Finland developed a nonfatal septicemic infection 1 day after consuming previously cooked but not reheated home-made salted mushrooms that were later found to contain 3.8×10^6 *L. monocytogenes* CFU/g (105). Both *Listeria* isolates from the patient's blood and a portion of the uneaten mushrooms were of serotype 4b and of the same phage type, thus confirming salted mushrooms as the vehicle of infection. According to the investigating team, the implicated home-grown mushrooms were washed, cooked, salted to a level of 7.5% NaCl, and then stored in a cold cellar for 5 months before consumption. Since this product, which was presumably contaminated after cooking, had a pH of 5.9 with visible mold growth on the surface, current information regarding behavior of *L. monocytogenes* under such conditions indicates that the pathogen probably grew in these mushrooms during the 5 months of storage. While the exact source of contamination was never determined, it is noteworthy that the man's wife did not become ill after consuming thoroughly reheated mushrooms from the same container. Hence, it appears that heavily contaminated vegetables also can be rendered safe by thorough cooking.

The final case of listeriosis directly linked to products of plant origin is markedly different in that consumption of alfalfa tablets, a dry product in which *L. monocytogenes* is presumably unable to grow, was directly responsible for a fatal case of listeric meningoencephalitis in a 55-year-old immunocompromised Canadian man (75). As in the two cases just discussed, *L. monocytogenes* strains of serotype 4b isolated from the victim's blood and cerebrospinal fluid as well as the remaining alfalfa tablets were all of the same electrophoretic enzyme type, thus confirming alfalfa tablets as the vehicle of infection in the only listeriosis case thus far linked to ingestion of a nearly completely dry product.

While not directly linking consumption of raw vegetables to listeric infection, several reports have provided additional circumstantial evidence for involvement of vegetables in cases of listeriosis. In one of these reports (43), a 74-year-old man contracted *L. monocytogenes* serotype 1/2c septicemia and meningitis 11 days after repair of his perforated duodenal ulcer in a London-area hospital. During the week before onset of illness, the patient reported consuming hospital food supplemented with high protein puddings and sandwiches containing various fillings, including cheese; however, hospital personnel failed to maintain an exact record of foods consumed. In conjunction with a survey to determine the incidence of listeriae in hospital-prepared foods, investigators isolated *L. monocytogenes* serotype 1/2a and *L. innocua* from 1 of 15 and 2 of 15 samples of washed English round lettuce but failed to detect *Listeria* spp. in 40 other food samples consisting primarily of dairy products and other raw vegetables. Most evidence suggests that listeriosis has an incubation period of 1 to several weeks; however, three of four patients in England with confirmed cases of foodborne listeriosis exhibited incubation periods of ≤1 week. Hence, while the incubation period observed in this 74-year-old man is compatible with a hospital-acquired listeric infection, isolation of different *L. monocytogenes* serotypes from the man and washed English round lettuce appears to preclude direct involvement of lettuce in this particular case of listeriosis. Nevertheless, since *L. monocytogenes* was recovered from washed lettuce but from no other hospital-prepared food, consumption of lettuce still appears to be a possible risk factor in development of hospital-acquired listeriosis.

During the previously discussed 1986–1987 case-control study in which consumption of uncooked frankfurters and undercooked chicken was epidemiologically associated with listeriosis, Schwartz et al. (161) isolated the same serotype and enzyme type of *L. monocytogenes* from five Hispanic listeriosis patients who resided in Los Angeles County. Of the four patients who voluntarily enrolled in the case-control study, all consumed lettuce as well as chicken and whole milk. Unfortunately, because matched controls consumed these products at rates similar to those of cases it was impossible to link consumption of lettuce as well as chicken or whole milk to listeriosis. Nevertheless, while epidemiological investigations alone can never prove causality, future studies similar to that just described will continue to play a vital role in elucidating possible relationships between listeriosis and consumption of vegetables as well as fruit, dairy, meat, poultry, seafood, and other foods not yet thought to be associated with this disease.

REFERENCES

1. Acheson,D. 1987. Food hazard warning: Vacherin Mont d'Or Swiss cheese. Department of Health and Social Security, London. Release PL/CMO(87)11.
2. Allerberger, F. 1988. Listeriosis in Austria—Report of an outbreak in Austria 1986. Tenth International Symposium on Listeriosis, Pecs, Hungary, Aug. 22–26, Abstr. 20.
3. Anonymous. 1976. Report of a WHO expert committee with the participation of the FAO—Microbiological aspects of food hygiene. *WHO Tech. Report Series 598*:1–103.
4. Anonymous. 1985. FDA is investigating deaths linked to Mexican-style cheese. *Food Chem. News 27*(15):42.
5. Anonymous. 1985. FDA still searching for source of Listeria in Mexican-style cheese. *Food Chem. News 27*(17):57.

6. Anonymous. 1985. Jalisco-brand Mexican style soft cheese recalled. FDA Enforcement Rep., June 26.
7. Anonymous. 1985. *Listeria. Food Chem. News 27*(23):2.
8. Anonymous. 1985. Second California firm recalls Mexican-style cheese because of *Listeria. Food Chem. News 27*(20):15.
9. Anonymous. 1986. FDA investigating three reports of *Listeria* contamination. *Food Chem. News 28*(22):24.
10. Anonymous. 1986. *Listeria* meningitis associated with soft imported cheese. *Communicable Disease Rep. 86*:8.
11. Anonymous. 1986. Listeriosis—Survey in French-speaking Switzerland. *Wkly. Epidem. Rec. 41*:317–318.
12. Anonymous. 1986. Mexican cheese maker receives 60-day jail sentence. *Food Chem. News 28*(12):51.
13. Anonymous. 1986. Sixty misdemeanor charges filed against maker of contaminated cheese. *Food Chem. News 28*(4):45–46.
14. Anonymous. 1987. CDC finds no food connection to *Listeria* cases in Philadelphia. *Food Chem. News 29*(16):13–14.
15. Anonymous. 1987. FDA, CDC investigate ice cream link to *Listeria* outbreak. *Food Chem. News 29*(8):3–4.
16. Anonymous. 1987. FDA finds no food link to *Listeria* deaths in Philadelphia. *Food Chem. News 29*(9):41.
17. Anonymous. 1987. Milk industry has spent $66 million on recalls and related expenses, Witte says. *Food Chem. News 29*(17):29–30.
18. Anonymous. 1987. *N.Y. Times* reports *Listeria* outbreak in Switzerland from soft cheese. *Food Chem. News 29*(40):18.
19. Anonymous. 1987. Swiss Vacherin Mont d'Or soft cheese. Department of Health and Social Security, London, Press Release 87/419.
20. Anonymous. 1988. AMI data show frankfurters most likely *Listeria* carrier in meat. *Food Chem. News 30*(16):37–39.
21. Anonymous. 1988. CDC listeriosis microbiology-vs.-epidemiology study hit at session. *Food Chem. News 30*(35):3–6.
22. Anonymous. 1988. Food analysis needed for "evidence" of listeriosis link, panel says. *Food Chem. News 30*(29):43–44.
23. Anonymous. 1988. Foodborne listeriosis-Switzerland. *J. Food Prot. 51*:425.
24. Anonymous. 1988. FSIS to expand *Listeria* testing to more products, plants. *Food Chem. News 30*(33):25–28.
25. Anonymous. 1988. *Listeria* destruction in cooked meat products ineffective: Hormel. *Food Chem. News 30*(15):32–34.
26. Anonymous. 1988. Listeriosis: Goats' milk cheese. Communicable Disease Rep., Feb. 12.
27. Anonymous. 1988. Uncooked hot dogs, undercooked chicken seen as listeriosis risk. *Food Chem. News 30*(26):11–14.
28. Anonymous. 1988. FSIS to expand *Listeria* testing to more products, plants. *Food Chem. News 30*(33):25–28.
29. Anonymous. 1989. Listeriosis from pre-cooked chicken reported in Britain. *Food Chem. News 30*(48):26–27.
30. Anonymous. 1989. Source of Washington state listeriosis cases remains unknown. *Food Chem. News 31*(38):33; *31*(41):40.
31. Anonymous. 1989. USDA to toughen regulatory policy on *Listeria* in meat, poultry. *Food Chem. News 31*(8):52–53.
32. Anonymous. 1990. CDC links Cajun pork sausage to listeriosis case: Product recalled. *Food Chem. News 32*(44):35.
33. Archer, D. L. 1988. Review of the latest FDA information on the presence of *Listeria* in foods. WHO Working Group on Foodborne Listeriosis, Geneva, Switzerland, Feb. 15–19.

34. Ashton, F. E., J. A. Ryan, and E. P. Ewan. 1988. Electrophoretic analysis of enzymes produced by *Listeria monocytogenes* serotype 4b. *Proceedings, Society for Industrial Microbiology-Comprehensive Conference on Listeria monocytogenes*, Rohnert Park, CA, Oct. 2–5, Abstr. P-11.

35. Ashton, F. E., J. A. Ryan, and E. P. Ewan. 1988. Enzyme electrophoretic analysis of *Listeria monocytogenes* serotype 4b associated with listeriosis in Canada. Tenth International Symposium on Listeriosis, Pecs. Hungary, Aug. 22–26, Abstr. P43.

36. Atkinson, E. 1917. Meningitis associated with gram-positive bacilli of diphtheroid type. *Med. J. Austral. 1*:115–118.

37. Audurier, A., A. G. Taylor, B. Carbonnelle, and J. McLauchlin. 1984. A phage typing system for *Listeria monocytogenes* and its use in epidemiological studies. *Clin. Invest. Med. 7*:229–232.

38. Azadian, B. S., G. T. Finnerty, and A. D. Pearson. 1989. Cheese-borne *Listeria* meningitis in immunocompetent patient. *Lancet i*:232–233.

39. Bannister, B. A. 1987. *Listeria monocytogenes* meningitis associated with eating soft cheese. *J. Infect. 15*:165–168.

40. Barnes, R., P. Archer, J. Stack, and G. R. Istre. 1989. Listeriosis associated with consumption of turkey franks. *Morbid. Mortal. Weekly Rep. 38*:267–268.

41. Beams, R. E., and K. F. Girard. 1958. The effect of pasteurization on *Listeria monocytogenes*. *Can. J. Microbiol. 4*:55–61.

42. Becroft, D. M. O., K. Farmer, R. J. Seddon, R. Sowden, J. H. Stewart, A. Vines, and D. A. Wattie. 1971. Epidemic listeriosis in the newborn. *Br. Med. J. 3*:747–751.

43. Bendig, J. W. A., and J. E. M. Strangeways. 1989. *Listeria* in hospital lettuce. *Lancet i*:616–617.

44. Berrang, M. E., J. F. Frank, and R. E. Brackett. 1988. Behavior of *Listeria monocytogenes* in chocolate milk and ice cream mix made from post-expiration date skim milk. *J. Food Prot. 51*:823 (Abstr.).

45. Bille, J. 1988. Anatomy of a foodborne listeriosis outbreak. *Foodborne Listeriosis—Proceedings of a Symposium*, Wiesbaden, West Germany, Sep. 7, pp. 30–35.

46. Bille, J. 1988. Epidemiology of human listeriosis in Europe with special reference to the Swiss outbreak. *Proceedings, Society for Industrial Microbiology-Comprehensive Conference on Listeria monocytogenes*, Rohnert Park, CA, Oct. 2–5, Abstr. I-11.

47. Bille, J., J. Rocourt, F. Mean, M. P. Glauser, and the Group "*Listeria*-Vaud." 1988. Epidemic food-borne listeriosis in Western Switzerland. II. Epidemiology, Interscience Conference on Antimicrobial Agents and Chemotherapy, Los Angeles, CA, Oct. 23–26, Abstr. 1107.

48. Bisping, W. von. 1957. Die Listeriose und ihre milchhygienische Bedeutung. *Kieler Milchwirtschaftliche Forschungsberichte 9*:595–606.

49. Blendon, D. C., and F. T. Szatalowicz. 1967. Ecological aspects of listeriosis. *J. Amer. Vet. Assoc. 151*:1761–1766.

50. Bojsen-Møller, J. 1972. Human listeriosis—diagnostic, epidemiological and clinical studies. *Acta Pathol. Microbiol. Scand. Section B. Suppl. 229*:1–157.

51. Borbély, E., and E. Méró. 1971. Isolation of *Listeria* in a meat combine. (In Hungarian). Meeting of the Hungarian Association of Hygienists, Siofok. (In Ralovich, B. S. 1975. Selective and enrichment media to isolate *Listeria*. In M. Woodbine (ed.) *Problems of Listeriosis—Proceedings of the Sixth International Symposium*, Leicester University Press, Leicester, pp. 286–294.)

52. Bowmer, E. J., J. A. McKiel, W. H. Cockcroft, N. Schmitt, and D. E. Rappay. 1973. *Listeria monocytogenes* infections in Canada. *Can. Med. Assoc. J. 109*:125–135.

53. Breer, C. 1987. *Listeria* in cheese. In A. Schoenberg (ed.), Listeriosis-Joint WHO/ROI Consultation on Prevention and Control, Berlin, West Germany, Dec. 10–12, pp. 106–109.

54. Bula, Ch., J. Bille, F. Mean, M. P. Glauser, and the Group "*Listeria*-Vaud." 1988. Epidemic food-borne listeriosis in Western Switzerland. I. Description of the 58 adult cases. Interscience Conference on Antimicrobial Agents and Chemotherapy, Los Angeles, CA, Oct. 23–26, Abstr. 1106.

55. Burn, C. G. 1936. Clinical and pathological features of an infection caused by a new pathogen of the genus *Listerella*. *Amer. J. Pathol. 12*:341–349.

56. Campbell, D. M. 1989. Listeriosis in Scotland, 1988. *Lancet i*:492.

57. Canfield, M. A., J. N. Walterspiel, M. S. Edwards, C. J. Baker, R. B. Wait, and J. N. Urteaga. 1984. An epidemic of perinatal listeriosis serotype 1b in Hispanics in a Houston hospital. *Pediatr. Infect. Dis. 4*:106.
58. Cantoni, C., C. Balzaretti, and M. Valenti. 1989. A case of *L. monocytogenes* human infection associated with consumption of "Testa in cascetta" (cooked meat pork product). *Archivo Veterinario Italiano 40*:141–142.
59. Carbonnelle, B., J. Cottin, F. Parvery, G. Chambreuil, S. Kouyoumdjian, M. Lirzin, and F. Vincent. 1978. Epidemic de listeriose dans l'ouest de la France (1975–1976). *Revue Epidémioloque et de Sante Publique* (Paris) *26*:451–467. (In McLauchlin, J. 1987. A review—*Listeria monocytogenes*, recent advances in the taxonomy and epidemiology of listeriosis in humans. *J. Appl. Bacteriol. 63*:1–11.)
60. Dedié, K. 1955. Beitrag zur Epizootologie der Listeriose. *Arch. Exp. Vet.-Med. 9*:251–264.
61. Dijkstra, R. G. 1976. *Listeria*-encephalitis in cows through litter from a broiler-farm. *Zbl. Bakteriol. Hyg. I Abt. Orig. B 161*:383–385.
62. Donnelly, C. W. 1989. Personal communication.
63. Donnelly, C. W., E. H. Briggs, and L. S. Donnelly. 1987. Comparison of heat resistance of *Listeria monocytogenes* in milk as determined by two methods. *J. Food Prot. 50*:14–17, 20.
64. Doyle, M. P. (ed.). 1989. *Foodborne Bacterial Pathogens*, Marcel Dekker, New York.
65. Doyle, M. P. 1990. Personal communication.
66. Doyle, M. P., K. A. Glass, J. T. Beery, G. A. Garcia, D. J. Pollard, and R. D. Schultz. 1987. Survival of *Listeria monocytogenes* in milk during high-temperature, short-time pasteurization. *Appl. Environ. Microbiol. 53*:1433–1438.
67. Eck, H. von. 1957. Encephalomyelitis listeriaca apostematosa. *Schweiz. Med. Wschr. 9*:210–214.
68. Elischerová, K., and S. Stupalová. 1972. Listeriosis in professionally exposed persons. *Acta Microbiol. Acad. Sci. Hung. 19*:379–384.
69. Elischerová, K., G. Havílková, and S. Stúpalová. 1976. *Listeria monocytogenes* isolation at work places in the meat industry. *Cs. Epidemiol. Mikrobiol. Imunol. 25*:326–332.
70. Elischerová, K., S. Stúpalová, R. Helbíchová, and J. Stepánek. 1979. Incidence of *Listeria monocytogenes* in faeces of employees of meat processing plants and meat shops. *Cs. Epidemiol. Mikrobiol. Imunol. 28*:97–102.
71. Embil, J. A., E. P. Ewan, and S. W. MacDonald. 1984. Surveillance of *Listeria monocytogenes* in human and environmental specimens in Nova Scotia, 1974 to 1981. *Clin. Invest. Med. 7*:325–327.
72. Evans, R. J., A. C. Allen, D. A. Stinson, R. Bortolussi, and L. J. Peddle. 1985. Perinatal listeriosis: Report of an outbreak. *Pediatr. Infect. Dis. 4*:237–241.
73. Facinelli, B., P. E. Varaldo, M. Toni, C. Casolari, and U. Fabio. 1989. Ignorance about *Listeria*. *British Med. J. 299*:738.
74. Faoagali, J. L., and M. Schousboe. 1985. Listeriosis in Christchurch 1967–1984. *N. Zeal. Med. J. 98*:64–66.
75. Farber, J. M., A. O. Carter, P. V. Varughese, F. E. Ashton, and E. P. Ewan. 1990. Listeriosis traced to the consumption of alfalfa tablets and soft cheese. *N. Engl. J. Med. 322*:338.
76. Felsenfeld, O. 1951. Disease of poultry transmissible to men. *Iowa State College Vet. 13*:89–92.
77. Fenlon, D. R. 1985. Wild birds and silage as reservoirs of *Listeria* in the agricultural environment. *J. Appl. Bacteriol. 59*:537–543.
78. Finle, G. G., and J. R. Long. 1977. An epizootic of listeriosis in chinchillas. *Can. Vet. J. 18*:164–167.
79. Fischer, M. 1962. Listeriose-Häufung in Raume Bremen in den Jahren 1960 und 1961. *Dtsch. med. Wochenschr. 87*:2682–2684.
80. Fleming, D. W., S. L. Cochi, K. L. MacDonald, J. Brondum, P. S. Hayes, B. D. Plikaytis, M. B. Homes, A. Audurier, C. V. Broome, and A. L. Reingold. 1985. Pasteurized milk as a vehicle of infection in an outbreak of listeriosis. *N. Engl. J. Med. 312*:404–407.
81. Foegeding, P. M., and S. B. Leasor. 1990. Heat resistance and growth of *Listeria monocytogenes* in liquid whole egg. *J. Food Prot. 53*:9–14.

82. Galsworthy, S. B. 1984. Immunomodulation by surface components of *Listeria monocytogenes*: A review. *Clin. Invest. Med.* 7:223–227.
83. Galsworthy, S. B., S. M. Gurofsky, and R. G. E. Murray. 1977. Purification of a monocytosis-producing activity from *Listeria monocytogenes*. *Infect. Immun.* 15:500–509.
84. Geurden, L. M. G., and A. Devos. 1952. Listerellose bij pluimvee. *Vlaams. Diergeneesk. Tijdschr.* 21:165–175.
85. Gilbert, R. J., S. M. Hall, and A. G. Taylor. 1989. Listeriosis update. *Public Health Laboratory Service Digest* 6:33–37.
86. Gray, M. L. 1958. Listeriosis in fowls—a review. *Avian Dis.* 2:296–314.
87. Gray, M. L. 1960. A possible link in the relationship between silage feeding and listeriosis. *J. Amer. Vet. Med. Assoc.* 136:205–208.
88. Gray, M. L., and A. H. Killinger. 1966. *Listeria monocytogenes* and listeric infections. *Bacteriol. Rev.* 30:309–382.
89. Gray, M. L., and F. Thorp, Jr. 1957. Perinatal infection in rabbits induced by *Listeria monocytogenes*. IV. Apparent transmission through dam's milk. *Zbl. Veterinärmed.* 4:405–414.
90. Gudkova, E. I., and T. P. Voronina. 1956. Diagnosis of listeric angina. *Zh. Mikrobiol. Epidemiol. Immunobiol.* 33:31–39.
91. Gudkova, E. I., K. A. Mironova, A. S. Kúzminskii, and G. O. Geine. 1958. A second outbreak of listeriotic angina in a single populated locality. *Zh. Mikrobiol. Epidemiol. Immunobiol.* 35:24–28.
92. Hall, S. M. 1988. The epidemiology of listeriosis in England and Wales. *Foodborne Listeriosis-Proceedings of a Symposium*, Wiesbaden, West Germany, Sept. 7, pp. 38–50.
93. Hayes, P. S., J. C. Feeley, L. M. Graves, G. W. Ajello, and D. W. Fleming. 1986. Isolation of *Listeria monocytogenes* from raw milk. *Appl. Environ. Microbiol.* 51:438–440.
94. Heisick, J. E., D. E. Wagner, M. L. Nierman, and J. T. Peeler. 1989. *Listeria* spp. found on fresh market produce. *Appl. Environ. Microbiol.* 55:1925–1927.
95. Hird, D. W. 1987. Review of evidence for zoonotic listeriosis. *J. Food Prot.* 50:429–433.
96. Ho, J. L., K. N. Shands, G. Friedland, P. Eckind, and D. W. Fraser. 1986. An outbreak of type 4b *Listeria monocytogenes* infection involving patients from eight Boston hospitals. *Arch. Intern. Med.* 146:520–524.
97. Hofer, E. 1983. Bacteriologic and epidemiologic studies on the occurrence of *Listeria monocytogenes* in healthy cattle. *Zbl. Bakteriol. Hyg. A* 256:175–183.
98. Hyslop, N. St. G. 1975. Epidemiologic and immunologic factors in listeriosis. In M. Woodbine (ed.), *Problems of Listeriosis*, Leicester University Press, Leicester, pp. 94–105.
99. Hyslop. N. St. G., and A. D. Osborne. 1959. Listeriosis: A potential danger to public health. *Vet. Rec.* 71:1082–1091.
100. Jacobs, M. R., H. Stein, A. Buqwane, A. Dubb, F. Segal, L. Rabinowitz, U. Ellis, I. Freman, M. Witcomb, and V. Vallabh. 1978. Epidemic listeriosis—Report of 14 cases detected in 9 months. *S. Afr. Med. J.* 54:389–392.
101. James, S. M., S. L. Fannin, B. A. Agree, B. Hall, E. Parker, J. Vogt, G. Run, J. Williams, L. Lieb, C. Salminen, T. Prendergast, S. B. Werner, and J. Chin. 1985. Listeriosis outbreak associated with Mexican-style cheese—California. *J. Amer. Med. Assoc.* 254:474.
102. James, S. M., S. L. Fanning, B. A. Agree, B. Hall, E. Parker, J. Vogt, G. Run, J. Williams, L. Lieb, C. Salminen, T. Prendergast, S. B. Werner, and J. Chin. 1985. Listeriosis outbreak associated with Mexican-style cheese—California. *Morbid. Mortal. Weekly Rep.* 34(24):357–359.
103. Jay, J. M. 1986. *Modern Food Microbiology*, 3rd ed., Van Nostrand Reinhold Co., New York.
104. Julianelle, L. A. 1940. The function of *Listerella* in infection. *Ann. Intern. Med.* 14:608–620.
105. Junttila, J., and M. Brander. 1989. *Listeria monocytogenes* septicemia associated with consumption of salted mushrooms. *Scand. J. Infect. Dis.* 21:339–342.
106. Kaczmarski, E. B., and D. M. Jones. 1989. Listeriosis and ready-cooked chicken. *Lancet* i:549.

107. Kampelmacher, E. H. 1962. Animal products as a source of listeric infection in man. In M. L. Gray (ed.)., *Second Symposium on Listeric Infection*, Montana State College, Bozeman, Montana, Aug. 29–31, pp. 146–151.

108. Kampelmacher, E. H., and L. M. van Noorle Jansen. 1969. Isolation of *Listeria monocytogenes* from faeces of clinically healthy humans and animals. *Zbl. Bakteriol. I Abt. Orig. 211*:353–359.

109. Kampelmacher, E. H., and L. M. van Noorle Jansen. 1980. Listeriosis in humans and animals in the Netherlands (1958–1977). *Zbl. Bakteriol. Hyg., I Abt. Orig. A 246*:111–227.

110. Kampelmacher, E. H., D. E. Maas, and L. M. van Noorle Jansen. 1976. Occurrence of *Listeria monocytogenes* in feces of pregnant women with and without direct animal contact. *Zbl. Bakteriol. Hyg. I Abt. Orig. A 234*:238–242.

111. Kaplan, M. M. 1945. Listerellosis. *N. Engl. J. Med. 232*:755–759.

112. Kerr, K. G., S. F. Dealler, and R. W. Lacey. 1988. Materno-fetal listeriosis from cook-chill and refrigerated food. *Lancet ii*:1133.

113. Khomenko, G. I., V. A. Matsievskii, and O. P. Lebedeva. 1953. Data to clinical picture and diagnosis of listerellosis. *Vrach. Delo. No. 12*:1099–1104. (In Ralovich, B. 1984. *Listeriosis Research—Present Situation and Perspective*, Akademiai Kiado, Budapest.)

114. Kúzminskii, A. S. 1956. Epidemiology of listerellosis outbreak. *Zh. Mikrobiol. Epidemiol. Immunobiol. 33*:25–30.

115. Kvenberg, J. E. 1988. Outbreaks of listeriosis/*Listeria*—contaminated foods. *Microbiol. Sci. 5*:355–358.

116. Lee, W. H. 1989. Personal communication.

117. Lennon, D., B. Lewis, C. Mantell, D. Becroft, B. Dove, K. Farmer, S. Tonkin, N. Yeates, R. Stamp, and K. Mickleson. 1984. Epidemic perinatal listeriosis. *Pediat. Infect. Dis. 3*:30–34.

118. Linnan, M. J., L. Mascola, X. D. Lou, V. Goulet, S. May, C. Salminen, D. W. Hird, M. L. Yonkura, P. Hayes, R. Weaver, A. Audurier, B. D. Plikaytis, S. L. Fannin, A. Kleks, and C. V. Broome. 1988. Epidemic listeriosis associated with Mexican-style cheese. *N. Engl. J. Med. 319*:823–828.

119. Lovett, J.,D. W. Francis, and J. M. Hunt. 1987. *Listeria monocytogenes* in raw milk: Detection, incidence, and pathogenicity. *J. Food Prot. 50*:188–192.

120. Malinverni, R., M. P. Glauser, J. Bille, and J. Rocourt. 1986. Unusual clinical features of an epidemic of listeriosis associated with a particular phage type. *Eur. J. Clin. Microbiol. 5*:169–171.

121. Malinverni, R., J. Bille, Cl. Perret, F. Regli, F. Tanner, and M. P. Glauser. 1985. Listériose épidémizue—Observation de 25 cas en 15 mois au centre hospitalier universitaire vaudois. *Schweiz. med. Wschr. 115*:2–10.

122. Mascola, L., S. L. Fannin, and M. Linnan. 1989. Epidemic listeriosis—response to letter. *N. Engl. J. Med. 320*:538.

123. Mascola, L., L. Chun, and J. Thomas. 1988. A case-control study of a cluster of perinatal listeriosis identified by an active surveillance system in Los Angeles County. *Proceedings, Society for Industrial Microbiology—Comprehensive Conference on Listeria monocytogenes*, Rohnert Park, CA, Oct. 2–5, Abstr. P-10.

124. Mascola, L., F. Sorvillo, J. Neal, K. Iwakoshi, and R. Weaver. 1989. Surveillance of listeriosis in Los Angeles County, 1985–1986. *Arch. Intern. Med. 149*:1569–1572.

125. Mascola, L., L. Chun, J. Thomas, W. F. Bibe, B. Schwartz, C. Salminen, and P. Heseltine. 1988. A case-control study of a cluster of perinatal listeriosis identified by an active surveillance system in Los Angeles County. *Proceedings, Society for Industrial Microbiology—Comprehensive Conference on Listeria monocytogenes*, Rohnert Park, CA, Oct. 2–5, Abstr. P-10.

126. McLauchlin, J., A. Audurier, and A. G. Taylor. 1986. Aspects of the epidemiology of human *Listeria monocytogenes* infections in Britain 1967–1984; the use of serotyping and phage typing. *J. Med. Microbiol. 22*:367–377.

127. McLauchlin, J., N. Crofts, and D. M. Campbell. 1989. A possible outbreak of listeriosis caused by an unusual strain of *Listeria monocytogenes*. *J. Infect. 18*:179–187.
128. McLauchlin, J. M. H. Greenwood, and P. N. Pini. 1990. The occurrence of *Listeria monocytogenes* in cheese from a manufacturer associated with a case of listeriosis. *Int. J. Food Microbiol.* (Accepted for publication.)
129. Méró, E., and B. Ralovich. 1972. Present situation of human listeriosis in Hungary. *Acta Microbiol. Acad. Sci. Hung. 19*:301–310.
130. Murray, E. G. D., R. A. Webb, and M. B. R. Swann. 1926. A disease of rabbits characterized by a large mononuclear leucocytosis, caused by a hitherto undescribed bacillus *Bacterium monocytogenes* (n. sp.). *J. Pathol. Bacteriol. 29*:407–439.
131. Nicolai-Scholten, M.-E., J. Potel, J. Natzschka, and St. Pekker. 1985. High incidence of listeriosis in Lower Saxony, 1983. *Immun. Infekt. 13*:76–77.
132. Nicholas, J.-A., and N. Vidaud. 1987. Contribution a l'étude des *Listeria* presentes dans les denrées d'origine animale destinées a la consommation humaine. *Recueil de Medecine Veterinaire 163*:283–285.
133. Nocera, D. A., M. H. Fonjallaz, E. Bannerman, J. C. Piffaretti, J. Rocourt, and J. Bille. 1989. Restriction endonuclease analysis of genomic DNA associated with multilocus enzyme electrophoresis for *Listeria monocytogenes* strains. Ann. Mtg., Amer. Soc. Microbiol., New Orleans, LA, May 14–18, Abstr. D-233.
134. Northolt, M. D., H. J. Beckers, U. Vecht, L. Toepoel, P. S. S. Soentoro, and H. J. Wissenlink. 1988. *Listeria monocytogenes*: Heat resistance and behavior during storage of milk and whey and making of Dutch types of cheese. *Neth. Milk Dairy J. 42*:207–219.
135. Olding, L., and L. Philipson. 1960. Two cases of listeriosis in the newborn, associated with placental infection. *Acta Pathol. Microbiol. Scand. 48*:24–30.
136. Olsen, J. A., A. E. Yousef, and E. H. Marth. 1988. Growth and survival of *Listeria monocytogenes* during making and storage of butter. *Milchwissenschaft 43*:487–489.
137. Ortel, S. 1968. Bakteriologische, serologishche und epidemiologische Untersuchungen während einer Listeriose-Epidemie. *Dtsch. Gesundheitwesen 23*:753–759.
138. Papageorgiou, D. K., and E. H. Marth. 1989. Fate of *Listeria monocytogenes* during the manufacture and ripening of blue cheese. *J. Food Prot. 52*:459–465.
139. Papageorgiou, D. K., and E. H. Marth. 1989. Fate of *Listeria monocytogenes* during the manufacture, ripening and storage of Feta cheese. *J. Food Prot. 52*:82–87.
140. Pierson, M. D., and N. J. Stern. 1986. *Foodborne Microorganisms and Their Toxins: Developing Methodology*, Marcel Dekker, New York.
141. Piffaretti, J.-C., H. Kressebach, M. Aeschbacher, J. Bille, E. Bannerman, J. M. Musser, R. K. Selander, and J. Rocourt. 1989. Genetic characterization of clones of the bacterium *Listeria monocytogenes* causing epidemic listeriosis. *Proc. Nat. Acad. Sci. USA 86*:3818–3822.
142. Piolino, M., and J.-P. de Kalbermatten. 1968. La listériose du systéme nerveux central. *Schweiz. med. Wschr. 98*:822–828.
143. Potel, J. 1952. Zur Granulomatosis-Infantiseptica. *Zbl. Bakteriol. Parasitenk. Abt. I Orig. 158*:329–331.
144. Potel, J. 1952/1953. Über die diaplazentare Übertragung von *Listeria* Infantiseptica. *Wiss. Z. Martin-Luther Univ. Halle-Wittenberg 2*:15–47.
145. Potel, J. 1953/1954. Aetiologic der Granulomatosis Infantiseptica. *Wiss. Z. Martin Luther Univ. 3*:341–354.
146. Pratt-Lowe, E. L., R. M. Geiger, T. Richardson, and E. L. Barrett. 1988. Heat resistance of alkaline phosphatase produced by microorganisms isolated from California Mexican-style cheese. *J. Dairy Sci. 71*:17–23.
147. Prentice, G. A., and P. Neaves. 1988. *Listeria monocytogenes* in food: Its significance and methods for its detection. *Bull. Int. Dairy Fed. 223*:1–6.
148. Ralovich, B. 1984. *Listeriosis Research—Present Situation and Perspective*, Akademiai Kiado, Budapest.
149. Ralovich, B., A. Forray, E. Méró, and H. Malovics. 1970. Additional data on diagnosis and epidemiology of *Listeria* infections. *Zbl. Bakteriol. I Abt. Orig. 214*:231–235.

150. Reiss, H. J., J. Potel, and A. Krebs. 1951. Granulomatosis Infantiseptica eine durch eine spezifischen Erreger hervorgerufene fetale Sepsis. *Klin. Wschr. 29*:29.
151. Riemann, H., and F. L. Bryan. 1979. *Foodborne Infections and Intoxications*, 2nd ed., Academic Press, New York.
152. Rothgardt, N. P., S. Samuelsson, A. Carvajal, and W. Fredericksen. 1988. Human listeriosis in Denmark 1981–1987. Tenth International Symposium on Foodborne Listeriosis, Pecs, Hungary, Aug. 22–26, Abstr. P27.
153. Ryser, E. T., and E. H. Marth. 1987. Behavior of *Listeria monocytogenes* during the manufacture and ripening of Cheddar cheese. *J. Food Prot. 50*:7–13.
154. Ryser, E. T., and E. H. Marth. 1987. Fate of *Listeria monocytogenes* during manufacture and ripening of Camembert cheese. *J. Food Prot. 50*:372–378.
155. Ryser, E. T., and E. H. Marth. 1989. Behavior of *Listeria monocytogenes* during manufacture and ripening of brick cheese. *J. Dairy Sci. 72*:838–853.
156. Samuelsson, S., N. P. Rothgardt, A. C. Christensen, and W. Fredericksen. 1988. An epidemiological study of human listeriosis in Denmark 1981–1987 including an outbreak November 1985–March 1987. Tenth International Symposium on Listeriosis, Pecs, Hungary, Aug. 22–26, Abstr. 19.
157. Schlech, W. F. 1984. New perspectives on the gastrointestinal mode of transmission in invasive *Listeria monocytogenes* infection. *Clin. Invest. Med. 7*:321–324.
158. Schlech, W. F., P. M. Lavigne, R. A. Bortolussi, A. C. Allen, E. V. Haldane, A. J. Wort, A. W. Hightower, S. E. Johnson, S. H. King, E. S. Nicholls, and C. V. Broome. 1983. Epidemic listeriosis: Evidence for transmission by food. *N. Engl. J. Med. 308*:203–206.
159. Schmidt, V., and A. Nyfeldt. 1938. Ueber Mononucleosis Infectiosa und Meningoencephalitis. *Acta Oto-Laryng. 26*:680–688.
160. Schwartz, B., D. Hexter, C. V. Broome, A. W. Hightower, R. B. Hirschhorn, J. D. Porter, P. S. Hayes, W. F. Bibb, B. Lorber, and D. G. Faris. 1989. Investigation of an outbreak of listeriosis: New hypothesis for the etiology of epidemic *Listeria monocytogenes* infections. *J. Infect. Dis. 159*:680–685.
161. Schwartz, B., C. V. Broome, G. R. Brown, A. W. Hightower, C. A. Ciesielski, S. Gaventa, B. G. Gellin, L. Mascola, and the Listeriosis Study Group. 1988. Association of sporadic listeriosis with consumption of uncooked hot dogs and undercooked chicken. *Lancet ii*:779–782.
162. Seeliger, H. P. R. 1961. *Listeriosis*, Hafner Publishing Co., New York.
163. Seeliger, H. P. R. 1972. New outlook on the epidemiology and epizoology of listeriosis. *Acta Microbiol. Acad. Sci. Hung. 19*:273–286.
164. Sipka, M., B. Stajner, and S. Zakula. 1973. Detection of *Listeria* in milk. *Wien tierärztl. Monatsschr. 60*(2/3):50–52.
165. Skalka, B., J. Smola, and K. Elischerová. 1982. Different haemolytic activities of *Listeria monocytogenes* strains determined on erythrocytes of various sources and exploiting the synergism of equi-factor. *Zbl. Vet. Med. B 29*:642–649.
166. Slade, P. J., and D. L. Collins-Thompson. 1988. Enumeration of *Listeria monocytogenes* in raw milk. *Lett. Appl. Microbiol. 6*:121–123.
167. Souëf, P., N. Le, and B. N. J. Walters. 1981. Neonatal listeriosis—A summer outbreak. *Med. J. Austral. 2*:188–191.
168. Todd, E. 1988. Cost of foodborne listeriosis. Tenth International Symposium on Listeriosis, Pecs, Hungary, Aug. 22–26, Abstr. P41.
169. Tulzer, G., R. Bauer, W. D. Daubek-Puza, F. Eitelberger, C. Grabner, E. Heinrich, L. Hohenauer, M. Stojakovic, and F. Wilk. 1987. A local epidemic of neonatal listeriosis in Austria—report of 20 cases. *Klin. Pädiat. 199*:325–328.
170. Urbach, H., and G. I. Schabinski. 1955. Zur Listeriose des Menschen. *Z. Hyg. 141*:239–248.
171. Vilde, J. L., A. Huchon, M. Mignon, H. Scherrer, E. Bergogne-Berezin, and J. Pierre. 1980. Infection d'allure typique due à *Listeria monocytogenes* aprés absorption d'huîtres. *La Nouvelle Presse Médicale 9*:3281.

172. Vizcaino, L. L., M.-J. Cubero, and A. Contreras. 1988. Listeric abortions in ewes and cows associated to orange peel and artichoke silage feeding. Tenth Int. Symposium on Listeriosis, Pecs, Hungary, Aug. 22–26, Abstr. P29.
173. Vlahovic, S. M., D. Pantic, M. Pavicic, and J. H. Bryner. 1988. Transmission of *Listeria monocytogenes* from mother's milk to her baby and to puppies. *Lancet ii*:1201.
174. Vries, J., and R. Strikwerda. 1957. Ein Fall klinishcher Euter-Listeriose beim Rind. *Zbl. Bakteriol. Abt. I Orig. 167*:229–232.
175. Watson, G. L., and M. G. Evans. 1985. Listeriosis in a rabbit. *Vet. Pathol. 22*:191–193.
176. Weis, J., and H. P. R. Seeliger. 1975. Incidence of *Listeria monocytogenes* in nature. *Appl. Microbiol. 30*:29–32.
177. WHO Working Group. 1988. Foodborne listeriosis. *Bull. WHO 66*:421–428.
178. Wilesmith, J. W., and M. Gitter. 1986. Epidemiology of ovine listeriosis in Great Britain. *Vet. Rec. 119*:467–470.
179. Winkenwerder, W. von. 1967. Das Vorkommen von *Listeria monocytogenes* bei Rindern in Neidersachsen. *Berl. Münch. tierärztl. Wschr. 23*:445–449.
180. Wramby, G. O. 1944. Ovn *Listerella monocytogenes* bokteriologi ach our forekomst av listerellainfection has djur. *Skandinavisk Veterinar Tidskrift 34*:278–290.
181. Wramby, G. O. 1944. Unpublished data.
182. Yersin, B. R., M. P. Glauser, and F. Regli. 1981. Infections à *Listeria monocytogenes* chez l'adulte—Etude de 10 cas et revue de la littérature. *Schweiz. med. Wschr. 111*:1596–1602.
183. Yousef, A. E., and E. H. Marth. 1988. Behavior of *Listeria monocytogenes* during the manufacture and storage of Colby cheese. *J. Food Prot. 51*:12–15.

9

Incidence and Behavior of *Listeria monocytogenes* in Unfermented Dairy Products

INTRODUCTION

Recognition of raw milk as a potential source of *L. monocytogenes* led to speculation that consumption of such milk was at least partly responsible for the previously described listeriosis outbreak in post–World War II Germany. After this listeriosis epidemic, only scattered reports of individuals drinking raw milk, along with assurances that raw milk was being properly pasteurized, virtually eliminated the threat of any further outbreaks of milkborne listeriosis. Consequently, research in this area also subsided. However, in 1983 concerns about the possibility of milkborne listeriosis were rekindled when consumption of pasteurized milk was epidemiologically linked to an outbreak of listeriosis in Massachusetts. Two events, namely, publication of an article in the *New England Journal of Medicine* describing details of this outbreak in Massachusetts and a report in June of 1985 that as many as 300 people in California had acquired listeriosis after eating Mexican-style cheese contaminated with *L. monocytogenes*, caused concern in the United States about presence of *L. monocytogenes* in dairy products. This problem has since taken on international proportions with the 1987 report of another cheese-related outbreak in which consumption of tainted Vacherin Mont d'Or soft-ripened cheese was directly linked to numerous cases of listeriosis in Switzerland.

In response to questions raised by milk producers, dairy processors, health officials, and the general public, numerous studies have been done since 1983 to examine the incidence and behavior of *L. monocytogenes* in unfermented (raw milk, pasteurized milk, chocolate milk, cream, butter, ice cream, other frozen dairy desserts) as well as fermented (cheese, yogurt, cultured milks) dairy products. The incidence and behavior of *L. monocytogenes* in unfermented dairy products will be dealt with in this chapter; similar information about fermented dairy products appears in Chapter 11.

INCIDENCE OF *LISTERIA* SPP. IN UNFERMENTED DAIRY PRODUCTS

The recent dairy-related listeriosis outbreaks (see Chapter 8) prompted scientists worldwide to determine the extent of *Listeria* contamination in raw milk and in pasteurized dairy products such as milk, ice cream, ice cream novelties, frozen desserts, nonfat dry milk, and casein. *Listeria monocytogenes* can readily enter dairy-processing facilities in the raw milk supply, which can in turn lead to contamination of the factory environment. The occasional appearance of listeriae in pasteurized dairy products nearly always has been associated with contamination of the product after pasteurization. Thus it is fitting to begin this discussion by examining the incidence of *Listeria* spp. in raw milk, which is one source of the bacteria in the environment of the dairy factory.

Raw Milk

As you will recall from the discussion of animal listeriosis in Chapter 3, dairy cattle can intermittently shed *L. monocytogenes* in their milk as a consequence of listeric mastitis, encephalitis, or a *Listeria*-related abortion. While milk from animals showing obvious signs of listeriosis is unlikely to reach consumers, the scientific literature contains numerous accounts in which mildly infected and apparently healthy dairy cattle have shed *L. monocytogenes* intermittently in their milk for many months. Thus it appears that asymptomatic cattle as carriers of listeriae pose the greatest threat to public health.

The 1983 listeriosis outbreak in Massachusetts that was supposedly associated with drinking a particular brand of pasteurized milk raised questions about the safety of pasteurized milk. The well-publicized outbreak of 1985 in which consumption of contaminated Mexican-style cheese was directly linked to at least 40 deaths in California raised additional concerns about the safety of dairy products manufactured in the United States. Since raw milk is a potential source of *L. monocytogenes*, this fact together with recalls of *Listeria*-contaminated pasteurized dairy products (i.e., milk, chocolate milk, ice cream) and imported soft-ripened cheeses prompted a series of surveys in the United States, Canada, New Zealand, and many European countries to determine the extent to which raw milk in these countries is contaminated with *Listeria* spp. Results of these surveys, which will now be described in some detail, have been summarized in Table 9.1.

The first large-scale survey of raw milk for *Listeria* spp. was prompted by the 1983 listeriosis outbreak in Massachusetts. During the 3-week period immediately following the outbreak, Fleming et al. and Hayes et al. (70,81) examined 121 raw milk samples collected from milk trucks (40 samples), milk cooperatives (72 samples), and bulk tanks from four farms on which bovine listeriosis was diagnosed (nine samples), as well as 14 milk socks (used to remove debris but not leukocytes from milk). All samples were analyzed for *L. monocytogenes* using the multiple two-stage enrichment procedure (see Figure 6.5). Although investigators at the Centers for Disease Control isolated the epidemic serotype along with other serotypes of *L. monocytogenes* from 15 of 121 (12.4%) (including 1 of 9 bulk tank samples) (80) and 2 of 14 (14%) raw milk and milk sock samples, respectively, the epidemic phage type was never detected.

Between October 1984 and August 1985, FDA officials made a survey in which 650 raw milk samples were obtained from bulk tanks in Massachusetts, Vermont, California, and the tri-state area of Kentucky, Ohio, and Indiana. The samples were examined for *Listeria* spp. using the original FDA method (see Fig. 6.14) (88). Low levels of various *Listeria* spp., including *L. monocytogenes*, were detected in raw milk samples obtained from all states except California. Overall, 82 of 650 (12.6%) samples contained *Listeria* spp., with *L. monocytogenes* being detected in 27 of 650 (4.2%) samples. Of the 27 *L. monocytogenes* strains isolated from raw milk, 16 were serotype 1,

10 were serotye 4, and one was nontypable. In addition, only 2 of the 27 *L. monocytogenes* strains proved to be nonpathogenic to mice, and both were of serotype 4.

In 1988, Donnelly et al. (54) reported using an automated flow cytometric procedure to analyze 939 samples of raw milk obtained from 54 farms in California. Unlike the FDA study just described (88), string samples (milk pooled from 25–40 cows), combination samples (milk pooled from ~200 cows), and samples of raw milk from bulk tanks were tested for *L. monocytogenes*. Using this novel method of analysis, *L. monocytogenes* was detected in 15 of 939 (1.5%) samples of raw milk.

Researchers in Minnesota (97) and Wisconsin (56,114) failed to detect *L. monocytogenes* in raw milk during three small surveys. However, this organism was found in 4.0 and 2.8% of raw milk samples obtained from bulk storage tanks and tank trucks in Nebraska (87) and Pennsylvania (55), respectively, with approximately equal numbers of *L. monocytogenes* isolates classified as serotype 1, 4, or nontypable (non–serotype 1 or 4) in the latter study. The overall findings from Table 9.1 indicate that *L. monocytogenes* was present in 0–12.4% of the U.S. raw milk samples examined. When the results are averaged, ~3.1% of all raw milk processed in the United States can be expected to contain low levels (i.e., <10 CFU/ml) of *L. monocytogenes* at any given time. Hence, it is imperative that all milk processors take special precautions to prevent the spread of *L. monocytogenes* from raw milk to production, packaging, and other sensitive areas within the factory.

Turning to the incidence of *Listeria* in raw milk in other countries (Table 9.1), Farber et al. (61) and Slade et al. (109), respectively, isolated *L. monocytogenes* from 6 of 445 (1.3%) and 17 of 315 (5.4%) raw milk samples obtained from bulk tanks located throughout the province of Ontario, Canada. Davidson et al. (49) also reported that a similar percentage of raw milk samples collected from four local dairies and 48 farms in Manitoba contained *L. monocytogenes*. In the study by Slade et al. (109), 14 of 17 (82%) *L. monocytogenes* isolates proved to be serotype 1 with the remaining three strains classified as serotype 4. While subsequent work (69) demonstrated that none of these *L. monocytogenes* strains harbored plasmid DNA, 8 of 22 (36%) strains of *L. innocua* did carry plasmids ranging in size from 10 to 44 megadaltons. Variation in the plasmid profiles of these isolates further suggests that contamination of raw milk on the farm is an ongoing process. Whereas these authors did not quantitate *L. monocytogenes* in any of the samples examined, Slade and Collins-Thompson (108) reported that positive raw milks from bulk tanks in southwestern Ontario always contained <5 *L. monocytogenes* CFU/ml when samples were analyzed by direct plating and an MPN enrichment procedure. Thus the positive raw milk samples encountered in the three Canadian studies likely contained only low levels of *L. monocytogenes*. As was true for the three FDA surveys (88) just discussed, *L. innocua* also was he most common *Listeria* sp. isolated from Canadian raw milk, with 8.2 and 9.7% of the samples being reported as positive. Overall, 11.4 and 12.4% of all Canadian raw milk samples examined by Slade et al. (109) and Farber et al. (61) contained *Listeria* spp. as compared to 12.6% of the raw milk samples analyzed in the United States by the FDA. Thus the incidence of listeriae in raw milk from both countries appears to be nearly identical.

Public concern and economic hardships brought about by several recalls of French Brie cheese imported into the United States prompted French scientists to begin surveying raw milk for *L. monocytogenes*. Results from three such surveys (41,42,77) con-

Table 9.1 Incidence of *Listeria* spp. in Raw Milk

Location	Number of samples	Number of positive samples (%)				Ref.
		L. monocytogenes	*L. innocua*	*L. welshimeri*	Others	
USA						
Massachusetts	121	15 (12.4)	ND	ND	ND	81
Ohio, Kentucky, and Indiana	350	13 (3.7)	27 (7.7)	6 (1.5)	3[a] (0.9)	88
California	100	0	4 (4.0)	0	1[b] (1.0)	88
Massachusetts, Vermont	939	15 (1.6)	ND	ND	ND	54
California	200	14 (7.0)	19 (9.5)	0	0	88
Minnesota	84	0	6 (7.1)	1 (1.2)	0	97
Wisconsin	50	0	ND	ND	ND	56
Wisconsin	55	0	ND	0	0	114
Nebraska	200	8 (4.0)	10 (5.0)	0	0	86
Pennsylvania	2511	79 (3.1)	ND	ND	ND	55
Canada						
Ontario	445	6 (1.3)	43 (9.7)	6 (1.3)	0	61
Ontario	315	17 (5.4)	26 (8.2)	1 (0.3)	0	109
Manitoba	256	4 (1.6)	ND	ND	ND	49
France	1409	85 (6.0)	ND	ND	ND	41
France	561	~21 (3.8)	ND	ND	ND	42
France	337	14 (4.2)	5 (1.5)	0	0	77, 78
France	51	10 (19.6)	10 (19.6)	18 (35.3)	9[c] (17.6)	77, 78
Great Britain	350	~13 (3.6)	ND	ND	ND	76
Scotland	~560	14 (2.5)	7 (1.3)	0	1[d] (0.2)	68
Hungary	50	2 (4.0)	ND	ND	ND	103
Ireland	50	4 (8.0)	ND	ND	ND	83
Netherlands	137	6 (4.4)	ND	ND	ND	44
West Germany	635	2 (0.3)	ND	ND	ND	75,112
New Zealand	71	0	10 (14.1)	1 (1.4)	7[e] (9.9)	111
Total	9837	342 (3.48)	167 (6.16)	33 (1.22)	21 (0.77)	

ND = Not determined (omitted from total).
[a]2 *L. ivanovii* and 1 *L. seeligeri*.
[b]*L. ivanovii*.
[c]8 *L. seeligeri* and 1 *L. grayi*.
[d]*L. seeligeri*.
[e]7 *L. grayi*

ducted between 1986 and 1988 indicated that 85 of 1409 (6.0%), ~21 of 561 (3.8%), and 14 of 337 (4.2%) raw milk samples from French bulk tanks were positive for *L. monocytogenes* with *L. innocua* being detected in about one-third as many samples in the latter study (77). During January of 1986, 51 raw milk samples were submitted to the French Central Laboratory of Food Hygiene. Both *L. monocytogenes* and *L. innocua* were found in 19.6% of these samples. The unusually high incidence of listeriae observed in this survey, as compared to other studies described thus far, may be the result of nonrandom sampling or seasonal variations, the latter of which will be discussed shortly.

The somewhat frequent isolation of *L. monocytogenes* from both European and American dairy products prompted additional surveys of raw milk, particularly in countries with sizable dairy industries. Results from two comprehensive year-long surveys in Great Britain (76) and Scotland (68) revealed an incidence of *L. monocytogenes* in raw milk similar to that observed in the United States and Canada with actual *Listeria* populations in positive samples again estimated to be extremely low. Several small-scale surveys have uncovered *L. monocytogenes* in 4 and 8% of the raw milk produced in Hungary (103) and Ireland (83), respectively. In 1987, Beckers et al. (44) reported culturing *L. monocytogenes* from 6 of 137 (4.4%) raw milk samples obtained from farms in the Utrecht region of The Netherlands. As was true for raw milk analyzed in the United States and Canada, samples from The Netherlands contained <100 *L. monocytogenes* CFU/ml of milk. In the only other European survey reported to date, Terplan (112) detected *L. monocytogenes* in only 2 of 635 (0.3%) raw milk samples obtained from farm bulk tanks in southern Württemberg, West Germany. Subsequent attempts to isolate the pathogen from 448 quarter-milk and 30 separator sludge samples failed, along with attempts to culture this organism from raw milk samples obtained from tank trucks and storage tanks.

Nearly halfway around the world, scientists determined the incidence of *L. monocytogenes* in raw milk produced in New Zealand (111). Between August of 1986 and March of 1987, 71 raw milk samples were obtained from tank trucks that delivered milk to a local dairy factory and were analyzed for *Listeria* spp. using both warm and cold enrichment. Although *L. monocytogenes* was not found in any of the raw milk samples examined, isolation of other *Listeria* spp. from 18 of 71 (25.4%) samples strongly suggests that raw milk produced in New Zealand is unlikely to be completely free of *L. monocytogenes*.

Further examination of data summarized in Table 9.1 indicates that ~3.1, 2.7, and 4.1% of the raw milk produced in the United States, Canada, and Europe, respectively, can be expected to contain low levels of *L. monocytogenes*. With the exception of European samples, *L. innocua* was isolated from raw milk more frequently than *L. monocytogenes* with the former found in 7.2, 9.1, and 2.3% of the samples analyzed for all *Listeria* spp. in the United States, Canada, and Europe, respectively. Although *L. innocua* is nonpathogenic, isolation of this organism and other listeriae from dairy products and dairy-processing facilities is taken very seriously in the United States since nonpathogenic listeriae and *L. monocytogenes* are assumed to occur in similar environmental niches. Use in the United States of *L. innocua* as a potential indicator of *L. monocytogenes* is supported by data from the raw milk surveys just described (Table 9.1) in that isolation of listeriae other than *L. monocytogenes* from dairy products and processing facilities suggests that the factory environment may be contaminated with

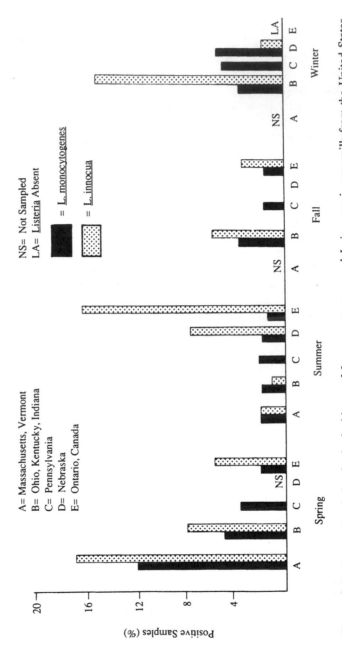

Figure 9.1 Seasonal variation in the incidence of *L. monocytogenes* and *L. innocua* in raw milk from the United States (55,81,86,88) and Canada (61).

raw milk, i.e., a product that can be expected to contain *L. monocytogenes* 3–4% of the time.

In addition to assessing the general incidence of listeriae in raw milk, several of the surveys just described also dealt with seasonal variations in the incidence of *L. monocytogenes* and *L. innocua* in raw milk produced in the United States (55,86,88) and Canada (61). However, since all of the aforementioned studies differ in numbers and sizes of samples analyzed as well as the *Listeria* isolation procedures employed, it is difficult to make any definitive statement concerning the seasonal occurrence of *Listeria* in raw milk (68,109). Nonetheless, several distinct trends can be observed from selected data in Fig. 9.1. First, the overall incidence of *L. monocytogenes* in raw milk was highest in spring (6.3%) followed by winter (5.0%), fall (2.8%), and summer (1.9%). Second, a somewhat similar seasonal variation also can be observed for the incidence of *L. innocua* in raw milk with the highest overall percentage of positive samples again occurring in spring (10.3%) followed by winter (8.5%), summer (6.8%), and fall (4.9%).

Using the following formula:

$$\frac{\text{Overall \% of samples containing } L.\ innocua}{\text{Overall \% of samples containing } L.\ monocytogenes} = \text{innocua/monocytogenes (IM) ratio}$$

IM ratios of 1.63, 3.37, 1.75, and 1.87 can be calculated for raw milk samples collected during spring, summer, fall, and winter, respectively. The higher incidence of *L. innocua* in summer samples from bulk tanks located throughout Ontario, Canada, is responsible for what appears to be an unusually high IM ratio during this period. An IM ratio of 1.83 is obtained when the Canadian data for summer are omitted from calculations. Thus, except for raw milk analyzed during the summer, the percentage of samples containing *L. innocua* outnumbered that of samples containing *L. monocytogenes* by IM ratios of 1.63–1.87. These findings again suggest the possibility of using *L. innocua* as a potential indicator for the presence of *L. monocytogenes*.

Although not fully understood, current herd management and feeding practices may be at least partly responsible for seasonal differences observed in isolation rates for *L. monocytogenes* and possibly *L. innocua*. During cold winter months, dairy cattle are normally fed silage as a major component of the diet. While investigating a listeriosis outbreak, Donnelly (52) observed that 8 of 44 Holstein cows fed *Listeria*-contaminated silage shed the organism in their milk. Furthermore, milk from these animals was free of *L. monocytogenes* 1 month after consumption of contaminated silage ceased. As you will recall from Chapter 3, ruminants that ingest contaminated silage may either succumb to infection or carry *L. monocytogenes* asymptomatically; however, if the animal lives, the organism can be shed for many months in feces and in milk if the animal is lactating. Extended survival of *L. monocytogenes* in fecal material, soil and grass can lead to perpetuation of the infectious cycle shown in Fig. 9.2, particularly when animals are wintered in cramped quarters. Once dairy cattle can resume grazing on pastures during late spring, summer, and early fall, *L. monocytogenes* becomes dispersed over a wide area, which, in turn, weakens the infectious cycle by decreasing the likelihood that animals will come in contact with contaminated material.

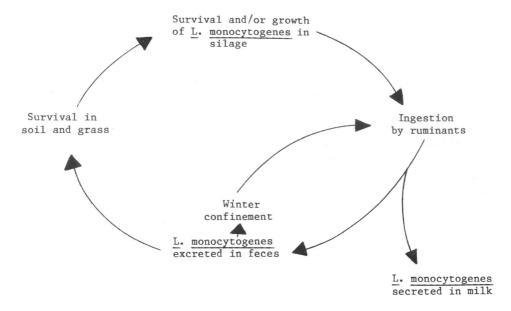

Figure 9.2 Infective cycle for maintaining *L. monocytogenes* in ruminants.

Seasonal differences in the incidence of *Listeria* spp. in raw milk also may be related to breeding practices. Dairy cattle typically bear their young in late winter or early spring. During winter gestation, dairy cattle develop a weakened immune system as a direct result of pregnancy, which, in turn, makes these animals more susceptible to listeric infections and abortions. These events can then culminate in the shedding of *L. monocytogenes* in milk and fecal material. Increased environmental stress and changes in habitat that occur during winter, along with increased difficulties in providing proper herd hygiene, all can serve to decrease the natural defense system in dairy cattle, which again increases the likelihood for listeric infections. Once an asymptomatic animal begins shedding *L. monocytogenes* in feces, the organism is likely to spread quickly to other animals that are housed in close proximity to the shedder. In this way, confinement of dairy cattle may play an important role in increasing the number of animals that shed *L. monocytogenes* in their milk during late winter and early spring.

Pasteurized Milk and Other Unfermented Dairy Products

The dairy industry has long been considered the most regulated food industry in the United States. The FDA was given responsibility under the Food, Drug and Cosmetic Act and the Public Health Service Act to assure the public that this country's milk supply is both uniformly safe and wholesome. Dairy sanitation laws and regulations, including microbiological criteria for some dairy products, enforced by the FDA and state agencies are based almost exclusively on the Public Health Service/FDA Grade A Pasteurized Milk Ordinance.

In the United States, pasteurized milk and other unfermented dairy products prepared from pasteurized milk, including ice cream, butter, and nonfat dry milk, generally have earned a reputation for being both safe and nutritious with one recent report indicating that consumption of pasteurized milk is responsible for ≤5% of all reported milk-related illnesses (92). Despite these impressive findings, public confidence in the safety of pasteurized milk began to erode in July of 1982 as the result of an outbreak of yersiniosis in Tennessee, Arkansas, and Mississippi, and again in 1983 when the CDC claimed that consumption of pasteurized milk was responsible for 49 cases of listeriosis in Massachusetts. In 1985 the dairy industry was dealt another blow when at least 16,000 culture-confirmed cases of salmonellosis were associated with drinking a particular brand of pasteurized milk produced in the Chicago area.

These three outbreaks, along with the previously discussed outbreak of listeriosis in California linked to consumption of contaminated Mexican-style cheese, prompted the FDA to take corrective action in the form of a large-scale testing program commonly referred to as the FDA Dairy Initiative Program (85) (Fig. 9.3). This program, begun in April of 1986 in cooperation with individual state agencies and members of the National Conference on Interstate Milk Shipments, was designed to examine every interstate milk shipment (IMS) pasteurization facility in the United States for potential safety problems related to pasteurization, postpasteurization contamination, cleaning and sanitizing regimens, equipment maintenance, and educational/training programs for dairy factory personnel. As part of the FDA Dairy Initiative Program, the FDA also established the Microbiological Surveillance Program, which was designed to detect *L. monocytogenes*, *Salmonella* spp., *Yersinia enterocolitica*, *Campylobacter jejuni*, and *Campylobacter coli* (*Campylobacter* omitted in 1987) as well as *Staphylococcus aureus*, which was added in 1987 for dry and fluid milk (14). Dairy products tested under this program included fluid milks, nonfat dry milk, cream, butter, ice cream, ice milk, and other dairy commodities over which the FDA has jurisdiction. Analysis of cheeses (except cottage cheese) was covered under a series of separate programs, which will be discussed in the next chapter dealing with fermented dairy products. Under provisions of this program, FDA inspectors collected 30 retail-sized containers of as many as five different products available from dairy factories at the time of inspection. Duplicate 25-g or 25-ml samples obtained after combining 30 retail-sized samples per product were then analyzed for *L. monocytogenes* and other listeriae using the original and later versions of the FDA procedure (see Figs. 6.14 and 6.15).

Since raw milk containing *L. monocytogenes* is likely to enter every dairy factory in the United States at one time or another, it is logical to assume that finished products also may become contaminated with this pathogen. During the first 2 years of the FDA Dairy Initiative Microbiological Surveillance Program (Table 9.2), *L. monocytogenes* was isolated from 2 of 350 samples of pasteurized whole milk and 5 of 415 samples of chocolate milk, which suggests that approximately 0.67% of the pasteurized milk available in the United States could contain this pathogen unless corrective measures in factories serve to reduce this value. In contrast, *L. monocytogenes* was isolated from 3 of 99, 23 of 659, and 30 of 351 samples of ice milk, ice cream, and novelty ice cream, respectively. Only two of the positive ice cream samples were analyzed quantitatively for *L. monocytogenes*. One contained an average of 15 *L. monocytogenes* CFU/g, whereas the other sample contained between 1 and 5 CFU/g. Thus during the time of this survey approximately 5% of frozen dairy products manufactured in the United States may have contained low levels of *L. monocytogenes*.

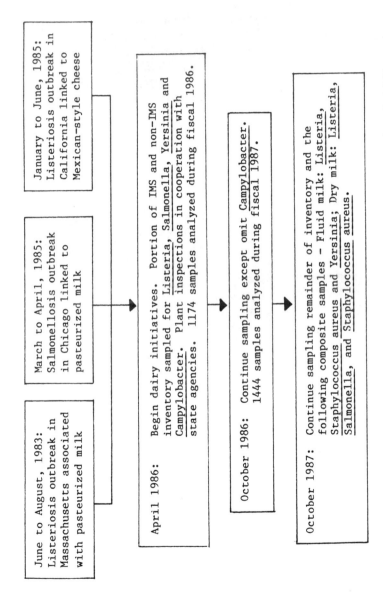

Figure 9.3 FDA Dairy Initiatives Program. IMS = Interstate Milk Shipment. (Adapted from Ref. 85.)

Table 9.2 Incidence of *Listeria* spp. in Unfermented Dairy Products Manufactured in the United States during 1986 and 1987

Product	Number of samples tested	Number of positive samples (%)	
		L. monocytogenes	*L. innocua*
Whole milk	350	2 (0.57)	0
Lowfat milk	182	0	2 (1.10)
Skim milk	98	0	0
Chocolate milk	415	5 (1.20)	1 (0.24)
Cream	52	0	0
Half and half	42	0	0
Ice milk	99	3 (3.03)	0
Ice cream	659	23 (3.03)	12[a] (1.82)
Novelty ice cream	351	30 (8.55)	10[b] (2.85)
Butter	30	0	0
Nonfat dry milk	44	0	0
Casein/Milk protein hydrolysate	15	0	0
Other products[c]	171	0	0
Total	2,518	63 (2.50)	25 (0.99)

[a]*L. seeligeri* also detected in 7 of 659 (1.06%) samples.
[b]*L. grayi* also detected in 1 of 351 (0.28%) samples.
[c]Dairy blend whey, eggnog.
Source: Ref. 43.

Furthermore *L. innocua* was isolated from 3 of 4 product categories (Table 9.2) which also contained samples positive for *L. monocytogenes*. Since both organisms likely occupy similar niches in the natural environment and dairy-processing facilities, isolation of *L. innocua* from a dairy product should raise immediate concerns about possible presence of *L. monocytogenes*.

Greater success in isolating *L. monocytogenes* from chocolate rather than whole milk is likely related to the organism's ability to grow better in this product than in other fluid dairy products. Reasons for enhanced growth of *Listeria* in chocolate milk will be discussed shortly in conjunction with the behavior of listeriae in autoclaved fluid dairy products.

The higher incidence of *L. monocytogenes* in frozen rather than fluid dairy products coincides with the relatively complex handling of ice milk, ice cream, and particularly ice cream novelties during manufacture and packaging. This, in turn, suggests that these products were most likely contaminated after pasteurization through either direct or indirect contact with listeriae within the dairy factory environment. This hypothesis is supported by frequent isolations of *L. monocytogenes* from many areas within dairy factories including floors, ceilings, drains, and coolers. In addition, this organism also has been found in air and condensate and on various pieces of equipment including conveyor belts. A detailed discussion of the incidence of *L. monocytogenes* in food-processing facilities, including dairy factories, can be found in Chapter 15.

Inability of the FDA to detect *L. monocytogenes* in skim and lowfat milk as well as half and half, cream, and butter may have resulted from the separation processes for adjustment of milkfat content that these products undergo. Such centrifugal separation processes tend to decrease levels of listeriae in these products, particularly if leukocytes containing the organism are still present after initial clarification of the milk.

Failure to isolate *L. monocytogenes* from nonfat dry milk and casein/protein hydrolysates may be partly related to the heat treatments necessary to manufacture these products. This theory is supported by the work of Doyle et al. (57), who demonstrated that populations of *L. monocytogenes* decreased ≥90% during conversion of skim milk into nonfat dry milk via spray drying. However, failure to isolate *L. monocytogenes* from dried dairy products also may result from the generally recognized inability of the FDA method to detect cells of *L. monocytogenes* that have been sublethally injured during thermal processing. Thus, as described in Chapter 6, the methodology employed to detect *L. monocytogenes* will predetermine whether or not the organism can be isolated from a particular food product.

According to the Food, Drug and Cosmetic Act of 1938, a food may be considered adulterated and therefore unfit for human consumption if the product contains poisons or other harmful substances (e.g., pathogenic microorganisms) at detrimental concentrations. Although the oral infective dose for *L. monocytogenes* is presently unknown, evidence from the California listeriosis outbreak involving Mexican-style cheese suggests that the number of *L. monocytogenes* cells needed to induce this life-threatening illness may be quite low—perhaps as few as several hundred to a few thousand total cells for certain segments of the population. While not directly applicable to the human population, several independent studies involving immunocompromised mice have demonstrated LD_{50} values (the dose of cells which is lethal to 50% of a given population) in the range of approximately 10 (79) and 4 to 480 (48,110) *L. monocytogenes* cells when the pathogen was administered orally and intraperitoneally, respectively. Consequently, because of a moral obligation to the public, the FDA has adopted and is continuing to uphold a policy of "zero tolerance" regarding presence of *L. monocytogenes* in ready-to-eat foods.

In accordance with Title 21 of the United States Code of Federal Regulations, Section 7.40 (71), the FDA can request that firms voluntarily recall any product that contains or is suspected of containing *L. monocytogenes*. These recalls can be classified into one of three categories: Class I, Class II, or Class III. A Class I recall, which is the most serious, is defined by the FDA as "a situation in which there is a reasonable probability that the use of or exposure to a violative product will cause serious adverse health consequences or death." Thus far, all recalls issued for products contaminated with *L. monocytogenes* have been categorized as Class I. In the unlikely event that a firm fails to comply with the FDA's request to recall a product contaminated with *L. monocytogenes*, FDA officials can (a) initiate a seizure request in the U.S. District Court to have the product removed from commerce (Title 21 Code of Federal Regulations, Section 334) or (b) obtain a legal injunction to halt production and distribution of the contaminated product (Title 21 Code of Federal Regulations, Section 332). In addition, the FDA also can take criminal action against individuals of a company who are responsible for commercial distribution of a contaminated product.

Adoption of the FDA Dairy Initiative Microbiological Surveillance Program in April of 1986 fostered the beginning of a series of recalls issued for milk and unfermented dairy products contaminated with *L. monocytogenes* (Table 9.3). Just one month after the surveillance program began, a California firm voluntarily recalled an unknown quantity of ice milk mix contaminated with *L. monocytogenes*. During the same month, approximately 1 million gallons of fluid dairy products comprised of milk, chocolate milk, half and half, whipping cream, ice milk mix, ice milk shake mix, and ice cream mix also were recalled in Texas (9,10). However, other than this single incident, the remaining 26 recalls issued before January 1990 have been confined almost exclusively to frozen dairy products such as ice cream, ice cream novelties, ice milk, and sherbet.

In July of 1986, a large recall of *Listeria*-contaminated ice cream bars received considerable media attention, which in turn did much to enhance the state of hysteria concerning presence of *L. monocytogenes* in dairy products (3). The following month another nationwide recall was issued for frozen dairy products. As a result of this recall, approximately 1 million gallons of products possibly contaminated with *L. monocytogenes* and including ice cream (132 flavors), ice milk (16 flavors), sherbet (9 flavors), and gelati-da products (6 flavors) were reportedly buried at a Minnesota landfill site. A similar recall also was issued in 1987 for contaminated ice cream, ice milk, and sherbet manufactured in Iowa (24,28). While well over 500 *Listeria*-contaminated dairy products have been voluntarily recalled in the United States at a total cost to the dairy industry of well over $70 million (27,91), corrective measures instituted by the dairy industry in response to governmental pressure have markedly reduced both the extent of *Listeria* contamination in processing facilities and the number of Class I recalls issued for *L. monocytogenes*-contaminated dairy products during 1988 and 1989 (42). However, product losses are likely to be substantially underreported since under certain circumstances, manufacturers can retrieve their own product without issuing a formal Class I recall. In one such instance, a manufacturer of *Listeria*-contaminated ice cream was not required to issue a formal recall because the product had not yet reached the consumer (32). Additional cases also likely occurred in which contaminated products moved only as far as the company's warehouse and were recalled internally by the manufacturer.

Despite millions of gallons of frozen dairy products that have been recalled both formally and internally, it must be stressed that no cases of listeriosis have yet been attributed to consumption of frozen dairy products contaminated with *L. monocytogenes*. On this basis, the International Ice Cream Association and the Milk Industry Foundation both contend that a Class I recall may be too harsh a response for a frozen dairy product containing presumably a very low level of *L. monocytogenes*. However, until the oral infectious dose for susceptible individuals can be firmly established, the FDA is likely to maintain a "zero tolerance" level for *L. monocytogenes* and continue requesting recalls of products containing this pathogen at any detectable level.

The United States government has developed one of the most stringent policies regarding presence of *L. monocytogenes* in ready-to-eat foods, whereas most other countries have adopted more relaxed policies, particularly where consumption of contaminated products that have not yet been firmly linked to cases of listeriosis is

Table 9.3 Chronological List of Voluntary Class I Recalls Issued in the United States During 1986 and 1987 for Milk and Unfermented Dairy Products Contaminated with *L. monocytogenes*

Type of dairy product	Month/year of recall	State of manufacture	Distribution	Quantity	Ref.
Ice milk mix	5/86	California	Arizona, Nevada, California	Unknown	7,9
Milk (2% & ½% fat), chocolate milk, chocolate milk (2% fat), half and half, whipping cream, vanilla and chocolate ice cream mix, ice milk shake mix, and ice cream mix	5/86	Texas	Texas	~1 million gal.	9,10
Ice cream bars	7/86	Virginia	Eastern United States	Large but unknown	3
Ice cream, sherbet	7/86	Wisconsin	Wisconsin	8,000 gal.	114
Ice cream (132 favors), ice milk (16 flavors), sherbet (9 flavors), gelati-da products (6 flavors)	8/86	Minnesota	Illinois, Indiana, Iowa, Kentucky, Michigan, Minnesota, North Missouri, North Dakota, Ohio, South Dakota, Wisconsin	~1 million gal.	6,8,11
Ice cream and ice cream novelties—bars, drumsticks, slices, sundaes	8/86	Iowa	Illinois, Iowa, Minnesota, Missouri, North Dakota, Wisconsin	Unknown	4
Ice cream	9/86	Wisconsin	Wisconsin	Unknown	5
Ice cream	12/86	New York	New York	~835 gal.	23,28
Ice cream	12/86	West Virginia	West Virginia, Ohio	450 gal.	13,24
Ice cream, ice milk, sherbet	1/87	Iowa	Arkansas, Delaware, Illinois, Iowa, Kansas, Maryland, Minnesota, Missouri, Nebraska, Oklahoma, Pennsylvania, South Dakota, Wisconsin	~1 million gal.	13,17,28
Ice cream	4/87	New York	New York, Pennsylvania	~316 gal.	25,28
Ice cream (48 flavors), ice milk (6 flavors), sherbet (5 flavors)	7/87	California	California, Oregon	~60,000 gal.	18,38

Product	Date	Origin	Distribution	Amount	Ref.
Ice cream nuggets	7/87	Maryland	Connecticut, Florida, Maryland, New Jersey, New York, North Carolina, Ohio, Pennsylvania, Virginia	20,400 boxes	19,26
Ice cream, ice milk	7/87	Nebraska	Colorado, Iowa, Kansas, Nebraska, North Dakota, South Dakota, Wyoming	~30,000 gal.	15
Ice cream sundae cones	8/87	Florida	Alabama, Arizona, British West Indies, Florida, Louisiana, Mississippi, North Carolina, Ohio, Puerto Rico, South Carolina, Tennessee, Virginia, West Virginia	Unknown	20
Chocolate ice cream	8/87	Kentucky	Florida, Puerto Rico	~956 gal.	12
Ice cream nuggets	9/87	Maryland	Nationwide	Unknown	21
Ice cream novelties—sandwiches, bars, pieces, slices, sundae cones	9/87	Ohio	Nationwide	Unknown	22
Ice cream bars	10/87	Ohio	Michigan, Ohio, Pennsylvania, West Virginia	51,780 bars	16
Chocolate ice cream	2/88	Georgia	Georgia, North Carolina	Unknown	30,33
Ice cream, sherbet, ice milk	7/88	Ohio	Ohio	>1,083 gal.	29
Ice cream	8/88	Connecticut	Connecticut, New York, Massachusetts	5.6–8.4 gal.	35
Ice cream	8/88	Connecticut	Connecticut	30 gal.	34
Ice cream pies	9/88	Connecticut	Connecticut, New York, Massachusetts	1,700 pies	31
Ice cream	9/88	Pennsylvania	Pennsylvania	215 gal.	36
Ice cream bars	12/88	New York	New York	~128 gal.	39
Ice cream	2/89	Connecticut	Connecticut	Unknown	40

concerned. Exemplary of the latter attitude, the Canadian government has decided to confine all formal recalls to only those foods that have been linked to major outbreaks of listeriosis, namely, coleslaw, soft cheese, and pasteurized milk, with the role of pasteurized milk in foodborne listeriosis still highly debatable (83). Hence, no recalls were issued when researchers at the Health Protection Branch of Health and Welfare Canada (analogous to the U.S. FDA) identified *L. monocytogenes* in 1 of 394 (0.25%) and 1 of 51 (2.0%) samples of ice cream and ice cream novelties, respectively (60), during their own federal inspection program. While subsequent investigations were presumably conducted to identify (a) the source of contamination, (b) proper corrective measures, and (c) possible links to human illness, Canadian officials maintained that recall of the two contaminated lots would be inappropriate without proof that consumption of *Listeria*-contaminated ice cream can lead to listeriosis. Many individuals and most manufacturers will undoubtedly argue in favor of the more relaxed Canadian position; however, it is our opinion that the presence of even small numbers of *L. monocytogenes* in any ready-to-eat food including ice cream constitutes a potential health risk to certain individuals including pregnant women, immunocompromised adults, and the elderly. Therefore, we believe that all governments should exercise their right and moral obligation to remove such potentially hazardous products from the hands of unsuspecting consumers.

As a result of several large recalls of French Brie cheese and a listeriosis outbreak in Switzerland that was traced to consumption of Vacherin Mont d'Or soft-ripened cheese, European scientists have logically focused their attention on the incidence of listeriae in cheese. However, numerous recalls of unfermented dairy products in the United States also have heightened public health concerns about the presence of listeriae in European dairy products other than cheese.

In one of the few European surveys reported thus far, researchers in Germany (112) failed to isolate *Listeria* spp. from pasteurized milk (39 samples), nonfat dry milk (11 samples), casein/caseinate (30 samples), and various dried products such as baby food (120 samples). Similar small surveys in Hungary (64) and The Netherlands (45) also failed to recover *L. monocytogenes* from 50 and 41 samples of pasteurized milk, respectively. However, *L. monocytogenes* was demonstrated as present in 12 of 1000 (1.2%) and 3 of 150 (2.0%) samples of pasteurized milk and ice cream, respectively, during a nationwide survey of dairy products produced in Great Britain (76). These latter findings are somewhat similar to those previously observed in the United States (Table 9.2). Although these preliminary results generally appear encouraging, the isolation methods used in most of these studies probably were unable to detect sublethally injured listeriae. To enhance recovery of injured cells, the International Dairy Federation has recommended that products such as pasteurized milk, nonfat dry milk, dried whey, dried buttermilk, casein, and caseinate undergo preenrichment in a nonselective medium (e.g., buffered peptone water) before subenrichment in various selective broths and plating on *Listeria*-selective media (113).

In response to the listeriosis outbreak linked to consumption of Vacherin Mont d'Or soft-ripened cheese, the Federal Dairy Research Institute in Switzerland began analyzing raw milk, pasteurized milk, dried milk, milk drinks, milk shakes, milk additives (i.e., fruits, chocolate powder, spices, cereals), raw cream, and all types of ice cream for listeriae (83,84). Members of the International Dairy Federation recently suggested

Table 9.4 Percentage of Pasteurized and Raw Milk
Samples from Spain Containing *Listeria* spp.

Species of *Listeria*	Positive samples (%)	
	Pasteurized milk[a,b]	Raw milk[c]
L. monocytogenes	21.4	45.3
L. grayi	89.2	89.5
L. innocua	10.7	15.8
L. welshimeri	3.6	3.1
L. seeligeri	0	1.1
L. ivanovii	0	0
L. murrayi	0	0
L. denitrificans	0	0

[a]$n = 28$.
[b]Commercially pasteurized at 78°C/15 sec.
[c]$n = 95$.
Source: Refs. 72, 104.

examining raw milk (from cows and other species), raw cream, pasteurized milk (cow
and other species), pasteurized cream, ice cream, milk shakes, dried milk, and other
refrigerated dairy products for *Listeria* spp. Results from these surveys will serve to more
accurately define the extent of *Listeria* contamination in unfermented European dairy
products and also will shed new light on the public health aspects of foodborne listeriosis
in Europe.

Thus far results from only one additional European survey dealing exclusively with
the incidence of listeriae in unfermented dairy products have been reported in the
literature. Working in Spain, Garayzabal et al. (72) examined pasteurized milk sold by
a milk-processing factory in central Madrid for listeriae. As shown in Table 9.4, 21.4%
of the samples contained strains of *L. monocytogenes*, all of which were pathogenic to
mice. In addition, 89.2 and 10.7% of the pasteurized milk samples contained *L. grayi*
and *L. innocua*, respectively, either alone or in combination with *L. monocytogenes*.

These data indicate that the incidence of *L. monocytogenes* in pasteurized milk is
considerably higher in Spain (21.4%) than in other parts of the world ($\leq1.2\%$). From
these results one can conclude that either *L. monocytogenes* was initially present in the
raw milk and survived pasteurization or that the pathogen entered the product after
pasteurization. In this study, pasteurized milk from which *L. monocytogenes* was isolated
was commercially processed using an HTST pasteurizer set to operate at 78°C/15
seconds. One year later, Garayzabal et al. (74) reported that *L. monocytogenes* would
not survive pasteurization when milk was inoculated to contain 3.2×10^6 to 1.2×10^8
freely suspended listeriae CFU/ml and processed in a pilot plant-sized pasteurizer at
≥73°C/15 seconds. Although there is some disagreement as to whether or not *L.
monocytogenes* is more heat resistant when in leukocytes than when freely suspended
in raw milk, the scientific community unanimously agrees that both intracellular and
freely suspended cells of *L. monocytogenes* will not survive pasteurization under the

conditions that were used to process raw milk at this Madrid dairy plant—78°C/15 seconds.

Hence, the only other explanation for the high incidence of *L. monocytogenes* in this pasteurized milk is that the product was contaminated after pasteurization. When Garayzabal et al. (72) surveyed pasteurized milk for listeriae, the same authors (104) also analyzed samples of commingled raw milk from the same dairy factory for *Listeria* spp. (Table 9.4). *Listeria monocytogenes* and *L. grayi* were found in 45.3 and 89.5% of the raw milk samples examined, respectively. If one assumes that the raw milk received by the dairy factory was of similar quality during both studies, it appears that pasteurization of raw milk at 78°C/15 seconds eliminated *L. monocytogenes* from only approximately 50% of the samples analyzed. Even more striking is the fact that approximately 89% of both raw and pasteurized milk samples contained *L. grayi*. In another survey by Garayzabal et al. (73) that was designed to examine the seasonal incidence of *L. monocytogenes* in raw milk, 30 of 67 (44.8%) samples that presumably came from the same dairy factory in Madrid also contained *L. monocytogenes*. Furthermore, these samples of raw milk had total mesophilic aerobic plate counts of 2.5×10^7 CFU/ml, well above the maximum allowable, 1×10^6 CFU/ml, for manufacturing grade milk in the United States. Milk of such quality cannot be used to produce pasteurized fluid milk in the United States and so is of reduced commercial value.

After weighing the evidence presented, one must conclude that the unusually high incidence of *L. monocytogenes* (and other *Listeria* spp.) in pasteurized milk processed at the dairy factory in Madrid, Spain, is the result of postpasteurization contamination. Numerous reports indicate that *L. monocytogenes* has been isolated from floors, drains, walls, ceilings, coolers, and other locations within dairy factories in the United States. Thus there is ample opportunity for this organism to enter dairy products after pasteurization. In addition to the milk becoming contaminated through direct contact with the dairy factory environment, Northolt et al. (94) also speculated that leaks in the pasteurizer plates may have been be responsible for the unusually high incidence of *L. monocytogenes* in pasteurized milk from this particular dairy factory.

According to results from an International Dairy Federation Survey published in March of 1989 (83), public health concerns regarding presence of listeriae in unfermented (and particularly fermented) dairy products are beginning to spread beyond the continental boundaries of Europe and North America. Following the 1987 discovery of *L. monocytogenes* in Australian ricotta cheese, New Zealand and Australia instituted *Listeria* monitoring programs for casein/caseinate products and high moisture cheese, pasteurized milk, ice cream, and milk powders, respectively. Results from one 10-month survey begun in April 1988 (115) revealed the presence of *L. monocytogenes* in 1 of 206 (0.48%) samples of pasteurized flavored/unflavored milk processed in and around Melbourne, Australia. Subsequent identification of the heat-labile alkaline phosphatase in the contaminated product (pasteurized milk to which a pasteurized flavored syrup was added) suggested that improper pasteurization was most likely responsible for presence of *L. monocytogenes* in the final product. However, unsatisfactory storage of the flavored syrup also may have contributed to contamination. In keeping with *Listeria* policies developed in the United States and Canada, Australian officials withdrew the affected product from the marketplace and prohibited the sale of all subsequently produced product until 12 consecutive lots of *Listeria*-free pasteurized flavored milk could be produced from the same product line.

BEHAVIOR OF *L. MONOCYTOGENES* IN UNFERMENTED DAIRY PRODUCTS

Although the psychrotrophic nature of *L. monocytogenes* and the ability of both normal and diseased animals to shed this pathogen in their milk have been recognized for many years, behavior of *L. monocytogenes* in raw milk and unfermented dairy products did not receive serious attention until 1983 when an outbreak of "milkborne" listeriosis was reported in Massachusetts. Research efforts prompted by this and two other dairy-related outbreaks in the United States and Switzerland have given us an understanding of the behavior of *L. monocytogenes* in raw and pasteurized milk as well as in chocolate milk, cream, nonfat dry milk, and butter. The remaining pages of this chapter will describe results from these studies along with preliminary data concerning behavior of this organism in ultrafiltered milk and ice cream mix.

Raw Milk

Despite long-time recognition of *L. monocytogenes* as a contaminant of raw milk, relatively few studies assessing the behavior of this organism in raw milk can be found in the literature. In 1958, Dedie (50) found that *L. monocytogenes* survived 210 days in naturally contaminated raw milk stored in an ice chest. Thirteen years later, Dijkstra (51) reported results from a much longer storage study in which 36 samples of naturally contaminated raw milk (obtained from cows that experienced *Listeria*-related abortions) were stored at 5°C and examined for viable *L. monocytogenes* over a period of 9 years. While 4 of 36 (11%) samples were free of *L. monocytogenes* within 6 months, the pathogen was still detected in 16 of 36 (44%) samples following 2 years of refrigerated storage. The number of samples from which listeriae could be isolated continued to decrease with 9 of 36 (25%) samples reported positive after 4 years of storage. However, the pathogen was still present in 4 of 36 (11%) raw milk samples after 8–9 years of refrigerated storage. These early findings emphasize the importance of establishing proper cleaning and sanitizing programs for all phases of milk production. If routinely used, such programs will likely prevent this organism from finding an appropriate niche within the farm or dairy factory environment and greatly reduce the threat of long-term survival by the pathogen.

The studies just described adequately demonstrate that *L. monocytogenes* can persist in raw milk for long periods; however, until several outbreaks of milkborne and cheeseborne listeriosis were reported in the 1980s, little attention had been given to the potential for growth of *L. monocytogenes* in raw milk.

In 1988 Northolt et al. (94) examined the behavior of listeriae in samples of freshly drawn raw milk that were inoculated to contain approximately 500 *L. monocytogenes* CFU/ml and incubated at 4 and 7°C. As shown in Figure 9.4, *Listeria* populations decreased approximately 4- and 8.5-fold in raw milk during the first 2 days of incubation at 4 and 7°C, respectively. These authors suggested that naturally occurring bacterial substances in raw milk (i.e., lactoperoxidase and lysozyme) may have partially inhibited

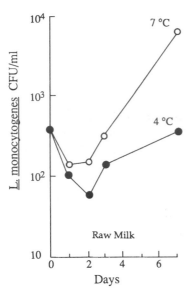

Figure 9.4 Growth of *Listeria monocytogenes* strains in raw milk incubated at 4 and 7°C (enumerated on Trypaflavine Nalidixic Acid Serum Agar). (Adapted from Ref. 94.)

growth of listeriae during the first 2 days of incubation. However, in a Canadian study which will be discussed shortly (62), no such decrease was observed when incubated samples of naturally contaminated raw milk were surface-plated on FDA Modified McBride Listeria Agar. Hence, a more likely explanation is that the plating medium (Trypaflavine Nalidixic Acid Serum Agar) used by Northolt et al. (94) was less than ideal for recovering listeriae, as also was observed during concurrent work with pasteurized milk. Although *L. monocytogenes* failed to grow in raw milk samples incubated at 4°C for up to 7 days, *Listeria* populations increased approximately 10-fold during this period when the incubation temperature was raised to 7°C. Following 3 days of incubation at 4 and 7°C, *Listeria* populations began doubling every 3.5 and 1 day, respectively.

Since *L. monocytogenes* failed to grow until the third day of incubation at 7°C, the authors concluded that the 3-day period during which raw milk is sometimes held in farm bulk tanks is insufficient to allow growth of the organism. However, the temperature of raw milk in farm bulk tanks will fluctuate every time freshly drawn raw milk at 37°C is commingled with milk tank milk at ~4°C from previous milkings. In 1985, Oz and Farnsworth (96) found that raw milk in farm bulk tanks attained temperatures of 30–31°C, 10–14°C, 12°C, and 9°C when freshly drawn raw milk was added after the first, second, third, and fourth milking periods, respectively. More important, 6 hours were generally needed for the milk to cool to 4°C after each milking period. In view of these findings, it appears that temperatures obtained after adding warm raw milk to farm bulk tanks may be sufficient to allow at least limited growth of *L. monocytogenes*, particularly when raw milk enters bulk tanks during early milking periods. While the temperature of bulk tank milk will eventually decrease to ~4°C, exposure to temperatures as high as 9°C when raw milk is trucked to processing facilities during summer (63) also may lead to some multiplication of the pathogen.

Discovery of a naturally infected cow in Canada that continuously shed freely suspended and phagocytized cells of *L. monocytogenes* in milk (maximum of 10^4 CFU/ml in milk from one of four quarters of the mammary gland) for nearly 3 years provided Farber et al. (62) with a unique opportunity to study growth of *L. monocytogenes* in naturally rather than artificially contaminated raw milk during extended storage at various temperatures. When raw milk from this cow was analyzed for numbers of *L. monocytogenes*, no appreciable growth of the pathogen was observed during the first 3 days and 1 day of incubation at 4 and 10°C, respectively (Fig. 9.5). The delay in onset of growth was less than 1 day at 15°C. Immunological staining of milk smears indicated that some multiplication of *L. monocytogenes* had occurred within macrophages after 1 and 2 days of incubation at 15 and 10°C, respectively, with 10–50% of the macrophages containing 1–20 intracellular listeriae. Nonetheless, as previously noted by Doyle et al. (58), rapid deterioration of macrophages shortly thereafter was followed by appearance of freely suspended listeriae in milk with few intact macrophages remaining after 5 days, regardless of incubation temperature. Following the lag phase, *L. monocytogenes* entered a period of logarithmic growth with generation or doubling times of 25.3, 10.8, and 7.4 hours calculated for raw milk samples held at 4, 10, and 15°C, respectively. Although maximum populations of *L. monocytogenes* were approximately 2×10^7 CFU/ml after 10, 7, and 3 days of incubation at 4, 10, and 15°C, respectively, the maximum achievable population in raw milk was independent of

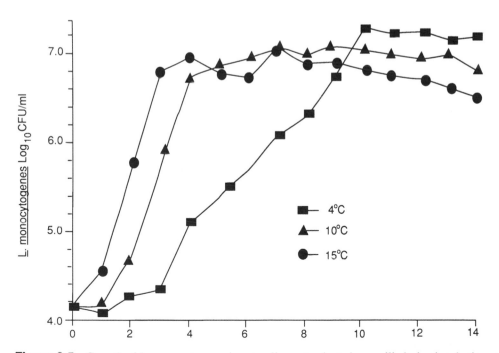

Figure 9.5 Growth of *L. monocytogenes* in naturally contaminated raw milk during incubation at 4, 10, and 15°C. (Adapted from Ref. 62.)

incubation temperature (Fig. 9.6). As in the previous study by Northolt et al. (94), these findings again stress the importance of maintaining raw milk at ≤4°C during storage and transport to milk-processing facilities.

Investigations dealing with behavior of listeriae in raw milk have not been limited to cow's milk. Reports of ovine listeriosis in Europe prompted Ikonomov and Todorov (82) to examine the behavior of *L. monocytogenes* in raw ewe's milk inoculated with the pathogen. Their results show that *L. monocytogenes* remained viable for long periods and persisted in the milk even after coagulation at 10 and 20°C. In 1987, a pregnant woman in the United States reportedly aborted after consuming feta cheese contaminated with *L. monocytogenes*. Since feta and other cheeses such as Roquefort, Manchego, Gjeost, and Chachcaval are traditionally manufactured from ewe's or goat's milk, interest in the behavior of listeriae in these milks as well as in ethnic-type cheeses manufactured from these milks will probably increase in the future.

Pasteurized and Intensively Pasteurized Milk

In addition to defining the growth pattern of *L. monocytogenes* in artificially contaminated raw milk (Fig. 9.4), Northolt et al. (94) also examined behavior of this organism in pasteurized (72°C/15 seconds) and intensively pasteurized whole milk (Fig. 9.6). Although *L. monocytogenes* failed to grow in raw milk incubated at 4°C (Fig. 9.4), *Listeria* populations in pasteurized milk increased nearly 10-fold during 7 days of incubation at the same temperature. The organism also grew markedly faster in pasteur-

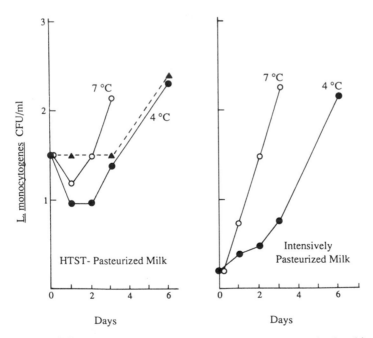

Figure 9.6 Growth of *L. monocytogenes* in HTST-pasteurized and intensively pasteurized milk incubated at 4 and 7°C. ——: Enumerated on Trypaflavine Nalidixic Acid Serum Agar; – – –: Enumerated on Nutrient Agar. (Adapted from Ref. 94.)

ized than in raw milk when both products were incubated at 7°C. In contrast to their data for raw and pasteurized milk, lag times for *L. monocytogenes* were reduced considerably when the organism was grown in intensively pasteurized milk incubated at 4 and 7°C. Furthermore, numbers of listeriae in intensively pasteurized milk increased approximately 100-fold following 3 and 6 days of incubation at 7 and 4°C, respectively. These results indicate that the growth rate for *L. monocytogenes* in milk is directly related to the degree of heat applied to milk. Further work is needed to more clearly define the effect of competing microorganisms on growth of listeriae in raw and pasteurized milk as compared to intensively pasteurized milk. However, biochemical changes that occur in milk during thermal processing (i.e., protein denaturation, enzyme inactivation, carmelization) also might influence growth of listeriae in this product.

Autoclaved Milk, Cream, and Chocolate Milk

Except for the two studies just described (62,94) and an initial attempt by Pine et al. (102) to follow growth of *L. monocytogenes* in inoculated samples of pasteurized milk, all remaining work dealing with behavior of *Listeria* in fluid dairy products has been done using autoclaved samples. While using such sterile products as growth media for listeriae offers several major advantages, including the ability to accurately quantitate both stressed and unstressed listeriae on nonselective plating media in the absence of other microbial contaminants, the reader should keep in mind that growth rates of *L. monocytogenes* are likely to be somewhat faster in autoclaved than in pasteurized or especially in raw milk products. Nevertheless, *L. monocytogenes* clearly can grow to dangerously high levels in all three types of milk during extended refrigeration.

In 1987, Rosenow and Marth (106) published results from a definitive study in which autoclaved (121°C/15 min) samples of whole, skim, and chocolate milk as well as whipping cream were each inoculated separately with four strains of *L. monocytogenes* (Scott A, V7, V37CE, or California), incubated at 4, 8, 13, 21, or 35°C and examined for numbers of listeriae at suitable intervals by surface plating appropriate dilutions on Tryptose Agar. Growth rates of *L. monocytogenes* were generally similar in all four products at a given temperature and increased with an increase in incubation temperature. At 4°C, listeriae began growing after an initial delay of approximately 5–10 days, depending on the bacterial strain and type of product (Fig. 9.7). All four strains generally attained maximum populations of $\geq 10^7$ CFU/ml after 30–40 days of incubation with little change in numbers occurring after 30–40 days of additional storage. Overall, chocolate milk supported development of the highest populations of *Listeria*, followed by skim milk, whole milk, and whipping cream. Generation times for growth at 4°C ranged between 28.16 and 45.55 hours. Average generation times for *L. monocytogenes* in all four products are shown in Table 9.5. While these results clearly demonstrate the ability of *L. monocytogenes* to grow to potentially hazardous levels in fluid dairy products held at 4°C, more recent data suggest that slow growth of this organism can even occur in milk held as low as 0°C. Thus the only way to avoid a public health problem with fluid dairy products is to prevent *L. monocytogenes* from entering such products before, during, and after manufacture.

Increasing the incubation temperature from 4 to 8°C decreased the lag period to 1.5–2 days (Fig. 9.8) and nearly tripled the growth rate for *L. monocytogenes* in all four

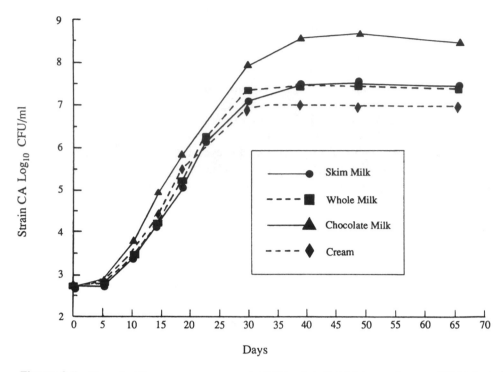

Figure 9.7   Growth of *L. monocytogenes* strain California in fluid dairy products at 4°C. (Adapted from Ref. 106.)

Table 9.5   Generation Times for *L. monocytogenes* in Autoclaved Samples of Various Dairy Products

Product	Generation time (h) at				
	4°C[a]	8°C[a]	13°C[a]	21°C[b]	35°C[b]
Whole milk	33.27	13.06	5.82	1.86	0.692
Skim milk	34.52	12.49	6.03	1.92	0.693
Chocolate milk	33.46	10.56	5.16	1.72	0.678
Whipping cream	36.30	11.93	5.56	1.80	0.683

[a]Average generation times for 4 strains of *L. monocytogenes*.

products (Table 9.5) (106). After 10–14 days of incubation, the growth curves at 4 and 8°C were similar with highest *Listeria* populations again found in chocolate milk. Theoretical calculations based on these data indicate that *Listeria* populations could increase from 10 to 4.2×10^6 organisms/quart (947 ml) of milk during 10 days of storage at 8°C (46°F), a temperature that commonly occurs in some home and commercial refrigerators. These findings raise additional safety concerns about reclaiming and reprocessing returned products that have likely undergone some degree of temperature abuse.

As is true for 8°C, 13°C (55°F) also represents a temperature that dairy products occasionally encounter during transportation and storage. Following a 12-hour lag period, all four *Listeria* strains grew nearly twice as fast at 13°C as at 8°C (Table 9.5) and generally attained levels of $\geq 10^6$ CFU/ml in all four products by the third day (106). These generation times are somewhat longer than those observed by Farber et al. (62) when naturally contaminated raw milk was incubated at 4 (25.3 h), 10 (10.8 h), and 15°C (7.4 h). *L. monocytogenes* also attained maximum populations that were approximately 10-fold lower in raw than in sterile milk, which in turn suggests possible depletion of essential nutrients by raw milk contaminants or production of substances inhibitory to growth of the pathogen. Maximum *Listeria* populations of $\sim 10^9$ CFU/ml were again observed in chocolate milk with numbers generally 10-fold lower in skim milk, whole

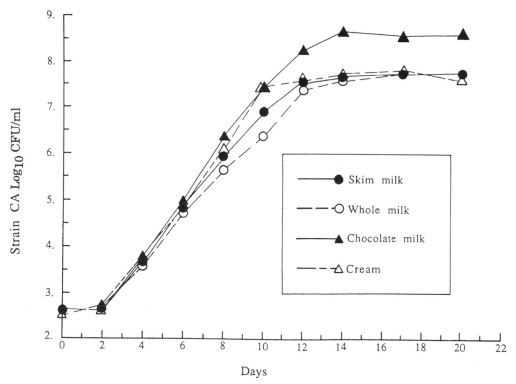

Figure 9.8 Growth of *L. monocytogenes* strain California in fluid dairy products at 8°C. (Adapted from Ref. 106.)

milk, and whipping cream (106). Increasing the incubation temperature to 21°C doubled the growth rate (Table 9.5) and led to maximum *Listeria* populations of 10^8–10^9 CFU/ml within 48 hours. As expected, *L. monocytogenes* grew most rapidly at 35°C with populations of 10^8–10^9 CFU/ml being observed after only 24 hours of incubation.

In another study examining the influence of temperature and milk composition on growth of listeriae, Donnelly and Briggs (53) found that five *L. monocytogenes* strains began growing in inoculated samples of autoclaved (121°C/10 min) whole, skim, and reconstituted nonfat dry milk (11% total solids) after approximately 24–48, 2–24, 4–12, and 0.5–4 hours of incubation at 4, 10, 22, and 37°C, respectively. Although growth rates for all *Listeria* strains were primarily determined by the incubation temperature, two strains of *L. monocytogenes* serotype 4b grew considerably faster in whole rather than skim or reconstituted nonfat dry milk during incubation at 4 and 10°C. These observations led Donnelly and Briggs (53) to suggest a possible relationship between levels of milkfat and the growth rate of *L. monocytogenes* in milk during refrigerated storage. Furthermore, these authors suggested that enhanced psychrotrophic growth in whole milk may be related to a listerial lipase produced by both β-hemolytic strains of *L. monocytogenes* serotype 4b. Unlike both of these strains, the three remaining *L. monocytogenes* strains of serotypes 1 and 3 failed to exhibit enhanced growth in whole milk at 10°C and had little if any hemolytic activity on McBride Listeria Agar containing sheep blood.

In contrast to what might be expected from the study just described, Rosenow and Marth (106) failed to observe any significant difference in growth rates among four strains of *L. monocytogenes* (two serotype 4b, two serotype 1) when they were incubated in autoclaved samples of whole and skim milk at 4, 8, 13, 21, and 35°C. The pathogen also attained lower maximum populations in whipping cream than in whole, skim, or chocolate milk at all incubation temperatures. In support of these findings, Marshall and Schmidt (89) failed to observe enhanced growth of *L. monocytogenes* strain Scott A (serotype 4b) in whole rather than skim milk during 8 days of incubation at 10°C. Finally, in a study to be discussed in greater detail in the next chapter (107), four strains of *L. monocytogenes* (three serotype 4b and one serotype 1) frequently attained higher maximum populations in whey samples that were defatted by centrifugation, filter sterilized, and incubated at 6°C than would be expected to occur in autoclaved skim milk, whole milk, or whipping cream after prolonged incubation at 8°C. While conflicting results between these three studies (89,106,107) and the work of Donnelly and Briggs (53) might be partly explained on the basis of different *L. monocytogenes* strains and milk sources, one must presently conclude that psychrotrophic growth of *L. monocytogenes* is not generally enhanced by the normal level of milk fat found in fluid milk.

Recognizing the vital importance of carbohydrates in microbial metabolism, researchers at the Centers for Disease Control (102) attempted to define growth of *Listeria* spp. in terms of sugar utilization. An initial experiment using aerobically incubated broth media indicated that five strains of *L. monocytogenes* and one strain each of *L. innocua*, *L. seeligeri*, and *L. ivanovii* utilized only the glucose moiety of lactose, whereas single strains of *L. grayi* and *L. murrayi* utilized both the glucose and galactose of lactose. Overall, maximum cell populations, as determined by optical density, were directly proportional to the concentration of glucose (≤0.125%) in the growth medium. However, marked differences were observed in the ability of *L. monocytogenes* and *L. innocua* to

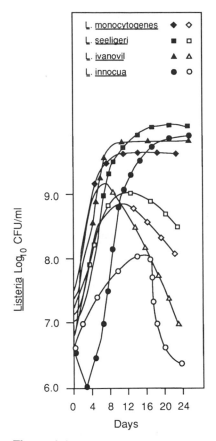

Figure 9.9 Growth of *Listeria* spp. in pasteurized (open symbols) and autoclaved whole milk (solid symbols) incubated at 5°C. (Adapted from Ref. 102.)

utilize lactose, with three strains of *L. monocytogenes* (isolated from Mexican-style cheese in connection with the 1985 listeriosis outbreak in California) unable to grow in a medium containing lactose as the only carbohydrate.

Growth of *L. monocytogenes* in autoclaved samples of whole and skim milk was generally similar to that previously observed by Rosenow and Marth (106) with maximum populations of $\leq 5 \times 10^8$ CFU/ml developing after extended incubation at 5 and 25°C. Except for *L. seeligeri*, the behavior of *L. innocua* and *L. ivanovii* did not differ markedly from that of *L. monocytogenes* in these samples (Fig. 9.9). However, as noted by Northolt et al. (94), higher maximum populations and increased survival rates were again observed when these organisms were grown in autoclaved rather than pasteurized whole milk. Examination of milk by gas-liquid chromatography indicated that lactic, acetic, isobutyric, isovaleric, and 2-hydroxy isocaproic acid were formed during incubation. Since this milk initially contained ~81–85 mg of glucose/L, the aforementioned acids likely resulted at least in part from fermentation of glucose. Since considerably lower populations of *L. monocytogenes* as well as *L. innocua*, *L. grayi*, and *L. murrayi* also developed in glucose oxidase–treated (an enzyme that degrades glucose) rather than

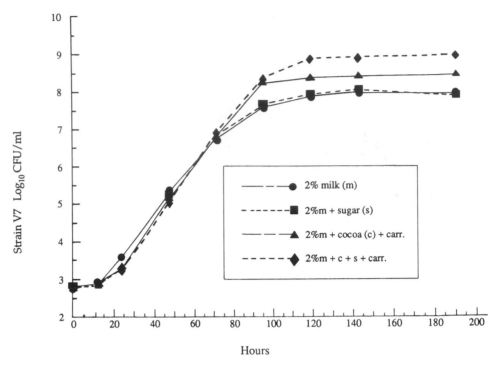

Figure 9.10   Growth of *L. monocytogenes* strain V7 in 2% fat milk with added sugar, cocoa, and carrageenan (carr.) at 13°C. (Adapted from Ref. 105.)

untreated milk during both aerobic and anaerobic incubation, it is evident that glucose is one of the major substrates for growth of listeriae in milk. However, when incubated anaerobically in glucose oxidase–treated milk, two lactose-negative *L. monocytogenes* isolates from Mexican-style cheese still attained final populations of ~10^8 CFU/ml, thus suggesting the involvement of other as yet unidentified growth factors.

In the aforementioned study by Rosenow and Marth (106), maximum populations of *L. monocytogenes* were usually approximately 10-fold higher in chocolate milk than in other fluid dairy products. To explain the enhanced growth of *L. monocytogenes* in chocolate milk, several investigators at the University of Wisconsin have examined the effect of major chocolate milk constituents (i.e., cocoa, sugar, and carrageenan) on growth of this organism in autoclaved skim milk and laboratory media. Rosenow and Marth (105) found that growth of *L. monocytogenes* at 13°C was only slightly enhanced in skim milk containing 5% cane sugar, and the organism attained higher final populations when commercial cocoa power (1.3%) and carrageenan stabilizer (0.5%) were used in place of cane sugar (Fig. 9.10). Carrageenan also enhanced the growth rate of *L. monocytogenes* in the presence of cocoa; however, the organism attained similar maximum populations regardless of the presence or absence of carrageenan. These findings suggest that carrageenan may be more important in increasing contact between cocoa particles and *Listeria* than as a source of nutrients. Highest final populations and shortest generation times were observed when *L. monocytogenes* was grown in skim milk containing cocoa, sugar, and carrageenan. In addition, maximum *Listeria* populations obtained in skim milk containing all three ingredients (Fig. 9.10) were similar to populations observed in initial work with commercially produced chocolate milk (Figs. 9.7 and 9.8).

Subsequently, Pearson and Marth (98) examined growth of *L. monocytogenes* strain V7 at 13°C in skim milk containing various concentrations of cocoa, sugar, and carrageenan. Since some *Listeria* strains can utilize sucrose, it is not surprising that *L. monocytogenes* developed significantly higher final populations (Fig. 9.11) and had shorter generation times (5.05 vs. 5.17 h) as the concentration of cane sugar (sucrose) in skim milk was increased from 0 to 12%. [Peters and Liewen (101) also reported that addition of 7% sucrose to ultrafiltered (concentrated) skim milk caused maximum *L. monocytogenes* populations to increase rather than decrease.] A near-linear relationship between increasing sugar concentration and maximum attainable populations of *L. monocytogenes* also was observed for all but one combination of sugar, cocoa, and carrageenan tested, i.e., 12% sugar and 0.03% carrageenan (Fig. 9.11). While addition of 0.03% carrageenan significantly lengthened generation time and decreased the maximum population compared to those observed in skim milk without carrageenan, *L. monocytogenes* achieved highest populations in skim milk containing 0.75% cocoa with or without carrageenan, which in turn indicates that the apparent ability of cocoa to stimulate growth of this organism in skim milk containing 0–12% sugar is independent of carrageenan. Since there are only trace amounts of fermentable carbohydrates in cocoa, these authors theorized that cocoa enhanced growth of *L. monocytogenes* in skim milk by providing increased levels of peptides and amino acids, particularly valine, leucine, and cysteine, which are reportedly essential for growth of this organism. Additional work showed that agitation, combined with the presence of cocoa, sugar,

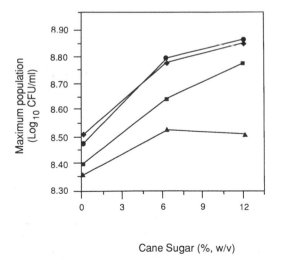

Cane Sugar (%, w/v)

Figure 9.11 Maximum *L. monocytogenes* populations in skim milk alone (■), skim milk + carrageenan (▲), skim milk + cocoa (●), and skim milk + cocoa + carrageenan (◆) with 0, 6.5, and 12.0% cane sugar after 36 hours of incubation at 13°C. Any two points differing by ≥ 0.07 $\log_{10}$ CFU/ml (length of bar) are significantly different ($p < 0.05$). (Adapted from Ref. 98.)

and/or carrageenan in skim milk, enhanced growth of the pathogen at 30°C when compared to growth in the same medium that was incubated quiescently. However, growth of *Listeria* in skim milk alone was better without rather than with agitation. Thus, agitation most likely increased the availability of extractable nutrients from cocoa, which in turn led to enhanced growth of the pathogen.

In 1968, anthocyanins in cocoa were reported to inhibit growth of salmonellae in laboratory media; however, the inhibitory effect of cocoa could be neutralized with casein (47). These early findings prompted Pearson and Marth (100) to investigate the effect of cocoa with and without casein on growth of *L. monocytogenes* strain V7. Using Modified Tryptose Phosphate Broth containing 0.2% tryptose, addition of 0.75–10% cocoa increased the generation time for *L. monocytogenes* at 30°C (1.02–1.12 h) as compared to samples without cocoa (0.94 h). However, the pathogen generally attained higher populations when grown in media with (1.1–1.5 × 10^9 CFU/ml) rather than without (6.4 × 10^8 CFU/ml) cocoa. Interestingly, when the same medium was inoculated to contain ~10^5 *L. monocytogenes* CFU/ml and agitated, the pathogen decreased to nondetectable levels in samples containing 5–10% cocoa after 15–24 hours of incubation at 30°C. Nonetheless, the organism readily grew in the presence of 0.75% cocoa and attained higher maximum populations in media with (1.9 × 10^9 CFU/ml) rather than without (7.6 × 10^8 CFU/ml) cocoa during agitated incubation at 30°C.

As previously reported for salmonellae, presence of 1.5 or 3.0% casein neutralized the inhibitory effect of cocoa toward *L. monocytogenes*, with the pathogen exhibiting shorter lag phases and higher maximum populations in media containing both casein and 5.0% cocoa rather than cocoa alone and incubated quiescently at 30°C. However, results obtained during agitated incubation of cultures containing 5.0% cocoa were far more dramatic with *L. monocytogenes* populations of 2.9 × 10^9 rather than <10 CFU/ml developing in samples with rather than without 2.5% casein. Hence, these findings suggest that the behavior of *L. monocytogenes* in laboratory media containing cocoa partially depends on the concentration of one or more inhibitory substances that can be neutralized by casein and that are more readily extracted during agitated rather than quiescent incubation.

Furthermore, Pearson and Marth (99) determined if theobromine and caffeine, i.e., two methylxanthine compounds in cocoa that reportedly possess different degrees of antimicrobial activity, were responsible for the previously observed antilisterial activity of cocoa. Overall, addition of 2.5% theobromine to both Modified Tryptose Phosphate Broth and autoclaved skim milk with and without 0.5% caffeine did not markedly influence the behavior of *L. monocytogenes* during incubation at 30°C. This suggests that theobromine is not responsible for suppressing or enhancing growth of listeriae in chocolate milk. Unlike theobromine, addition of 0.5% caffeine to Modified Tryptose Phosphate Broth doubled or tripled the length of the organism's lag phase, nearly doubled the organism's generation time, and led to maximum *Listeria* populations approximately 10-fold lower than those obtained in caffeine-free media. Similar trends also were observed when autoclaved skim milk instead of Modified Tryptose Phosphate Broth served as the growth medium. Thus, while caffeine within cocoa may contribute to inhibition of *L. monocytogenes* in a broth medium, failure of casein within skim milk to neutralize the inhibitory effect of cocoa indicates that caffeine also is not responsible for inhibition of listeriae as observed in the previous study. Such efforts to identify

Listeria-active components within cocoa should be continued to better understand the behavior of this pathogen in chocolate milk.

Sweetened Condensed and Evaporated Milk

To our knowledge, *Listeria* spp. have not yet been isolated from commercially produced sweetened condensed milk (i.e., a nonsterile concentrated fluid milk product containing approximately 64% sucrose or glucose in the water phase, 8.5% milk fat, and 28% total milk solids) or evaporated milk (an unsweetened commercially sterile concentrated fluid milk product containing approximately 7.9% milk fat and 25.9% total milk solids). However, given the widespread incidence of *Listeria* in food-processing facilities, it is conceivable that listeriae could enter both of these products as postprocessing contaminants. Such concerns prompted Farrag et al. (67) to examine the fate of three *L. monocytogenes* strains in samples of commercially produced sweetened condensed and evaporated milk that were inoculated to contain three different levels ($\sim$$10^3$–$10^7$ CFU/ml) of the pathogen.

Regardless of initial inoculum, *Listeria* populations in sweetened condensed milk decreased $\leq$1.2 and 1.6–3.4 orders of magnitude following 42 days of storage at 7 and 21°C, respectively. This behavior was not surprising since addition of sugar to this product during manufacture reduces its water activity (a_w) to $\sim$0.83, well below the minimum a_w value of 0.932 reported for growth of *L. monocytogenes*. Unlike sweetened condensed milk, the relatively high a_w value for evaporated milk ($\sim$0.986) allowed profuse growth of listeriae with lowest inoculum levels increasing approximately 4 orders of magnitude after 7 and 14 days of incubation at 21 and 7°C, respectively. In addition, no decrease in numbers of listeriae was noted during continued incubation at either temperature. [Preliminary results obtained by El-Gazzar et al. (59) also indicate that *L. monocytogenes* behaves similarly in unsweetened milk concentrated 5-fold by ultrafiltration.] Thus, since *L. monocytogenes* can survive >42 days in sweetened condensed milk and grow rapidly in evaporated milk, special precautions should be taken to prevent listeriae from entering these products during packaging, storage, and subsequent use.

GROWTH OF *L. MONOCYTOGENES* IN MIXED CULTURES

Except for several early works assessing the behavior of *L. monocytogenes* in raw and pasteurized milk, all studies described thus far have dealt with growth of *L. monocytogenes* in the absence of competitive microorganisms. While results from these studies have been of great value to the dairy industry, one should remember that pasteurized dairy products are not sterile. Psychrotrophic bacteria, mostly in the genus *Pseudomonas*, are normally present in raw milk and, like *L. monocytogenes*, can grow in milk at refrigeration temperatures both before and after milk is pasteurized. Although pseudomonads are readily destroyed during pasteurization, these organisms universally appear in pasteurized dairy products as postpasteurization contaminants, often at levels > 100 CFU/ml. Since *L. monocytogenes* is thought to enter dairy products primarily after pasteurization, products that contain low levels of listeriae (probably <10 CFU/ml) will likely contain higher populations of other psychrotrophs. Although the ability of psy-

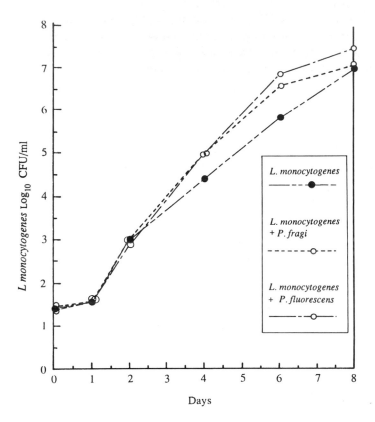

Figure 9.12 Growth of *Listeria monocytogenes* at 10°C in whole milk preincubated for 3 days with selected *Pseudomonas* spp. (Adapted from Ref. 89.)

chrotrophic pseudomonads to stimulate growth of nonpathogenic as well as pathogenic bacteria in dairy products has been recognized for more than 25 years, until recently no information was available on behavior of *L. monocytogenes* in mixed cultures.

After initial work (65) with Tryptose Broth demonstrated that growth of *L. monocytogenes* was slightly inhibited by the presence of *Pseudomonas fluorescens* (see Chapter 5), Farrag and Marth (66) examined associative growth of *L. monocytogenes* (strains Scott A, CA, and V7) with *P. fluorescens* (strains P26 and B52) in autoclaved (121°C/15 min) skim milk that was inoculated to contain equal populations ($\sim 10^5$ CFU/ml) of both organisms and incubated at 7 or 13°C for 56 days. Growth of *L. monocytogenes* was generally enhanced by the presence of *P. fluorescens* after 7 days of incubation with the pathogen attaining populations of $\sim 10^7$ CFU/ml in mixed cultures. However, continued incubation at 7°C led to lower numbers of listeriae in mixed rather than pure cultures with populations of strain V7 inhibited approximately 8-fold by *P. fluorescens* B52 following 56 days of storage. When the incubation temperature was increased to 13°C, growth of *L. monocytogenes* was neither enhanced nor inhibited by either *Pseudomonas* strain during the first 7 days of incubation. However, after 56 days of incubation final populations of *Listeria* were up to 20-fold lower in mixed rather than pure culture. While these overall findings indicate that *P. fluorescens* was more detrimental to survival of listeriae in skim milk stored at 13 than 7°C, growth and survival of *P. fluorescens* was not appreciably affected by presence of *L. monocytogenes* with pseudomonads consistently reaching populations of 10^8–10^9 CFU/ml. In a similar study, Marshall and Schmidt (89) found that growth of *L. monocytogenes* strain Scott A (used in the previous study) in autoclaved skim and whole milk was not enhanced by the presence of *Pseudomonas fragi* during 8 days of incubation at 10°C. Similarly, growth of *P. fragi* also was unaffected by *L. monocytogenes*.

Some researchers have speculated that psychrotrophic pseudomonads may be able to utilize some of the nutrients in milk faster than *L. monocytogenes*, thus suppressing growth of listeriae in milk during refrigerated storage. Marshall and Schmidt (89) investigated this theory by inoculating samples of autoclaved whole milk, skim milk, and reconstituted nonfat dry milk (10% solids) with *P. fragi* or *P. fluorescens* (strain T25, P26, or B52); incubating the samples for 3 days at 10°C to obtain $\sim 10^6$–10^7 *P. fragi* CFU/ml or 10^4–10^6 *P. fluorescens* CFU/ml; inoculating these *Pseudomonas* cultures with *L. monocytogenes* and then incubating the samples for an additional 8 days at 10°C. Throughout this study, addition of listeriae to all milks preincubated with *P. fluorescens* or *P. fragi* did not significantly affect growth or survival of either pseudomonad. However, as shown in Fig. 9.12, *L. monocytogenes* grew faster and attained higher final populations in samples of whole milk that were preincubated with either of the two pseudomonads than in whole milk that was not treated with pseudomonads. *L. monocytogenes* behaved similarly in both whole and skim milk with average generation times of approximately 7 and 8 hours in milks preincubated with *P. fluorescens* and *P. fragi*, respectively (Fig. 9.13). Although accelerated growth of *Listeria* was observed in reconstituted nonfat dry milk preincubated with either pseudomonad, generation times for listeriae in either of the two mixed cultures generally did not differ significantly. As was true for whole and skim milk, *L. monocytogenes* attained populations of 1×10^7 to 5×10^7 CFU/ml in reconstituted nonfat dry milk with highest numbers occurring in milk preincubated with *P. fluorescens* rather than *P. fragi*.

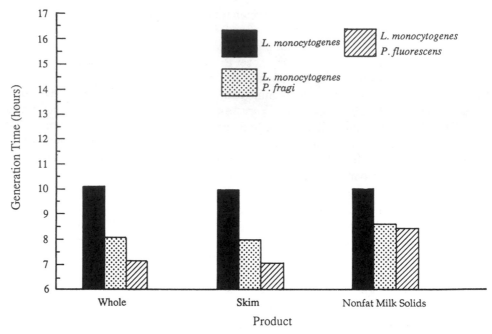

Figure 9.13   Generation times of *Listeria monocytogenes* at 10°C in various milks preincubated for 3 days with *P. fragi* or *P. fluorescens* spp. (Adapted from Ref. 89.)

These results dispel the previous theory and indicate that *L. monocytogenes* can readily compete with both *P. fragi* and *P. fluorescens* for nutrients in milk and at the same time can outgrow these pseudomonads at refrigeration temperatures even if the ratio of *L. monocytogenes* to pseudomonads is on the order of 1:100,000. Enhanced growth of microorganisms, including *L. monocytogenes*, in the presence of psychrotrophic *Pseudomonas* spp. is generally thought to be related to increased levels of nutrients that occur in milk as a result of proteolytic enzymes produced by pseudomonads. Since many of these enzymes are heat stable and able to survive pasteurization, raw milk must be handled properly and pasteurized within a reasonable time (i.e., 3–4 days) to prevent conditions that may favor growth of listeriae. As previously noted (94), enhanced growth of listeriae in intensively pasteurized as compared to HTST-pasteurized and raw milk also might be related to this phenomenon.

NONFLUID DAIRY PRODUCTS

While the aforementioned studies demonstrate the ability of *L. monocytogenes* to grow to potentially hazardous levels in fluid dairy products held at refrigeration temperatures, concern about the behavior of this organism in dairy products extends well beyond fluid milks and cream. As you will recall from Table 9.3, at least 26 recalls have been issued in the United States for *Listeria*-contaminated ice cream. These recalls, along with FDA reports suggesting that about 3.5% of the ice cream and 8.5% of the ice cream novelties produced in the United States may be contaminated with presumably low levels of *L.*

monocytogenes, have prompted research on the fate of listeriae in frozen dairy products. Additionally, the behavior of *Listeria* during manufacture and storage of nonfat dry milk and butter also has been investigated in the event that these products are inadvertently prepared from skim milk and cream, respectively, that have been contaminated after pasteurization.

Ice Cream

Frequently, pasteurized milk that has not been sold in retail stores is returned to dairy factories and reprocessed into chocolate ice cream. Since large commercial refrigeration units often fail to maintain a constant temperature of 4°C, virtually all reclaimed milk has undergone some degree of temperature abuse during the period in which the product was on sale. In addition to possible growth of *L. monocytogenes* during this 2-week period of "cold enrichment," pseudomonads also can grow in milk and produce an environment that is more favorable for growth of *Listeria*, even after pasteurization.

These observations led Berrang et al. (46) to investigate the behavior of *L. monocytogenes* in inoculated samples of chocolate ice cream (and chocolate milk as discussed earlier) prepared from fresh skim milk and commercial skim milk that was held beyond the expiration date. While growth of listeriae was certainly not expected in ice cream stored at −18 to −24°C, preliminary results indicate that the pathogen survived equally well in both types of chocolate ice cream. Hence, use of returned milk in chocolate ice cream did not appear to enhance survival of *L. monocytogenes* in this product.

In addition to this study, Amelang and Doores (1,2) recently determined generation times for *L. monocytogenes* in nine formulations of commercially produced ice cream mix that varied in type and level of fat (cream, butter), sugar (cane sugar, corn sweetener), and milk solids (condensed milk, skim milk, whey powder). To simulate postprocessing contamination, all samples were inoculated to contain ~10^3 *L. monocytogenes* strain Scott A or V7 CFU/ml and incubated at 4, 21, and 35°C. Overall, *L. monocytogenes* had average generation times of 21.6, 1.08, and 0.79 hours in ice cream mixes incubated at 4, 21, and 35°C, respectively, with similar growth rates occurring in mixes containing 10, 14, and 15% fat and held at the same temperature. It is noteworthy that these generation times are markedly shorter than those calculated by Rosenow and Marth (137) for growth of the same strains in whole milk, skim milk, chocolate milk, and whipping cream (Table 9.5). Although *L. monocytogenes* generally behaved similarly in all ice cream mixes incubated at 4 and 21°C, differences in generation times were noted at 35°C when the pathogen was cultured in ice cream mixes made with alternative fat and milk solids. At 35°C, growth of listeriae was somewhat enhanced in mixes containing butter rather than cream, skim milk powder or whey powder rather than condensed skim milk, and egg yolk as an additional source of solids. While the pathogen grew most rapidly in ice cream mix containing a 50:50 ratio of cream to butter, partial replacement of cane sugar (sucrose: glucose + fructose) with corn sweetener (glucose and maltose) or high fructose corn syrup failed to significantly shorten generation times.

Butter

In 1988 Olsen et al. (95) examined the fate of *L. monocytogenes* during manufacture and storage of butter in the event that the product is prepared from contaminated cream.

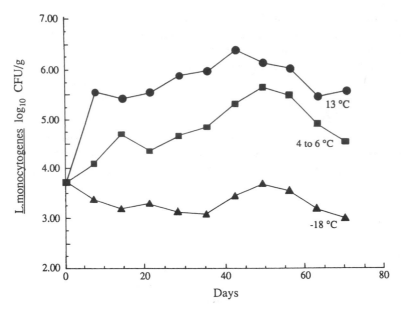

Figure 9.14   Survival of *L. monocytogenes* in butter manufactured from artificially contaminated cream and stored at 12, 4–6, and –18°C. Each line represents the average of 4 trials. (Adapted from Ref. 95.)

According to their report, pasteurized cream was inoculated to contain 10^4–10^5 *L. monocytogenes* CFU/g and churned into butter. After removing the buttermilk, washed butter grains were salted to a level of 1.2% and resultant butter was analyzed weekly for listeriae during 10 weeks of storage at –18, 4–6, and 13°C. During manufacture ~95% of the *L. monocytogenes* population was lost in buttermilk with the remaining 5% of the population appearing in butter. The pathogen was present at levels of 1.7×10^4 to 1.8×10^5 CFU/g in cream as compared to 1.5×10^3 to 1.6×10^4 CFU/g in butter, indicating that like *Staphylococcus aureus* (93), *L. monocytogenes* also favors the water, rather than lipid phase during butter making. As shown in Fig. 9.14, *Listeria* populations increased 1.9 and 2.7 orders of magnitude in butter stored at 4–6 and 13°C, with maximum numbers observed after 49 and 42 days of storage, respectively. These results indicate that enough milk solids were trapped in the water phase (containing ~6% salt) to support growth of listeriae at refrigeration temperatures. Numbers of listeriae then began to decrease; however, the organism was still present at levels $>10^4$ CFU/g following 70 days of refrigerated storage. While freezing the contaminated butter prevented growth of *L. monocytogenes*, the organism was still present at levels of ~10^3 CFU/g after 70 days of storage at –18°C. When considering these data, it must be remembered that Olsen et al. (95) dealt with laboratory-produced butter, which probably had larger moisture droplets than does commercially produced butter. This may have contributed to growth of *L. monocytogenes* in the experimental butter.

Thus far *L. monocytogenes* has not been isolated from pasteurized cream manufactured in the United States; however, given the massive *Listeria* recall of Texas-produced fluid dairy products, including half and half and whipping cream, in May of 1986

(Table 9.3), one cannot assume that all pasteurized cream and butter manufactured in the United States and elsewhere will be universally free of listeriae. As you will recall from Chapter 8, one recent cluster of listeriosis cases in southern California has already been attributed to consumption of contaminated butter (90). Hence, since growth of *L. monocytogenes* has been demonstrated experimentally in both cream and butter during refrigerated storage, it is necessary to ensure that cream is pasteurized and that recontamination of pasteurized cream is prevented before and during its churning into butter.

Nonfat Dry Milk

Dried dairy products, including nonfat dry milk, whey, and casein, also may become contaminated with pathogenic microorganisms, both before and after drying. Such concerns have been raised most recently in Australia and New Zealand (83). Although all dry dairy products examined thus far have been *Listeria*-free, methods used to detect listeriae in these surveys were generally unable to recover cells that may have been injured during the drying process.

Two factors, namely the unusual thermal resistance of *L. monocytogenes* and the report of a milkborne listeriosis outbreak in Massachusetts during 1983, prompted Doyle et al. (57) to examine behavior of *L. monocytogenes* during manufacture and storage of nonfat dry milk. Samples of concentrated (30% solids) and unconcentrated (10% solids) skim milk were inoculated to contain ~10^5–10^6 *L. monocytogenes* (strain Scott A or V7) CFU/ml and dried to moisture contents of 3.6–6.4% in a gas-fired pilot-plant–sized spray dryer with inlet and outlet air temperatures of 165 ± 2 and $67 \pm 2°C$, respectively. All samples of nonfat dry milk were stored at 25°C for up to 16 weeks and periodically analyzed for listeriae using both direct-plating on McBride Listeria Agar (detects uninjured cells) and cold enrichment in Tryptose Broth (detects injured and uninjured cells). *Listeria* populations decreased approximately 1–1.5 orders of magnitude during spray drying, regardless of whether or not nonfat dry milk was prepared from concentrated or unconcentrated skim milk. Strain V7 was generally hardier than strain Scott A during both spray drying and storage of nonfat dry milk. Twelve to 16 weeks of storage at room temperature were required to decrease populations of strain V7 >1000-fold in nonfat dry milk, whereas only 6 weeks of storage were necessary to obtain similar decreases in numbers of strain Scott A. Overall, strains Scott A and V7 survived a maximum of 8 and 12 weeks in nonfat dry milk, respectively. While strain Scott A generally survived equally well in nonfat dry milk prepared from concentrated and unconcentrated skim milk, strain V7 survived 2 weeks longer in nonfat dry milk manufactured from concentrated rather than unconcentrated skim milk. The higher moisture content of nonfat dry milk (i.e., 5.7 and 6.4%) prepared from concentrated skim milk may have enhanced survival of listeriae in this product during extended storage. Overall, populations of *L. monocytogenes* decreased >10,000-fold in nonfat dry milk during 16 weeks of storage at room temperature. Hence, if commercially produced nonfat dry milk is ever found to contain *L. monocytogenes*, presumably at very low levels, it may be possible to eliminate this pathogen by holding the product at room temperature for several months.

REFERENCES

1. Amelang, J., and S. Doores. 1989. The effect of ingredients in ice cream formulations on the growth of *Listeria monocytogenes*. Ann. Mtg., Inst. Food Technol., Chicago, IL, June 25–29, Abstr. 468.
2. Amelang, J., and S. Doores. 1989. The effect of medium, growth phase and temperature on the growth of *Listeria monocytogenes* in ice cream mix. Ann. Mtg., Inst. Food Technol., Chicago, IL, June 25–29, Abstr. 469.
3. Anonymous. 1986. Ice cream bars recalled. FDA Enforcement Report, July 16.
4. Anonymous. 1986. Ice cream recalled. FDA Enforcement Report, Oct. 22.
5. Anonymous. 1986. Ice cream recalled. FDA Enforcement Report, Oct. 29.
6. Anonymous. 1986. Ice cream, sherbet and glacee recalled. FDA Enforcement Report, Sept. 3.
7. Anonymous. 1986. Ice milk mix recalled. FDA Enforcement Report, June 25.
8. Anonymous. 1986. Large class I recall made of ice cream because of *Listeria*. *Food Chem. News* 28(24):11–12.
9. Anonymous. 1986. *Listeria* causes class I recalls of ice milk mix, milk. *Food Chem. News* 28(16):22.
10. Anonymous. 1986. Milk, chocolate milk, half and half, cultured buttermilk, whipping cream, ice milk, ice milk mix and ice milk shake mix recalled. FDA Enforcement Report, June 25.
11. Anonymous. 1986. Sherbets, non-dairy products, ice milk products, gelati-da products and ice cream recalled. FDA Enforcement Report, Aug. 27.
12. Anonymous. 1987. Chocolate ice cream recalled. FDA Enforcement Report, Sept. 16.
13. Anonymous. 1987. Class I recall made of cheese because of *Listeria*. *Food Chem. News* 28(50):52.
14. Anonymous. 1987. FDA launching two-year pathogen surveillance program. *Food Chem. News* 29(31):10–12.
15. Anonymous. 1987. Ice cream and ice milk recalled. FDA Enforcement Report, Aug. 26.
16. Anonymous. 1987. Ice cream bars recalled. FDA Enforcement Report, Nov. 4.
17. Anonymous. 1987. Ice cream, ice milk and sherbet recalled. FDA Enforcement Report, Feb. 11.
18. Anonymous. 1987. Ice cream, ice milk and sherbet recalled. FDA Enforcement Report, Aug. 19.
19. Anonymous. 1987. Ice cream nuggets recalled. FDA Enforcement Report, Aug. 5.
20. Anonymous. 1987. Ice cream products recalled. FDA Enforcement Report, Sept. 2.
21. Anonymous. 1987. Ice cream products recalled. FDA Enforcement Report, Sept. 16.
22. Anonymous. 1987. Ice cream products recalled. FDA Enforcement Report, Sept. 23.
23. Anonymous. 1987. Ice cream recalled. FDA Enforcement Report, Jan. 28.
24. Anonymous. 1987. Ice cream recalled. FDA Enforcement Report, Feb. 11.
25. Anonymous. 1987. Ice cream recalled. FDA Enforcement Report, May 27.
26. Anonymous. 1987. Ice cream recalled because of *Listeria*, pottery because of lead. *Food Chem. News* 29(21):16–17.
27. Anonymous. 1987. Milk industry has spent $66 million on recalls and related expenses, Witte says. *Food Chem. News* 29(17):29–30.
28. Anonymous. 1987. More ice cream recalled because of *Listeria*. *Food Chem. News* 28(48):33.
29. Anonymous. 1988. Frozen dessert products recalled. FDA Enforcement Report, July 27.
30. Anonymous. 1988. Ice cream, cheese recalled because of *Listeria*. *Food Chem. News* 30(6):27.
31. Anonymous. 1988. Ice cream pies recalled. FDA Enforcement Report, Dec. 28.
32. Anonymous. 1988. Ice cream products, cheese recalled because of *Listeria*. *Food Chem. News* 30(9):47.
33. Anonymous. 1988. Ice cream recalled. FDA Enforcement Report, April 6.
34. Anonymous. 1988. Ice cream recalled. FDA Enforcement Report, Sept. 7.
35. Anonymous. 1988. Ice cream recalled. FDA Enforcement Report, Sept. 14.
36. Anonymous. 1988. Ice cream recalled. FDA Enforcement Report, Nov. 2.
37. Anonymous. 1988. International Dairy Federation: Group E64—Detection of *Listeria monocytogenes*—sampling plans for *Listeria monocytogenes* in foods, Feb. 9. Brussels, Belgium.

38. Anonymous. 1988. More cheese, ice cream linked to possible *Listeria*. *Food Chem. News* 29(11):37–38.
39. Anonymous. 1989. Ice cream bars recalled. FDA Enforcement Report, Feb. 15.
40. Anonymous. 1989. Ice cream recalled. FDA Enforcement Report, April 19.
41. Anonymous. 1989. Le contrôle des résidus dans les produits laitiers. *Bull. Inf.-Minist. Agric., France 1273*:22–24.
42. Anonymous. 1990. USDA, FDA officials report apparent decrease in *Listeria* isolations. *Food Chem. News 32*(1):12–15.
43. Archer, D. L. 1988. Review of the latest FDA information on the presence of *Listeria* in foods. WHO Working Group on Foodborne Listeriosis, Geneva, Switzerland, Feb. 15–19.
44. Beckers, H. J., P. S. S. Soentoro, and E. H. M. Delfgou-van Asch. 1987. The occurrence of *Listeria monocytogenes* in soft cheeses and raw milk and its resistance to heat. *Intern. J. Food Microbiol. 4*:249–256.
45. Beckers, H. J., P. H. in't Veld, P. S. S. Soentoro, and E. H. M. Delfgou-van Asch. 1988. The occurrence of *Listeria* in food. *Foodborne Listeriosis—Proceedings of a Symposium*, Wiesbaden, West Germany, Sept. 7, pp. 84–97.
46. Berrang, M. E., J. F. Frank, and R. E. Brackett. 1988. Behavior of *Listeria monocytogenes* in chocolate milk and ice cream mix made from post-expiration date skim milk. *J. Food Prot. 51*:823 (Abstr.).
47. Busta, F. F., and M. L. Speck. 1968. Antimicrobial effect of cocoa on salmonellae. *Appl. Microbiol. 16*:424–425.
48. Conner, D. E., V. N. Scott, S. S. Sumner, and D. T. Bernard. 1989. Pathogenicity of foodborne, environmental and clinical isolates of *Listeria monocytogenes* in mice. *J. Food Sci. 54*:1553–1556.
49. Davidson, R. J., D. W. Sprung, C. E. Park, and M. K. Rayman. 1989. Occurrence of *Listeria monocytogenes*, *Campylobacter* spp., and *Yersinia enterocolitica* in Manitoba raw milk. *Can. Inst. Food Sci. Technol. J. 22*:70–74.
50. Dedie, K. 1958. Weitere experimentelle Untersuchungsbefunde zur Listeriose bei Tieren. In R. Roots and D. Strauch (eds.), *Listeriosen*, Zbl. Veterinärmed. Beiheft, pp. 99–109.
51. Dijkstra, R. G. 1971. Investigations on the survival times of *Listeria* bacteria in suspensions of brain tissue, silage and faeces and in milk. *Zbl. Bakteriol. I Abt. Orig. 216*:92–95.
52. Donnelly, C. W. 1986. Listeriosis and dairy products: Why now and why milk? *Hoards Dairyman 131*(14):663, 687.
53. Donnelly, C. W., and E. H. Briggs. 1986. Psychrotrophic growth and thermal inactivation of *Listeria monocytogenes* as a function of milk composition. *J. Food Prot. 49*:994–998.
54. Donnelly, C. W., G. J. Baignet, and E. H. Briggs. 1988. Flow cytometry for automated analysis of milk containing *Listeria monocytogenes*. *J. Assoc. Off. Anal. Chem. 71*:655–658.
55. Doores, S., and J. Amelang. 1990. Incidence of *Listeria monocytogenes* in the raw milk supply in Pennsylvania. *J. Food Prot.* (submitted).
56. Doyle, M. P., and J. L. Schoeni. 1986. Selective-enrichment procedure for isolation of *Listeria monocytogenes* from fecal and biologic specimens. *Appl. Environ. Microbiol. 51*:1127–1129.
57. Doyle, M. P., L. M. Meske, and E. H. Marth. 1985. Survival of *Listeria monocytogenes* during the manufacture and storage of nonfat dry milk. *J. Food Prot. 48*:740–742.
58. Doyle, M. P., K. A. Glass, J. T. Beery, G. A. Garcia, D. J. Pollard, and R. D. Schultz. 1987. Survival of *Listeria monocytogenes* in milk during high-temperature, short-time pasteurization. *Appl. Environ. Microbiol. 53*:1433–1438.
59. El-Gazzar, F. E., H. F. Bohner, and E. H. Marth, 1991. Growth of *Listeria* monocytogenes at 4, 32 and 40°C in skim milk and in retentate and permeate from ultrafiltered skim milk. *J. Food Prot. 54* (accepted).
60. Farber, J. M., G. W. Sanders, and M. A. Johnston. 1989. A survey of various foods for the presence of *Listeria* species. *J. Food Prot. 52*:456–458.
61. Farber, J. M., G. W. Sanders, and S. A. Malcom. 1988. The presence of *Listeria* spp. in raw milk in Ontario. *Can. J. Microbiol. 34*:95–100.

62. Farber, J. M., G. W. Sanders, and J. I. Speirs. 1990. Growth of *Listeria monocytogenes* in naturally-contaminated raw milk. *Lebensm. Wiss. Technol. 23*:252–254.
63. Farber, J. M., G. W. Sanders, J. I. Speirs, J.-Y. D'Aoust, D. B. Emmons, and R. McKellar. 1988. Thermal resistance of *Listeria monocytogenes* in inoculated and naturally contaminated raw milk. *Intern. J. Food Microbiol. 7*:277–286.
64. Farkas, G. Y., S. Szakaly, and B. Ralovich. 1988. Occurrence of *Listeria* strains in a Hungarian dairy plant—Pecs. 10th International Symposium on Listeriosis, Pecs, Hungary, Aug. 22–26, Abstr. P59.
65. Farrag, S. A., and E. H. Marth. 1989. Behavior of *Listeria monocytogenes* when incubated together with *Pseudomonas* species in tryptose broth at 7 and 13°C. *J. Food Prot. 52*:536–539.
66. Farrag, S. A., and E. H. Marth. 1989. Growth of *Listeria monocytogenes* in the presence of *Pseudomonas fluorescens* at 7 or 13°C in skim milk. *J. Food Prot. 52*:852–855.
67. Farrag, S. A., F. E. El-Gazzar, and E. H. Marth. 1990. Fate of *Listeria monocytogenes* in sweetened condensed and evaporated milk during storage at 7 or 21°C. *J. Food Prot. 53*:747–750.
68. Fenlon, D. R., and J. Wilson. 1989. The incidence of *Listeria monocytogenes* in raw milk from farm bulk tanks in North-East Scotland. *J. Appl. Bacteriol. 66*:191–196.
69. Fistrovici, E., and D. L. Collins-Thompson. 1990. Use of plasmid profiles and restriction endonuclease digest in environmental studies of *Listeria* spp. from raw milk. *Intern. J. Food Microbiol. 10*:43–50.
70. Fleming, D. W., S. L. Cochi, K. L. MacDonald, J. Brondum, P. S. Hayes, B. D. Plikaytis, M. B. Holmes, A. Audurier, C. V. Broome, and A. L. Reingold. 1985. Pasteurized milk as a vehicle of infection in an outbreak of listeriosis. *N. Engl. J. Med. 312*:404–407.
71. Food and Drug Administration. 1989. Code of Federal Regulations, Title 21, Code Fed. Reg., U.S. Dept. Health Human Services, Washington, DC.
72. Garayzabal, J. F. F., L. D. Rodriguez, J. A. V. Boland, J. L. B. Cancelo, and G. S. Fernandez. 1986. *Listeria monocytogenes* dans le lait pasteurisé. *Can. J. Microbiol. 32*:149–150.
73. Garayzabal, J. F. F., L. D. Rodriguez, J. A. V. Boland, E. Gomez-Lucia, E. R. Ferri, and G. S. Fernandez. 1987. Occurrence of *Listeria monocytogenes* in raw milk. *Vet. Rec. 120*:258–259.
74. Garayzabal, J. F. F., L. D. Rodriguez, J. A. V. Boland, E. R. Ferri, V. B. Dieste, J. L. B. Cancelo, and G. S. Fernandez. 1987. Survival of *Listeria monocytogenes* in raw milk treated in a pilot plant size pasteurizer. *J. Appl. Bacteriol. 63*:533–537.
75. Gasparovic, E. von, M. Sabolic, W. Unglaub, and G. Terplan. 1989. Untersuchungen über das Vorkommen von *Listeria monocytogenes* in Rohmilch in Südwürttemberg. *Tierärztl. Umschau 44*:783–790.
76. Gilbert, R. J. 1990. Personal communication.
77. Gledel, J. 1986. Epidemiology and significance of listeriosis in France. In A. Schönberg (ed.), Listeriosis-Joint WHO/ROI Consultation on Prevention and Control, West Berlin, December 10–12, 1986, pp. 9–20. Institut für Veterinärmedizin des Bundesgesundheitsamtes, Berlin.
78. Gledel, J. 1988. *Listeria* and the dairy industry in France. *Foodborne Listeriosis—Proceedings of a Symposium*, Wiesbaden, West Germany, Sept. 7, pp. 72–82.
79. Golnazarian, C. A., C. W. Donnelly, S. J. Pintauro, and D. B. Howard. 1989. Comparison of infectious dose of *Listeria monocytogenes* F5817 as determined for normal versus compromised C57B1/6J mice. *J. Food Prot. 52*:696–701.
80. Hayes, P. S. 1988. Personal communication.
81. Hayes, P. S., J. C. Feeley, L. M. Graves, G. W. Ajello, and D. W. Fleming. 1986. Isolation of *Listeria monocytogenes* from raw milk. *Appl. Environ. Microbiol. 51*:438–440.
82. Ikonomov, L., and D. Todorov. 1964. Studies of the viability of *Listeria monocytogenes* in ewe's milk and dairy products. *Vet. Med. Nauki, Sofiya 7*:23–29.
83. International Dairy Federation. 1989. Pathogenic *Listeria*—Abstracts of replies from 24 countries to questionnaire 1288/B on pathogenic *Listeria*. Circular 89/5, March 31, Intern. Dairy Fed., Brussels.
84. Kaufmann, V. 1988. Personal communication.
85. Kozak, J. J. 1986. FDA's dairy program initiatives. *Dairy Food Sanit. 6*:184–185.

86. Liewen, M. B., and M. W. Plautz. 1988. Occurrence of *Listeria monocytogenes* in raw milk in Nebraska. *J. Food Prot. 51*:840–841.

87. Liewen, M. B., D. L. Peters, and M. W. Plautz. 1987. Incidence of *L. monocytogenes* in raw milk in Nebraska. Ann. Mtg., Inst. Food Technol., Las Vegas, NV, June 16–19, Abstr. 118.

88. Lovett, J., D. W. Francis, and J. M. Hunt. 1987. *Listeria monocytogenes* in raw milk: detection, incidence, and pathogenicity. *J. Food Prot. 50*:188–192.

89. Marshall, D. L., and R. H. Schmidt. 1988. Growth of *Listeria monocytogenes* at 10°C in milk preincubated with selected pseudomonads. *J. Food Prot. 51*:277–282.

90. Mascola, L., L. Chun, J. Thomas, W. F. Bibe, B. Schwartz, C. Salminen, and P. Heseltine. 1988. A case-control study of a cluster of perinatal listeriosis identified by an active surveillance system in Los Angeles County. Society for Industrial Microbiology—Comprehensive Conference on *Listeria monocytogenes*, Rohnert Park, CA, Oct. 2–5, Abstr. P-10.

91. Mattingly, J. A., B. T. Butman, M. C. Plank, R. J. Durham, and B. J. Robison. 1988. Rapid monoclonal antibody-based enzyme-linked immunosorbant assay for detection of *Listeria* in food products. *J. Assoc. Off. Anal. Chem. 71*:679–681.

92. McBean, L. D. 1988. A perspective on food safety concerns. *Dairy Food Sanit. 8*:112–118.

93. Minor, T. E., and E. H. Marth. 1972. *Staphylococcus aureus* and enterotoxin A in cream and butter. *J. Dairy Sci. 55*:1410–1414.

94. Northolt, M. D., H. J. Beckers, U. Vecht, L. Toepoel, P. S. S. Soentoro, and H. J. Wisselink. 1988. *Listeria monocytogenes*: Heat resistance and behavior during storage of milk and whey and making of Dutch types of cheese. *Neth. Milk Dairy J. 42*:207–219.

95. Olsen, J. A., A. E. Yousef, and E. H. Marth. 1988. Growth and survival of *Listeria monocytogenes* during making and storage of butter. *Milchwissenschaft 43*:487–489.

96. Oz, H. H., and R. J. Farnsworth. 1985. Laboratory simulation of fluctuating temperature of farm bulk tank milk. *J. Food Prot. 48*:303–305.

97. Patterson, R. L., D. J. Pusch, and E. A. Zottola. 1989. The isolation and identification of *Listeria* spp. from raw milk. *J. Food Prot. 52*:745.

98. Pearson, L. J., and E. H. Marth. 1990. Behavior of *Listeria monocytogenes* in the presence of cocoa, carrageenan, and sugar in a milk medium incubated with and without agitation. *J. Food Prot. 53*:30–37.

99. Pearson, L. J., and E. H. Marth. 1990. Behavior of *Listeria monocytogenes* in the presence of methylxanthines-caffeine and theobromine. *J. Food Prot. 53*:47–50, 55.

100. Pearson, L. J., and E. H. Marth. 1990. Inhibition of *Listeria monocytogenes* by cocoa in a broth medium and neutralization of this effect by casein. *J. Food Prot. 53*:38–46.

101. Peters, D. L., and M. B. Liewen. 1988. Growth and survival of *Listeria monocytogenes* in unfiltered milk. Ann. Mtg., Inst. Food Technol., New Orleans, LA, June 19–22, Abstr. 326.

102. Pine, L., G. B. Malcolm, J. B. Brooks, and M. I. Daneshvar. 1989. Physiological studies on the growth and utilization of sugars by *Listeria* species. *Can. J. Microbiol. 35*:245–254.

103. Rodler, M., and W. Körbler. 1988. Examination of *Listeria monocytogenes* in milk products. 10th International Symposium on Listeriosis, Pecs, Hungary, Aug. 22–26, Abstr. 47.

104. Rodriguez, L. D., J. F. F. Garayzabal, J. A. V. Boland, E. R. Ferri, and G. S. Fernandez. 1985. Isolation de micro-organismes du genre listeria à partir de lait cru destiné à la consommation humaine. *Can. J. Microbiol. 31*:938–941.

105. Rosenow, E. M., and E. H. Marth. 1987. Addition of cocoa powder, cane sugar, and carrageenan to milk enhances growth of *Listeria monocytogenes*. *J. Food Prot. 50*:726–729, 732.

106. Rosenow, E. M., and E. H. Marth. 1987. Growth of *Listeria monocytogenes* in skim, whole and chocolate milk, and in whipping cream during incubation at 4, 8, 13, 21, and 35°C. *J. Food Prot. 50*:452–459.

107. Ryser, E. T., and E. H. Marth. 1988. Growth of *Listeria monocytogenes* at different pH values in uncultured whey or in whey cultured with *Penicillium camemberti. Can. J. Microbiol. 34*:730–734.

108. Slade, P. J., and D. L. Collins-Thompson. 1988. Enumeration of *Listeria monocytogenes* in raw milk. *Lett. Appl. Microbiol. 6*:121–123.

109. Slade, P. J., D. L. Collins-Thompson, and F. Fletcher. 1988. Incidence of *Listeria* species in Ontario raw milk. *Can. Inst. Food Sci. Technol. J. 21*:425–429.
110. Stelma, G. N. Jr., A. L. Reyes, J. T. Peeler, D. W. Francis, J. M. Hunt, P. L. Spaulding, C. H. Johnson, and J. Lovett. 1987. Pathogenicity test for *Listeria monocytogenes* using immunocompromised mice. *J. Clin. Microbiol. 25*:2085–2089.
111. Stone, D. L. 1987. A survey of raw whole milk for *Campylobacter jejuni*, *Listeria monocytogenes* and *Yersinia enterocolitica*. *New Zealand J. Dairy Sci. Technol. 22*:257–264.
112. Terplan, G. 1988. Factors responsible for the contamination of food with *Listeria monocytogenes*. WHO Working Group on Foodborne Listeriosis. Geneva, Switzerland, Feb. 15–19.
113. Terplan, G. 1988. Provisional IDF-recommended method: Milk and milk products—Detection of *Listeria monocytogenes*. International Dairy Federation, Brussels, Belgium.
114. Vassau, N. 1988. Personal communication.
115. Venables, L. J. 1989. *Listeria monocytogenes* in dairy products—the Victorian experience. *Food Australia 41*:942–943.

10

Incidence and Behavior of *Listeria monocytogenes* in Cheese and Other Fermented Dairy Products

INTRODUCTION

On June 14, 1985, *L. monocytogenes* emerged from relative obscurity to the front page of many American newspapers as the result of a large listeriosis outbreak in California that was directly linked to consumption of Mexican-style cheese manufactured in metropolitan Los Angeles. By the time this outbreak subsided in August, as many as 300 cases of listeriosis were reported, including 85 deaths—at least 40 of which were traced to the tainted cheese. In response to this foodborne outbreak of listeriosis, FDA officials added *L. monocytogenes* to their list of pathogenic organisms that should be of concern to cheesemakers and began surveying a variety of soft domestic cheeses for listeriae.

Approximately 6 months later, isolation of *L. monocytogenes* from several imported Brie cheeses purchased at a supermarket led to the eventual recall of approximately 300,000 tons of Brie cheese imported from France and to a real concern about the incidence of this pathogen in other European cheeses. Recall of the Brie cheese prompted two corrective measures: (a) adoption of a cheese certification program by the United States and France to prevent importation of *Listeria*-contaminated cheese and (b) initiation of numerous large-scale surveys to determine the extent of *Listeria* contamination in virtually all types of cheese manufactured in the United States, Canada, and Western Europe.

Throughout 1986 and most of 1987, the impact of *Listeria* on European cheesemakers was primarily in the form of economic losses from destruction of contaminated product. However, *L. monocytogenes* struck again late in 1987 with the report of a large listeriosis outbreak in Switzerland (see Chapter 8) in which Vacherin Mont d'Or soft-ripened cheese was incriminated as the vehicle of infection.

These two cheeseborne listeriosis outbreaks prompted scientists on both sides of the Atlantic Ocean to determine the incidence of *Listeria* spp. in a variety of cheeses and examine the behavior of *L. monocytogenes* during manufacture and storage of fermented dairy products. The first portion of this chapter summarizes *Listeria*-related recalls of cheese in the United States and results from surveys dealing with the incidence of listeriae in domestic and imported fermented dairy products. The second half deals with the fate of *L. monocytogenes* during manufacture and storage of buttermilk, yogurt, and a variety of cheeses (including whey) and the potential for cheese ingredients such as rennet, salt brine, and coloring agents to serve as vehicles of contamination during cheesemaking.

UNITED STATES SURVEILLANCE PROGRAMS AND RECALLS FOR *L. MONOCYTOGENES* IN DOMESTIC AND IMPORTED CHEESE

Domestic Cheese

The concept of listeriosis as a foodborne illness is not new. As you will recall from Chapter 8, consumption of contaminated raw milk was believed to have caused several cases of listeriosis in post–World War Two Germany. In 1961, Seeliger (141) also suggested sour milk, cream, and cottage cheese as possible vehicles of infection in this outbreak. While results from two Yugoslavian studies concerned with behavior of *L. monocytogenes* in various fermented dairy products (i.e., cultured cream, unsalted skim milk cheese, Kachkaval cheese, and yogurt) were published in 1964 (109) and 1981 (148), no surveys dealing with the incidence of listeriae in fermented dairy products were made before contaminated Mexican-style cheese was linked to the California listeriosis outbreak in June of 1985.

Public health concerns about presence of *L. monocytogenes* in domestic and imported fermented dairy products as well as other foods such as meat, poultry, seafood, fruits, and vegetables can be traced either directly or indirectly to the 1985 listeriosis outbreak in California. Less than one month after the first nationwide Class I *Listeria*-associated recall was issued for 22 varieties of Mexican-style cheese contaminated with *L. monocytogenes* (Table 10.1), the FDA developed a series of programs designed to prevent the reoccurrence of such an outbreak (147) (Fig. 10.1).

The Domestic Soft Cheese Surveillance Program—the first of the dairy factory initiative programs—was instituted by the FDA in July of 1985 and involved on-site inspection of firms manufacturing soft cheese (9). Priority was given to manufacturers of Mexican-style soft cheese, followed by firms that produced other ethnic-type soft cheeses such as Edam, Gouda, Liederkranz, Limburger, Monterey Jack, Muenster, and Port du Salut from raw, heat-treated [<71.7°C (161°F)/15 sec] or pasteurized (≥71.7°C (161°F)/15 sec] milk. In addition to determining the firm's compliance with good manufacturing practices (i.e., use of proper pasteurization, cleaning, and sanitizing procedures), FDA inspectors collected cheese samples to be analyzed for *L. monocytogenes* by the original FDA procedure (see Fig. 6.14). Cheese samples also were tested for presence of enteropathogenic strains of *E. coli* and for activity of the enzyme phosphatase, which if present generally indicates improper pasteurization of cheesemilk and/or its contamination with raw milk. However, suitability of the phosphatase test for cheese has since been questioned.

Less than 2 months into this program, FDA officials isolated a pathogenic strain of *L. monocytogenes* from one sample of domestically produced Liederkranz cheese (Table 10.1). The manufacturer subsequently recalled the product nationwide. Following preliminary FDA reports of further *Listeria* contamination, this recall was extended to include all lots of Brie and Camembert cheese manufactured at the same facility (3,7). However, final laboratory reports indicated that both Brie and Camembert cheese were contaminated with *L. innocua*, a nonpathogenic *Listeria* sp., rather than *L. monocytogenes*. Although the Domestic Soft Cheese Surveillance Program also was responsible for temporarily closing two soft cheese factories in California that produced

Table 10.1 Chronological List of Class I Recalls in the United States for Domestic Cheese Contaminated with *L. monocytogenes*

Type of cheese	Date recall initiated	Origin	Distribution	Quantity (lb.)	Ref.
Jalisco brand soft Mexican-style: Cotija, Queso Fresco, and 20 other varieties	06/13/85	California	Arizona, Arkansas, California, Colorado, Georgia, Guam, Hawaii, Idaho, Illinois, Kansas, Louisiana, Marshall Islands, Massachusetts, Nevada, New Jersey, New Mexico, New York, Oklahoma, Oregon, Rhode Island, Samoa, Texas, Utah, Washington	Unknown	5,6
Liederkranz [Brie,[a] Camembert]	08/14/85	Ohio	Nationwide, Puerto Rico	~10,000	3,4,7
Soft Mexican-style: Queso Fresco and 5 other varieties	03/05/86	California	Arizona, California, Oregon, Texas	127,607	15,33
Semi-soft Salvador-style white	09/11/86	Virginia	Virginia, Washington, DC	10,850	37,49
Soft-ripened: Old Heidelberg	04/17/87	Illinois	Illinois, North Carolina, Ohio, Pennsylvania	1,150	47
Soft-ripened: Bonbel and Gouda	05/06/87	Kentucky	Nationwide	~13,800	46
Raw milk sharp Cheddar	08/21/87	Wisconsin	California, Washington	~1,400	48,147
Soft Mexican-style: Cotija, Queso Fresco, and 8 other varieties + Baby Jack and Monterey Jack	01/29/88	California	Arizona, California, Florida, Texas, Washington	Unknown	59

[a]Later found to contain only *L. innocua*.

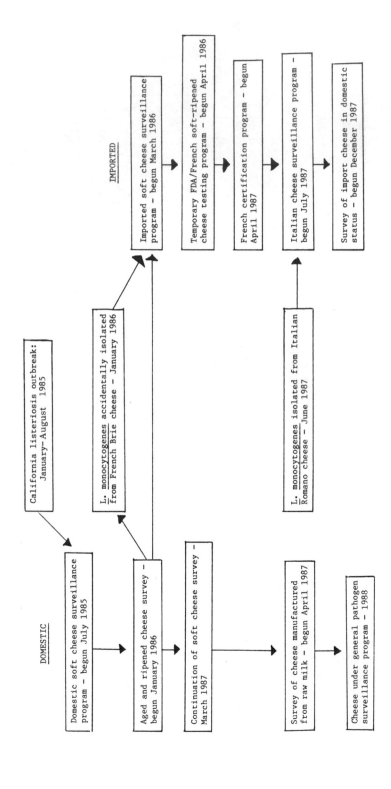

Figure 10.1 Surveillance programs for *Listeria* spp. in domestic and imported cheese. (Adapted from Ref. 72.)

phosphatase-positive cheese (4), it must be stressed that *L. monocytogenes* was never isolated from cheeses produced at either facility.

In general, FDA inspections of other soft cheese factories uncovered problems similar to those encountered during inspections of Grade A fluid milk factories: (a) potential bypasses of the pasteurizer, (b) postpasteurization blending of product, and (c) a general lack of education and/or training of plant personnel (115). Items of particular concern to cheesemakers and that were not generally found during visits to Grade A milk factories include defects in the pasteurization process, discrepancies in pasteurization/production records, and a higher incidence (than in Grade A milk factories) of pathogenic microorganisms (including *L. monocytogenes*) on environmental surfaces in production and storage areas.

Inspections of domestic cheese factories continued throughout 1986, 1987, and 1988 under four separate programs (Fig. 10.1) with FDA officials reaching nearly half of the 400 soft cheese factories in the United States by April of 1986 and the remaining factories (including follow-up inspections of problem factories) by late 1987 (41). Since January of 1986, six additional Class I recalls were issued for various ethnic-type soft and semi-soft cheeses contaminated with *L. monocytogenes* (Table 10.1). According to FDA records (72), *L. monocytogenes* was confirmed in 12 of 658 (1.82%) domestic cheese samples analyzed during 1986. As previously mentioned, while all products contaminated with *L. monocytogenes* must be retrieved from the marketplace, formal Class I recalls do not have to be issued for contaminated products that have not yet reached retail stores. Since such situations typically lead to nonpublished "internal recalls" issued by the manufacturer, more cheese was likely destroyed during this 3-year period than has actually been reported. Several such informal recalls involved a part-skim milk cheese manufactured in California (52) as well as ricotta, Parmesan, and mozzarella cheese of uncertain origin (118).

Following a report by Ryser and Marth (130) that *L. monocytogenes* can survive more than 1 year in Cheddar cheese (i.e., well beyond the mandatory 60-day aging period for Cheddar cheese manufactured from raw milk), the FDA modified its Domestic Cheese Program in August of 1987 to include cheese prepared from unpasteurized milk (41). Between April and October of 1987, 181 samples of domestic aged [held a minimum of 60 days at $\geq 1.7°C$ (35°F)] natural cheese manufactured from raw milk, as well as similar imported cheeses in domestic status, were collected from retail stores by FDA field personnel and analyzed for *L. monocytogenes* (Table 10.2). These efforts uncovered one positive sample—a sharp Cheddar cheese manufactured in Wisconsin, which was subsequently recalled from the market in July of 1987 (Table 10.1).

Late in 1987, the FDA announced plans for a 2-year pathogen surveillance program (38) which was designed to examine domestic and imported cheese as well as other high-risk foods (i.e., milk, vegetables, and seafood) for presence of *L. monocytogenes* and other selected pathogens including *Vibrio cholerae*, *Vibrio parahaemolyticus*, *E. coli*, enteropathogenic *E. coli*, *Staphylococcus aureus*, *Salmonella* spp., *Yersinia enterocolitica*, *Campylobacter jejuni*, and *Campylobacter coli*. Under this program, samples of soft-ripened and raw milk cheese, as well as imported hard and artificial blended cheese were examined for all of the above organisms except *Vibrio* spp. Domestic cheeses were collected at the wholesale level, whereas samples of imported cheese were obtained from retail stores. Results from this 2-year study should be forthcoming.

Table 10.2   Incidence of *L. monocytogenes* in
"Domestic" Cheese Manufactured from Raw Milk—
FDA 1987[a]

Type of cheese	Number of samples analyzed	Number of positive samples (%)
Blue	18	0
Brick	5	0
Cheddar	71	1[b] (1.4)
Colby	8	0
Edam	4	0
Goat	6	0
Gouda	1	0
Monterey Jack	9	0
Swiss	42	0
Other	17	0
Total	181	1 (0.55)

[a]Includes imported cheese in domestic status.
[b]2 samples with *L. innocua*.
Source: Adapted from Ref. 72.

Several other fermented dairy products also were examined for *L. monocytogenes* in conjunction with the FDA Dairy Initiative Program (72) (see Chapter 9). In 1986, 10 samples of cottage cheese were found to be free of listeriae. Other than cheese, 1% fat cultured buttermilk (28,30) and frozen yogurt (68) are the only other domestically produced, fermented dairy products known to have been contaminated with *L. monocytogenes*. The first of these products was included in a 1986 Class I recall involving approximately 1 million gallons of dairy foods (fluid milk, chocolate milk, half-and-half, whipping cream, ice milk, ice milk mix, ice milk shake mix, ice cream, and ice cream mix), all of which presumably contained *L. monocytogenes*. Three years later, officials from the Wisconsin Department of Agriculture, Trade and Consumer Protection issued a statewide recall for one particular brand of frozen yogurt after routine testing revealed presence of *L. monocytogenes* in one sample of mandarin orange frozen yogurt (68). Both of these products were retrieved from the marketplace without incident.

Imported Cheese

France

International concern over the potential health hazard of consuming *Listeria*-contaminated cheese also is rooted in the California listeriosis outbreak of 1985. This outbreak and an earlier link between consumption of French Brie and/or Camembert cheese and several outbreaks of foodborne illness in the United States and Europe caused by enterotoxigenic and/or enteropathogenic *E. coli* (113,119,156) prompted a meeting in September of 1985 between FDA officials and representatives of the French Embassy/French Delegation on Food Safety and Food Distribution to discuss the FDA's plans for inspecting imported soft cheese (8). Late in September, representatives from the Code Committee on Food Hygiene and the International Dairy Federation agreed with FDA officials that a "Code of Hygienic Practices" should be developed for manufacture of fresh and soft cheese (2). Use of raw milk (a known source of *L. monocytogenes*) to improve organoleptic properties of certain cheeses was cited as a particular area of concern. Although a basic certification program for soft cheese produced in France was in operation for some time, agreement on a general "Code of Hygienic Practices" for manufacture of soft cheese was not reached during the remainder of 1985.

In January of 1986, as part of a research effort to enhance recovery of listeriae from cheese, FDA officials inadvertently isolated a pathogenic strain of *L. monocytogenes* from two uninoculated control samples of French Brie cheese purchased at a local supermarket (14,72). Ironically, both cheeses were prepared from pasteurized milk in a cheese factory certified by the French government under the existing soft-ripened cheese agreement. In response to these findings, the first in a series of six nationwide recalls was issued on February 12, 1986, for *Listeria*-contaminated French Brie cheese (Table 10.3). The following week, the French firm that manufactured the tainted cheese agreed to cease all production (14). Shipment of additional cheese that was previously certified as "*Listeria*-free" by an independent French laboratory (certification by the French Ministry of Agriculture began January 1, 1986) was also stopped pending identification of the contamination source. In addition, all suspect lots of French Brie cheese en route to the United States were detained upon entry and tested for *Listeria* by the FDA before being released. Shortly thereafter, sampling was extended to include virtually all lots of French Brie cheese produced by this manufacturer.

The French cheese industry was dealt its most serious blow on March 14, 1986 when approximately 660 million pounds of Brie cheese produced by five different manufacturers were recalled in the United States (Table 10.3). This recall, which involved nearly 60% of all Brie cheese marketed in the United States, immediately raised the possibility of block-listing French firms that produced contaminated cheese (16). Consequently, in March of 1986 FDA officials began testing all shipments of French soft-ripened cheese as well as 20% of French soft/semi-soft cheese and 20% of all other imported soft cheeses for presence of *Listeria*, *E. coli*, and phosphatase (Fig. 10.1) (19).

Recognizing the danger of contracting listeriosis from consuming contaminated French soft-ripened cheese, FDA officials drafted the following proposal to detain, test, and certify all French soft-ripened cheeses exported to the United States (67):

> FDA intends to detain any entry that is found to be *Listeria*-positive, regardless of the species of *Listeria* found. French soft-ripened cheese without a certificate indicating negative results for the *Listeria* analysis or with a positive analysis for *Listeria* will be detained. . . . In addition, all French soft-ripened cheeses are to be sampled and analyzed for the presence of *Listeria*. [Under the previous agreement, cheeses were shipped with a certificate of analysis which only indicated the level of *E. coli* and the absence of phosphatase.] The analysis may be carried out by a private laboratory after the cheese has arrived in the United States, or alternatively the analysis may be conducted so that the availability of the results will coincide with the arrival of the shipment in the United States. The timing of the analysis is important to insure that the nature of the cheese tested, particularly the pH, is identical to that examined by the FDA, if we decide to perform an

Table 10.3 Chronological List of Class I Recalls in the United States for Imported Cheese Contaminated with *L. monocytogenes*

Type of cheese	Date recall initiated	Country of manufacture	Distribution	Quantity	Ref.
Brie	02/24/86	France	Illinois, Minnesota, New Jersey	909 cases	12,34
Brie	02/12/86	France	Bermuda, Nationwide	57,000 2–6-lb. wheels	12,14,21,24
Brie	02/14/86	France	Georgia, New Jersey	40 cases	11
Brie	02/14/86	France	Colorado, Connecticut, Florida, Louisiana, Maryland, Massachusetts, New Jersey, New York, Ohio, Washington, DC	100 cases	11
Brie	02/14/86	France	Florida, New York, Washington, DC	10 cases	11
Brie	02/14/86	France	Nationwide	Unknown	11,32
Brie	02/21/86	France	Oregon, Washington	Unknown	10,32
Brie	03/14/86	France	Nationwide	~660 million lb.	31,35
Brie	04/01/86	France	Colorado, Connecticut, Georgia, New Jersey, New York, North Carolina, Texas, Washington, DC	~230 lb.	22,31
Soft-ripened: Tourre de l'Aubier and Fromage des Burons	06/23/86	France	New York, Ohio, Pennsylvania	Unknown	23,26

Product	Date	Country	Distribution	Quantity	Reference
Soft-ripened: Tourre de l'Aubier	08/13/86	France	California, Illinois, Maine, Massachusetts, New Jersey, New York, Oregon	1056 lb.	27
Semi-soft: Morbier Rippoz	08/18/86	France	Illinois, Massachusetts, Michigan	~1600 lb.	23,25,29
Soft-unripened, full fat	04/16/87	France	New Jersey, New York, Texas	15 wheels	42,43
Semi-soft	01/27/88	Italy	Nationwide	410 cartons	54
Semi-soft: L'Amulette Danish Esrom	02/11/88	Denmark	California	Unknown	51,52,55
Semi-soft: L'Amulette Danish Esrom	02/12/88	Denmark	East, Midwest, North, South	~11,500 lb.	51,52,56
Semi-soft: L'Amulette Danish Esrom	02/18/88	Denmark	Florida, New Jersey, New York, Massachusetts	~1,150 lb.	51–53,57
Blue	04/06/88	Denmark	California, Florida, Illinois, Massachusetts, Michigan, Minnesota, New Jersey, New York, North Carolina, Oregon, Pennsylvania, Texas	~5,000 lb.	50,51
Anari	05/26/89	Cyprus	New York	50 cases	63
Anari	07/27/89	Cyprus	Illinois, Texas	79 cases	64
Anari	08/09/89	Cyprus	New York	80 cases	65
Halloumi	09/15/89	Cyprus	Florida, New Jersey, New York	14,400 lb.	70

audit on the entry. Thus, importers of French soft-ripened cheese should provide FDA with certificates indicating the dates testing was initiated and completed. Cheese shipments will not be released without a certificate indicating negative results for *Listeria* analysis. . . .

In this proposal, FDA officials stressed that other methods used to detect *Listeria* in cheese should conform to the 7-day FDA method described in Chapter 6 and also suggested that 1/16-inch-thick slices from the cheese surface (sample with highest pH) be analyzed for listeriae rather than cross-sectional plugs of cheese.

Following FDA threats to halt importation of soft-ripened cheese, the French Ministry of Agriculture agreed to begin lot-by-lot testing on April 21, 1986, as outlined in the FDA proposal of March 25 (20). However, French authorities stressed that such a program would not be practical on a long-term basis and hoped that the FDA would accept an expansion of the existing factory/product certification program to include *Listeria* testing in the near future. Beginning May 7, 1986, FDA officials announced that all shipments of French soft-ripened cheese lacking certification of analysis for *Listeria* would be detained (18). Inspections during the next 2 months uncovered *L. monocytogenes* in two French cheeses—a noncertified Brie and a 6-lb. certified lot of Muenster (18)—both of which were presumably recalled internally.

Continued problems with *Listeria*-contaminated French soft-ripened cheeses prompted FDA officials to revise the imported cheese surveillance program in August of 1986 (13). These changes allowed immediate detention of French cheeses that were: (a) manufactured at a non–government-certified factory, (b) unaccompanied by a *Listeria*-free government certificate, (c) positive for phosphatase, or (d) manufactured by one of several firms that were block-listed for *Listeria*. While these changes made importation of French cheeses more difficult, sampling of cheeses that were manufactured at certified factories and accompanied by *Listeria*-free certificates was decreased to the 20% level.

Between June and August of 1986, four additional Class I recalls were issued for French semi-soft/soft-ripened cheese contaminated with *L. monocytogenes* (Table 10.3). Two of three firms involved in these recalls were previously block-listed by the FDA (13). An additional Class I recall issued for semi-soft Morbier Rippoz cheese (Table 10.3) was accompanied by the following press release (29):

> Although *Listeria* is a rare cause of human illness, it can be life-threatening to pregnant women and their fetuses, frail elderly persons or other persons with weakened immune systems. In healthy adults, it is a transient illness with such mild-to-moderate flu-like symptoms as fever, headaches, and/or gastrointestinal tract distress.

The language used in such press releases also has received considerable attention. These messages to the public must be firm enough to accomplish the goals of the recall but not so alarming as to create a nationwide panic.

After considerable consultation on both sides of the Atlantic Ocean, the governments of France and the United States reached agreement on a French certification program for soft cheese (44,72). Under this program, which began February15, 1987, cheeses are to be tested before shipping using methods that are mutually acceptable by both governments. French cheeses manufactured at certified factories would be sampled at the 5% level, whereas other French cheeses (and cheeses manufactured in other countries without certification programs) would be analyzed at the 20% level. In the event of a *Listeria*-positive shipment, personnel at the French cheese factory would be required to investigate the potential source of contamination and analyze every lot of cheese for listeriae in at least the next 20 consecutive shipments destined for the United States. Although a positive finding will not automatically result in suspension of the certified status for a cheese factory under this program, FDA officials reserve the right to initiate detentions and/or recalls if a product is found to contain *L. monocytogenes*. After this certification program was accepted, only one additional recall involving a French soft-ripened full-fat cheese has been reported (Table 10.3).

Other Western European Countries

Despite the adverse publicity that the French cheese industry received throughout 1986 and 1987, it must be recognized that the problem of *Listeria*-contaminated cheese was not limited to France. Between October and December of 1986, FDA inspectors isolated *Listeria* spp. from 4 of 74 (5.4%) cheeses imported from Italy, two cheeses of which also contained high levels of phosphatase (40). After finding similar percentages of positive samples during January, February, and March of 1987, FDA officials told representatives of the Italian government to either submit a draft for a certification program (or recommend an alternate solution) or face a ban on importation of potentially hazardous cheeses into the United States. As of April 30, 1987, only 13 of all Italian cheese samples analyzed complied with current FDA safety standards: free of *Listeria*, phosphatase, and enteropathogenic strains of *E. coli*. Additionally, 144 cheese samples examined as part of an import alert were suspected of containing *L. monocytogenes* (39).

After isolating listeriae, in June of 1987, from Italian Pecorino Romano cheese prepared from goat's milk (Fig. 10.1) (147), the previous import alert was extended to include both soft and hard varieties of Italian cheese (45). (This was the first instance in which *L. monocytogenes* was isolated from hard cheese.) Subsequently, the FDA ordered intensified sampling of soft and hard cheese for the next 2 months (39).

Late in 1987, FDA officials also increased the number of cheeses sampled from Austria, Denmark, Germany, Italy, and Switzerland as part of the agency's ongoing imported cheese surveillance program (Fig. 10.1) (52). While this action prompted the recall of several Danish cheeses in early 1988 (Table 10.3), no additional Class I recalls were issued during the remainder of 1988 for imported cheese contaminated with *L. monocytogenes*. Heightened concern over the presence of this pathogen in European cheeses (which stems from the 1987 cheeseborne outbreak of listeriosis in Switzerland) and subsequent initiation of corrective action are probably both responsible for the lack of Class I recalls issued during the remainder of 1988 and early 1989. However, during the latter half of 1989, FDA officials issued (a) four separate Class I recalls for *Listeria*-contaminated soft cheeses manufactured in Cyprus (Table 10.3) and (b) an import alert for contaminated soft and hard cheeses produced by two Italian firms (98). Thus, while the overall situation regarding presence of *L. monocytogenes* in imported (and domestic) cheese has greatly improved since 1986 (71), sporadic detection of listeriae in imported cheeses suggests that limited surveillance of such products is still necessary to safeguard public health.

SURVEYS AND MONITORING PROGRAMS
FOR *LISTERIA* SPP. IN CHEESE PRODUCED
OUTSIDE THE UNITED STATES

In response to the 1985 cheeseborne listeriosis outbreak in California, scientists around the world began analyzing many types of cheese for *Listeria* spp. Given the possible ramifications of selling *Listeria*-contaminated cheese and the fact that large quantities of European specialty cheeses are exported to the United States and Canada, high priority was given to determining the incidence of listeriae in cheeses manufactured in Western Europe.

Since 1986, numerous surveys have been made and they have generated considerable information concerning the incidence of *Listeria* spp. in a variety of cheeses. However, since sampling designs [i.e., number and size of sample, site of sample collection (cheese factory or retail store), age of sample, portion of cheese analyzed (surface, interior, or both)] and methods for detecting and identifying listeriae vary widely among different surveys, many of the Western European studies to be discussed need to be interpreted with some caution.

Canada

Limited reports from federal monitoring programs in both Canada and the United States (52,110) suggest that the incidence of listeriae in Canadian cheese (and nonfermented dairy products as described in Chapter 9) is relatively low. In the only Canadian survey thus far recorded in the literature, Farber et al. (99) examined 182 samples of soft and semi-soft cheeses for listeriae using the original FDA Method (see Fig. 6.14). The cheeses analyzed in this survey were produced at 61 different cheese factories, most of which were located in the provinces of Ontario and Quebec. While all cheeses examined were *Listeria*-free, 19 of 79 samples (24.0%) were positive for phosphatase, which suggests that these cheeses may have been prepared, at least in part, from raw milk. The only additional information concerning Canadian cheese is the unconfirmed isolation of *L. monocytogenes* from Cheddar and Colby cheeses (112), both of which were manufactured from raw milk and held a minimum of 60 days at $\geq 1.7^{\circ}$C ($\geq 35^{\circ}$F) as required by the Canadian government.

While the incidence of *L. monocytogenes* in Canadian-produced cheese appears to be low, the pathogen has been detected in cheese exported to Canada from several Western European countries including Denmark, France, Switzerland, and West Germany (61,110). In conjunction with the Canadian survey just discussed, Farber et al. (99) also examined 187 samples of Western European soft and semi-soft cheese (98 different brands from 12 different countries) that were regularly exported to Canada. Three soft and semi-soft cheeses produced by the same manufacturer in France were positive for *Listeria* spp. (Table 10.4). Two cheeses contained *L. monocytogenes* alone, whereas the third contained both *L. monocytogenes* and *L. innocua*. In keeping with the previously described 1988 policy regarding foods that have been directly linked to major listeriosis outbreaks (see Chapter 9), Canadian officials immediately recalled the contaminated cheese. While some of the tainted cheese was likely consumed before the recall, no cases of listeriosis linked to consumption of this cheese were reported.

Despite being labeled as manufactured from pasteurized milk, the three French cheeses from which listeriae were isolated yielded positive results with the phosphatase

Table 10.4 Incidence of *Listeria* spp. in Soft/Semi-Soft European Cheeses Exported to Canada Between October 1985 and March 1987

Country of origin	Number of samples analyzed	*L. monocytogenes*	*L. innocua*	Other *Listeria* spp.
Austria	2	0	0	0
Denmark	43	0	0	0
Finland	1	0	0	0
France	104	3 (2.9)	1 (1.0)	0
Greece	2	0	0	0
Italy	3	0	0	0
Netherlands	2	0	0	0
Norway	7	0	0	0
Portugal	2	0	0	0
Sweden	2	0	0	0
Switzerland	3	0	0	0
West Germany	16	0	0	0
Total	187	3 (1.60)	1 (0.53)	0

Column header spanning: "Number of positive samples (%)"

Source: Adapted from Ref. 99.

test as did other cheese imported from Denmark, Finland, and Switzerland. Such findings, along with unpublished reports of phosphatase in pasteurized dairy products, have raised serious questions as to the validity of the phosphatase test. Results from a recent study (125) demonstrated that certain heat-labile, microbially produced alkaline phosphatases can mimic the natural phosphatase found in milk and produce false-positive results in the Scharer test. Hence the ability of the phosphatase test to determine whether or not a dairy product such as cheese was made from pasteurized milk (or from pasteurized milk contaminated with raw milk) may have to be reexamined.

France

Beginning in early 1986, sporadic *Listeria*-contamination problems have been associated with French soft cheeses exported to the United States and Canada as well as England (110), the Netherlands (77), Norway (110,164), Sweden (110), West Germany (69), and Australia (108). Hence, in an effort to bolster public confidence in the safety of cheeses produced in France, the French government, in cooperation with the Veterinary Service for Food Hygiene in France, conducted a series of systematic surveys for incidence of *Listeria* spp. in French cheeses destined for domestic and foreign markets (Table 10.5) (80,104). Overall, 1.34% of predominantly soft, 30-day-old French cheeses examined during 1986 and 1987 contained detectable levels of both *L. monocytogenes* and other *Listeria* spp., with little if any difference between cheeses destined for domestic or foreign consumption. It also is noteworthy that comparable levels of contamination were observed in soft cheeses prepared from raw and pasteurized milk. These findings agree with those of most other surveys which suggest that soft cheeses are most likely to become contaminated with *L. monocytogenes* during the latter stages of manufacture and ripening.

While *L. monocytogenes* also was recovered from 8.3% of unspecified French

Table 10.5 Incidence of *Listeria* spp. in French Cheese Destined for Domestic (France) and Foreign Markets during 1986 and/or 1987

Market	Type of cheese	Number of samples analyzed	Number of positive samples (%)	
			L. monocytogenes	Other *Listeria* spp.
Domestic[a]	Soft	192	2(1.0)	3(1.6)
	Other	135	0	1(0.7)
Foreign[b]	Soft (pasteurized milk)	736	11(1.5)	10(1.4)
	Soft (raw milk)	355	6(1.7)	5(1.4)
Total		1418	19(1.34)	19 (1.34)

[a]Results from January to November 1987.
[b]Results from January 1986 to September 1987.
Source: Adapted from Ref. 80.

cheeses examined during another survey in the Fall of 1988 (129), most surveys have suggested contamination rates ranging from approximately 1 to 3%.

In a similar survey conducted in France during 1986 (103), workers at the Veterinary Service for Food Hygiene recovered *L. monocytogenes* as well as *L. innocua* and other *Listeria* spp. from 0.3 to 3.5% of cottage, soft-ripened, and semi-hard cheeses examined (Table 10.6), with comparable contamination rates again observed for soft-ripened cheese prepared from raw and pasteurized milk.

Additional efforts in France have focused on characterization of listeriae isolated from cheese and other milk products. *Listeria* spp. isolated from French dairy products during 1986 included *L. monocytogenes* (370 strains), *L. innocua* (134 strains), *L. seeligeri* (17 strains), and *L. ivanovii* (1 strain), with 299 of 370 (80.0%) and 48 of 370 (13.0%) *L. monocytogenes* strains being of serotypes 1/2 and 4b, respectively. Additional surveys made in France during 1986 and 1987 (80,104) also indicated that a disproportionately large number of *L. monocytogenes* strains isolated from cheese and other dairy products were of serotype 1/2. This situation appears to be reversed in the United States, with isolates of serotype 4b typically outnumbering those of serotype 1/2.

Phage-typing has become a useful means of characterizing particular *L. monocytogenes* strains isolated from dairy products and of tracking the probable source of foodborne listeriosis outbreaks. Although only 33.8% of all *L. monocytogenes* strains isolated from French dairy products during 1986 and 1987 were typable using the currently available set of phages, some phage types appeared to be unique to particular regions within France (80). In some instances, excellent correlations were observed between specific phage types and certain varieties of cheese, with some phage types even specific to a particular dairy. Such findings may lead to better control of the listeriosis problem within the dairy industry in the future.

The inadvertent isolation of *L. monocytogenes* from French soft-ripened cheese by FDA officials in January of 1986 prompted several additional surveys of French cheese exported to other Western European countries. Working in The Netherlands, Beckers et al. (77) examined 69 samples of French soft cheese (i.e., Brie and Camembert) for *L. monocytogenes* using both direct plating and cold enrichment. The pathogen was recovered from 7 of 69 (10.1%) cheeses at levels ranging between 10^3 and 10^6 CFU/g. Cold enrichment uncovered three additional cheeses with *L. monocytogenes* for a total of 10 positive samples. Although all 10 *Listeria*-positive cheeses were prepared from raw milk, comparable rates of contamination have frequently been reported for cheese manufactured from raw and pasteurized milk (80,103).

Italy

Public health concerns raised in the United States following the isolation of *L. monocytogenes* from imported cheese prompted four surveys (80,85,87,99) which included cheeses manufactured in Italy (Tables 10.4 and 10.6). Working in Italy, Cantoni et al. (83) conducted a much broader survey of Italian cheeses during 1988. These researchers isolated *L. monocytogenes* from 14 of 375 (3.73%), 14 of 216 (6.48%), and 5 of 95 (5.30%) samples of Gorgonzola (blue-veined), Tallegio (soft, surface-ripened), and other Italian cheeses, respectively. However, the pathogen was never recovered from

Table 10.6 Incidence of *Listeria* spp. in European Cheeses

Country of origin	Type of cheese	Number of samples analyzed	Number of positive samples (%)			Ref.
			L. monocytogenes	L. innocua	Other Listeria spp.	
Belgium	Not specified	37	0	0	0	80
Denmark	Not specified	25	8 (32.0)	ND[a]	8 (32.0)	80
England and Wales	Soft	222	23 (10.4)	ND	ND	124
	Soft (ripened)	750	62 (8.2)	NR[b]	NR	102
	Soft (unripened)	350	4 (1.1)	NR	NR	102
	Goat's milk	450	18 (4.1)	NR	NR	102
France	Soft-ripened (raw milk)	330	3 (0.9)	6 (1.8)	1 (0.3)	103
	Soft-ripened (pasteurized milk)	873	12 (1.4)	5 (0.6)	3 (0.3)	103
	Semi-hard	289	10 (3.5)	1 (0.3)	1 (0.3)	103
	Bleu	126	0	0	0	103
	Cottage	149	2 (1.3)	0	0	103
	Not specified	242	20 (8.3)	NR	61	129
Greece	Not specified	1	0	0	0	80
	Soft	40	1 (2.5)	NR	NR	110
Ireland	Not specified	52	4 (7.7)	0	0	80
Italy	Soft	400	8 (2.0)	ND	ND	85
	Soft (unripened)	18	0	ND	ND	87
	Soft/Semi-soft	64	0	ND	ND	87
	Hard	10	0	ND	ND	87
	Goat's milk	21	1 (4.8)	ND	ND	87
Spain	Not specified	~100	0	NR	NR	110
Switzerland	Not specified	17	0	ND	1 (5.9)	80
	Soft	604	40 (6.6)	38 (6.3)	0	82
	Soft (mold-ripened)	54	0	ND	ND	36
	Soft (smear-ripened)	18	4 (22.2)	3 (16.7)	ND	36
	Semi-soft	205	4 (1.9)	0	0	82
	Semi-soft (mold-ripened)	261	7 (27)	ND	ND	82
	Semi-soft (smear-ripened)	343	33 (9.6)	ND	ND	82
	Semi-soft (smear-ripened)	69	6 (8.7)	13 (18.8)	ND	36
	Hard	88	0	0	0	82

West Germany					
Soft	712	33 (4.6)	58 (8.1)	4[c] (0.6)	149
Soft	166	7 (4.2)	ND	ND	152
Soft	248	3 (1.2)	16 (6.4)	0	140
Soft (mold-ripened)	117	4 (3.4)	5 (4.3)	0	59
Soft (smear-ripened)	41	3 (7.3)	5 (12.2)	0	59
Soft (unripened)	8	0	0	0	59
Soft/Semi-soft	256	23 (9.0)	ND	7 (2.7)	80
Semi-soft	268	9 (3.4)	7 (2.6)	8[c] (3.0)	149
Semi-soft	45	0	1 (2.2)	0	140
Semi-soft (mold ripened)	12	0	0	0	59
Semi-soft (smear-ripened)	7	2 (28.6)	0	0	59
Semi-soft (unripened)	89	4 (4.5)	1 (1.1)	3[c] (3.4)	59
Semi-hard	237	7 (3.0)	14 (5.9)	0	149
Semi-hard	108	6 (5.6)	ND	ND	152
Hard	42	2[d] (4.8)	0	1[c] (2.4)	21
Acid	61	2 (3.3)	22 (36.1)	1[c] (1.6)	21
Acid	48	1 (2.1)	ND	ND	152
Fresh	149	0	0	0	21
Processed	21	0	0	0	21
Total	8,848	376 (4.25)	179 (3.72)	22 (0.46)	

[a]Not determined.
[b]Not reported.
[c]All isolates of *L. seeligeri*.
[d]Both isolates from ewe's milk cheese.

1150 samples of soft, semi-soft, semi-hard, or hard cheese or from 72 samples of pasta filata-type cheese such as provolone and mozzarella.

Between January 1987 and September 1988, Massa et al. (114) also examined 54 soft rindless (i.e., Mascarpone, mozzarella, Crescenza) and 67 soft thin-rind (i.e., Italico, Caciotta) cheeses produced by both large and small northern Italian factories for listeriae and *E. coli*. *Listeria monocytogenes* was detected in only 2 of 47 (4.2%) rind samples from thin-rind cheeses manufactured by one small factory with core samples from these two positive cheeses proving negative for the pathogen. While all other samples from thin-rind and rindless soft cheeses were free of *L. monocytogenes*, two mozzarella cheeses contained detectable levels of *L. innocua*. According to these investigators, *E. coli* populations in these cheeses ranged from <10 to 8×10^5 CFU/g with the two *L. monocytogenes*-positive cheeses containing $\geq 10^4$ *E. coli* CFU/g. However, since 14 similar *Listeria*-free cheeses also contained $\geq 10^3$ *E. coli* CFU/g, *E. coli* is clearly a poor choice as an organism to indicate possible presence of listeriae.

Switzerland

While several major Western European countries have experienced various degrees of economic loss from *Listeria*-contaminated cheese, thus far only Switzerland and the United States have been forced to deal with major outbreaks of cheeseborne listeriosis. Well before the 1987 listeriosis outbreak in Switzerland linked to consumption of Vacherin Mont d'Or soft-ripened cheese, Swiss officials began examining various cheeses for listeriae. Although these surveys apparently were prompted by the 1985 listeriosis outbreak in California, an unusually high incidence of listeriosis in certain areas of Switzerland which could not yet be explained may have provided added incentive to initiate these surveys. A two-stage *Listeria* monitoring program has since been established for cheese and other dairy products with random testing of 10-g samples obtained at both the factory and retail level (110). According to the Federal Bureau of Health, such samples must be completely free of *L. monocytogenes* before the product is deemed acceptable.

Working in Switzerland, Breer (82) examined 799 domestic and imported cheese samples for listeriae during the winter of 1985/1986. Various *Listeria* spp. were detected in 19.2% of the soft surface-ripened cheeses, all of which were traced to 10 Swiss and a few foreign manufacturers. During follow-up investigations of these 10 cheese factories in Switzerland, *Listeria* spp. were isolated from surfaces of various cheeses and also from curing and smearing brines, waste-water sinks, and surfaces of wooden boards used in cheese ripening. In addition, identical serotypes of *L. monocytogenes* (1/2b and/or 4b) and/or *L. innocua* were isolated repeatedly from the same cheese factories. These findings demonstrate that ample opportunity existed for cheese to become contaminated with listeriae during the later stages of manufacture and ripening.

Subsequently, Breer (82) reported that 4.9 and 4.7% of all cheeses sold in Switzerland contained *L. monocytogenes* or *L. innocua*, respectively (Table 10.6). Of equal importance is the fact that both *Listeria* spp. were isolated more frequently from soft (6.6, 6.3%) than semi-soft cheese (1.9, 0%) and that neither organism was detected in 88 samples of hard cheese.

During 1986 Breer (81) also found that 12.9 and 10.0% of soft surface-ripened

Table 10.7 Incidence of *Listeria* spp. in Soft Mold- and Smear-Ripened Cheeses Manufactured in Switzerland During 1986 from Pasteurized and Raw Milk

Type of cheese	Number of samples analyzed	Number of positive samples (%)	
		L. monocytogenes	*L. innocua*
Mold-ripened			
Raw milk	22	2 (9.1)	0
Pasteurized milk	9	0	1 (11.1)
Smear-ripened			
Raw milk	17	3 (17.6)	4 (23.5)
Pasteurized milk	22	4 (18.2)	2 (9.1)
Total	70	9 (12.9)	7 (10.0)

Source: Adapted from Ref. 81.

cheeses manufactured in Switzerland were contaminated with *L. monocytogenes* and *L. innocua*, respectively (Table 10.7). The incidence of both *Listeria* spp. was generally twice as high in smear- rather than mold-ripened cheese. As in previous studies, the rate of *Listeria* contamination was typically independent of the type of milk (raw or pasteurized) from which smear-ripened cheeses were manufactured.

These Swiss studies, along with several West German surveys to be discussed shortly, indicate a greater likelihood of isolating *L. monocytogenes* and *L. innocua* from high rather than low moisture cheese, with special emphasis on mold- and smear-ripened varieties. In support of this observation, Bannerman and Bille (74) found that 110 of 449 (24.5%) rinds from soft cheese produced in Switzerland were contaminated with *Listeria* spp., including a high percentage of samples with *L. monocytogenes*. During an additional survey made between October 1986 and September 1987 (36), *L. monocytogenes* was detected in 4 of 18 (22.2%) and 6 of 67 (8.7%) smear-ripened soft (i.e., Limburger, Romadur, Muenster, Reblochon) and semi-soft (i.e., St. Paulin, Tilsiter, Mutschli, Raclette) cheeses, respectively, with many cheeses also containing *L. innocua*. From the apparent widespread distribution of *Listeria* within some cheese factory environments, it follows that cheeses prepared from raw and pasteurized milk are equally likely to contain listeriae. Additional information concerning the incidence and control of listeriae in dairy factories and other food-processing facilities is given in Chapter 15.

West Germany

As mentioned in Chapter 8, Germany experienced a major outbreak of listeriosis shortly after World War II. This outbreak, which may have resulted from consuming contaminated raw milk, led to an increased interest in listeriosis research, and this in turn prompted Prof. H. P. R. Seeliger to publish his time-honored monograph *Listeriosis* in 1961. During the last 40 years, Dr. Seeliger has emerged as one of the world's leading authorities on listeriosis. In addition, he has been operating a listeriosis research center at the Institut für Hygiene und Mikrobiologie der Universität Würzburg to which *Listeria* isolates can be sent for biochemical and serological confirmation. Hence, it is not surprising to learn that the incidence of listeriae in cheese has received considerable attention in West Germany.

Although spared from the heavy economic losses experienced by the United States and France, West Germany and most other European countries have not escaped the *Listeria* problem completely unscathed. Despite rigorous testing, *Listeria*-laden West German blue-veined cheese was recalled from France (110), with a similar recall issued for sour milk cheese exported to Canada (61,110) and The Netherlands (110). Consequently, a series of *Listeria*-monitoring programs were introduced for West German soft, semi-soft, semi-hard, and hard cheeses as well as cultures, cheese byproducts, and the general environment within cheese factories. As of December 1990, West German officials were enforcing a policy similar to that adopted in Canada in which only contaminated foods previously associated with foodborne listeriosis outbreaks would be recalled from the marketplace.

Results from various surveys made since 1986 (Table 10.6) indicate that 0–7.3% (average of 3.9%) and 0–28.6% (average of 3.6%) of the soft and semi-soft cheeses marketed in Germany contained *L. monocytogenes*, respectively, with the highest incidence of listeriae generally occurring in smear-ripened varieties. With few exceptions, *L. innocua* was isolated more frequently from soft and semi-soft cheese than was *L. monocytogenes*. While somewhat similar average percentages were reported for the incidence of *L. monocytogenes* in semi-hard (3.8%) and hard cheese (4.8%), the two hard cheeses that contained *L. monocytogenes* were reportedly manufactured from ewe's rather than cow's milk. Overall, it appears that the *Listeria* contamination rate for hard cheeses prepared from cow's milk may still be relatively low, as also observed in Switzerland (Table 10.6). Hence, these results from West Germany generally agree with those from other surveys in that *L. monocytogenes* was found more frequently in high rather than low moisture cheese.

Of the three remaining categories of West German cheese shown in Table 10.6, only acid curd cheese was positive for listeriae. The apparent absence of *Listeria* spp. from samples of fresh (i.e., cottage) and processed cheese is not entirely unexpected since procedures used to manufacture these cheeses include relatively severe heat treatments. Even if a few listeriae survived the manufacturing process, most, if not all, of the survivors would have been sublethally injured during exposure to heat and/or acid and would therefore be unable to grow in most selective enrichment broths that are commonly used for examining cheese.

In the only other study thus far reported, Weber et al. (159) examined a variety of West German cheeses, including 11 types manufactured from ewe's and goat's milk, for listeriae (Table 10.8). While all cheeses prepared from ewe's or goat's milk were free of *L. monocytogenes*, *L. innocua* was detected in one sample of fresh goat's milk cheese.

Despite the ability of lactating sheep and goats to shed *L. monocytogenes* in their milk, as further evidenced by the recent isolation of *L. monocytogenes* from approximately 4 of 450 (0.8%) samples of raw goat's milk in England (102), relatively few additional studies have dealt with the incidence of listeriae in ewe's and goat's milk cheese. Nevertheless, in addition to the aforementioned survey of German hard cheese produced from ewe's milk (149), Tham (153) also recently reported isolating *L. monocytogenes* from one sample of 8-week-old goat cheese marketed in Sweden.

The incidence of *L. monocytogenes* in the remaining cheeses prepared from cow's

Table 10.8   Incidence of *Listeria* spp. in Domestic and Imported Cheese Analyzed in West Germany Between October 1987 and June 1988

Type of cheese/milk[a]	Number of samples analyzed	Number of positive samples (%)	
		L. monocytogenes	*L. innocua*
Fresh/Cow	21	2 (9.5)	0
Fresh/Goat	1	0	1 (100.0)
Soft/Cow	307	8 (2.6)	11 (3.6)
Soft/Goat	1	0	0
Soft/Ewe	3	0	0
Semi-soft/Cow	144	19 (13.2)	8 (5.6)
Semi-soft/Ewe	6	0	0
Semi-hard/Cow	22	0	11 (50.0)
Hard/Cow	4	0	0

[a]Milk from which cheese was manufactured.
Source: Adapted from Ref. 159.

milk was similar to those values obtained in other studies (Table 10.6), with the pathogen detected in 2.6 and 13.2% of the soft and semi-soft (presumably mold- and smear-ripened varieties) cheeses examined, respectively. The unusually high incidence of *L. monocytogenes* in fresh curd cheese (9.5%) is probably the result of contamination during later stages of manufacture and/or packaging as well as the small number of samples examined. As was true for surveys of French soft and soft-ripened cheese discussed earlier in this chapter, most *L. monocytogenes* isolates were of serotype 1/2 (22 strains), with the remaining seven isolates classified as 4ab or 4b. However, since most clinical *L. monocytogenes* isolates from West Germany have been identified as being of serotype 4b, it appears that some questions may remain concerning the ability of present isolation methods to recover *L. monocytogenes* serotype 4b, as compared to other serotypes, from various foods, including cheese.

Other European Countries

As already implied, recent *Listeria* problems that have affected the European cheese industry are not limited to France, Italy, Switzerland, and West Germany. Other European nations including Austria, Belgium, Denmark, England, Finland, Greece, Hungary, The Netherlands, Spain, and Sweden also expressed concern in a March 1989 poll conducted by the International Dairy Federation (110). According to the survey, *L. monocytogenes* has been isolated from domestic cheese sold in Austria (soft cheese), Belgium (rind-type cheese), Denmark (various soft cheeses), England (various cheeses), Ireland (soft farm-house cheese), The Netherlands (young farm-house Gouda), and Sweden (goat's milk cheese), with Denmark, England, and Sweden also experiencing problems with soft or semi-soft cheeses imported from Denmark, France, and/or West Germany. In contrast, Norway (110,161) and Spain (110) have thus far only been affected by imported soft and/or blue-veined cheeses that contained detectable levels of *L. monocytogenes*. Thus, in addition to France, Italy, Switzerland, and West Germany, Austria, Belgium, Denmark (62), England, Finland, Greece, Hungary, The Netherlands, and Sweden also have developed programs to actively monitor the incidence of listeriae in domestic/imported cheese (especially soft surface-ripened varieties) and/or manufacturing environments within cheese factories.

According to the March 1989 survey (110), Austria, Denmark, France, Greece, Hungary, Italy, Sweden, Switzerland, and West Germany presumably have enacted regulations regarding the sale of cheese and other foods contaminated with *L. monocytogenes*, with most countries attempting to prevent distribution and sale of cheese (and in some instances other ready-to-eat foods associated with listeriosis) in which the pathogen is detected in 10–30 g of product. Since these observations along with the 1987 listeriosis outbreak in Switzerland involving Vacherin Mont d'Or cheese both support the widespread notion that *L. monocytogenes* poses a significant health threat to certain segments of the population, the European Economic Community Consumers Association has published a list of soft and semi-soft cheeses manufactured in France and Switzerland that should be avoided by susceptible individuals—pregnant women, immunocompromised adults, and the elderly. This highly controversial list of cheeses (and brands when applicable) included Brie (La Renommee), Muenster (Ermitage), Crème de Bleu (Diapason), Lys Bleu, Camembert (I Signy), Tilsit, Fourme de Bresse, Bleu de Bresse, Reblochon, Pont L'Eveque, Gruyère, and Vacherin Mont d'Or.

In February of 1988, a case of cheeseborne listeriosis was reported in England in which a 40-year-old woman contracted meningitis shortly after consuming Anari-type soft goat's milk cheese that contained *L. monocytogenes* at levels > 10^7 CFU/g (see Chapter 8). During follow-up investigations at the factory (116), the same *L. monocytogenes* strain also was isolated from 8 of 11, 4 of 8, 1 of 1, and 1 of 1 factory and/or retail samples of Halloumi, Cheddar, Gjestost, and soft chive cheese, respectively. In addition, *L. innocua* also was isolated from several samples of Halloumi and Cheddar cheese. As in the previously described studies by Pini and Gilbert (124) and Massa et al. (114), no clear relationship was observed between the presence of *L. monocytogenes/L. innocua* and coliforms/*E. coli*, which again suggests that coliforms are poor indicators of *Listeria* contamination.

More recently, the Public Health Laboratory Service in London coordinated a large-scale survey in which various dairy products produced in England and Wales were sent to 46 laboratories throughout the country for *Listeria* testing. Preliminary results from this comprehensive survey (Table 10.6) indicated that 8.2, 1.1, and 4.1% of the soft-ripened, soft-unripened, and goat's milk cheese manufactured in England and Wales contained *L. monocytogenes*, with strains of serotype 1 presumably predominating. These incidence rates for *L. monocytogenes* in soft-ripened and unripened cheese are similar to those that have been observed in most other European countries.

As just suggested, numerous surveys for incidence of listeriae in cheese also have been completed in many of these aforementioned countries which, with the exception of Denmark, have not experienced major economic problems associated with *Listeria*-contaminated cheese. Following the 1986 report of an English woman who contracted listeriosis after consuming French soft cheese (75), two English researchers (124) examined 45 domestic soft cheeses as well as 177 soft cheeses imported from France, Italy, Cyprus, West Germany, Denmark, and Lebanon for *Listeria* spp. and *E. coli*. (Table 10.9). Overall, *L. monocytogenes* was isolated from 2 of 45 (4.4%) English cheeses and 21 of 177 (11.9%) soft cheeses imported from France, Italy, and Cyprus.

Table 10.9 Incidence of *L. monocytogenes* and *E. coli* in Soft Cheese Sampled in England During 1987

Country of origin	Number of samples analyzed	L. monocytogenes			Number of samples with >10 E. coli CFU/g (%)
		Number of positive samples (%)	Level/g		
England	85	12 (14.1)	$<10^2-10^5$		32 (37.6)
France	45	2 (4.4)	$<10^4$		14 (31.1)
Italy	44	7 (15.9)	$<10^2-10^4$		12 (27.3)
Cyprus	20	2 (10.0)	$<10^2$		3 (15.0)
West Germany	17	0	ND^a		9 (52.9)
Denmark	6	0	ND		2 (33.3)
Lebanon	5	0	ND		1 (20.0)
Total	222	23 (10.4)	$ND-10^5$		73 (32.9)

[a]Not detected.
Source: Adapted from Ref. 124.

Populations of *L. monocytogenes* in contaminated cheese ranged from $<10^2$ to 10^5 CFU/g with 9 of 12 French cheeses containing $\geq 10^4$ CFU/g. Despite differences in media and methods used in various surveys, the contamination rate of 14.1% for soft French cheeses calculated in this study was close to the 14.5% previously observed for French soft cheese exported to The Netherlands. As was true for previous surveys of French dairy products, all strains of *L. monocytogenes* (except one nontypable strain) were of serotypes 1/2 or 4b with the former predominating. *Listeria innocua*, the only other *Listeria* sp. detected during this survey, was isolated from 9 of 85 (10.6%), 7 of 44 (15.9%), 2 of 45 (4.4%), and 1 of 6 (16.7%) soft cheeses produced in France, Italy, England, and Denmark, respectively, with 6 of 222 (2.7%) cheeses containing both *Listeria* spp. Although *E. coli* populations exceeded 10 CFU/g in 73 of 222 (32.9%) cheeses examined, no correlation was observed between the presence of *L. monocytogenes* or *L. innocua* and contamination with *E. coli*. In fact, *E. coli* was detected at >10 CFU/g in only 10 of 23 (43.5%) cheeses that contained the pathogen. In this study, 10 of 23 (43.5%) cheeses contaminated with *L. monocytogenes* were prepared from pasteurized milk, whereas two and 11 of the remaining positive cheeses were manufactured from raw milk and milk of undetermined processing, respectively. Thus, as in previous studies, the type of milk (i.e., raw or pasteurized) from which cheese is made appears to be a poor indicator of possible *Listeria* contamination.

Problems regarding occasional presence of *L. monocytogenes* in soft cheese also have surfaced in the Scandinavian countries with the pathogen being identified in Danish Esrom and Blue Costello cheese that was exported to Norway (110,164), Sweden (110), and the United States. While four Class I recalls were issued for Danish Esrom and Blue Costello cheese in the United States (Table 10.3), both of these cheeses (~20% of which were contaminated) were on sale for up to 2 months in Norway before being removed from the market, apparently without incident (161). Danish officials also took steps to prevent unsold cheese from reaching consumers and have since developed a *Listeria* surveillance program (62) similar to that instituted in the United States with routine testing of various cheeses as well as cheesemaking facilities.

Additional concern over the microbiological safety of various cheeses also led to isolation of *L. monocytogenes* serotype 1/2b from two soft-ripened cheeses presumed to be from France (one prepared from raw milk and one from pasteurized milk) and that were exported to Norway and Sweden (154). Surface and interior samples from the raw milk cheese contained 7.5×10^5 and 1.0×10^2 *L. monocytogenes* CFU/g, respectively, whereas corresponding samples from the pasteurized milk cheese contained 4.0×10^6 and 1.0×10^6 *L. monocytogenes* CFU/g. The reasons for nonuniform distribution of listeriae in soft-ripened cheese will be explored in the second half of this chapter. Although cheese prepared from raw milk contained 3×10^6 to 7×10^6 coliform bacteria/g, coliform tests indicated that the remaining cheese manufactured from pasteurized milk was fit for consumption. These findings reinforce the fact that coliform-free cheese may not necessarily be free of *L. monocytogenes*.

Other Countries

While primarily undocumented in the scientific literature, reports of *Listeria*-contaminated cheese in countries outside of North America and Europe also are beginning to surface. In 1987, *L. monocytogenes* was recovered from ricotta cheese manufactured in Melbourne, Australia (158). This event, along with identification of *L. monocytogenes* in the same imported brands of Danish blue and French blue cheese that were recalled in the United States (108) prompted Venables (158) to determine the incidence of listeriae in Camembert, blue vein, ricotta, cottage, pasta filata, high moisture, low acid, and other varieties of cheese manufactured in and around Melbourne, Australia. Overall, *L. monocytogenes* was recovered from 6 of 338 (1.8%) cheeses produced by five different manufacturers, with the pathogen identified as present in pasta filata (three samples), ricotta (two samples), and shredded (one sample) cheese. One cheese also contained *L. seeligeri*. Simultaneous identification of *L. monocytogenes* in environmental samples from all factories producing *Listeria*-positive cheese strongly suggests that these cheeses were contaminated during manufacture and/or ripening. In keeping with United States policies, attempts were made to remove tainted cheese from the marketplace. Furthermore, after thoroughly cleaning and sanitizing the factory, government officials required that *Listeria*-free cheese be produced for 12 consecutive days before being released to the public. Recent discovery of nonpathogenic listeriae in raw milk from neighboring New Zealand also has prompted authorities in that country to institute a similar environmental monitoring program for all cheesemakers who export their products.

While information regarding presence of listeriae in dairy products produced elsewhere is particularly scant, results from the March 1989 IDF Survey (110) indicate that *L. monocytogenes* has not yet been isolated from any dairy products manufactured in South Africa, Israel, and the Soviet Union. Consequently these countries have not yet expressed any major concern over presence of listeriae in dairy products or other ready-to-eat foods. Although *Listeria* spp. also have not yet been identified in any domestic or imported foods sold in Japan, government officials in Japan are well aware of the problems that have been associated with consumption of *Listeria*-contaminated cheese elsewhere and therefore have begun to monitor both domestic and imported cheese for listeriae.

Given the enormous volume of dairy products exported to other countries and the fact that *L. monocytogenes* has been isolated from the natural environment of all seven continents except Antarctica, it appears that other developed countries are unlikely to remain completely untouched by the problems associated with *Listeria*-contaminated foods. Consequently, interest in the incidence of listeriae in dairy products and other ready-to-eat foods is likely to increase in the years ahead.

BEHAVIOR OF *L. MONOCYTOGENES* IN FERMENTED MILKS

Before the well-known 1985 outbreak of cheeseborne listeriosis occurred in California, very little information was available about the behavior of *L. monocytogenes* in fermented milks and cheese. In fact, at the time of this outbreak, a search of the scientific literature uncovered only four such studies, which were reported from Bulgaria (109,155) and Yugoslavia (145,148) between 1965 and 1979. Hence, in addition to prompting numerous surveys for *Listeria* spp. in cheese, discovery of cheese as an important vehicle in foodborne listeriosis has thus far (May 1990) led to over 30 publications addressing the fate of *L. monocytogenes* in fermented dairy products during manufacture and storage.

As described elsewhere in this book, cows, sheep, and goats can shed *L. monocytogenes* naturally in their milk during lactation. According to results from recent environmental surveys of dairy-processing facilities, ample opportunity exists for this pathogen to enter pasteurized milk as a postpasteurization contaminant before the fermentation process begins as well as afterward as a contaminant of the finished product. Thus far most studies have dealt with behavior of *L. monocytogenes* in fermented dairy products inoculated with the pathogen either before or after fermentation, with relatively few studies addressing the fate of listeriae in fermented dairy products manufactured from naturally contaminated raw milk.

Although the extent to which *L. monocytogenes* survives in cultured dairy products is partly dictated by whether or not the pathogen enters the product before or after fermentation, viability of *Listeria* in fermented dairy products, particularly cheese, depends on the type of product in which the pathogen is found. Hence, to better understand the complex interactions between the various factors that affect viability of listeriae in cheese (i.e., amount, activity and type of starter culture, a_w, pH, salt content, temperature during manufacture and storage), it is appropriate to begin this section by first discussing the behavior of *L. monocytogenes* in milk fermented with mesophilic and thermophilic lactic starter cultures. Commingled with this information will be recent data concerning the fate of this foodborne pathogen during manufacture and storage of cultured buttermilk, cream, and yogurt. The viability of *L. monocytogenes* in coagulants (e.g., calf rennet, microbial rennet, and bovine-pepsin rennet extract), coloring agents (e.g., annatto), and starter distillates (e.g., natural flavor compounds derived from cultured milk) used in cheesemaking also will be considered before our discussion of natural cheeses and cold-pack cheese food. Two additional areas of concern to cheesemakers, namely the fate of *L. monocytogenes* in whey and salt brine solutions, will be examined in the final pages of this chapter.

Starter Cultures, Cultured Milks, and Cream

Fermented or cultured buttermilk, cream, and yogurt were among the first dairy products to be mass-produced commercially using pure bacterial starter cultures. Today, two mesophilic (optimal growth at 30°C) lactic acid bacteria starter cultures, namely *Streptococcus lactis* and *Streptococcus cremoris* (recently reclassified as *Lactococcus lactis* ssp. *lactis* and *Lactococcus lactis* ssp. *cremoris*, respectively), are commonly used either alone or in combination to manufacture cultured buttermilk and cream, whereas a mixture of two thermophilic (optimal growth at or above 37°C) lactic acid bacteria, namely *Streptococcus thermophilus* and *Lactobacillus bulgaricus* (recently reclassified as *Streptococcus salivarius* ssp. *thermophilus* and *Lactobacillus delbrückii* ssp. *bulgaricus*, respectively) is used to produce yogurt. These same mesophilic and thermophilic starter cultures also are used to produce over 400 varieties of cheese that are currently recognized by the United States Department of Agriculture (157). (Worldwide there are probably more than 1200 varieties of cheese.) The variety of cheese to be produced depends, in part, on which of the lactic acid bacteria are used, either alone or in combination, as the starter culture.

Mesophilic Starter Cultures

Viability of *L. monocytogenes* in the presence of mesophilic lactic acid bacteria was first examined by Schaack and Marth (138). Samples of autoclaved skim milk were inoculated to contain approximately 10^3 *L. monocytogenes* CFU/ml along with 0.1, 0.5, 1.0, or 5.0% of a *S. cremoris* or *S. lactis* milk culture and then fermented at 21 or 30°C for 15 hours.

As shown in Figure 10.2, *L. monocytogenes* grew to some extent in all samples during fermentation, regardless of the species of lactic acid bacterium, inoculum level, or incubation temperature. Maximum *Listeria* populations after 15 hours of incubation at 21°C were ~1.0–2.3 orders of magnitude lower in skim milk containing 0.1–5.0% of either starter culture than in control samples without starter culture. Increasing the incubation temperature to 30°C led to final *Listeria* populations that were ~2.5–4.0 orders of magnitude lower than in controls. As expected, growth of *L. monocytogenes* increased as the starter culture inoculum level decreased from 5.0 to 0.1%. Although acid production by the starter culture played a major role in limiting multiplication of *Listeria* with the pathogen never growing at pH < 5.0, two situations were reported in which the organism was almost completely inhibited at pH 5.6–6.0—well above the minimum pH value generally required for growth.

Results obtained with a commercially prepared starter culture medium with internal pH control prompted Wenzel and Marth (160) to speculate that factors other than pH (e.g., nisin, volatile compounds) may be responsible for at least partial inhibition of *L. monocytogenes* during a 30-hour fermentation with *S. lactis* at 21 and 30°C. However, these results do not negate the importance of using an active starter culture, normally at

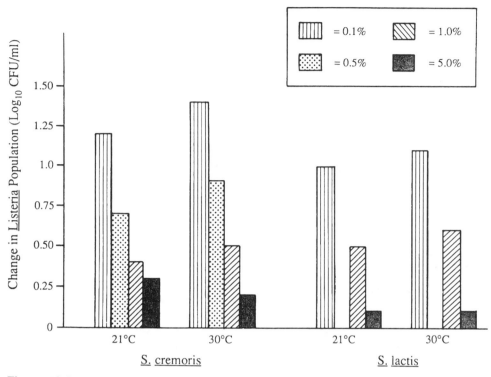

Figure 10.2 Changes in populations of *L. monocytogenes* in skim milk following a 15-hour fermentation at 21 and 30°C with 0.1, 0.5, 1.0, or 5.0% (v/v) added *S. cremoris* or *S. lactis*. (Adapted from Ref. 138.)

the 1.0% inoculum level, to help control growth of listeriae and other microbial contaminants during manufacture of fermented milks and cheese.

Cultured Buttermilk

Cultured buttermilk is essentially pasteurized skim milk that has undergone a 12- to 15-hour fermentation at 20°C with *S. cremoris* or *S. lactis* (0.5% initial inoculum) and certain flavor-enhancing lactic acid bacteria such as *Leuconostoc cremoris* or *Leuconostoc dextranicum*. After fermentation, the final product is packaged and refrigerated until consumed.

As part of a follow-up study (139), all 15-hour-old fermented milk samples from the aforementioned study by Schaack and Marth (138) were stored at 4°C and examined for *L. monocytogenes*. Survival of the pathogen ranged from an average of 5 weeks in skim milk fermented at 30°C with a 5.0% inoculum of *S. cremoris* to 12.5 weeks in skim milk fermented at 21°C with a 0.1% inoculum of *S. cremoris* (Table 10.10). Similarly, *Listeria* viability averaged 2.5–13.0 weeks in skim milk previously fermented at 30 and 21°C with 5.0 and 0.1% *S. lactis*, respectively. Slower inactivation of the organism in skim milks fermented at 21 rather than 30°C may be related to the rate of acid production during fermentation since pH values for fermented milks ranged between 4.3–6.0 and

Table 10.10 Weeks of Survival of *L. monocytogenes* in Skim Milks Fermented with *S. cremoris* or *S. lactis* at 21 and 30°C for 15 Hours and Then Stored at 4°C

| | *S. cremoris* | | *S. lactis* | |
Inoculum (%)	21°C	30°C	21°C	30°C
0.1	12.5[a]	6.5	13.0	2.0
0.5	10.5	6.0	ND[b]	ND
1.0	8.0	4.5	8.5	3.0
5.0	9.0	5.0	6.0	2.5

[a]Average of 2 trials.
[b]Not determined.
Source: Adapted from Ref. 139.

4.2–4.6 immediately after 15 hours of incubation at 21 and 30°C, respectively. The fact that *L. monocytogenes* can survive 10.5 weeks in a refrigerated product similar to cultured buttermilk (fermented 15 hours at 21°C with 0.5% *S. cremoris*) emphasizes the importance of maintaining sanitary conditions during manufacture of cultured buttermilk.

In addition to entering pasteurized skim milk as a postpasteurization contaminant, *L. monocytogenes* also can be introduced into cultured buttermilk as a postfermentation contaminant. Choi et al. (84) studied the second of these scenarios. Samples of commercially produced, cultured buttermilk (pH 4.21) were inoculated separately with each of four strains to contain an average of 3.5×10^3 *L. monocytogenes* CFU/ml and stored at 4°C. Under these conditions, the pathogen survived an average of 22.8 days (Table 10.11) with populations of three of four *Listeria* strains decreasing more than 100-fold during the first 8–12 days of refrigerated storage. It is important to realize that while *L. monocytogenes* was inactivated faster when added directly to cultured buttermilk than when skim milk was fermented into a "buttermilk-like" product in the previous study

Table 10.11 Survival of *L. monocytogenes* in Inoculated Samples of Commercially Produced Buttermilk and Yogurt Stored at 4–5°C

| Product | *L. monocytogenes* inoculum ($\log_{10}$ CFU/ml) | pH | | Survival (days) |
		Initial	Final	
Buttermilk	3.55	4.21	4.38	22.8
Plain yogurt				
Brand D[a]	4.26	4.02	4.08	21.2
Brand Y[b]	4.36	4.03	4.09	24.7
Vanilla-flavored yogurt				
Brand D	4.21	4.03	4.10	24.7
Brand Y	4.70	4.03	4.10	22.3
Plain low fat yogurt	2.10	4.10	4.10	3
Plain low fat yogurt	7.10	4.10	4.10	9

[a]Custard-style
[b]Fluid-style.
Source: Adapted from Refs. 84, 146.

(139), the pathogen still survived throughout the normal shelf life of the product. Furthermore, results from an earlier study (105) demonstrating that *E. coli* and *Enterobacter aerogenes* are inactivated faster than *L. monocytogenes* in cultured buttermilk imply that coliform-free buttermilk may not necessarily be free of listeriae. These findings again emphasize the importance of good sanitation in producing *Listeria*-free buttermilk.

Cultured Cream

Unlike cultured buttermilk, far less is known about the viability of *L. monocytogenes* in cultured cream. In the only study reported thus far, Stajner et al. (148) manufactured cultured cream from naturally contaminated raw cow's milk containing approximately 5×10^5 *L. monocytogenes* CFU/ml. According to these Yugoslavian authors, viable listeriae were detected in the finished product throughout 7 days of storage at 3–5°C.

Thermophilic Starter Cultures

Practically speaking, thermophilic fermentations used to produce yogurt and certain cheeses (e.g., Swiss, Parmesan, mozzarella, and Romano) are not normally continued beyond 4–6 hours. The only two exceptions are in production of Bulgarian buttermilk and acidophilus milk, which require thermophilic fermentations of 10–12 and 18–24 hours, respectively. Therefore, primary emphasis will be placed on the behavior of *Listeria* during the first 6 hours of incubation.

In addition to determining the fate of *L. monocytogenes* in the presence of mesophilic starter cultures (138), Schaack and Marth (137) also investigated the ability of this organism to grow during fermentation of skim milk with thermophilic lactic acid bacteria. As in the previous study, samples of autoclaved skim milk were inoculated to contain ~10^3 *L. monocytogenes* CFU/ml. After adding 0.1, 1.0, or 5.0% *Streptococcus thermophilus*, *Lactobacillus bulgaricus*, or a mixture of the two species, all samples were examined for numbers of listeriae during 15 hours of incubation at 37 and 42°C.

Limited growth of *L. monocytogenes* occurred in all samples with the organism generally attaining maximum populations after 6 hours of incubation at either temperature (Fig. 10.3). At this point, *Listeria* populations were generally 1.0–1.5 orders of magnitude lower in fermented than in unfermented control samples, indicating that growth of the pathogen was markedly suppressed by the thermophilic starter culture, particularly when used at inoculum levels of 5%. In addition, greater inhibition of listeriae was consistently observed in milks fermented at 42 rather than 37°C.

Listeria monocytogenes behaved similarly in milks fermented with *S. thermophilus*, *L. bulgaricus*, and a mixture of both starter cultures during the initial 6 hours of incubation; however, viability of the pathogen in milks fermented beyond 6 hours varied with the species of lactic acid bacterium used in the fermentation. While populations of listeriae remained relatively unchanged in all milks fermented 6–15 hours with *S. thermophilus*. (final pH of 4.55–4.90), the pathogen frequently survived only 9–15 hours in milks fermented with *L. bulgaricus* alone. Rapid inactivation of the pathogen coincided with pH values ≤ 4.0 which developed in milks fermented 9–15 hours with *L. bulgaricus*. The combination of *L. bulgaricus* and *S. thermophilus* was more inhibitory to *Listeria* than was *S. thermophilus* alone, but less inhibitory than was *L. bulgaricus* alone. Although populations of listeriae failed to decrease in milks fermented at 37°C

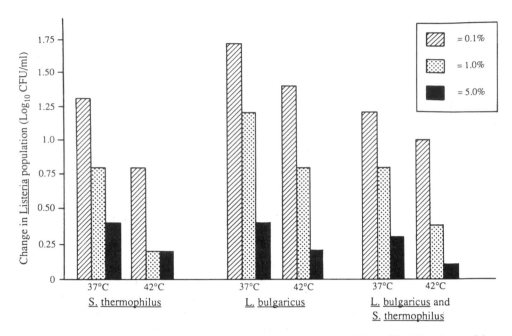

Figure 10.3 Changes in populations of *L. monocytogenes* in skim milk following a 6-hour fermentation at 37 and 42°C with 0.1, 1.0, and 5.0% (v/v) added *Lactobacillus bulgaricus*, *Streptococcus thermopilus*, or *L. bulgaricus* + *S. thermopilus*. (Adapted from Ref. 137.)

Table 10.12 Weeks of Survival[a] of *L. monocytogenes* in Skim Milks Fermented with *S. thermophilus* or *S. thermophilus* + *L. bulgaricus* (LBST) at 37 and 42°C for 15 Hours and Then Stored at 4°C

Inoculum (%)	*S. thermophilus*		LBST	
	37°C	42°C	37°C	42°C
0.1	28.5	15.0	7.5	1.5
1.0	32.0	8.5	1.5	12 h
5.0	21.0	5.0	1.0	15 h

[a]Average of 2 trials.
Source: Adapted from Ref. 135.

with the mixed starter culture, some inactivation was noted in all corresponding samples incubated at 42°C. As was true when *L. bulgaricus* was used alone, inactivation of listeriae by the mixed starter culture again was most pronounced in samples having pH values ≤ 4.0.

Following 15 hours of incubation, all fermented milks in this study were stored at 4°C and monitored for listeriae by Schaack and Marth (139). Using *S. thermophilus* alone, *L. monocytogenes* survived 21–32 and 5–15 weeks in milks fermented at 37 and 42°C, respectively (Table 10.12). Failure of these milks to attain pH values ≤ 4.0 after fermentation with *S. thermophilus* helps explain the unusually long survival of listeriae. As expected, *L. bulgaricus* was most detrimental to listeriae with the pathogen surviving beyond 15 hours only in samples fermented with the lowest inoculum. With 0.1% *L. bulgaricus* inoculum the pathogen was eliminated from milks fermented at 37 and 42°C following 7 and 3 days of refrigerated storage, respectively. Milks cultured with a combination of *S. thermophilus* and *L. bulgaricus* yielded results that were between both extremes observed when the two starter cultures were used separately (Table 10.12). Once again, *L. monocytogenes* survived longer in refrigerated milks fermented at 37 than 42°C, with slower inactivation in the former attributed to slightly higher pH values.

Yogurt

As previously mentioned, *L. monocytogenes* can enter yogurt either before the fermentation as a contaminant of the milk or afterward as a contaminant of the finished product. Schaack and Marth (137,139) examined the behavior of *Listeria* under the first of these conditions by inoculating yogurt mix to contain ~10^3–10^4 *L. monocytogenes* (strains V7, OH, Scott A, and CA) CFU/ml and 2% of a commercial starter culture containing *S. thermophilus*, *L. bulgaricus*, and *Lactobacillus acidophilus*. Yogurt mix was fermented at 45°C for 5 hours and then stored at 4°C. Populations of all four *Listeria* strains increased an average of 2.5- to 10.0-fold in yogurt mix during the fermentation. After finished yogurt at pH 4.75 was refrigerated at 4°C, numbers of listeriae decreased with strains V7, OH, Scott A, and CA surviving 7–12, 7–12, 4–12, and 1–5 days, respectively. The pH of yogurts in which listeriae were last detected ranged from 3.88 to 4.11. These findings are further supported by a similar French study (89) in which highly acidic yogurt (pH 3.5) prepared from yogurt mix inoculated to contain 10^2–10^7 *L. monocytogenes* CFU/ml was free of listeriae following 1–2 days of storage at 4°C. While both of these studies clearly show that acid development plays a major role in inactivating listeriae, other factors including production of antilisterial compounds (bacteriocins) by certain strains of *L. acidophilus* (127) also may contribute to the rapid demise of *Listeria* in yogurt, provided this lactic acid bacterium is in the product.

Although nearly all yogurt currently produced in the United States is prepared from cow's milk, this product is sometimes manufactured from ewe's and/or goat's milk, particularly in Eastern Europe and the Middle East. Hence, in 1964 two Bulgarian researchers (109) studied the viability of *L. monocytogenes* in yogurt prepared from naturally contaminated ewe's milk. After fermenting the milk with a mixture of *S. thermophilus* and *L. bulgaricus*, the finished product was stored at 10 and 18–22°C and was periodically analyzed for listeriae. Viability of *L. monocytogenes* was markedly influenced by the storage temperature with the pathogen surviving <24–40 hours and >6 days in yogurt held at 18–22 and 10°C, respectively. Faster demise of listeriae in yogurt stored at the higher rather than lower temperature again was at least partly related to acid production by the starter culture.

Many in the dairy industry believe that contamination of yogurt is more likely to occur after rather than before fermentation. Choi et al. (84) simulated postfermentation contamination of yogurt by inoculating two commercial brands of plain and vanilla-flavored custard- and fluid-style yogurt to contain ~10^4–10^5 *L. monocytogenes* CFU/ml. The pathogen survived an average of 21.2–24.7 days in yogurt held at 4°C (Table 10.11), with most listeriae being inactivated during the first 8–12 days of refrigerated storage. After inoculating various formulations of experimentally produced yogurt to contain ~10^6 *L. monocytogenes* CFU/ml, Griffith and Deibel (107) also detected the pathogen in yogurt samples having a pH value of 4.3 following 28 days of storage at 4°C. While the type of yogurt had no apparent effect on *Listeria* survival in either of these two studies, the point at which yogurt became contaminated greatly influenced survival of listeriae, with Schaack and Marth (139) showing that the pathogen survived only 1–12 days when added to yogurt mix before fermentation.

Siragusa and Johnson (146) conducted a similar study in which three different brands of commercial, unflavored, low-fat yogurt were inoculated to contain approximately 10^2 and 10^7 *L. monocytogenes* CFU/g and then stored at 5°C. Listeriae survived <3 days in yogurt inoculated with low levels of the pathogen, even though pH values of yogurt were similar to those in the study by Choi et al. (Table 10.11). Using the high inoculum, viable listeriae were found for only 9 days with populations decreasing approximately 100-fold each after 3 and 6 days of refrigerated storage. Griffith and Deibel (107) also found that *L. monocytogenes* populations decreased approximately four orders of magnitude in artificially acidified (pH 4.2) rather than fermented yogurt during the first 6 days of storage at 4°C. Hence, decreased tenacity of *L. monocytogenes* in inoculated yogurt samples in these two studies as compared to the work by Choi et al. (84) again demonstrates that factors other than pH likely contribute to the demise of *Listeria* in such fermented products.

Many yogurts and cultured buttermilks marketed today have pH values of approximately 4.0 and 4.3, respectively. Since large populations of *L. monocytogenes* were inactivated faster in yogurt than in buttermilk during refrigerated storage, one would expect a lower incidence of listeriae in commercial yogurt. Evidence from FDA surveys discussed earlier in this chapter supports this view since thus far the pathogen has been detected in commercial buttermilk but not yogurt. However, as was true for buttermilk, *E. coli* and *Enterobacter aerogenes* are also inactivated faster than *L. monocytogenes* in yogurt during refrigerated storage (105). Hence, coliform-free yogurt may not necessarily be free of *Listeria*. This is important to remember when results of coliform tests on these products are interpreted. It is evident from this discussion that good sanitation practices are of utmost importance in producing *Listeria*-free yogurt, buttermilk, and other fermented milk products.

Since yogurt is occasionally used as an ingredient in other foods, Sikes (144) recently investigated the fate of *L. monocytogenes* in low moisture (1.9% water), medium acid (pH 4.9) yogurt-based dairy bars supplied to the United States military. These bars, which contained ~34% heavy cream, 27.5% yogurt, 27.5% cream cheese, and 11% of other ingredients (i.e., sugar, sunflower oil, whey), were inoculated to contain approximately 1×10^5 *L. monocytogenes* strain Scott A CFU/g and then periodically examined for numbers of listeriae during extended storage at 25°C. Preliminary results indicated that *Listeria* populations decreased only approximately 100-fold after 40 days of incubation, thus demonstrating the ability of this organism to persist in low moisture, medium acid foods. As will soon be discussed, similar behavior has been reported for *L. monocytogenes* in semi-hard cheeses such as Cheddar, Colby, and Gouda which also have pH values near 5.0.

BEHAVIOR OF *L. MONOCYTOGENES* IN CHEESE

Considerable work has been done at the University of Wisconsin-Madison and elsewhere to define the behavior of *L. monocytogenes* during manufacture and ripening of various types of cheese. Most of these studies describe what might happen if cheese is prepared from contaminated milk. Since North American and European surveys have indicated that soft/semi-soft cheeses ripened with mold or bacteria are most frequently contaminated with *L. monocytogenes*, research dealing with such varieties of cheese will be discussed first, followed by data on ripened cheeses of progressively lower moisture content, unripened cheese, goat's milk cheese, and cold-pack cheese food. Whereas this chapter concludes with a discussion of the behavior of *L. monocytogenes* in whey and brine solutions, we will begin this section by first examining the viability of listeriae in coagulants, coloring agents, and starter distillates, all three of which are commonly used in cheesemaking.

Coagulants

To produce cheese curd, milk must first be coagulated or clotted, which can be done either by acidification or addition of a coagulating enzyme. In the first method, an active lactic starter culture is used to lower the pH of the milk to 4.6–4.7 (isoelectric point of casein) at which point the casein micelles in the milk precipitate and form a coagulum. Alternatively, coagulation is occasionally accomplished by adding food-grade acids directly to milk. Coagulation of milk by either means of acidification is primarily confined to the manufacture of cottage cheese and a few ethnic varieties of fresh cheese.

The second method, in which a coagulating enzyme is added to destabilize the casein micelles and clot milk at a near-neutral pH, is used to manufacture virtually all other types of cheese. Coagulants presently used in cheesemaking include calf rennet extract, bovine pepsin-rennet extract, and microbial rennet. Traditionally, calf rennet is extracted from the lining of the abomasum (fourth stomach) of suckling calves and contains two enzymes—pepsin and chymosin (the latter is most important for coagulation of milk). Shortage of calf rennet following World War II led to the use of bovine pepsin-rennet, an extract obtained from the abomasum of somewhat older calves, that can be substituted for calf rennet. Increased production costs of both calf rennet and bovine pepsin-rennet have in turn prompted development of several rennets of microbial origin. Thus far enzyme preparations obtained from molds belonging to the genus *Mucor* (particularly *M. miehei*) have proven to be the most satisfactory substitutes for animal rennet.

Since two of three coagulants used in cheesemaking are of animal origin and since these animals sometimes carry *L. monocytogenes*, this pathogen might occasionally appear in both crude enzyme preparations and finished coagulant at the time of shipping. While microbial rennet should be free of *Listeria* spp. when manufactured, presence of

Table 10.13 Survival of *L. monocytogenes* Strain California in Three Milk Coagulants Stored at 7°C

Product	Number/ml after days of storage						
	0	7	14	28	42	56	70
Calf rennet extract	2.5×10^3	1.5×10^2 (+)[a]	<10 (−)[b]	<10 (−)	<10 (−)	—	—
	1.1×10^4	3.5×10^2 (+)	<10 (−)	<10 (−)	<10 (−)	—	—
	3.0×10^5	6.0×10^4 (+)	1.2×10^3 (+)	30 (+)	<10 (−)	—	—
	2.0×10^6	6.0×10^4 (+)	4.5×10^3 (+)	2.0×10^2 (+)	<10 (−)	—	—
Bovine pepsin-rennet extract	9.5×10^3	10	<10 (−)	<10 (−)	<10 (−)	<10 (−)	—
	2.0×10^4	30	<10 (−)	<10 (−)	<10 (−)	<10 (−)	—
	7.5×10^5	1.0×10^3	1.0×10^2	<10 (+)	<10 (+)	<10 (−)	—
	1.0×10^6	2.0×10^4	1.0×10^2	<10 (+)	<10 (+)	<10 (−)	—
Microbial rennet	6.0×10^3	1.5×10^3	7.6×10^2	2.8×10^2	3.3×10^2	1.2×10^2	40
	7.0×10^3	1.7×10^3	1.0×10^3	2.2×10^2	4.4×10^2	1.4×10^2	90
	2.0×10^5	1.7×10^4	2.3×10^4	2.5×10^4	2.3×10^4	1.6×10^4	8.5×10^3
	1.0×10^6	1.5×10^5	4.0×10^4	3.6×10^4	9.3×10^4	7.0×10^3	9.0×10^3

[a] (+) Positive result by cold enrichment.
[b] (−) Not detected after 6 weeks of cold enrichment.
Source: Adapted from Refs. 93, 94, 96.

listeriae within the rennet-manufacturing facility or the cheese factory environment could lead to contamination of all three products if mishandled. Hence the possible presence of *L. monocytogenes* in coagulants should be of concern to cheesemakers. In fact, in 1989 the International Dairy Federation was considering a proposal to add rennet to its list of cheesemaking ingredients to be examined for *Listeria* spp. (150).

During 1988 and 1989, El-Gazzar and Marth published results from three studies examining the viability of listeriae in calf (93), bovine pepsin (94), and microbial rennet (96). In each of these studies, commercially produced, *Listeria*-free rennet was inoculated to contain approximately 10^3, 10^4, 10^5, or 10^6 *L. monocytogenes* CFU/ml and analyzed for listeriae during 56–70 days of storage at 7°C using both direct plating and cold enrichment.

All samples of calf and bovine pepsin-rennet inoculated with the two lowest levels of *Listeria* were free of the pathogen after 14–28 days of storage at 7°C (Table 10.13). Even though 42–56 days of storage were required to eliminate the pathogen from samples containing initial inocula of approximately 10^5 and 10^6 *L. monocytogenes* CFU/ml, the reader is reminded that all four inoculum levels used in these studies were many times greater than levels that might occur naturally in commercially produced coagulants. Hence, barring contamination in the cheese factory, these findings suggest that calf and bovine pepsin-rennet are normally held long enough in distribution channels to ensure cheesemakers that both coagulants are *Listeria*-free. Inactivation of *L. monocytogenes* in both calf rennet and pepsin-rennet probably results from the combined effects of 5% propylene glycol, 2% sodium propionate, 0.1% (or more) sodium benzoate, 14–21% salt, and a relatively low pH of 5.6. Results from several studies assessing the viability of *L. monocytogenes* in the presence of benzoic acid and sodium propionate are discussed in Chapter 5.

Unlike calf and bovine pepsin-rennet, more than 70 days of storage were required to eliminate *L. monocytogenes* at even the lowest inoculum level from microbial rennet (Table 10.13). Enhanced survival of listeriae in microbial rennet may be related to the nature of the coagulant itself as well as the presence of fewer preservatives. While *L. monocytogenes* is unlikely to gain entrance to microbial rennet during manufacture, the relatively high incidence of listeriae in cheese factories may lead to inadvertent contamination of the coagulant during cheesemaking. Considering the tenacity of *L. monocytogenes* in microbial rennet and the long shelf life of this product, it may be prudent for cheesemakers to periodically verify that the microbial rennet they are using is indeed *Listeria*-free.

Coloring Agents and Starter Distillates

Depending on local preference, various yellow-orange colorants such as annatto [an extract from annatto seed (*Bixia orellana*)] and turmeric [an extract from the turmeric root (*Curcuma longa*)] can be added to milk at the beginning of cheesemaking, with annatto most commonly used in the manufacture of Cheddar, Colby, Muenster, and brick cheese. While freshly prepared colorants are unlikely to contain microbial pathogens, inadvertent exposure of these coloring agents to *L. monocytogenes* in the cheese factory could lead to production of a contaminated product. Thus, in addition to the aforementioned coagulants, El-Gazzar and Marth (95) also investigated the fate of listeriae in five commercially available annatto/turmeric extracts that were inoculated to contain approximately 10^3–10^7 *L. monocytogenes* strain California/ml and stored at 22°C. Regardless of the initial inoculum level, populations of listeriae immediately decreased ≥4 orders of magnitude in all colorants, with the pathogen completely inactivated immediately after addition to three of five extracts. The almost instantaneous demise of *Listeria* in these three colorants was attributed to the presence of propylene glycol and a pH of 13.3 (one extract). While *Listeria* populations of ≤800 CFU/ml were observed in the two remaining colorants immediately after inoculation with the highest level of listeriae, these samples were free of the pathogen following 7 days of ambient storage. Overall, these findings indicate that the length of time that these colorants spend at ambient temperatures during distribution and before use at the cheese factory is more than adequate to inactivate small numbers of listeriae that might enter as chance contaminants.

Small levels of starter distillates, i.e., mixtures of natural flavor compounds such as diacetyl obtained by distilling specially cultured milks, are frequently used to enhance the flavor of cottage and processed cheese as well as ice cream, margarine, butter, yogurt, snack foods, and certain types of candy. Hence, in connection with the study just described, El-Gazzar and Marth (95) also examined the fate of listeriae in a commercially available starter distillate that was inoculated to contain 10^2–10^6 *L. monocytogenes* strain California, Scott A, or V7 CFU/ml and held at 7°C. Overall, strain California decreased to nondetectable levels in all samples after 2–7 days of storage, depending on the initial inoculum, whereas 7–28 days of incubation were required to eliminate strains Scott A and V7 from similar samples. Therefore, barring inadvertent contamination in the cheese factory, the time involved in shipping and distributing these starter distillates should be more than sufficient to eliminate any inadvertent *Listeria* contaminants.

Mold-Ripened Cheeses

Mold-ripened cheeses can be divided into two categories: (1) white mold cheeses, which are surface-ripened by either *Penicillium camemberti* or *Penicillium caseicolum* (i.e., Brie and Camembert), and (b) blue mold or blue-veined cheeses in which ripening results from growth of *Penicillium roqueforti* or *Penicillium glaucum* throughout the cheese (i.e., Roquefort, blue, Gorgonzola). The relatively high moisture content of the surface-ripened cheeses, along with a nearly neutral pH in fully ripened cheese, allows rapid growth of *L. monocytogenes* as well as other foodborne pathogens that would normally be inhibited in more acidic cheeses. Since mold-ripened cheeses also are highly susceptible to surface contamination during ripening, it is not surprising that Brie and Camembert were among the first varieties of cheese in which *L. monocytogenes* was detected and the behavior of the organism studied.

Camembert Cheese

Pasteurized milk was inoculated to contain approximately 500 *L. monocytogenes* (four strains evaluated separately) CFU/ml and manufactured into Camembert cheese by Ryser and Marth (131). Following 10 days of storage at ~15°C/95% R.H. to permit proper growth of *P. camembert* on the cheese surface, all cheeses were wrapped in foil and ripened at 6°C. Wedge (pie-shaped), surface, and interior samples of the cheese were diluted in Tryptose Broth and analyzed for listeriae at appropriate intervals using both direct plating and cold enrichment.

Populations of *L. monocytogenes* increased 5- to 10-fold during the first 24 hours after manufacture; however, this increase probably did not result from growth of the organism during cheesemaking. Numerous studies have shown that bacterial populations typically increase 5- to 10-fold during curd formation as a direct result of entrapment of organisms in curd particles, with the exact level of increase dependent upon the moisture content of the cheese. In all likelihood, *L. monocytogenes* was similarly concentrated during formation of Camembert cheese curd. That *L. monocytogenes* was trapped in curd particles is further supported by the fact that in this study, only 1.3% of the original *Listeria* inoculum in the milk was lost in the whey. Yousef et al. (164) later demonstrated that the failure to observe *L. monocytogenes* population increases of approximately 5- to 10-fold after formation of Camembert as well as Cheddar and cottage cheese curd was probably related to the method of sample preparation. Their improved procedure in which curd samples were homogenized in warm (45°C) Tryptose Broth containing 2% trisodium citrate was subsequently used to examine behavior of *L. monocytogenes* during manufacture and storage of brick (135), Colby (162), feta (123), blue (122), and Parmesan cheese (163).

During the initial 17 days of ripening, the first 10 days of which the Camembert cheese was held at ~15°C, populations of 3 of 4 *L. monocytogenes* strains decreased 10- to >1000-fold, with lowest numbers generally observed in surface samples (Fig. 10.4). Upon further ripening at 6°C, all four *Listeria* strains grew (particularly between 25 and 30 days of storage) and attained maximum populations of 10^6–10^8 CFU/g in wedge and surface samples from fully ripened cheese; however, maximum listeriae populations were generally 10- to 100-fold lower in interior samples from the same cheeses. While growth of *L. monocytogenes* clearly paralleled the increase in pH of the cheese during ripening with growth usually commencing after the cheese attained a pH value of 5.75–6.25, decreased viability of three of four *Listeria* strains in surface samples having pH values of 6.25–6.50 suggests that factors other than pH are also involved in controlling growth of this pathogen in Camembert cheese.

Results from a subsequent study by Ryser and Marth (133) showed greater growth of *L. monocytogenes* in filter-sterilized Camembert cheese whey previously cultured with *P. camemberti* than in uncultured whey adjusted to pH values of 5.60–6.80 and thus suggest that *P. camemberti* is not involved in reducing *Listeria* populations on the surface of Camembert cheese. In support of these findings, Geisen et al. (101) also failed to observe any antilisterial activity among several strains of *P. camemberti* that were tested against *L. monocytogenes* in vitro. However, in the work by Ryser and Marth (131) possible antilisterial activity from yeasts and non–lactic acid bacteria (i.e., micrococci, coryneforms) that are naturally present on the cheese surface during initial stages of ripening was not precluded.

To simulate contamination of cheese in the ripening room, Ryser and Marth (131) also inoculated surfaces of 10-day-old wheels of *Listeria*-free Camembert cheese to contain 2–40 *L. monocytogenes* (four strains tested separately) CFU/20 cm². All cheeses were then ripened at 6°C for 60 days during which time 10-g surface samples were analyzed for listeriae. Three of four *L. monocytogenes* strains grew on the surface of the

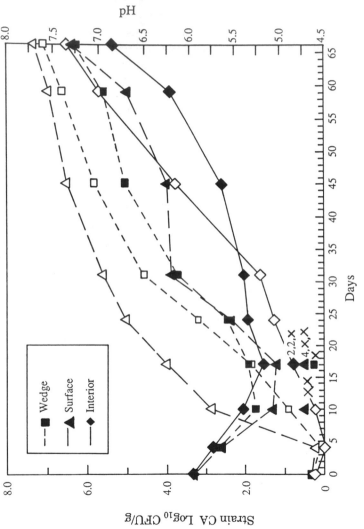

Figure 10.4 Behavior of *L. monocytogenes* strain CA (solid symbols) and pH (open symbols) during ripening of Camembert cheese. Solid symbols at <1.0 $\log_{10}$ strain CA/g indicate results for cold enrichment. Numbers indicate the week at which strain CA was found, whereas an "x" signifies that the pathogen was not detected after 8 weeks of cold enrichment. (Adapted from Ref. 131.)

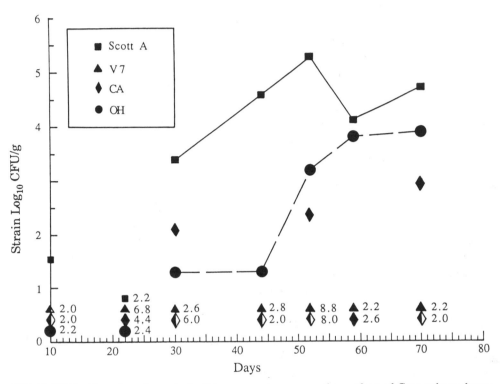

Figure 10.5 Growth and survival of *L. monocytogenes* on the surface of Camembert cheese. Half-solid and solid symbols at <1 log₁₀ *Listeria*/g indicate that the organism was detected in 1 of 2 or 2 of 2 samples, respectively, using cold enrichment. Numbers indicate the week at which *L. monocytogenes* was found. (Adapted from Ref. 131.)

cheese and attained maximum populations of ~10^3–10^5 CFU/g (Fig. 10.5). Although the remaining *Listeria* strain failed to grow on the cheese surface after 60 days of storage, the pathogen was routinely detected throughout the ripening period using cold enrichment. These findings, along with the unfortunate recall of over 300,000 tons of French Brie cheese, stress the importance of manufacturing surface-ripened soft cheeses from high quality, *Listeria*-free milk and observing good sanitary practices in the ripening room. Nonetheless, even under ideal manufacturing and ripening conditions, such cheeses may still inadvertently become contaminated with listeriae.

Since there are public health hazards associated with rapid growth of *L. monocytogenes* on surface-ripened cheeses, researchers on both sides of the Atlantic Ocean are exploring various means to eliminate this pathogen from such cheeses that are surface-ripened with mold as well as bacteria. According to one report (90), addition of lactoperoxidase system components to the surface of soft bacterial smear-ripened French cheese containing 10^2–10^6 *L. monocytogenes* CFU/g led to complete inactivation of the pathogen following 4 days of storage at 15°C. In 1989, Johnson (111) showed that lysozyme was only bacteriostatic to *L. monocytogenes* in Camembert cheese. While initial attempts failed (73), results from several additional studies exploring the possibility of employing nisin, nisin-producing starter cultures, and/or listeriocin-producing cheese surface flora to eliminate chance *Listeria* contaminants from soft, surface-ripened cheeses should be forthcoming.

In 1986, Terplan et al. (151) reported results from a study conducted in West Germany in which Camembert cheese was prepared from pasteurized milk inoculated to contain 95 *L. monocytogenes* CFU/ml. These researchers obtained results similar to those of Ryser and Marth (91) in that (a) *L. monocytogenes* failed to grow during cheesemaking, (b) low numbers of listeriae were recovered during the period of rapid growth of *Penicillium candidum* on the cheese surface, (c) populations of listeriae in cheese increased >10-fold between 21 and 28 days of ripening at 5°C, and (d) maximum *Listeria* populations of 9.5×10^6 CFU/g were detected in surface slices from fully ripened (pH > 7.0) 70-day-old cheese. In contrast to cheese prepared by Ryser and Marth (131), interior samples from 4- to 56-day-old Camembert cheese ripened at 5°C consistently contained <100 *L. monocytogenes* CFU/g and never attained pH values > 5.6, even after 56 days of ripening. Hence, under these conditions, growth of the pathogen was probably suppressed or severely retarded. However, some cells may have been sublethally injured during continuous exposure to this acidic environment, which in turn would have probably decreased the number of *Listeria* colonies observed on selective plating media.

Current evidence suggests that this pathogen behaves similarly in naturally contaminated, commercially produced soft and semi-soft mold-ripened cheese. While conducting a survey of soft/semi-soft cheese sold in Canada, Farber et al. (99) uncovered eight 4-month-old French cheeses, presumably of the Brie/Camembert variety, that contained ~10^4–10^5 *L. monocytogenes* CFU/g. Following one year of continuous storage at 4°C, *Listeria* populations remained constant in one cheese and decreased only 10- to 100-fold in the seven remaining cheeses. In view of these results, it is easy to understand why this pathogen has been most frequently detected in soft/semi-soft cheeses that have been surface-ripened by molds.

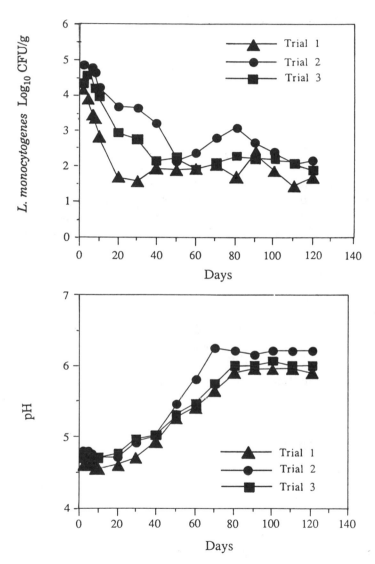

Figure 10.6 Changes in population of *L. monocytogenes* strain Scott A and pH during ripening of blue cheese. (Adapted from Ref. 122.)

Blue Cheese

Blue-veined cheeses such as blue, Roquefort, and Gorgonzola that are ripened internally and sometimes externally with *P. roqueforti* or *P. glaucum* also have been examined for their ability to support growth and survival of listeriae. Papageorgiou and Marth (122) used the modified Iowa method to manufacture blue cheese from pasteurized milk inoculated to contain approximately 1000 *L. monocytogenes* (strains Scott A or CA) CFU/ml. All cheeses were ripened 84 days at 9–12°C (90–98% R.H.) and then held an additional 36 days at 4°C.

Numbers of listeriae increased by an average of 1.50 $\log_{10}$ CFU/g during the first 24 hours of manufacture with increases of 0.62 and 0.71 $\log_{10}$ CFU/g attributed to entrapment of the organism within curd particles and growth, respectively. Growth of *L. monocytogenes* occurred primarily during the first 9 hours of manufacture and ceased when the pH of the cheese dropped below 5.0. As expected, somewhat less growth occurred in two lots of cheese with particularly rapid acid production.

Unlike the behavior of *L. monocytogenes* in Camembert cheese, the pathogen not only failed to grow during ripening of blue cheese, but decreased in numbers by two to nearly three orders of magnitude during the first 56 days of storage at 5°C (Fig. 10.6). These decreases, which occurred in spite of favorable pH values that developed during ripening from growth of *P. roqueforti*, may have resulted partly from the reported ability of eight different *P. roqueforti* strains to produce listeriocins in laboratory media (101). Nonetheless, combined effects of a relatively high pH and low storage temperature were probably responsible for both *Listeria* strains surviving at least 120 days in all lots of blue cheese. While additional tests showed that strain Scott A was evenly distributed throughout blocks of 120-day-old blue cheese, strain CA was far less tolerant to environmental conditions on the cheese surface and was detected in such samples only after cold enrichment. The lengthy survival of *L. monocytogenes* in blue cheese, coupled with the recall of Danish Bleu cheese and isolation of *L. monocytogenes* from Italian Gorgonzola cheese, all stress the importance of preparing blue mold cheeses from properly pasteurized milk under good hygienic conditions to prevent a possible public health problem involving *Listeria*.

Bacterial Surface-Ripened Cheeses

This group of cheeses consists of soft and semi-soft varieties that are ripened under conditions which induce a progression of microbial growth on the cheese surface. Examples of such cheeses include brick and Liederkranz from the United States, Port Salut and Saint Paulin from France, Tilsiter from Germany, Bel Paese from Italy, and Limburger from Belgium. Differences between these varieties result from the shape of the cheese as well as the amount and/or type of surface growth. Microorganisms are not normally added as pure cultures, but rather develop naturally on the cheese surface since ripening conditions promote growth of organisms that are normally present in the ripening room.

Proper aging of these surface- or smear-ripened cheeses results from the sequential growth of halotolerant yeast, lactic acid–metabolizing bacteria (*Micrococcus* spp.), and *Brevibacterium linens*, the last-named organism being essential for proper flavor development. As in mold-ripened cheeses, a pH gradient also develops during aging of bacterial surface-ripened cheeses, which in turn creates a more favorable environment for growth of contaminating microorganisms, including *Listeria*.

Using the washed curd procedure, Ryser and Marth (135) prepared brick cheese from pasteurized milk inoculated to contain ~10^2–10^3 *L. monocytogenes* (strain OH, Scott A, V7, or CA) CFU/ml. Following manufacture, cheeses were smeared with a culture of *B. linens* and ripened at 15°C/95% R.H. for 2, 3, and 4 weeks to simulate production of mild, aged, and "Limburgerlike" brick cheese, respectively. Since a natural pH gradient develops as brick cheese ripens, three types of cheese samples—surface, interior, and slice (surface and interior)—were analyzed for numbers of listeriae during 20–22 weeks of additional storage at 10°C.

Populations of strains OH, Scott A, CA, and V7 increased approximately 64.6-, 37.2-, 7.4-, and 6.8-fold, respectively, upon completion of brining approximately 32 hours after the start of cheesemaking. Since a population increase of approximately 10-fold can be attributed to entrapment of listeriae within curd particles with relatively few organisms appearing in the whey, growth of *L. monocytogenes* during the latter stages of cheesemaking before brining was confined to strains OH and Scott A. Numbers of listeriae remained relatively stable at 10^3–10^4 CFU/g of cheese during brining; however, a few organisms were leached from the cheese into the 22% NaCl brine solution. Information on behavior of *Listeria* in salt brine solutions appears at the end of this chapter.

Strains OH (isolated from Liederkranz cheese produced in Ohio) and Scott A grew rapidly during the initial 2 weeks of smear development required to manufacture mild brick cheese and generally attained maximum populations of approximately 6.20 and 6.60, 6.90 and 7.00, and 5.10 and 5.60 $\log_{10}$ CFU/g in 4-week-old slice (pH 6.0–6.5), surface (pH 6.5–6.9), and interior (pH 5.6–6.2) samples, respectively. During the remaining 20 weeks of ripening at 10°C, numbers of strains OH and Scott A generally decreased only 1- to 7-fold in mild brick cheese. Both strains also behaved similarly in aged and "Limburger-like" cheese during smear development and extended storage at 10°C.

In contrast, strains CA and V7 failed to grow appreciably during or after smear development, despite favorable pH values of 6.8–7.4 in fully ripened cheese. While strains CA and V7 were detected only sporadically in 4- to 26-week-old samples of mild, aged, and "Limburger-like" cheese at levels ranging between 2.70 and 4.60 $\log_{10}$ CFU/g, both strains were routinely recovered from 24- to 26-week-old slice, surface, and interior samples after cold enrichment. Hence, all four *L. monocytogenes* strains survived beyond the normal shelf life of brick cheese. Subsequent experiments dealing with possible antilisterial effects of several sulfur compounds (i.e., methyl sulfide, dimethyl disulfide, and methyl trisulfide) produced during ripening of brick cheese failed to explain the inability of strains CA and V7 to grow in mild, aged, and "Limburger-like" brick cheese. (Details of this experiment are in Chapter 5.)

In conjunction with the previously mentioned European study involving Camembert cheese, Terplan et al. (151) also assessed the behavior of *Listeria* during manufacture and ripening of red smear-ripened ("brick-like") cheese. When this cheese was produced from pasteurized milk inoculated to contain 95 *L. monocytogenes* CFU/ml, numbers of listeriae increased 10-fold after the coagulum was cut as a result of entrapment within the curd; however, no growth of the pathogen was detected during the remainder of cheese manufacture. In fact, unlike the study by Ryser and Marth (135), *Listeria* populations decreased 10-fold by the time the cheese at pH 4.9 was ready for brining, with the cheese containing only 9 *L. monocytogenes* CFU/g after brining. Following 8 days of smear development at 16.5°C/93% R.H., all cheeses were ripened at 5°C for an additional 62 days. *Listeria* populations close to the cheese surface increased from 2.5×10^1 CFU/g immediately after smear development to 1.5×10^4 CFU/g in 14-day-old cheese, during which time the pH increased from 4.9 to 5.1. Continued ripening of "brick-like" cheese at 5°C led to development of stable *L. monocytogenes* populations of 2.5×10^5 CFU/g in 1-cm thick surface slices of 42-day-old cheese. However, unlike the study by Ryser and Marth (135), the pathogen was never detected in interior cheese samples that were more than 4 days old, despite pH values of 5.7 in interior samples of 56-day-old cheese. While results of Ryser and Marth (135) suggest that *L. monocytogenes* should at least have been isolated occasionally from interior samples of "brick-like" cheese, the FDA procedure used in this study was unable to detect listeriae in these samples, possibly because of acid injury which may have occurred during exposure to pH values ≤ 5.2 for as long as 6 months.

Semi-Soft and Hard Cheeses

By definition, hard cheeses are those which contain $\leq 40\%$ moisture. Cheeses in this category include such varieties as Edam and Gouda (which can also be classified as semi-soft cheeses) as well as Colby, Cheddar, Swiss, Emmentaler, Gruyere, Romano, and Parmesan, the last two of which are very hard grating cheeses. Transformation of chalky, acid-tasting curd into a ductile, full-flavored cheese is accomplished during ripening through the action of milk enzymes, rennet, and various microorganisms in the cheese, including the starter culture. The biochemical changes which occur during cheese ripening are complex and involve hydrolysis of fats and proteins with subsequent decarboxylation, deamination, and/or dehydrogenation as well as production of carbonyls, nitrogenous compounds, fatty acids, and sulfur compounds, all of which contribute to the overall flavor of the final product. The amount of aging needed to obtain a fully ripened cheese is directly related to moisture content with a minimum of 2 and 10 months of ripening required for Edam (~40% moisture) and Parmesan cheese (~30% moisture), respectively. The current popularity of many of these cheeses, along with the ability of *L. monocytogenes* to survive in acidic environments during refrigerated storage, has prompted a series of studies examining the behavior of *L. monocytogenes* during manufacture and storage of seven semi-soft and hard cheese varieties.

Gouda and Maasdam Cheeses

Beginning with semi-soft/hard cheeses, Northolt et al. (120) prepared Gouda and Maasdam cheese in The Netherlands from pasteurized milk inoculated to contain approximately 500 *L. monocytogenes* CFU/ml. Gouda cheese was manufactured according to standard procedures with the exception that one lot was prepared using 0.3 rather than 0.6% starter culture to obtain a cheese with an unusually high moisture content of ~45%. Maasdam cheese was prepared using a culture of propionic acid bacteria in combination with 0.6% mesophilic lactic starter. After brine salting, Gouda cheese was ripened 6 weeks at 13°C, whereas Maasdam cheese was ripened 2 weeks at 13°C, 2 weeks at 18°C, and then stored at 4°C for an additional 2 weeks.

As in previous studies, entrapment of listeriae within curd particles during cheese-making resulted in population increases of approximately 10-fold as compared to the original level in pasteurized milk. However, some *Listeria* growth was noted during manufacture with populations increasing an additional 4-fold in normal Gouda and Maasdam cheese before brining. Six hours after manufacture, slightly higher *Listeria* populations were detected in Gouda cheese of high rather than normal moisture. Although numbers of listeriae in interior samples from both Gouda and Maasdam cheese remained relatively constant at ~10^4 CFU/g during the first 2 weeks of ripening, the pathogen was not detected in cheese samples taken at or near the surface. After 6 weeks of ripening, *L. monocytogenes* reappeared in surface samples from all cheeses at levels between 10^2 and 10^4 CFU/g. In contrast, numbers of listeriae in interior samples from 6-week-old cheese were only 4- to 8-fold lower than populations in the same cheeses immediately after brining. While *L. monocytogenes* survived best in high moisture Gouda cheese which had a pH of 6.0, the selective plating medium used in this study (Trypaflavine Nalidixic Acid Serum Agar) proved to be less than optimal for recovery of stressed or acid-injured listeriae that probably were present in fully ripened Gouda and Maasdam cheese having pH values of 5.48 and 5.44, respectively.

Colby Cheese

Yousef and Marth (162) prepared Colby cheese from pasteurized milk inoculated to contain 10^2–10^3 *L. monocytogenes* (strain V7 or CA) CFU/ml. Following manufacture, all blocks of cheese were held at 4°C for 140 days.

During cheesemaking, most *Listeria* cells were trapped in curd with an average of

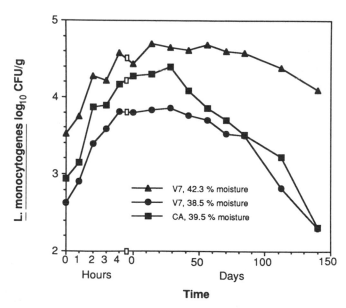

Figure 10.7   Behavior of *L. monocytogenes* during manufacture and ripening of Colby cheese. (Adapted from Ref. 162.)

only 2.4% of the original inoculum escaping in whey. Populations of *L. monocytogenes* in cheese increased an average of 1.27 orders of magnitude after pressing—about 29 hours after the start of manufacture (Fig. 10.7). Since an increase of no more than one order of magnitude can be attributed to entrapment of listeriae within curd particles after cutting, these findings suggest that slight growth of the organism did occur, particularly during the later stages of cheesemaking and pressing. Numbers of both *Listeria* strains remained relatively constant in cheese during the first 40 days of ripening, after which populations of listeriae decreased almost linearly (Fig. 10.7). Viability of *L. monocytogenes* was strongly influenced by moisture content of cheese with strain V7 decreasing more than twice as fast in cheese containing 38.5% (D-value of 54 days) rather than 42.3% (D-value of 124 days), which is well above the maximum allowable moisture content of 40.0% for Colby cheese.

Behavior of *L. monocytogenes* in cheese of normal moisture content also was strain-dependent, with strain CA being less stable than strain V7. However, strains V7 and CA were still detected in 140-day-old Colby cheese by direct plating, with cold enrichment results from a follow-up study (164) indicating that both strains were still viable in 5- to 8-month-old Colby cheese stored at 4°C. According to the FDA, Colby and other selected cheeses can be manufactured from raw or heat-treated (subpasteurization) milk, provided that the finished cheese is held a minimum of 60 days at or above 1.7°C (35°F) before sale in an attempt to eliminate pathogenic microorganisms. These results (and those for Cheddar cheese to follow) suggest it may be necessary to reconsider the adequacy of this aging requirement for cheeses prepared from raw milk.

Cheddar Cheese

Normal stirred-curd Cheddar cheese, which has a moisture content only slightly less than Colby (i.e., 36–38%), was manufactured by Ryser and Marth (130) from pasteurized whole milk inoculated to contain approximately 5×10^2 *L. monocytogenes* (strain Scott A, V7, or CA) CFU/ml. The resulting 4.5-kg (10 lb.) blocks of cheese were ripened at 6 and 13°C and assayed for numbers of listeriae at appropriate intervals.

All curd samples examined during manufacture contained approximately 5×10^2 *L. monocytogenes* CFU/g, which indicates that the organism was only minimally concentrated in the curd and failed to grow during cheesemaking. However, since only 6.4% of the initial *Listeria* inoculum was recovered in the whey, the expected 10-fold increase from entrapment of the organism in curd particles probably went unnoticed because inadequate sample preparation methods were used; the methods have since been improved in our laboratory (164). Numbers of listeriae increased slightly in cheese during pressing, with all three strains attaining maximum populations of ~3.50–3.75 $\log_{10}$ CFU/g after 14–35 days of ripening at 13 (Fig. 10.8) and 6°C (Fig. 10.9). This population increase, which was approximately 10-fold higher than that of the original inoculum in milk, probably resulted because of enhanced recovery of the pathogen from older cheese which was easier to homogenize rather than from actual growth, as shown by Yousef et al. (164). After 35 days of storage at either temperature, *Listeria* populations in cheese began to decrease, with all cheeses maintaining pH values of 5.04–5.09 throughout ripening. Strains Scott A, V7, and CA survived 70–224, 126–196, and 70–126 days in cheese ripened at 13°C, respectively, whereas the same strains remained viable for 70–154, 126–434, and 70–154 days in cheese aged at 6°C. Thus, except for

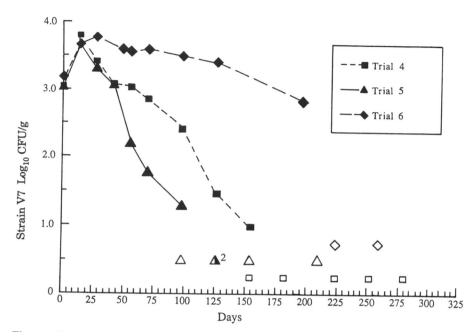

Figure 10.8 Survival of *L. monocytogenes* strain V7 in Cheddar cheese ripened at 13°C. Open symbols at <1 $\log_{10}$ *Listeria*/g indicate that the organism was not detected after 8 weeks of cold enrichment, whereas half-solid or solid symbols at <1 $\log_{10}$*Listeria*/g indicate that the pathogen was detected in 1 of 2 or 2 of 2 samples, respectively, using cold enrichment. Numbers indicate the week at which *L. monocytogenes* was found. (Adapted from Ref. 130.)

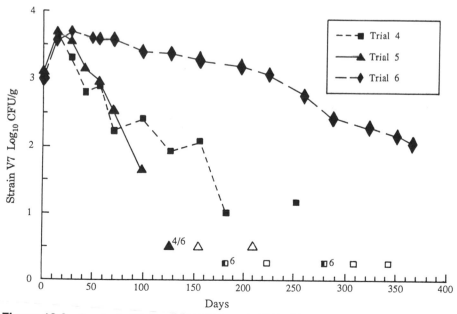

Figure 10.9 Survival of *L. monocytogenes* strain V7 in Cheddar cheese ripened at 6°C. See Fig. 10.8 for explanation of symbols. (Adapted from Ref. 130.)

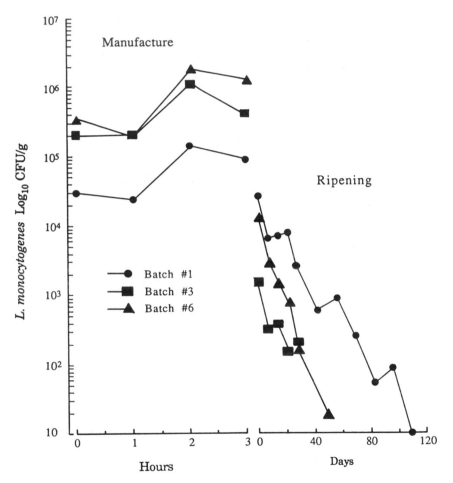

Figure 10.10 Survival of *Listeria monocytogenes* strain V7 during manufacture and ripening of Parmesan cheese. (Adapted from Ref. 162.)

strain V7, which was still present in one block of 434-day-old cheese at a level of 30 CFU/g, the remaining two strains survived equally well in cheeses ripened at either temperature. Additional experiments with strains V7 and CA demonstrated that *L. monocytogenes* was uniformly distributed in Cheddar cheese during at least the first 98 days of ripening at 6°C. These data currently provide the strongest evidence for the inadequacy of the 60 day/$\geq$1.7°C minimum holding period for cheeses manufactured from raw or subpasteurized milk.

Parmesan Cheese

Parmesan cheese, a hard cheese with a low moisture content, was prepared by Yousef and Marth (163) from pasteurized milk inoculated to contain ~10^4–10^5 *L. monocytogenes* (strains V7 or CA) CFU/ml. Unlike the cheeses discussed previously, a lipolytic enzyme (lipase) is sometimes added to cheesemilk to produce the characteristic flavor of fully ripened Parmesan cheese. In addition, the coagulum is cut into very small particles which are cooked at ~52°C (125°F) for 45 minutes until the pH decreases to 6.1. This step serves to expel whey, thus producing a dry, rice-like curd which can be pressed to form a very dense, low moisture cheese. Following manufacture, the cheese produced in this study was brine-salted (22% NaCl) for 7 days at 13°C, dried 4–6 weeks in a humidity-controlled chamber at 13°C, vacuum-packaged, and ripened at 13°C for a minimum of an additional 9 months.

During the first 2 hours of cheesemaking, populations of both *Listeria* strains increased approximately 6- to 10-fold, largely from entrapment of the organism within curd particles (Fig. 10.10). While *Listeria* counts remained relative stable during cooking of the curd at 52°C (125°F) for 45 minutes, populations decreased appreciably during pressing of the curd. During brining, drying, and ripening at 13°C numbers of both *Listeria* strains decreased almost linearly with estimated D-values ranging between 8 and 36 days. Using direct plating, strains V7 and CA were no longer detected in cheese after 21–112 and 14–63 days of ripening at 13°C, respectively. Despite large differences in survival of *L. monocytogenes* between different batches of cheese, both *Listeria* strains decreased at a faster rate in Parmesan than in Gouda, Maasdam, Cheddar, and Colby cheese during ripening. Decreased viability of the pathogen in Parmesan cheese is probably related to a combination of factors including (a) action of lipase added to the milk, (b) heat treatment that the curd receives during cheesemaking, and (c) lower moisture content (and water activity) of the fully ripened cheese. To decrease the moisture content and develop proper flavor, the present regulation in the United States requires that Parmesan cheese be aged a minimum of 10 months, regardless of whether or not the cheese is prepared from raw or pasteurized milk. According to the results of this study, such an aging process should be sufficient to produce Listeria-free Parmesan cheese.

Hard Italian-Type Cheese

Working in Italy, Comi and Valenti (86) inoculated the surface and interior of three freshly prepared hard Italian-type cheeses (a_w 0.95–0.98, pH 5.2–5.5) to contain 10^4–10^5 *L. monocytogenes* CFU/g. As was true for Parmesan cheese, the pathogen failed to grow in this relatively hard cheese, with *Listeria* populations decreasing 10- to 100–fold in both surface and interior samples from all three cheeses during the first 28 days of ripening at 4°C. Although the pH of surface and interior samples increased to 5.4–5.5 and 5.8–6.0, respectively, after 35 days ripening, *Listeria* populations continued to decrease with the pathogen only detectable by cold enrichment (i.e., populations $< 10^2$ CFU/g) in samples from 35-day-old cheeses. Results from composition analysis of these cheeses suggest that loss of moisture after 35 days of ripening (a_w 0.95–0.96) may have offset the benefit for *Listeria* growth caused by the increase in pH.

Pickled Cheeses

The terms "pickled" and "white-brined" are often used to describe a group of soft/semi-soft, white curd cheeses to which large quantities of salt are added as a preservative. Cheeses belonging to this group are principally manufactured in countries bordering the Mediterranean Sea and include such varieties as feta (Greece), Teleme (Bulgaria), Domiati (Egypt), and Kareish (Egypt). Some of these types of cheese are frequently prepared from ewe, goat, or buffalo milk. Depending on the variety of cheese, salt either can be added directly to the milk or curd, or the finished cheese can be stored in salt brine, salted whey, salted skim milk, or dry salt. The extreme tolerance of *L. monocytogenes* to high concentrations of salt, along with the organism's ability to grow at refrigeration temperature, has made these cheeses of particular interest to food microbiologists working with *Listeria*.

Feta Cheese

In 1989, Papageorgiou and Marth (123) described the fate of *L. monocytogenes* during manufacture, ripening, and storage of feta cheese. During the course of this work, there was an unconfirmed report of a woman in New York who delivered a stillborn infant in December of 1987 after consuming feta cheese contaminated with *L. monocytogenes*. Hence this study, which will now be discussed, has taken on added importance.

According to these authors, cow's milk was inoculated to contain approximately 5×10^3 *L. monocytogenes* (strain Scott A or CA) CFU/ml. After warming milk to 35°C, a 1% commercial starter culture of *S. thermophilus/L. bulgaricus* was added. Forty minutes after addition of rennet, the coagulum was cut and the resulting curd was transferred to metal hoops. Following 6 hours of draining, cheeses were removed from the hoops and placed in a 12% salt brine solution for 24 hours. The following day, all cheeses were transferred to 6% salt brine at 22°C for 4 days until the cheese attained a pH of 4.3–4.4. Finally, cheese in the same 6% brine solution was moved to storage at 4°C.

Cells of *L. monocytogenes* were entrapped in the curd during cheesemaking with populations nearly 10-fold greater in curd than in inoculated milk. Only about 3.2% of the original inoculum was lost in the whey. During whey drainage and the first 1–2 days of ripening at 22°C, numbers of listeriae increased ~1.5 $\log_{10}$ CFU/g with both strains attaining maximum populations of approximately 1×10^6 CFU/g (Fig. 10.11). Although growth of both *Listeria* strains generally ceased at pH values between 4.6 and 5.0, numbers of listeriae remained virtually constant in cheese during 2–5 days of storage at 22°C in 6% brine solution. Both salt brines in which feta cheese was ripened and/or stored were positive for listeriae (the details of this appear in our discussion of brine

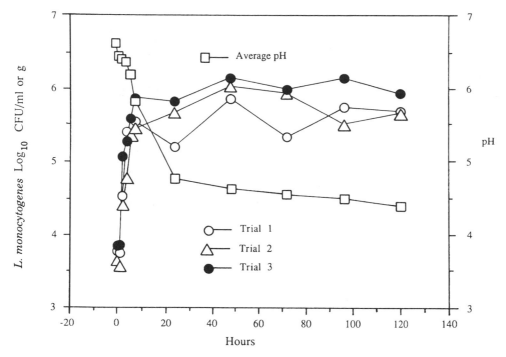

Figure 10.11   Fate of *L. monocytogenes* strain Scott A during manufacture and early brining of feta cheese. (Adapted from Ref. 123.)

solutions at the end of this chapter). Although all feta cheeses older than 5 days maintained a pH of 4.3, both *L. monocytogenes* strains survived >90 days in finished cheese stored at 4°C (Fig. 10.12). However, differences between the two *Listeria* strains were noted with populations of strains Scott A and CA decreasing 1.28 and 3.07 $\log_{10}$ CFU/g in 90- as compared to 2-day-old feta cheese, respectively. While feta cheese can be prepared from raw milk, ripening such cheese at or above 1.7°C for 60 days will not guarantee that the cheese is *Listeria*-free. Hence, it appears prudent to manufacture feta cheese only from pasteurized milk under good hygienic conditions to decrease the chance of a public health problem involving *Listeria*.

Bulgarian White-Pickled Cheese

As early as 1964, Ikonomov and Todorov (109) reported manufacturing white-pickled cheese from ewe's milk containing 10^2–10^3 *L. monocytogenes* CFU/ml. A mixture of 0.1% *S. lactis* and *Lactobacillus casei* served as the starter culture. Although *L. monocytogenes* survived 15–30 days in white-brined cheese ripened at 18–22°C, the pathogen survived twice as long when the same cheese was ripened at 12–15°C. In addition to storage temperature, *Listeria* viability also was partly dependent on the amount of acid produced in the cheese during ripening, with pH values of approximately 4.3 and 4.6 reported as lethal to listeriae in cheese ripened at 12–15 and 18–22°C, respectively.

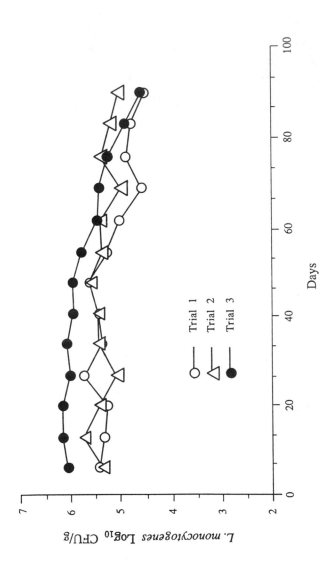

Figure 10.12 Survival of *L. monocytogenes* strain Scott A during storage of feta cheese. (Adapted from Ref. 123.)

Yugoslavian White-Brined Cheese

Ten years later, Sipka et al. (145) published results from another study in which white-brined cheese was prepared from naturally infected cow's milk containing 240 *L. monocytogenes* CFU/ml. Following manufacture, the pathogen grew rapidly in cheese, reaching populations of 7.8×10^5 and 1.0×10^6 CFU/g after 7 and 14 days of brining, respectively. Although maximum *Listeria* populations were similar to those observed in feta cheese (123), the pathogen appeared to be less hardy in white-brined than in feta cheese with populations decreasing to 1.3×10^5 and 1.2×10^2 CFU/g in 24- and 42-day-old fully ripened cheese, respectively. Increased inactivation of listeriae in white-brined rather than feta cheese apparently is not entirely related to acid development since the pH of the former cheese, 4.5–5.1, was higher than that of the latter, 4.3.

Ewe's and Goat's Milk Cheese

In areas of the world where cows are not plentiful (i.e., northern Scandinavia, Eastern Europe, Mediterranean, Middle East, and India), ewe's and goat's milks have been adapted for use either alone or in combination with cow's milk to manufacture different types of cheese. Representative cheeses in this group include such well-known varieties as French Roquefort and Greek feta cheese, both of which are traditionally prepared from ewe's milk. Lesser known cheeses typically prepared from ewe's and/or goat's milk include Egyptian Kachkaval, Italian fontina, Spanish Manchego, and Italian Pecorino Romano as well as many varieties of white-brined and goat's milk cheese, the latter of which are often produced in mountainous areas of Central Europe and Scandinavia. The occasional presence of *L. monocytogenes* in milk from healthy ewes and goats has prompted several studies dealing with behavior of this pathogen during manufacture and ripening of some of these less common cheeses.

Kachkaval Cheese

Work with this group of cheeses dates back to 1964 when Ikonomov and Todorov (109) examined the behavior of *L. monocytogenes* in Kachkaval cheese (a relatively soft, brine-salted cheese manufactured from ewe's milk in Eastern Europe and the Middle East, pH $\cong$ 5.0–5.8) prepared from raw ewe's milk inoculated with the pathogen. According to these investigators, *L. monocytogenes* survived in curd immersed in 5–6% salt brine at 71–76°C during cheesemaking and was still present in Kachkaval cheese (pH 5.0–5.4) after 30–50 days of ripening at 18–22°C.

Manchego Cheese

The next such study did not appear in the literature until 1987 when Dominguez et al. (91) reported manufacturing four lots of Manchego cheese (a hard aromatic cheese traditionally prepared from ewe's milk in Spain, pH $\cong$ 5.8) from a blend of pasteurized ewe's, goat's, and cow's milk (15:35:50) inoculated to contain either 4.0×10^3 or 1.9×10^5 *L. monocytogenes* CFU/ml. To assess growth of listeriae in cheeses having different rates of acid development, milks were inoculated with either 0.1 or 1.0% of a starter culture consisting of mesophilic lactic acid bacteria. The coagulum was cut approximately 45 minutes after addition of rennet; the resulting curd was drained, hooped, and pressed for approximately 10 hours. The finished cheese was then brine-salted overnight, ripened 10 days at 15°C/85–90% R.H., covered with paraffin, and aged an additional 50 days at 15°C.

Numbers of *L. monocytogenes* increased ≤10-fold in all cheeses during the first 10 hours of manufacture, primarily from entrapment of the organism within curd particles. The fact that cheeses prepared with either 0.1 or 1.0% starter culture contained similar *Listeria* populations indicates that behavior of the pathogen was not greatly influenced by the rate of acid production during cheesemaking. After the cheese was brined overnight, populations of listeriae decreased approximately 3- to 100-fold with additional small decreases observed during ripening of unparaffined cheese at 15°C. However, numbers of listeriae remained relatively constant in cheese at pH 5.1–5.8 after paraffining, with populations in 60-day-old cheese approximating the original inoculum in milk from which the cheese was manufactured.

Goat's Milk Cheese

Working in Sweden, Tham (153) examined the viability of *Listeria* in cheese prepared from raw goat's milk inoculated to contain 10^5–10^6 *L. monocytogenes* CFU/ml. A mixture of mesophilic lactic acid bacteria served as the starter culture. Approximately 45 minutes after addition of rennet, the coagulum was cut into cubes which were cooked at 37°C, drained, hooped, pressed for 1 hour, and brine-salted for 10 hours. The finished cheese was then ripened at 12°C for 22 weeks.

Actual numbers of *L. monocytogenes* could be determined in cheeses from only 2 of 6 lots using a blood agar/pour plate method. As shown in Fig. 10.13, *Listeria* populations decreased approximately 10-fold in goat's milk cheese during the first 14 weeks of ripening at 12°C. Extended survival, along with slight growth of listeriae in cheeses ripened longer than 14 weeks, probably is related to an increase in pH from 5.55 to 6.20 during ripening as well as a decrease in numbers of competitive microorganisms that were initially present in the raw milk. Although large numbers of enterococci and other microbial competitors interfered with the quantitative recovery of *L. monocytogenes* in the remaining four cheeses, the pathogen survived 10–16 weeks in three of these cheeses as determined by cold enrichment.

As you will recall from Chapter 8, a middle-aged English woman reportedly developed listeric meningitis in February of 1988 after consuming 2–3 ounces of commercially produced Anari-type goat's milk cheese containing 3–5×10^7 *L. monocytogenes* CFU/g (58). During a series of follow-up investigations (116), *L. monocytogenes* populations of <10 CFU/g were discovered in one 2- to 3-day-old Anari cheese and in three 2- to 3-day-old Halloumi cheeses produced by the same manufacturer. After these naturally contaminated cheeses were stored at 4°C for 4–5 weeks, *Listeria* populations as high as 8×10^4 and 1×10^6 CFU/g developed in Anari (pH 5.0–6.0) and Halloumi cheese (pH 6.0), respectively. Assuming a lag time of zero and an original *L. monocytogenes* population of 1–9 CFU/g, these authors calculated generation times of 47–56 and 32–37 hours for this pathogen in Anari and Halloumi cheese, respectively. Both of these generation times are similar to those previously reported for *L. monocytogenes* in refrigerated fluid milks (see Table 9.5). Since these cheeses would have been on sale for up to 3 months after distribution, there would have been ample time for potentially hazardous levels of listeriae to develop in such products during retail storage. Hence, as with cow's milk

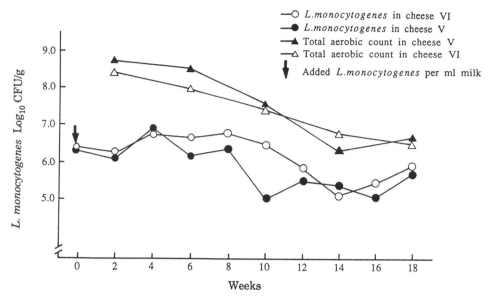

Figure 10.13 Survival of *L. monocytogenes* and total aerobic flora during manufacture and ripening of raw goat's milk cheese. (Adapted from Ref. 153.)

cheeses, it also is imperative that goat's milk and ewe's milk cheeses be manufactured from high quality pasteurized milk under the best possible hygienic conditions.

Soft Unripened Cheese

Soft unripened cheeses include such high moisture, white-curd varieties as cottage, baker's, cream, and American-type Neufchatel cheese. Unlike the groups of cheeses discussed thus far, milk to be manufactured into soft unripened cheese is coagulated through production of acid by the starter culture (or alternatively, by direct acidification of milk to pH 4.6–4.7 with gluconic acid, glucono-delta-lactone, or a mineral acid plus the lactone) rather than by the addition of rennet. Hence, these products are sometimes referred to as acid-curd cheese. Since the refrigerated shelf life of most soft unripened cheeses is typically less than 60 days, these varieties must be prepared from pasteurized milk or cream in the event cream cheese is made. Although pH values of 4.6–5.0 provide an unfavorable environment for microorganisms that may contaminate soft unripened cheese before, during, or after manufacture, the fact that these cheeses can be consumed immediately after production may pose a public health risk, particularly if psychrotrophic, acid-tolerant organisms such as *L. monocytogenes* are present.

Cottage Cheese

Nearly one year before the famed cheeseborne listeriosis outbreak in California, Ryser et al. (136) used the short-set procedure to prepare cottage cheese from pasteurized skim milk inoculated to contain 10^4–10^5 *L. monocytogenes* CFU/ml. Following manufacture, half the curd was creamed to contain ≥4% milkfat and half remained uncreamed. Both products were stored at 3°C and examined for numbers of listeriae for 28 days.

Numbers of *L. monocytogenes* remained relatively constant during the initial 5–6 hours of cheesemaking, during which the pH of milk decreased from 6.65 to 4.70. These findings are in agreement with those of Schaack and Marth (138), who later demonstrated that growth of *L. monocytogenes* in skim milk at 30°C is completely suppressed by a 5% inoculum of *S. cremoris*. After increasing the temperature of the curd/whey mixture to 57.2°C (135°F) over 90 minutes and cooking the curd at this temperature for an additional 30 minutes, *L. monocytogenes* was not detected in samples of curd or whey that were directly plated on McBride Listeria Agar. However, following cold enrichment in Tryptose Broth *L. monocytogenes* was detected in 4 of 8, 2 of 8, 1 of 8, and 2 of 8 samples of cooked curd, whey, wash water, and washed curd, respectively, which suggests that some *Listeria* cells were only sublethally injured during cooking of the curd at pH 4.6–4.7. As indicated in Chapter 6, such injury may preclude growth on McBride Listeria Agar which contains both lithium chloride and phenylethanol as selective agents.

Examination of the finished product indicated that *L. monocytogenes* survived in both creamed and uncreamed cottage cheese at levels generally < 100 CFU/g during 28 days of refrigerated storage. While there was no evidence for growth of listeriae in either cheese during refrigerated storage, probably because of pH values generally < 5.5, the pathogen was recovered more frequently and at higher numbers in creamed rather than uncreamed cottage cheese. Higher pH values in 3-day-old creamed (pH 5.32–5.45) rather than uncreamed (pH 5.12–5.22) cottage cheese may have been responsible for increasing the repair rate of injured cells, thereby increasing recovery of listeriae on McBride Listeria Agar.

Although behavior of *L. monocytogenes* in cheese failed to gain widespread attention until 1985, a search of the scientific literature has uncovered an earlier study by Stajner et al. (148) which examined the viability of *Listeria* in small unsalted skim milk cheese (similar to uncreamed cottage cheese) manufactured from naturally infected milk containing approximately 5×10^5 *L. monocytogenes* CFU/ml. Results from these Yugoslavian investigators support the findings of Ryser and Marth (136) in that the pathogen survived at least 7 days in finished cheese (pH 4.55–4.75) stored at 3–5°C.

Alternatively, El-Shenawy and Marth (97) recently studied the behavior of listeriae in cottage cheese prepared from pasteurized skim milk that was inoculated to contain 10^6 *L. monocytogenes* CFU/ml and then coagulated over a period of 3 hours using hydrochloric acid, gluconic acid, or bovine rennet rather than a lactic acid bacteria starter culture during which time the temperature of the milk was gradually increased from 2 to 32°C. The resulting coagulum was then cut and cooked using the aforementioned procedure of Ryser et al. (136).

As might be expected, acidification of the milk to a pH of 4.7–4.8 followed by heating again was detrimental to survival of listeriae during manufacture of cottage cheese. Overall, *L. monocytogenes* populations decreased ~4.5 and >6 orders of magnitude in fully cooked (57.2°C/30 min) curd obtained by addition of hydrochloric and gluconic acid, respectively (Figure 10.14). However, using cold enrichment, *Listeria* was recovered from samples of fully cooked gluconic acid curd. Numbers of listeriae decreased faster in acidified whey than curd, with cold enrichment results indicating that the pathogen was eliminated from gluconic but not hydrochloric acid whey after 30

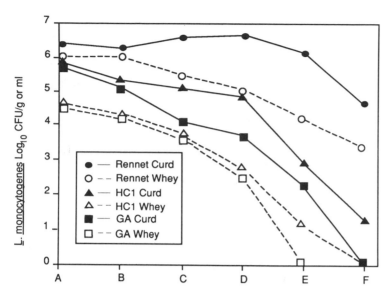

Figure 10.14 Survival of *L. monocytogenes* in curd and whey obtained during preparation of cottage cheese made with rennet, HCl, or gluconic acid (GA). A: Immediately after cutting; B: after temperature was increased to 48.9°C; C: after temperature was increased to 54.4°C; D: after temperature was increased to 57.2°C; E: after 15 minutes of cooking; and F: after 30 minutes of cooking. (Adapted from Ref. 97.)

minutes of cooking at 57.2°C. Nonetheless, direct acidification of milk (pH 4.7–4.8) for cottage-cheesemaking followed by cooking of the resultant curd at 57.2°C for 30 minutes should be more than sufficient to eliminate expected numbers of listeriae (<10 CFU/ml) that might inadvertently enter pasteurized milk as postprocessing contaminants.

In contrast to acid curd/whey, populations of listeriae in freshly cut rennet curd and whey were virtually identical to those initially observed in milk (Figure 10.14). Furthermore, slight increases in numbers of listeriae were noted midway through manufacture with fully cooked rennet curd (pH 6.6) and whey still containing nearly 10^5 and 10^6 *L. monocytogenes* CFU/g or ml, respectively. Thus, listericidal effects associated with cooking were greatly enhanced under acidic conditions. Subsequent experiments with selective plating media confirmed that substantial numbers of *L. monocytogenes* cells were sublethally injured during manufacture of cottage cheese, as was suggested by Ryser and Marth (136) 5 years earlier. Sublethal injury was far more evident in whey rather than curd samples, probably because curd afforded some thermal protection to listeriae. Not surprisingly, the degree of sublethal injury was also closely related to coagulant type (i.e., acidity) and cooking temperature, with less injury observed in rennet rather than acid curd/whey and partially rather than fully cooked samples of curd and whey. Heat alone was primarily responsible for rennet-associated injury, whereas the combined effects of heat and acid led to injury of listeriae in acid curd and whey.

With the exception of cottage cheese prepared from milk acidified with gluconic acid, both of these studies demonstrated limited survival of *L. monocytogenes* in cottage cheese. However, the fact that the pathogen failed to grow in the product and decreased drastically in numbers during manufacture suggests that cottage cheese poses far less of a health threat to the general public than do hard cheeses or those varieties that are surface-ripened with molds or bacteria. Lower health risks associated with consumption of cottage cheese are also supported by the extremely low incidence of *L. monocytogenes* in commercially produced cottage cheese examined in recent American and European surveys.

Since the likelihood of *L. monocytogenes* contaminating cottage cheese is greater from creaming and/or packaging operations than from its presence in pasteurized milk and survival in cooked curd, addition of various bacteriocins, including PA-1 (a recently discovered inhibitory substance produced by one strain of *Pediococcus acidilactici*) and nisin (produced by certain strains of *S. lactis*), has been examined as one means of ridding cottage cheese of viable listeriae that may have inadvertently entered the product after cooking. Using commercially prepared dry cottage cheese curd to which 7.5×10^3 *L. monocytogenes* CFU/g were added during creaming, Pucci et al. (126) found that the product (pH 5.1) still contained 1×10^2 *L. monocytogenes* CFU/g after 7 days of storage at 4°C. In contrast, addition of bacteriocin PA-1 powder to identical samples led to complete inactivation of the pathogen within 24 hours. However, inability of bacteriocin PA-1 to prevent growth of the pathogen in commercially prepared cheese sauce (pH 6.0) and half and half (pH 6.6) shows that listericidal activity of this bacteriocin is strongly dependent upon the pH of the food system.

Using a different brand of dry cottage cheese curd that was inoculated to contain 3×10^5 *L. monocytogenes* CFU/g during creaming, Benkerroum and Sandine (79) detected very few viable listeriae in the product (pH 4.9–5.0) after 1 or more days of storage at 4°C. This antagonistic effect of cottage cheese (presumably from natural flora or byproducts in cottage cheese) toward listeriae was enhanced by addition of nisin (2.5×10^3 IU/g) with viable cells of the pathogen completely eliminated from such cheese after 1 day of refrigerated storage.

In both of these studies nisin and bacteriocin PA-1 remained active in creamed cottage cheese (pH 4.9–5.1) during extended refrigerated storage. Thus it appears that these bacteriocins may also prove useful in protecting other fermented dairy products including natural cheeses, cold-pack cheese food, and various cheese spreads (60,67) against *Listeria* contamination during the normal shelf life of these products.

Cream Cheese

In the only other study dealing with the behavior of listeriae in soft unripened cheese, Cottin et al. (89) recently prepared cream cheese from a chemically acidified mixture of milk and cream that was inoculated to contain 10^1–10^7 *L. monocytogenes* CFU/ml. Using the lowest inoculum, *Listeria* grew in the finished product (pH ≤ 6.0) and attained a stable population of ~10^3 CFU/g within 2 days of storage at 4°C. Thus, unlike cottage cheese, the pH and moisture content of cream cheese are apparently both high enough to permit limited growth of listeriae in the product during refrigeration.

Cold-Pack Cheese Food

Unlike the natural cheeses discussed thus far, cold-pack cheese food is typically prepared by comminuting and blending aged Cheddar cheese (or another variety) with nonfat dry milk, dried whey, water, cream, plastic cream (composition similar to butter), salt, acidulants (i.e., lactic and/or acetic acid), preservatives (i.e., potassium sorbate and/or sodium propionate), and other optional ingredients into a homogeneous mass without the use of heat. Since all of the dairy ingredients and some of the optional ingredients used in manufacturing cold-pack cheese food can potentially harbor *L. monocytogenes*, Ryser and Marth (134) investigated the behavior of this pathogen in nine different formulations of cold-pack cheese food inoculated to contain approximately 500 *L. monocytogenes* (four strains analyzed separately) CFU/g of finished product.

During 182 days of storage at 4°C, populations of all four *Listeria* strains decreased less than 10-fold in nonacidified cheese food (pH 5.20) prepared without preservatives (Fig. 10.15). Thus the pathogen survived throughout the product's entire 6-month shelf life.

In sharp contrast to these findings, addition of preservatives with or without acidifying agents led to the eventual demise of listeriae in cheese food stored at 4°C (Fig. 10.16). In nonacidified cheese food (pH 5.20) preserved with 0.3% sodium propionate, *L. monocytogenes* survived an average of 142 days as compared to 118, 103, and 98 days in the same product adjusted to pH 5.0 to 5.1 with lactic, lactic plus acetic, and acetic acid, respectively. Using 0.3% sorbic acid in place of sodium propionate, the pathogen survived an average of 130 days in nonacidified cheese food (pH 5.45) as compared to 112, 93, and 74 days in cheese food acidified to pH 5.0 to 5.1 with lactic, lactic plus

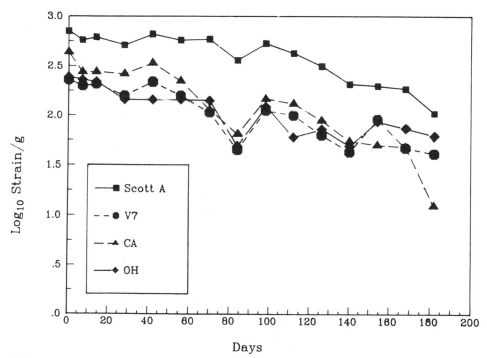

Figure 10.15 Survival of four strains of *L. monocytogenes* in nonacidified cold-pack cheese food manufactured without preservatives. (Adapted from Ref. 134.)

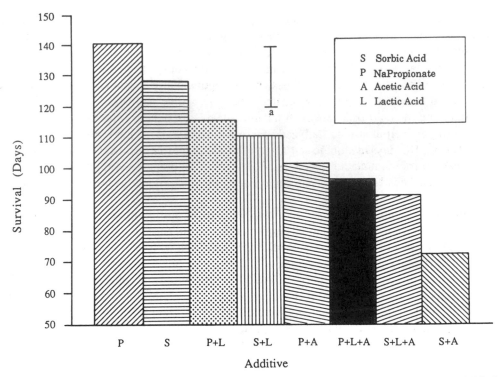

Figure 10.16 Maximum length of survival of *L. monocytogenes* in acidified and nonacidified cold-pack cheese food containing preservatives. Each bar represents the average maximum length of survival of all four *Listeria* strains in 1 of 8 different formulations of cheese food manufactured in duplicate. Any two differing by >20.24 days (length of bar) are significantly different ($p < 0.05$). (Adapted from Ref. 134.)

acetic, and acetic acid, respectively. Thus, sorbic acid was consistently more antagonistic to listeriae than sodium propionate. In addition, antilisterial effects of both preservatives were more pronounced in cheese food acidified with acetic rather than lactic acid. Since organic acids are far more bactericidal in the undissociated than dissociated state, increased inactivation of listeriae in the presence of acetic acid probably resulted from the higher proportion of undissociated acetic (~36%) rather than lactic acid (~5.9%) in cheese food acidified to pH 5.0–5.1. These findings indicate that it would be prudent to consider (a) adding preservatives, particularly sorbic acid, to cold-pack cheese food and (b) reducing the pH of the product to 5.0 by adding small amounts of lactic and/or acetic acid to decrease the chances for survival of *L. monocytogenes* in the finished product. Additional information on conditions leading to inhibition and/or inactivation of this pathogen by sorbic, propionic, lactic, and acetic acid can be found in Chapter 5.

Behavior of *L. monocytogenes* in Cheese as Affected by Cheese Composition

As suggested earlier, the fate of *L. monocytogenes* and other foodborne pathogens during ripening of cheese is determined by the microbiological, biochemical, and physical properties of the particular cheese. Thus cheese is a very complex system with the following factors acting simultaneously to determine the behavior of *L. monocytogenes* during cheese ripening: (a) type, amount and activity of the starter culture, (b) pH as determined by concentrations of lactic, acetic, formic, and other acids, (c) presence of hydrogen peroxide, diacetyl, and various antimicrobial agents (i.e., nisin, diplococcin, bacteriocins), (d) levels of nutrients, salt, moisture, and oxygen, and (e) the temperature at which the cheese is ripened.

While all of these factors act together to produce a particular outcome, a few conclusions concerning the ability of *L. monocytogenes* to grow and/or survive in some of the aforementioned cheeses can be drawn by examining the behavior of this pathogen in relation to the combined effects of moisture content, water activity (a_w), and salt in the moisture phase as well as the pH of the cheese and the temperature(s) at which the cheese is ripened (Table 10.14).

Except that fully ripened Camembert and feta cheese had pH values of 7.5 and 4.4, respectively, both cheeses were very similar in terms of moisture content, water activity, percentage of salt in the water phase, and ripening temperature. Thus rapid growth of *L. monocytogenes* in Camembert cheese can be largely attributed to the increase in pH of the cheese during ripening, whereas a pH value of 4.4 appears to be responsible for preventing growth of the bacterium during ripening of feta cheese.

Inability of *L. monocytogenes* to multiply in blue cheese during ripening and storage is probably related to the high concentration of salt in the water phase (which results in a low a_w), since other workers have confirmed that this organism will not grow in laboratory media (142) and skim milk (121) containing >10 and 12% salt, respectively.

As with Camembert cheese, growth of two of four *L. monocytogenes* strains in brick cheese appears to be directly related to the high pH that the cheese attained during extended ripening. However, a general inability of the remaining two strains to grow in brick cheese of similar composition is as yet unexplained.

When comparing the behavior of *L. monocytogenes* in Cheddar and Colby cheese, we find that the initial inactivation rate for the pathogen was somewhat slower in the latter cheese. At first glance, it appears that increased viability of *Listeria* in Colby cheese during the early stages of ripening may be related to the lower percentage of salt in the water phase in this cheese than in Cheddar cheese. However, data in Table 10.14 show that *L. monocytogenes* was inactivated at similar rates in Colby cheese and cold-pack cheese food, the latter is compositionally is similar to Colby cheese with the exception of a higher concentration of salt in the water phase. Hence, factors other than a low concentration of salt in the water phase also must be involved in enhancing the viability of listeriae during ripening of Colby cheese.

Lack of growth and decreased survival of *L. monocytogenes* in Parmesan and in an unidentified hard Italian cheese as compared to other varieties in Table 10.14 correlates well with the lower moisture content/water activity of these cheeses during ripening. Barring thermal and/or acid injury of *L. monocytogenes*, which is likely to occur during manufacture of cottage cheese and possibly other varieties that undergo substantial heat treatments during manufacture (i.e., mozzarella, Swiss), factors outlined in Table 10.14 may be useful in predicting whether or not this pathogen will grow in other cheeses having similar microbiological, biochemical, and physical characteristics.

Table 10.14 Behavior of *L. monocytogenes* During Cheese Ripening as Affected by Cheese Composition

Cheese	Moisture (%)	Estimated a_w	Estimated salt in water phase (%)	pH Initial[a]	pH Final	Ripening temp. (°C)	Log$_{10}$ of *L. monocytogenes* CFU/g Initial[a]	Maximum	Final	Survival (days)	Ref.
Camembert	54.4	0.975	4.72	4.6	7.5	15/6	3.1–3.6	6.7–7.5	6.7–7.5	65	131
Blue	38.9	0.950	11.52	4.6	6.3	9–12/4	4.0–5.0	4.0–5.0	1.0–2.3	120	122
Brick	43.0	0.990	1.89	5.3	7.3	15/10	3.0–4.7	4.6–6.7	2.7–6.1	168	135
Feta	54.7	0.975	4.57	4.7	4.4	22/4	5.2–6.2	5.7–6.2	2.8–4.6	90	123
Cheddar	37.2	0.975	4.61	5.1	5.1	6	2.5–3.2	2.6–3.8	0–1.5	70–434	130
Cheddar	37.2	0.975	4.61	5.1	5.1	13	2.6–3.4	3.0–3.7	0	70–224	130
Colby	40.0	0.975	3.91	5.1	5.1	4	3.5–4.5	3.6–4.6	2.3–4.1	112–140	162
Parmesan	32.0	0.935	4.96	5.1	5.1	13	3.3–4.3	3.3–4.3	1.0–1.3	21–112	163
Hard Italian	NR[c]	0.950	2.12[d]	5.3	5.7	4	4.5–5.1	4.5–5.6	2.0	35	86
Cold-pack cheese food[b]	41.4	0.975	4.90	5.3	5.1	4	2.4–2.8	2.4–2.8	1.1–2.0	180	134

[a] Approximately 24 hours after the start of cheesemaking.
[b] Prepared without preservatives or acidifying agents.
[c] Not reported.
[d] Percent salt in solid and water phase.

Feasibility of Preparing Cheese from Raw Milk

According to current FDA regulations in the United States, milk pasteurization or use of a similar heat treatment during cheesemaking is required for the manufacture of 16 cheese varieties including cottage, cream, Neufchatel, Monterey, mozzarella, Muenster, Gammelost, Koch Kaese, and Sapsago. Seven varieties of manufacturing cheese (i.e., for use in pasteurized processed cheese, cheese foods, cheese spreads) require neither pasteurization of the cheesemilk nor a 60-day minimum ripening at ≥1.7°C (≥35°F), whereas the 34 remaining varieties of cheese recognized under current standards of identity must either be manufactured from pasteurized milk or held a minimum of 60 days at ≥1.7°C (≥35°F) to eliminate pathogenic microorganisms. While no statistics on milk pasteurization for cheesemaking are available, current evidence indicates that a major portion of the natural cheeses sold in the United States are prepared from pasteurized milk (117).

The mandatory holding period of 60 days at ≥1.7°C (≥35°F) for cheeses manufactured from raw milk was adopted in 1949 (1) after researchers demonstrated that viable *Brucella abortus*, the causative agent of brucellosis, was eliminated from cheese using such an aging process. While this 60-day holding period was generally deemed adequate to eliminate most foodborne pathogens, later studies demonstrated that *Salmonella typhimurium* can survive such a cheese-ripening process (106). Furthermore, results in Table 10.14 indicate that *L. monocytogenes* can survive well beyond 60 days in many natural cheeses held at ≥1.7°C (≥35°F).

In keeping with the grave nature of listeriosis as compared to most other foodborne illnesses, the FDA has adopted a policy of "zero tolerance" for *L. monocytogenes* in all ready-to-eat foods. Thus far no well-documented cases of listeriosis have been associated with consumption of cheeses that were legally prepared from raw milk and held a minimum of 60 days at ≥1.7°C (≥35°F). In spite of this, since ~4% of the raw milk supply can be expected to contain *L. monocytogenes*, it would be prudent to manufacture cheeses from pasteurized milk whenever possible. Although Yousef and Marth (163) recently demonstrated that ripening Parmesan cheese for 10 months, as legally required, is sufficient to produce a high quality, *Listeria*-free product, desirable flavor and texture characteristics are not easily attainable in sharp Cheddar and Swiss cheese prepared from pasteurized milk. Hence, alternative means would be helpful in enhancing the safety of these products. Such methods might include cold sterilization of the milk via microfiltration or addition of various flavor- and texture-enhancing enzymes (or microorganisms) to pasteurized milk, which would allow the cheesemaker to obtain a higher quality product. However, as important as it is to manufacture cheese from *Listeria*-free milk, it is equally important to prevent contamination of the product during manufacture, ripening, and storage by using good manufacturing practices. Information concerning problem areas and safeguards during manufacture of dairy products and other foods can be found in Chapter 15.

Whey

To our knowledge, *L. monocytogenes* has not yet been isolated from commercially produced cheese whey. However, studies have shown that when various cheeses were

Table 10.15 Number of Listeriae Recovered from Whey During Manufacture of Various Cheeses Prepared from Pasteurized Milk Inoculated to Contain ~500–5000 *L. monocytogenes* CFU/ml

Cheese	*L. monocytogenes* CFU/ml of whey	Percent of original inoculum in whey	Ref.
Camembert	8	1.3	132
Blue	43	3.6	122
Brick	12	2.5	135
Feta	15	3.2	123
Gouda	5	1.0	120
Colby	21	2.4	162
Cheddar	22	5.0	130
Average	18	2.7	

experimentally produced from pasteurized milk inoculated with *L. monocytogenes*, between 1.0 and 5.0% of the original inoculum was lost in the whey during cheesemaking (Table 10.15). These findings again demonstrate that the pathogen is concentrated 8- to 10-fold in curd during milk coagulation. Unlike other wheys, populations of *L. monocytogenes* in acid whey (pH 4.6) obtained from the manufacture of cottage cheese were reduced more than 10,000-fold after cooking the curd/whey mixture at 57.2°C (135°F) for 30 minutes. However, as previously noted, the organism was detected in several whey samples after 6 weeks of cold enrichment (136) which, in turn, suggests that the pathogen was only sublethally injured during cooking of the curd/whey mixture.

These observations prompted Ryser and Marth (133) to examine the behavior of *L. monocytogenes* in wheys from Camembert cheese that were filter-sterilized and adjusted to pH values of 5.0–6.8. All whey samples were then inoculated to contain ~100–500 *L. monocytogenes* (four strains analyzed separately) CFU/ml and incubated at 6°C.

Although the four *L. monocytogenes* strains failed to grow in wheys having pH values ≤ 5.4, the pathogen survived in all samples with populations decreasing ≤10-fold during 35 days of refrigerated storage. In contrast, *L. monocytogenes* grew in all remaining samples after a 3-day lag period and attained average maximum populations of 7.48, 7.87, and 7.84 $\log_{10}$ CFU/ml in wheys adjusted to pH 5.6, 6.2, and 6.8, respectively, following 35 days of incubation. As previously noted, these *Listeria* populations in whey were slightly higher than those that would be expected to develop in skim or whole milk during refrigerated storage. Generation times of *L. monocytogenes* in wheys adjusted to pH 5.6, 6.2, and 6.8 ranged between 25.2 and 31.6 hours, 14.8 and 21.1 hours, and 14.0 and 19.4 hours, respectively, depending on the individual strain. While doubling times were similar for all strains at the same pH value, generation times were significantly longer at pH 5.6 than at pH 6.2 and 6.8. Interestingly, Johnson (111) observed that *L. monocytogenes* could be inactivated in similar samples of demineralized whey by adding lysozyme. However, this enzyme did not decrease viability of the pathogen in normal whey, which in turn suggests that lysozyme activity is neutralized by whey minerals and/or proteins.

Using a different approach to examine the behavior of *Listeria* in whey, Northolt et al. (120) inoculated heat-treated (68°C/10 sec) wheys (pH 6.5) to contain 500–1000 *L. monocytogenes* CFU/ml and incubated the samples at temperatures between 7 and 30°C. Following a 6- to 24-hour lag period, the pathogen grew in all samples with doubling times of 12 hours, 6 hours, 4 hours, and 40 minutes in wheys incubated at 7, 12, 20, and 30°C, respectively. Although incubation of all samples was terminated before *L. monocytogenes* reached the stationary growth phase, the pathogen did attain populations of 10^4–10^6 CFU/ml of whey at the conclusion of the experiment.

In the only study thus far reported dealing with nonsterile whey, researchers in France (76) produced whey containing 2–7 *L. monocytogenes* CFU/ml from previously inoculated milk and examined samples for listeriae after 101, 156, and 251 days of storage at 4°C. Moderate growth and extended survival of the pathogen were observed in whey collected immediately after coagulation of the milk (pH 5.4) with 156- and 251-day-old whey samples at pH 4.8 containing 2.5×10^4 and 7.0×10^2 *L. monocytogenes* CFU/ml, respectively. As predicted by Ryser and Marth (133), the pathogen also failed to grow in more acidic wheys (pH 5.2–5.3) collected after hooping with listeriae no longer observed in 101- and 156-day-old wheys having pH values of 3.28 and 4.26, respectively. Not surprisingly, increasing the incubation temperature to 6, 14, and 20°C led to faster demise of listeriae in 21 similar wheys (pH 3.75–5.72) initially containing 60–96 *L. monocytogenes* CFU/ml, with the pathogen eliminated from all but one sample (pH 5.72) examined after 114 days of incubation at 6°C. These research findings demonstrate that *L. monocytogenes* can grow to high numbers in fluid wheys having pH values of ≥5.4 and remain viable in more acidic wheys during many months of refrigerated storage.

Given results of a study described in Chapter 9 in which numbers of *L. monocytogenes* decreased only 1–5 orders of magnitude during manufacture of nonfat dry milk (92), it appears that this organism also is likely to survive the spray-drying process used in converting fluid whey into whey powder. However, to our knowledge no *Listeria* spp. have yet been isolated from dried whey manufactured commercially in Europe or the United States. Although Gabis et al. (100) failed to find any *Listeria* spp. in 23 environmental samples from whey-processing factories, these authors did isolate *L. monocytogenes* from a floor drain that was located within a raw milk receiving room of a dry milk–processing factory. Additionally, *Listeria* spp. other than *L. monocytogenes* were isolated from several drains and trenches in the powder production area of a second factory that manufactured dry milk products. Considering the widespread use of dried whey (and nonfat dried milk) as an ingredient in cheese food, ice cream, and sherbet, as well as candy, beverages, and baked goods, strict enforcement of good manufacturing practices for dried whey and nonfat dry milk should be continued to prevent a possible public health problem involving listeriae.

Brine Solutions

Since *L. monocytogenes* is quite halotolerant, it is not surprising to learn that brine solutions in which cheeses are salted and/or ripened also can serve as potential reservoirs for this organism. Current evidence suggests that these brine solutions may become contaminated with *L. monocytogenes* through direct/indirect contact with the cheese factory environment (i.e., equipment, condensate on walls, floors, and ceilings) as well as actual shedding of *L. monocytogenes* into the brine solution from Listeria-contaminated cheese. Recently, Breer (82) and Terplan (149) reported isolating *L. monocytogenes* from commercial brine solutions in Europe. In one instance, the pathogen was detected in brine tanks 4 days after soft/semi-soft cheeses were removed from the salt brine. Such reports are likely to increase in Europe and spread to the United States as increased attention is given to the incidence of listeriae in brine solutions.

Migration of *L. monocytogenes* into brine solutions during salting of artificially contaminated cheese has been well documented. Ryser and Marth (135) brine-salted brick cheese containing ~10^3–10^4 *L. monocytogenes* CFU/g at 10°C. Cold enrichment of membrane filters through which 50-ml portions of 22% brine solution were filtered indicated that the pathogen leached from the cheese into the salt solution during 24 hours of brining. Furthermore, viable listeriae were detected in samples of 22% brine solution stored at 10°C at least 5 days after blocks of cheese were removed from the brine.

In conjunction with their study on the fate of *L. monocytogenes* during manufacture, ripening, and storage of feta cheese, Papageorgiou and Marth (123) also examined the viability of *Listeria* in the brine solution in which cheese was salted and stored. After 1 day of salting, a 12% brine solution contained an average *Listeria* population of 2.63 $\log_{10}$ CFU/g, which again indicates that the pathogen leached from cheese into the brine solution (Fig. 10.17). However, no growth of *L. monocytogenes* was observed in the 12% brine solution despite ample migration of cheese nutrients into salt brine as well as favorable values for temperature and pH. After transferring feta cheese to a 6% brine solution, the pathogen leached from cheese into salt brine and grew rapidly with similar populations observed in both cheese and 6% brine solution after 6 days of incubation at 22°C (Fig. 10.17). Although numbers of listeriae decreased in both cheese and salt brine during 90 days of refrigerated storage, the pathogen was inactivated slower in 6% salt brine than in feta cheese.

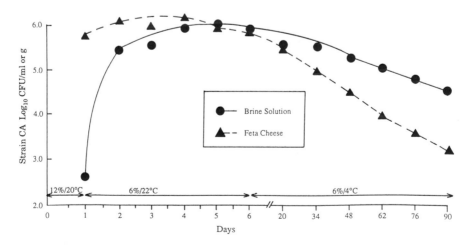

Figure 10.17 Average populations of *L. monocytogenes* strain CA in 12 and 6% salt brine during ripening and storage of feta cheese. (Adapted from Ref. 123.)

Since feta and other white-pickled cheeses such as Teleme, Halloumi, and Domiati are frequently cured in whey or skim milk containing 6 or 12% salt, Papageorgiou and Marth (121) examined behavior of *Listeria* in salted whey and skim milk. Autoclaved samples of skim milk (pH 6.0–6.2) and deproteinated whey (pH 5.5–5.7) containing 6 and 12% NaCl were inoculated to contain ~10^3 *L. monocytogenes* (strains Scott A or CA) CFU/ml and incubated at 4 and 22°C.

After a lag period of 5–10 days, *L. monocytogenes* grew rapidly in both 6% salted whey and skim milk with the pathogen attaining maximum populations of 10^7–10^8 CFU/ml following 50–55 days of refrigerated storage (Table 10.16). In the study discussed earlier, Ryser and Marth (133) reported that these same *Listeria* strains had shorter lag periods and generation times, but achieved similar maximum populations in unsalted, filter-sterilized whey (pH 5.6) after 24 days of incubation at 6°C. Hence these findings suggest that addition of 6% salt to whey played a major role in decreasing the growth rate of *Listeria*.

Increasing the incubation temperature to 22°C resulted in lag periods of 6–12 hours for both *Listeria* strains in whey and skim milk containing 6% salt. Generation times were similarly reduced with both strains exhibiting faster growth rates and higher maximum populations in salted whey rather than salted skim milk (Table 10.16). These findings agree with those of other researchers who also observed that *L. monocytogenes* grew faster and attained higher maximum populations in unsalted whey (133) than in skim milk (128).

Unlike the previous findings obtained with 6% salt, growth of *L. monocytogenes* was completely inhibited in 12% salted whey and skim milk with populations of both strains decreasing <10-fold during 130 days of storage at 4°C. Although strain Scott A also persisted >130 days in 12% salted whey and skim milk incubated at 22°C, strain CA proved to be less salt tolerant, surviving only 80 and 105 days in 12% salted skim milk and whey, respectively (Fig. 10.18). Increased destruction of *L. monocytogenes* in salt solutions held at ambient rather than refrigeration temperatures has been well documented. Results from several of these studies dealing with viability of listeriae in salted Tryptose Broth (143) and cabbage juice (88) are discussed in Chapter 5. Based on these observations, acidification of brine solutions used in cheesemaking to pH values

Table 10.16 Generation Times (G.T.) and Maximum Populations (M.P.) of *L. monocytogenes* Strains Scott A and CA in 6% Salted Whey and Skim Milk Incubated at 4 and 22°C

Strain	Product	G.T. (h)	M.P. (log_{10} CFU/ml)
Incubation at 4 °C			
Scott A	whey	46.81	7.97
Scott A	skim milk	45.23	7.58
CA	whey	37.49	8.04
CA	skim milk	49.43	7.69
Incubation at 22 °C			
Scott A	whey	3.67	8.02
Scott A	skim milk	4.31	7.70
CA	whey	3.56	8.10
CA	skim milk	4.42	7.89

Source: Adapted from Ref. 121.

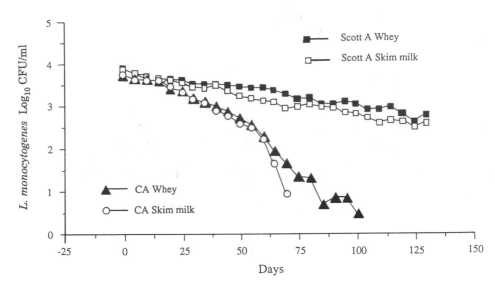

Figure 10.18 Behavior of *L. monocytogenes* strains Scott A and CA in 12% salted whey and skim milk during extended storage at 4°C. (Adapted from Ref. 121.)

<5.0 has been recommended to prevent growth of *L. monocytogenes*, particularly if such solutions contain ≤10% salt. In 1989, Johnson (111) also noted that addition of 0.35% H_2O_2 to a 23% brine solution caused numbers of *L. monocytogenes* to decrease by six orders of magnitude within 24 hours. However, unlike organic acids, the bactericidal activity of H_2O_2 dissipates fairly rapidly. Hence addition of H_2O_2 to salt brine provides only temporary protection against listeriae that might be present within the cheesemaking environment.

REFERENCES

1. Anonymous. 1949. Cheeses, processed cheeses, cheese foods, cheese spreads, and related foods, definitions and standards of identity. *Fed. Reg.* April 22:1960–1992.
2. Anonymous. 1985. Code of hygienic practices for soft cheeses to be elaborated. *Food Chem. News* 27(31):12.
3. Anonymous. 1985. FDA finds *Listeria* in 3 brands of General Foods soft cheeses. *Food Chem. News* 27(25):33.
4. Anonymous. 1985. FDA is checking facilities of cheese plant after finding *Listeria*. *Food Chem. News* 27(24):25.
5. Anonymous. 1985. FDA is investigating deaths linked to Mexican-style cheese. *Food Chem. News* 27(15):42.
6. Anonymous. 1985. Jalisco-brand Mexican style soft cheese recalled. FDA Enforcement Report, June 26.
7. Anonymous. 1985. Liederkranz, Camembert and Brie cheese recalled. FDA Enforcement Report, Sept. 4.
8. Anonymous. 1985. Planning program for inspection of imported soft cheese. *Food Chem. News* 27(30):35.

9. Anonymous. 1985. Soft cheese manufacturers to be inspected under FDA priority program. *Food Chem. News* 27(18):22.

10. Anonymous. 1986. Brie cheese recalled. FDA Enforcement Report, April 2.

11. Anonymous. 1986. Brie cheese recalled. FDA Enforcement Report, April 9.

12. Anonymous. 1986. Cheese recalls extended by General Foods, U.S. importer. *Food Chem. News* 27(52):25–26.

13. Anonymous. 1986. FDA advises import alert on imported soft cheese. *Food Chem. News* 28(23):22–23.

14. Anonymous. 1986. FDA finds *Listeria* in Brie from French certified plant. *Food Chem. News* 27(50):35.

15. Anonymous. 1986. FDA finds *Listeria* in Mexican-style soft cheese. *Food Chem. News* 28(1):54.

16. Anonymous. 1986. FDA may block list all soft-ripened cheeses from France. *Food Chem. News* 28(2):64–65.

17. Anonymous. 1986. FDA proposes soft-ripened cheese testing program to France. *Food Chem. News* 28(4):3–4.

18. Anonymous. 1986. FDA to detain all soft-ripened French cheese lacking certification. *Food Chem. News* 28(10):9–10.

19. Anonymous. 1986. FDA to sample 20% of soft cheeses from all foreign countries. *Food Chem. News* 28(6):27–28.

20. Anonymous. 1986. France agrees to temporary FDA soft-ripened cheese testing program. *Food Chem. News* 28(7):24–26.

21. Anonymous. 1986. French Brie cheese recalled. FDA Enforcement Report, March 12.

22. Anonymous. 1986. French Brie cheese recalled. FDA Enforcement Report, May 14.

23. Anonymous. 1986. French cheeses recalled because of *Listeria*. *Food Chem. News* 28(24):12.

24. Anonymous. 1986. French firm agrees to stop shipments of Brie cheese. *Food Chem. News* 27(51):12–14.

25. Anonymous. 1986. French semi-soft cheese recalled. FDA Enforcement Report, August 20.

26. Anonymous. 1986. French soft-ripened cheese recalled. FDA Enforcement Report, August 13.

27. Anonymous. 1986. French soft-ripened cheese recalled. FDA Enforcement Report, Sept. 24.

28. Anonymous. 1986. *Listeria* causes class I recalls of ice milk mix, milk. *Food Chem. News* 28(16):22.

29. Anonymous. 1986. Listeriosis hazard still being evaluated, FDA tells France. *Food Chem. News* 18(26):29–32.

30. Anonymous. 1986. Milk, chocolate milk, half and half, cultured buttermilk, whipping cream, ice milk, ice milk mix and ice milk shake mix recalled. FDA Enforcement Report, June 25.

31. Anonymous. 1986. More recalls made of French cheese, animal feeds. *Food Chem. News* 28(7):52–53.

32. Anonymous. 1986. Recall of Brie cheese is extended by FDA. *Food Chem. News* 28(1):54.

33. Anonymous. 1986. Soft Mexican-style cheeses recalled. FDA Enforcement Report, April 9.

34. Anonymous. 1986. Soft, ripened Brie cheese recalled. FDA Enforcement Report, April 9.

35. Anonymous. 1986. Soft-ripened French Brie cheese recalled. FDA Enforcement Report, April 23.

36. Anonymous. 1987. Annual Report, Swiss Institute for Dairy Research, Liebefeld-Berne, pp. 344–353.

37. Anonymous. 1987. Class I recall made of cheese because of *Listeria*. *Food Chem. News* 28(50):52.

38. Anonymous. 1987. FDA launching two-year pathogen surveillance program. *Food Chem. News* 29(31):10–12.

39. Anonymous. 1987. FDA orders sampling of Italian hard cheese for microorganisms. *Food Chem. News* 29(22):36.

40. Anonymous. 1987. FDA renews threat of automatic detention for Italian soft cheese. *Food Chem. News* 29(6):3–4.

41. Anonymous. 1987. FDA sets separate program for cheese from unpasteurized milk. *Food Chem. News 29*(8):17–18.
42. Anonymous. 1987. French full fat soft cheese recalled. FDA Enforcement Report, May 13.
43. Anonymous. 1987. French full fat cheese recalled because of *Listeria*. *Food Chem. News 29*(9):16.
44. Anonymous. 1987. French soft cheese certification to be in place Feb. 15. *Food Chem. News 28*(50):36.
45. Anonymous. 1987. Hard cheese from Italian firm blocklisted. *Food Chem. News 29*(23):19.
46. Anonymous. 1987. Mini Bonbel and Gouda semi-soft cheese recalled. FDA Enforcement Report, June 3.
47. Anonymous. 1987. Old Heidelberg soft-ripened cheese recalled. FDA Enforcement Report, June 3.
48. Anonymous. 1987. Raw milk sharp Cheddar cheese recalled. FDA Enforcement Report, Aug. 19.
49. Anonymous. 1987. Salvador-style white semi-soft cheese recalled. FDA Enforcement Report, Feb. 11.
50. Anonymous. 1988. Blue Castello Danish blue cheese recalled. FDA Enforcement Report, May 4.
51. Anonymous. 1987. Danish cheese recalled because of *Listeria*. *Food Chem. News 30*(4):42.
52. Anonymous. 1988. FDA finds *Listeria* in foreign soft cheeses. *Food Chem. News 29*(49):36–37.
53. Anonymous. 1988. Ice cream, cheese recalled because of *Listeria*. *Food Chem. News 30*(6):27.
54. Anonymous. 1988. Italian semi-soft cheese recalled. FDA Enforcement Report, March 30.
55. Anonymous. 1988. L'Amulette Danish Esrom cheese recalled. FDA Enforcement Report, March 23.
56. Anonymous. 1988. L'Amulette Danish Esrom cheese recalled. FDA Enforcement Report, March 30.
57. Anonymous. 1988. L'Amulette Danish Esrom cheese recalled. FDA Enforcement Report, April 6.
58. Anonymous. 1988. Listeriosis: Goats' milk cheese. Communicable Disease Report, Feb. 12.
59. Anonymous. 1988. Mexican-style, baby Jack and Monterey Jack cheese recalled. FDA Enforcement Report, March 9.
60. Anonymous. 1988. Nisin preparation affirmed as GRAS for cheese spreads. *Food Chem. News 30*(6):37–38.
61. Anonymous. 1988. Soft cheese warning because of *Listeria monocytogenes*. *Food Chem. News 29*(49):2.
62. Anonymous. 1989. Controlling *Listeria*-the Danish solution. *Dairy Indust. Intern. 54*(5):31–32, 35.
63. Anonymous. 1989. Cyprus Anari cheese recalled. FDA Enforcement Report, July 12.
64. Anonymous. 1989. Cyprus Anari cheese recalled. FDA Enforcement Report, Sept. 27.
65. Anonymous. 1989. Cyprus Anari cheese recalled. FDA Enforcement Report, Nov. 1.
66. Anonymous. 1989. Frozen yogurt recalled. FDA Enforcement Report, Nov. 7.
67. Anonymous. 1989. Pasteurized process cheese spread: Amendment of standard of identity. *Fed. Reg. 54*:6120–6121.
68. Anonymous. 1989. Salmon recalled because of *Listeria*; blocklist covers hard cheeses. *Food Chem. News 31*(37):27–28.
69. Anonymous. 1989. Umweltministerium warnt vor zwei Weichkäsesorten. *Deutsche Molkerei Zeitung 110*:898.
70. Anonymous. 1990. Cyprus Halloumi cheese recalled. FDA Enforcement Report, Jan. 17.
71. Anonymous. 1990. USDA, FDA officials report apparent decrease in *Listeria* isolations. *Food Chem. News 32*(1):12–15.
72. Archer, D. L. 1988. Review of the latest FDA information on the presence of *Listeria* in foods. WHO Working Group on Foodborne Listeriosis. Geneva, Switzerland, Feb. 15–19.
73. Asperger, H., B. Url, and E. Brandl. 1989. Interactions between *Listeria* and the ripening flora of cheese. *Neth. Milk Dairy J. 43*:287–298.

74. Bannerman, E. S., and J. Billie. 1988. A selective medium for isolating *Listeria* spp. from heavily contaminated material. *Appl. Environ. Microbiol. 54*:165–167.

75. Bannister, B. A. 1987. *Listeria monocytogenes* meningitis associated with eating soft cheese. *J. Infect. 15*:165–168.

76. Barnier, E., J. P. Vincent, and M. Catteau. 1988. Survie de *Listeria monocytogenes* dans les saumures et sérum de fromagerié. *Sci. Aliments 8*:175–178.

77. Beckers, H. J., P. S. S. Soentoro, and E. H. M. Delfgou-van Asch. 1987. The occurrence of *Listeria monocytogenes* in soft cheeses and raw milk and its resistance to heat. *Int. J. Food Microbiol. 4*:249–256.

78. Beckers, H. J., P. H. in't Veld, P. S. S. Soentoro, and E. H. M. Delfgou-van Asch. 1988. The occurrence of *Listeria* in food. *Foodborne Listeriosis—Proceedings of a Symposium*, Wiesbaden, West Germany, Sept. 7, pp. 84–97.

79. Benkerroum, N., and W. E. Sandine. 1988. Inhibitory action of nisin against *Listeria monocytogenes. J. Dairy Sci. 71*:3237–3245.

80. Bind, J.-L. 1988. Review of latest information concerning data about repartition of *Listeria* in France. WHO Working Group on Foodborne Listeriosis, Geneva, Switzerland, February 15–19.

81. Breer, C. 1986. The occurrence of *Listeria* spp. in cheese. In *Proc. 2nd World Congress on Foodborne Infections and Intoxications*, Inst. Vet. Med., Robert von Ostertag Inst., West Berlin, pp. 230–233.

82. Breer, C. 1988. Occurrence of *Listeria* spp. in different foods. WHO Working Group on Foodborne Listeriosis, Geneva, Switzerland, Feb. 15–19.

83. Cantoni, C., M. Valenti, and G. Comi. 1988. *Listeria* in formaggi e in salumi. *Ind. Alimentari 27*:859–861.

84. Choi, H. K., M. M. Schaack, and E. H. Marth. 1988. Survival of *Listeria monocytogenes* in cultured buttermilk and yogurt. *Milchwissenschaft 43*:790–792.

85. Comi, C., and C. Cantoni. 1988. Alcuni aspetti della presenza di *L. monocytogenes* nei formaggi. *Ind. Alimentari 27*:104–106.

86. Comi, G., and M. Valenti. 1988. Survival and growth of *Listeria monocytogenes* in Italian type cheese. *Latte 13*:956–958.

87. Comi, G., C. Cantoni, and S. d'Aubert. 1987. Indagine sulla presenza di *Listeria monocytogenes* nei formaggi. *Ind. Alimentari 26*:216–218.

88. Conner, D. E., R. E. Brackett, and L. R. Beuchat. 1986. Effect of temperature, sodium chloride, and pH on growth of *Listeria monocytogenes* in cabbage juice. *Appl. Environ. Microbiol. 52*:59–63.

89. Cottin, J., F. Picard-Bonnaud, and B. Carbonnelle. 1988. Study of *Listeria monocytogenes* survival during the preparation and the conservation of two kinds of dairy products. 10th International Symposium on Listeriosis, Pecs, Hungary, Aug. 22–26, Abstr. 52.

90. Denis, F., and J.-P. Ramet. 1989. Antibacterial activity of the lactoperoxidase system on *Listeria monocytogenes* in trypticase soy broth, UHT milk and French soft cheese. *J. Food Prot. 52*:706–711.

91. Dominguez, L., J. F. F. Garayzabal, J. A. Vazquez, J. L. Blanco, and G. Suarez. 1987. Fate of *Listeria monocytogenes* during manufacture and ripening of semi-hard cheese. *Lett. Appl. Microbiol. 4*:125–127.

92. Doyle, M. P., L. M. Meske, and E. H. Marth. 1985. Survival of *Listeria monocytogenes* during the manufacture and storage of nonfat dry milk. *J. Food Prot. 48*:740–742.

93. El-Gazzar, F. E., and E. H. Marth. 1988. Loss of viability by *Listeria monocytogenes* in commercial calf rennet extract. *J. Food Prot. 51*:16–18.

94. El-Gazzar, F. E., and E. H. Marth. 1988. Loss of viability of *Listeria monocytogenes* in commercial bovine pepsin-rennet extract. *J. Dairy Sci. 72*:1098–1102.

95. El-Gazzar, F. E., and E. H. Marth. 1989. Fate of *Listeria monocytogenes* in some food colours and starter distillate. *Lebensm. Wiss. Technol. 22*:406–410.

96. El-Gazzar, F. E., and E. H. Marth. 1989. Loss of viability by *Listeria monocytogenes* in commercial microbial rennet. *Milchwissenschaft 44*:83–86.

97. El-Shenawy, M. A., and E. H. Marth. 1990. Behavior of *Listeria monocytogenes* in the presence of gluconic acid and during preparation of cottage cheese curd using gluconic acid. *J. Dairy Sci. 73*:1429–1438.
98. Farber, J. M., G. W. Sanders, and S. A. Malcom. 1988. The presence of *Listeria* spp. in raw milk in Ontario. *Can. J. Microbiol. 34*:95–100.
99. Farber, J. M., M. A. Johnston, U. Purvis, and A. Loit. 1987. Surveillance of soft and semi-soft cheeses for the presence of *Listeria* spp. *Int. J. Food Microbiol. 5*:157–163.
100. Gabis, D. A., R. S. Flowers, D. Evanson, and R. E. Faust. 1989. A survey of 18 dry dairy product processing plant environments for *Salmonella, Listeria* and *Yersinia. J. Food Prot. 52*:122–124.
101. Geisen, R., E. Glenn, and L. Leistner. 1988. Effects of *Penicillium roquefortii, P. camemberti* and *P. nalgiovense* on growth of *Listeria monocytogenes* in vitro. *Mitteilungsblatt der Bundesanstalt fuer Fleischforschung, Kulmbach 101*:8088–8092.
102. Gilbert, R. J. 1990. Personal communication.
103. Gledel, J. 1986. Epidemiology and significance of listeriosis in France. In A. Schönberg (ed.), Listeriosis-Joint WHO/ROI Consultation on Prevention and Control, West Berlin, December 10–12, pp. 9–20. Institut für Veterinarmedizin des Bundesgesundheitsamtes, Berlin.
104. Gledel, J. 1988. *Listeria* and the dairy industry in France. *Foodborne Listeriosis—Proceedings of a Symposium*, Wiesbaden, West Germany, Sept. 7, pp. 72–82.
105. Goel, M. C., D. C. Kulshrestha, E. H. Marth, D. W. Francis, J. G. Bradshaw, and R. B. Read, Jr. 1971. Fate of coliforms in yogurt, buttermilk, sour cream, and cottage cheese during refrigerated storage. *J. Milk Food Technol. 34*:54–58.
106. Goepfert, J. M., N. F. Olson, and E. H. Marth. 1968. Behavior of *Salmonella typhimurium* during manufacture and curing of Cheddar cheese. *Appl. Microbiol. 16*:862–866.
107. Griffith, M., and K. Deibel. 1988. Survival of *Listeria monocytogenes* in yogurt and acidified milk. Ann. Mtg., Amer. Soc. Microbiol., Miami Beach, FL, May 8–13, Abstr. P-21.
108. Hapke, B. 1989. Personal communication.
109. Ikonomov, L., and D. Todorov. 1964. Studies of the viability of *Listeria monocytogenes* in ewe's milk and dairy products. *Vet. Med. Nauki, Sofiya 7*:23–29.
110. International Dairy Federation. 1989. Pathogenic *Listeria*—Abstracts of replies from 24 countries to questionnaire 1288/B on pathogenic *Listeria*. Circular 89/5, March 31, International Dairy Federation, Brussels.
111. Johnson, E. A. 1989. Personal communication.
112. Lafaivre, J. 1988. Personal communication.
113. Marier, R., J. G. Wells, R. C. Swanson, W. Callahan, and I. J. Mehlman. 1973. An outbreak of enteropathogenic *Escherichia coli* foodborne disease traced to imported French cheese. *Lancet ii*:1376–1378.
114. Massa, S., D. Cesaroni, G. Poda, and L. D. Trovatelli. 1990. The incidence of *Listeria* spp. in soft cheeses, butter and raw milk in the province of Bologna. *J. Appl. Bacteriol. 68*:153–156.
115. McBean, L. D. 1988. A perspective on food safety concerns. *Dairy Food Sanit. 8*:112–118.
116. McLauchlin, J., M. H. Greenwood, and P. N. Pini. 1990. The occurrence of *Listeria monocytogenes* in cheese from a manufacturer associated with a case of listeriosis. *Int. J. Food Microbiol.* (accepted).
117. Nelson, J. H. 1988. Should pasteurization of milk for cheesemaking be mandatory? *J. Food Prot. 51*:826. (Abstr.)
118. Nichols, J. G. 1987. Personal communication.
119. Nooitgedagt, A. J., and B. J. Hartog. 1988. A survey of the microbiological quality of Brie and Camembert cheese. *Neth. Milk Dairy J. 42*:57–72.
120. Northolt, M. D., H. J. Beckers, U. Vecht, L. Toepoel, P. S. S. Soentoro, and H. J. Wisselink. 1988. *Listeria monocytogenes*: Heat resistance and behavior during storage of milk and whey and making of Dutch types of cheese. *Neth. Milk Dairy J. 42*:207–219.
121. Papageorgiou, D. K., and E. H. Marth. 1989. Behavior of *Listeria monocytogenes* at 4 and 22°C in whey and skim milk containing 6 or 12% sodium chloride. *J. Food Prot. 52*:625–630.
122. Papageorgiou, D. K., and E. H. Marth. 1989. Fate of *Listeria monocytogenes* during the manufacture and ripening of blue cheese. *J. Food Prot. 52*:459–465.

123. Papageorgiou, D. K., and E. H. Marth. 1989. Fate of *Listeria monocytogenes* during the manufacture, ripening and storage of feta cheese. *J. Food Prot. 52*:82–87.
124. Pini, P. N., and R. J. Gilbert. 1988. The occurrence in the U.K. of *Listeria* species in raw chickens and soft cheeses. *Int. J. Food Microbiol. 6*:317–326.
125. Pratt-Lowe, E. L., R. M. Geiger, T. Richardson, and E. L. Barrett. 1988. Heat resistance of alkaline phosphatase produced by microorganisms isolated from California Mexican-style cheeses. *J. Dairy Sci. 71*:17–23.
126. Pucci, M. J., E. R. Vedamuthu, B. S. Kunka, and P. A. Vandebergh. 1988. Inhibition of *Listeria monocytogenes* by using bacteriocin PA-1 produced by *Pediococcus acidilactici* PAC 1.0. *Appl. Environ. Microbiol. 54*:2349–2353.
127. Raccach, M., R. McGrath, and H. Daftarian. 1989. Antibiosis of some lactic acid bacteria including *Lactobacillus acidophilus* toward *Listeria monocytogenes*. *Int. J. Food Microbiol. 9*:25–32.
128. Rosenow, E. M., and E. H. Marth. 1987. Growth of *Listeria monocytogenes* in skim, whole and chocolate milk, and in whipping cream during incubation at 4, 8, 13, 21 and 35°C. *J. Food Prot. 50*:452–459.
129. Rousset, A., and M. Rousset. 1989. *Listeria monocytogenes* isolées de fromages prélevés au niveau différents points de vente. *Sci. Aliments 9*:129–131.
130. Ryser, E. T., and E. H. Marth. 1987. Behavior of *Listeria monocytogenes* during the manufacture and ripening of Cheddar cheese. *J. Food Prot. 50*:7–13.
131. Ryser, E. T., and E. H. Marth. 1987. Fate of *Listeria monocytogenes* during manufacture and ripening of Camembert cheese. *J. Food Prot. 50*:372–378.
132. Ryser, E. T., and E. H. Marth. 1987. Unpublished data.
133. Ryser, E. T., and E. H. Marth. 1988. Growth of *Listeria monocytogenes* at different pH values in uncultured whey or whey cultured with *Penicillium camemberti*. *Can. J. Microbiol. 34*:730–734.
134. Ryser, E. T., and E. H. Marth. 1988. Survival of *Listeria monocytogenes* in cold-pack cheese food during refrigerated storage. *J. Food Prot. 51*:615–621, 625.
135. Ryser, E. T., and E. H. Marth. 1989. Behavior of *Listeria monocytogenes* during manufacture and ripening of brick cheese. *J. Dairy Sci. 72*:838–853.
136. Ryser, E. T., E. H. Marth, and M. P. Doyle. 1985. Survival of *Listeria monocytogenes* during manufacture and storage of cottage cheese. *J. Food Prot. 48*:746–750, 753.
137. Schaack, M. M., and E. H. Marth. 1988. Behavior of *Listeria monocytogenes* in skim milk and in yogurt mix during fermentation by thermophilic lactic acid bacteria. *J. Food Prot. 51*:607–614.
138. Schaack, M. M., and E. H. Marth. 1988. Behavior of *Listeria monocytogenes* in skim milk during fermentation with mesophilic lactic starter cultures. *J. Food Prot. 51*:600–606.
139. Schaack, M. M., and E. H. Marth. 1988. Survival of *Listeria monocytogenes* in refrigerated cultured milks and yogurt. *J. Food Prot. 51*:848–852.
140. Schoen, R., and G. Terplan. Personal communication.
141. Seeliger, H. P. R. 1961. *Listeriosis*, Hafner Publishing Co., New York.
142. Seeliger, H. P. R., and D. Jones. 1987. *Listeria*. In *Bergy's Manual of Systematic Bacteriology*, 9th ed. Williams and Wilkins, Baltimore, pp. 1235–1245.
143. Shahamat, M., A. Seaman, and M. Woodbine. 1980. Survival of *Listeria monocytogenes* in high salt concentrations. *Zbl. Bakteriol. Hyg. I Abt. Orig. A 246*:506–511.
144. Sikes, A. 1989. Fate of *Staphylococcus aureus* and *Listeria monocytogenes* in certain low moisture military rations during processing and storage. Ann. Mtg., Inst. Food Technol., Chicago, IL, June 25–29, Abstr. 466.
145. Sipka, M., S. Zakula, I. Kovincic, and B. Stajner. 1974. Secretion of *Listeria monocytogenes* in cow's milk and its survival in white brined cheese. *19th International Dairy Congress IE*:157.
146. Siragusa, G. R., and M. G. Johnson. 1989. Persistence of *Listeria monocytogenes* in yogurt as determined by direct plating and cold enrichment methods. *Int. J. Food Microbiol. 7*:147–160.
147. Skinner, K. J. 1989. *Listeria*—Battling back against one "tough bug." *Dairy, Food Environ. Sanit. 9*:23–24.

148. Stajner, B., S. Zakula, I. Kovincic, and M. Galic. 1979. Heat resistance of *Listeria monocytogenes* and its survival in raw milk products. *Vet. Glasnik 33*:109–112.
149. Terplan, G. 1988. Factors responsible for the contamination of food with *Listeria monocytogenes*. WHO Working Group on Foodborne Listeriosis, Geneva, Switzerland, Feb. 15–19.
150. Terplan, G. 1988. Personal communication.
151. Terplan, G., R. Schoen, W. Springmeyer, I. Degle, and H. Becker. 1986. *Listeria monocytogenes* in Milch und Milchprodukten. *Deutsche Molkerei Zeitung 41*:1358–1368.
152. Terplan, G., R. Schoen, W. Springmeyer, I. Degle, and H. Becker. 1986. *Listeria monocytogenes* in Milch und Milchprodukten. In 27th Arbeitstagung des Arbeitsgebietes "Lebensmittelhygiene" von 9–12, September in Garmisch-Partenkirchen. Giessen/Lahn, German Federal Republic; Deutsche Veterinärmedizinische Gesellschafte V.
153. Tham, W. 1988. Survival of *Listeria monocytogenes* in cheese made of unpasteurized goat milk. *Acta Vet. Scand. 29*:165–172.
154. Tham, W. A., and V. M.-L. Danielsson-Tham. 1988. *Listeria monocytogenes* isolated from soft cheese. *Vet. Rec. 122*:539–540.
155. Toschkoff, Al., A. Lilova-Popova, and D. Veljanov. 1975. Dynamics of multiplication and changes in the virulence of some pathogenic microorganisms in milk and milk products. *Acta Microbiol. Virol. Immunol. 1*:40–45.
156. Tulloch, E. F., Jr., K. J. Ryan, S. B. Formal, and F. A. Franklin. 1973. Invasive enteropathogenic coli dysentery. *Ann. Intern. Med. 79*:13–17.
157. United States Department of Agriculture. 1978. Cheese varieties and descriptions. Agricultural Handbook No. 54. Agricultural Research Service, Washington, DC (Reprinted by National Cheese Institute, Alexandria, VA.)
158. Venables, L. J. 1989. *Listeria monocytogenes* in dairy products—the Victorian experience. *Food Australia 41*:942–943.
159. Weber, A. von, C. Baumann, J. Potel, and H. Friess. 1988. Nachweis von *Listeria monocytogenes* und *Listeria innocua* in Käse. *Berl. Münch. tierärztl. Wschr. 101*:373–375.
160. Wenzel, J. M., and E. H. Marth. 1988. 1990. Behavior of *Listeria monocytogenes* in the presence of *Streptococcus lactis* in a medium with internal pH control. *J. Food Prot. 53*:918–923.
161. Yndestad, M. 1988. Personal communication.
162. Yousef, A. E., and E. H. Marth. 1988. Behavior of *Listeria monocytogenes* during the manufacture and storage of Colby cheese. *J. Food Prot. 51*:12–15.
163. Yousef, A. E., and E. H. Marth. 1990. Fate of *Listeria monocytogenes* during the manufacture and ripening of Parmesan cheese. *J. Dairy Sci. 73*:3351–3356.
164. Yousef, A. E., E. T. Ryser, and E. H. Marth. 1988. Methods for improved recovery of *Listeria monocytogenes* from cheese. *Appl. Environ. Microbiol. 54*:2643–2649.

11

Incidence and Behavior of *Listeria monocytogenes* in Meat Products

INTRODUCTION

Recognition of *L. monocytogenes* as a serious foodborne pathogen has raised concerns about the possible role of meat products as vehicles of listeric infections. However, thus far repeated efforts have failed to conclusively link consumption of meat products to a single case of human listeriosis. While this apparent absence of any recorded cases of meatborne (excluding poultry products) listeriosis in years past may have resulted from a combination of inadequate methods to detect *L. monocytogenes* in meat and a general lack of awareness of foodborne listeriosis, these conditions no longer exist. Thus, in all probability, current epidemiological investigations and follow-up laboratory studies will uncover evidence for transmission of listeriosis through consumption of contaminated meat. Such efforts have already implicated home-made Italian pork sausage (62) and cooked Cajun pork sausage (42) as presumptive infectious vehicles in two isolated cases of listeriosis (see Chapter 8).

Given the psychrotrophic nature of *L. monocytogenes*, the ubiquity of this pathogen within slaughterhouse and meat-packing environments, and a heightened awareness of foodborne listeriosis, it is not surprising that the incidence and behavior of *L. monocytogenes* in meat products are receiving considerable attention in North America and Europe. The initial pages of this chapter trace the development of the United States Department of Agriculture–Food Safety Inspection Service (USDA-FSIS) *Listeria*-testing program for raw, cooked, and ready-to-eat meat products, after which results from this effort will be summarized along with findings from similar independent surveys of various meat products marketed in the United States, Canada, Western Europe, and elsewhere. Information regarding behavior of *L. monocytogenes* in raw meat, cooked meat, and various sausage products can be found in the second half of this chapter.

INCIDENCE OF *LISTERIA* IN MEAT PRODUCTS

Development of Various USDA-FSIS *Listeria*-Monitoring/Verification Programs

Public health concern about presence of *L. monocytogenes* in meat and other foods sold in the United States is directly related to the June 1985 listeriosis outbreak in California that was linked to consumption of contaminated Mexican-style cheese. Two factors,

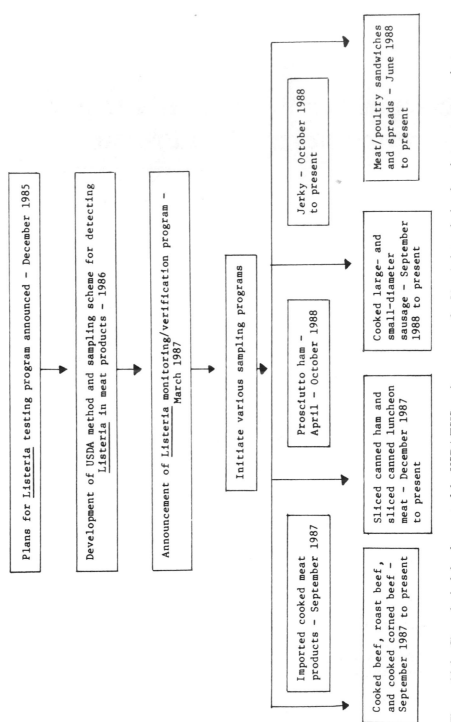

Figure 11.1 Chronological development of the USDA/FSIS testing programs for *Listeria* in cooked and ready-to-eat meat products. (Adapted from Refs. 64, 84.)

namely (a) heightened awareness of foodborne listeriosis resulting from this outbreak and (b) the realization that humans are likely to at least occasionally consume *Listeria*-contaminated meat products, prompted a December 1985 announcement by the USDA-FSIS indicating that a *Listeria*-testing program would be developed for cooked and ready-to-eat meat products (3) (Fig. 11.1).

Government officials were immediately faced with several problems regarding their proposed testing program, the most serious of which was lack of a reliable method to detect *L. monocytogenes* in meat products. At least 1 year of experimentation was required to develop two enrichment broths and one selective plating medium along with methodology for the original USDA procedure (see Fig. 6.19), which was subsequently accepted for isolating *L. monocytogenes* from meat and poultry products. During initial testing of the USDA procedure, McClain and Lee (111) recovered *L. monocytogenes* from 20 of 41 (40%) samples of frozen ground beef and 12 of 23 (52%) samples of pork sausage. These findings led to concerns about possible widespread contamination of raw and ready-to-eat meat products and also prompted a serious dilemma about regulatory policies for *Listeria*-contaminated meat since at that time consumption of these products was not yet proven to constitute any threat to public health.

Despite many problems still facing the USDA-FSIS, the agency made public its plan to initiate *Listeria* testing of various meat products. According to the formal announcement in the March 11, 1987, issue of the *Federal Register* (88), USDA-FSIS officials were to immediately begin phasing in a testing/monitoring program for *L. monocytogenes* in domestic and imported cooked/ready-to-eat meat and poultry products with special emphasis on ready-to-eat items such as dry-cured pork, fermented sausage and luncheon meats, and cooked/ready-to-eat products that were returned to the manufacturer for reprocessing. This program has undergone several major changes which will be discussed in due course; however, when this program was first announced, USDA-FSIS officials considered seizing and/or recalling a product only if one or more follow-up samples contained *L. monocytogenes*. Affected firms were (and still are) strongly encouraged to carefully review their manufacturing operations for conditions that might allow growth of *L. monocytogenes* and, where possible, reduce the potential for this pathogen to contaminate products by implementing Hazard Analysis Critical Control Point (HACCP) principles along with Good Manufacturing Practices. A detailed discussion of the incidence and control of listeriae in meat-processing facilities can be found in Chapter 15.

One month later, USDA-FSIS officials yielded to pressure from the meat industry and agreed to delay the start of their planned *L. monocytogenes* monitoring/verification program for at least 90 days. Among considerations responsible for this delay were (a) arguments that the *Listeria*-detection method may be inadequate, (b) fear that enforcement of the proposed policy would lead to widespread disruption of the processed meat industry (8,9), (c) concern that anticipated seizures and recalls of contaminated product would not withstand legal challenges since consumption of such products was not yet linked to any case of listeriosis, (d) lack of data concerning the oral dose of *L. monocytogenes* needed to induce illness, and (e) a need for USDA-FSIS officials to identify and recommend specific means by which manufacturers can avoid producing *Listeria*-contaminated products (11,13).

After considerable debate by government officials and representatives of the meat industry, the USDA-FSIS established a zero–tolerance policy for *L. monocytogenes* in processed meat and poultry products, which was still in effect as of January 1991 (30,31,44). Although this decision was based more on an inability to arrive at a "permissible level" of *L. monocytogenes* in ready-to-eat meat and poultry products than on scientific evidence concerning the oral infective dose (15), authorities at CDC and FDA maintained that consumption of any food product contaminated with even a very low level of *L. monocytogenes* may pose a significant threat to pregnant women and immunocompromised individuals (7,13). Furthermore, the possibility of *Listeria* growing in ready-to-eat foods during extended refrigerated storage could increase the risk to consumers of contracting listeriosis. Hence, even though consumption of meat products has not yet been positively linked to listeric infections, USDA-FSIS officials had no choice but to adopt a zero-tolerance policy for *L. monocytogenes* in ready-to-eat meat and poultry products. This decision basically agrees with the FDA's policy regarding presence of *L. monocytogenes* in food products under its jurisdiction (5).

The USDA-FSIS monitoring/verification program for *L. monocytogenes* in meat products finally began in September of 1987 with sampling of domestic corned beef, roast beef, cooked corned beef, and massaged corned beef as well as imported cooked meats. This program was later expanded to include a much wider range of products (Fig. 11.1) with meat/poultry sandwiches and spreads added most recently following the inadvertent discovery of *L. monocytogenes* in such products in March 1989 (24).

According to the original regulatory policy adopted in September 1987, 25-g monitoring samples were collected from the firm's current production and diluted in 225 ml of enrichment broth. However, unlike the FDA procedure in which 50 g of product is normally analyzed for listeriae, only 10 ml of the 1:10 dilution (1 g of product) was examined using the USDA-FSIS protocol. [The smaller sample size used by USDA-FSIS officials obviously reduced the chances of finding *L. monocytogenes* in meat products (37).] Although prudent to do so, manufacturers were not required to hold sampled lots until *Listeria* test results became available. In the event that *L. monocytogenes* was detected in a monitoring sample, the manufacturer was notified of the results so that "like-product" [i.e., "product that is produced with the same species of raw material identified with the same name" (46)] could be held. However, unlike the current USDA-FSIS (and FDA) policy regarding *Listeria*, the firm was under no obligation to recall the contaminated lots (4,27) since it was believed that monitoring samples from which subsamples were taken for other microbiological analyses (*Salmonella*) could have been inadvertently contaminated with *L. monocytogenes* in the laboratory (12), thus leading to obvious legal disputes regarding the source of contamination. After allowing 5 days for factory clean-up and development of a corrective action plan (4,10), government inspectors were instructed to collect, freeze, and analyze six verification samples from intact packages of currently produced "like-product." If any of these six verification samples contained *L. monocytogenes*, USDA-FSIS officials requested a voluntary Class I recall only if the sampled *Listeria*-positive lots had entered commerce (4,14,27). However, assuming that the firm retained all lots from which verification samples were taken, these products could then be recalled internally, thus avoiding the adverse publicity associated with a formal Class I recall. Nevertheless, in either situation government officials initiated (a) a hold-test program for all "like-product" produced by the firm until five consecutive production lots were *Listeria*-free and (b) a Microbiological Incident

Surveillance Sampling Program in which inspectors sampled a wide range of cooked and/or ready to eat products manufactured over a period of 5 months (10,14,27).

Although this policy was enforced throughout the remainder of 1987 and all of 1988, USDA-FSIS officials dramatically changed their stance regarding *Listeria*-contaminated meat and poultry products in 1989 after an Oklahoma breast cancer patient contracted listeriosis from consuming turkey frankfurters that were contaminated with *L. monocytogenes* (40,53). In the light of this direct evidence linking a cooked poultry product to a case of listeriosis, USDA-FSIS officials revised the previously discussed policy regarding presence of *L. monocytogenes* in cooked/ready-to-eat meat and poultry products prepared at federally inspected facilities and certified foreign establishments.

Under the revised *Listeria* policy (Fig. 11.2), which appeared in the May 23, 1989, issue of the *Federal Register* (70), 25-g rather than 1-g monitoring samples (29,39) obtained from intact retail packages (e.g., frankfurters, luncheon meat, sausages) will be examined for *L. monocytogenes* using the revised USDA procedure (see Fig. 6.20). If any of these samples contain *L. monocytogenes*, the entire lot manufactured on the day or during the shift the positive monitoring sample was taken will be considered adulterated. Unlike the previous policy, which required identification of *L. monocytogenes* in one or more verification samples before initiation of further action, the present policy grants USDA-FSIS officials power to request firms to issue an immediate Class I recall for all tainted lots in the marketplace. (However, manufacturers again can avoid a formal recall by holding all sampled lots until results of *Listeria* testing are known.) In either event, government officials also will (a) initiate a hold-test program until consistent production of *Listeria*-free product has been achieved, (b) collect and analyze other potentially contaminated products manufactured at the same facility, (c) encourage firms to review their operations for conditions that may allow growth of listeriae, and (d) take any additional appropriate in-factory action to prevent production of contaminated product.

The current policy regarding large products that are not normally available in retail-sized packages (e.g., roast beef, corned beef) (Fig. 11.2) more closely resembles the September 1987 version of the monitoring/verification program in that USDA-FSIS officials will not request an immediate Class I recall if *L. monocytogenes* is detected in one or more monitoring samples. In such instances, verification samples (intact samples from subsequent lots) will be collected and analyzed for *L. monocytogenes* using current USDA methodology (39). Any verification sample that is positive for *L. monocytogenes* will automatically trigger action similar to that just described for products in intact retail-sized packages weighing ≤3 pounds (46); included is issuance of an immediate Class I recall in the unlikely event that the firm failed to hold all sampled lots until results of *Listeria* testing became known.

In addition to the federal inspection program just described, the state of Wisconsin attempted to initiate a more rigorous *Listeria*-testing program on June 1, 1988, for ready-to-eat processed meat products (e.g., frankfurters, sausage) produced at state-inspected facilities (21,22). Under this program, which was similar to that adopted by the FDA for dairy products, intact packages of processed meat products obtained from the state's meat-processing plants and retail stores would have been examined for *L. monocytogenes* using the USDA method. More important, any positive finding would have prompted an immediate recall of the product along with issuance of a press release

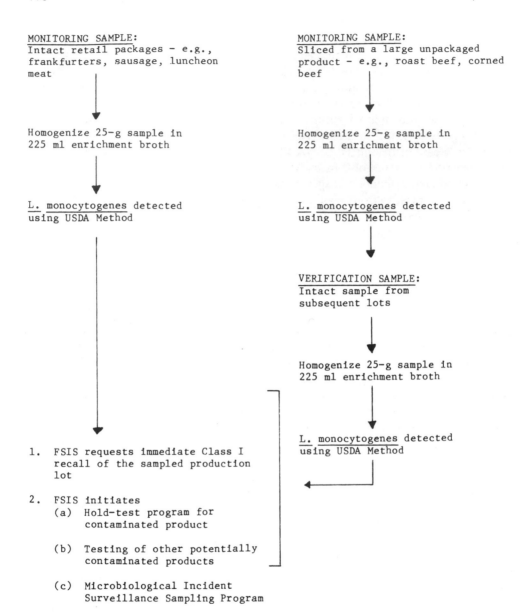

Figure 11.2 USDA-FSIS Monitoring/Verification Program for *L. monocytogenes* in cooked and ready-to-eat meat products, May 1989. (Adapted from Ref. 70.)

by the state. However, state officials agreed to delay the start of this program after industry representatives argued that recalls based on single samples would unduly harm the processed meat industry in Wisconsin. This policy was subsequently modified after consultation with USDA-FSIS officials. According to the revised state program, state inspectors may take several actions if *L. monocytogenes* is found in a product in which no USDA-inspected ingredients are suspected as the source of contamination. These actions may include (a) further testing of meat products, (b) issuing a statewide recall for all intact packages from the affected lot, and/or (c) ordering destruction of remaining inventory held by retail stores within Wisconsin (26). However, USDA-FSIS officials will retain the legal right to use their own policy in dealing with *Listeria*-contaminated products manufactured and sold in Wisconsin if USDA-inspected ingredients in such products are suspected as the source of contamination.

Results from Various USDA-FSIS *Listeria*-Monitoring/Verification Programs

Raw Meat

In January 1987, the USDA-FSIS began a monitor-sampling program to determine incidence of *L. monocytogenes* in domestic raw beef. This program was not undertaken to initiate regulatory action against particular firms but rather to provide the agency with critical background information. During the 26-month period from January 1987 to February 1990, *L. monocytogenes* was isolated from 122 of 1726 (7.1%) 25-g monitor-

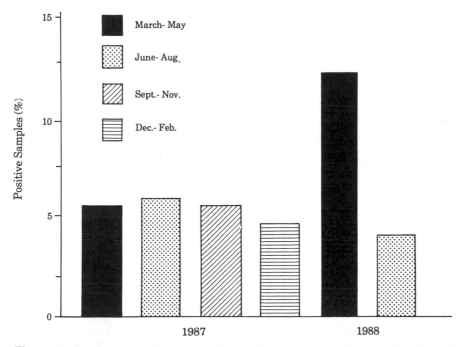

Figure 11.3 Seasonal variation in incidence of *L. monocytogenes* in raw beef. (Adapted from Ref. 64.)

ing samples of domestically produced raw beef (52). While the percentage of *Listeria*-positive samples remained virtually constant throughout all of 1987, a dramatic increase in the incidence of *Listeria*-contaminated raw beef was observed during the spring of 1988 (Fig. 11.3). Such an increase might be attributable to higher numbers of silage-fed animals shedding listeriae in feces along with increased growth of the pathogen in wet farm environments, as was previously suggested to have caused the higher incidence of *L. monocytogenes* in raw milk samples obtained during late winter and early spring compared to other seasons. Grouping these data according to bovine type showed that the highest percentage of positive samples was associated with cows (9.6%), followed by bulls (7.6%), steers (5.9%), heifers (4.5%), and calves (1.8%). Thus, at least in this study, the incidence of *L. monocytogenes* appears to be age-related with raw beef from older animals most frequently contaminated with the pathogen.

Cooked Beef, Roast Beef, and Cooked Corned Beef

Beginning in September 1987, USDA-FSIS officials initiated the first of a series of ongoing monitoring/verification programs (Fig. 11.1) designed to determine the extent of *L. monocytogenes* contamination in cooked beef, roast beef, and cooked corned beef. As of October 1988, the pathogen was detected in 14 of 49 (28.6%) domestic and 0 of 26 1-g samples of imported cooked beef, roast beef, and cooked corned beef (6,64). However, more recent results (Table 11.1) indicate that *L. monocytogenes* was present in only 30 of 1102 (2.7%) samples of domestic/imported cooked beef, roast beef, and cooked corn beef, with most positive samples being cooked beef (28). In most instances, these products were removed from their packages after cooking and then repackaged for sale, thus suggesting that the pathogen most likely entered the product through direct contact with the factory environment, knives, and/or gowns worn by workers. At least two other firms handled raw and finished product in the same production area of the factory but at different times, which, in turn, indicates the possibility of cross-contamination between raw and finished product.

To our knowledge, this program has uncovered only one firm that was producing contaminated product after having been given an opportunity for clean-up and modification of manufacturing/sanitizing procedures (20,64). In this instance, *L. monocytogenes* was detected in six of six verification samples of cooked corned beef after initial monitoring samples were positive for the pathogen. Fortunately, all lots awaiting verification of *L. monocytogenes* were withheld from the retail market, thus avoiding a formal recall of the product. In accordance with USDA-FSIS policy, all lots of contaminated product were reprocessed and retested before release to consumers. Subsequently this firm cleared the hold-test phase of the regulatory program and has since encountered no further problems with *Listeria*-contaminated products.

Sliced Canned Ham and Luncheon Meats

In December 1987, USDA-FSIS officials began another monitoring/verification program in which sliced canned ham and luncheon meat were examined for presence of *L. monocytogenes* (Fig. 11.1). As of September 1989, the pathogen was detected in only 1 of 278 (0.36%) samples examined (Table 11.1).

Table 11.1   Incidence of *L. monocytogenes* in USDA-FSIS
Monitoring Samples of Cooked and Ready-to-Eat Meat Products,
September 1987 to September 1989

Meat product	Number of samples examined	Number of positive samples (%)
Domestic/imported cooked beef, roast beef, and cooked corned beef	1102	30 (2.7)
Sliced canned ham and sliced canned luncheon meat	278	1 (0.36)
Prosciutto ham	136	3 (2.2)
Cooked large- and small-diameter sausage	1036	9 (0.87)
Jerky	264	0

Source: Adapted from Refs. 64, 65.

Prosciutto Ham

In April 1988, prosciutto ham, a raw pork product which must be heavily salted and air-dried for 6 months before consumption, was added to the list of ready-to-eat meat products to be examined for *L. monocytogenes* (Fig. 11.1). During this 7-month-long testing program, the organism was detected in 3 of 136 (2.2%) monitoring samples (Table 11.1), all three of which came from one of nine U.S. firms that manufacture prosciutto ham (64). *L. monocytogenes* was later detected in verification samples from the same firm, which, in turn, led to condemnation of the affected product along with initiation of a hold-test program by USDA-FSIS officials. As of October 1988, this was only the second time that *L. monocytogenes* was identified in verification samples of ready-to-eat meat products, the first being the incident involving cooked corned beef described earlier.

Large/Small-Diameter Sausage and Jerky

Testing programs for two additional products, cooked large/small-diameter sausage (including products prepared from both meat and poultry) and jerky, were initiated in September and October 1988, respectively (Fig. 11.1). As of September 1989, *L. monocytogenes* has been recovered from 9 of 1036 (0.87%) monitoring samples of cooked large/small-diameter sausage (Table 11.1) with 7 of these 9 positive samples identified as red meat frankfurters (3 samples), poultry frankfurters, poultry/red meat frankfurters, poultry/red meat bologna, and turkey sausage (28). However, to our knowledge, *L. monocytogenes* has not yet been isolated from jerky.

Recalls and Other Regulatory Actions

As of July 1990, the aforementioned USDA-FSIS monitoring/verification programs (Fig. 11.1) have resulted in at least 12 separate Class I recalls of cooked/ready-to-eat meat and related products contaminated with *L. monocytogenes* (Table 11.2). While the

Table 11.2 Chronological List of Class I Recalls Issued in the United States for Cooked/Ready-to-Eat Meat and Related Products Contaminated with *L. monocytogenes*

Type of product	Date recall initiated	Origin	Distribution	Quantity	Ref.
Beef, sausage, and ham salad sandwiches—6 varieties	05/03/89	Virginia	Alabama, Florida, Georgia, Ohio, Louisiana, North Carolina, South Carolina, Virginia	372,000 sandwiches	33,41
Ham salad	08/04/89	West Virginia	Kentucky, Ohio, Virginia, West Virginia	2,220 lb.	38,113
Frozen meat patties	08/22/89	Virginia	Alabama, Florida, Georgia, Indiana, Louisiana, Michigan, North Carolina, Ohio, South Carolina, Virginia	73,080 sandwiches	32
Sausage sandwiches	10/20/89	Tennessee	Ohio	1,500 sandwiches	35
Meat salad	10/23/89	North Carolina	North Carolina, South Carolina, Virginia	848 lb.	113
Frozen chili dogs, chili and cheese dog sandwiches	10/23/89	Texas	Mississippi, Tennessee, Texas	642 cases	25
Refrigerated/frozen beef, corned beef, pork sausage, chicken, turkey, cheese, fish, and other sandwiches —133 varieties	10/24/89	Minnesota	California, Colorado, Georgia, Illinois, Iowa, Kentucky, Michigan, Minnesota, New Jersey, New York, North Dakota, Ohio, Tennessee, Texas, Wisconsin	~100,000 sandwiches	34
Beef, corned beef, pork, sausage, chicken, turkey, cheese, fish, and other sandwiches—66 varieties	11/08/89	Missouri	Kansas, Missouri	~900 sandwiches	43,49
Smoked pork sausage	11/14/89	Massachusetts	Massachusetts, Rhode Island	13 lb.	36,113
Meat salad	11/28/89	Connecticut	Not reported	3,825 lb.	113
Luncheon meat	12/06/89	South Carolina	South Carolina	222 lb.	113
Processed pork	12/15/89	Louisiana	Arizona, California, Florida, Louisiana, Texas	5,221 lb.	113

first of these recalls was issued in May 1989 for 372,000 sausage and ham salad sandwiches, the first recall of a product under the USDA's jurisdiction occurred several weeks earlier and involved turkey frankfurters that were directly linked to a case of listeriosis in Oklahoma (see Chapters 8 and 12). Thus far half of all recalls issued for cooked/ready-to-eat meat products have involved prepared sandwiches and meat spreads with well over 500,000 sandwiches removed from the marketplace. However, actual product losses are undoubtedly somewhat higher since firms holding tested products until results of *Listeria* analyses become known can "recall" all contaminated lots internally, thereby avoiding a formal Class I recall.

Considering the wide variety of tainted sandwiches that have been withdrawn from sale, it appears that *L. monocytogenes* entered these products during cutting, slicing, and/or packaging rather than being initially present in the many different types of sandwich fillings. This conclusion is further supported by the fact that this pathogen was widespread within the working environment of one large sandwich factory that was cited in the May 1989 recall as well as for ongoing production of *Listeria*-contaminated sandwiches since January 1989 (50). Following continued unsuccessful efforts to clean this factory, government officials filed for a court-ordered injunction in May 1989 (48,50) which would effectively close this facility until *L. monocytogenes* is completely eliminated from the factory environment and all manufacturing equipment.

To our knowledge, the only other USDA-initiated action regarding cooked/ready-to-eat meat products has been the November 2, 1989, block-listing of *Listeria*-contaminated frozen cooked beef imported from Argentina (45). This action currently (July 1990) requires import inspectors to submit intact samples of Argentinian beef for *Listeria* analysis and retain all product until test results become known (113). As a consequence of this action, it appears that USDA officials will soon require exporters of cooked/ready-to-eat meat (and poultry) products to develop *Listeria* monitoring programs that are equivalent to those used in the United States.

Other Nonregulatory United States Surveys

In addition to the various USDA-FSIS *Listeria*-monitoring/verification programs just discussed, Buchanan et al. (60) made a limited nonregulatory survey of raw and cured meat products to (a) compare the ability of two selective plating media to recover *Listeria* spp. from various meats and (b) test a three-tube MPN (most probable number) enrichment procedure for quantitating listeriae in meat products. (Isolation, detection, and quantitation methods used in this study are described in Chapter 6.) Overall, low levels of *Listeria* spp. (generally <1 CFU/g) were detected in 11 of 21 (52.4%) raw meat samples (Table 11.3). It is noteworthy that multiple *Listeria* spp. were identified in 5 of the 11 positive samples with 9 of 21 (42.9%), 6 of 21 (28.6%), and 1 of 21 (4.8%) samples containing *L. monocytogenes*, *L. innocua*, and *L. welshimeri*, respectively. Unlike results from the previously described USDA-FSIS raw beef–monitoring program, 72.2% of all *Listeria*-positive raw meat samples originated from young animals, i.e., calves and lambs. Presently it is unclear whether results from this study represent a statistical anomaly (nonuniform and/or small number of samples) or an actual predisposition for *Listeria* contamination among younger animals, which, in turn, may be related to current animal-rearing, slaughtering, and/or processing methods.

Table 11.3 Limited Survey of Raw and Cured Retail Meats for *Listeria* spp.

Product	Number of samples analyzed	Number of positive samples	Level of *Listeria* spp. (CFU/g)[a]	*Listeria* spp. identified[b]
Raw meats				
Sausage	3	1	0.03	M, I
Pork sausage	1	1	0.03	M
Hamburger	4	1	0.92	M, I, W
Veal (ground)	4	3	0.62–0.74	2M[c], 2I
Veal patties (ground)	1	1	0.36	M
Veal sausage	1	1	0.36	W
Beef liver	2	0	ND[d]	–
Calf liver	1	0	ND	–
Lamb (ground)	3	3	2.10–4.27	3M, 2I
Lamb kidney	1	0	ND	–
Cured meats				
Corned beef	1	0	ND	–
Salami	2	1	0.36	I
Bologna	2	0	ND	–
Ham and cheese loaf	1	0	ND	–
Luncheon meat	1	0	ND	–
Olive loaf	1	0	ND	–
Liver sausage	1	0	ND	–
Pepperoni	1	0	ND	–
Lebanon bologna	1	0	ND	–

[a]Minimum detectable level = 0.03 *Listeria* spp. CFU/g using an MPN procedure.
[b]M = *L. monocytogenes*; I = *L. innocua*; W = *L. welshimeri*.
[c]Number of samples (1) containing a particular *Listeria* sp.
[d]Not detected.
Source: Adapted from Ref. 60.

In contrast to results for raw meat, isolation of listeriae from various cured meats was limited to detection of a low level of *L. innocua* in a single sample of salami (Table 11.3), with all test samples being free of *L. monocytogenes*. While these results imply that *Listeria* populations are markedly reduced when raw meats are made into ready-to-eat products, isolation of *L. innocua* from one salami sample suggests that *Listeria* spp. are most likely to enter such products late in manufacture and/or during packaging.

Data gathered by a major commercial meat producer also show that raw sausage mix can contain *Listeria* spp.; however, populations were usually higher (~0.93 *Listeria* spp. CFU/g) than levels previously detected by Buchanan et al. (60) in finished sausage products. The same firm also isolated listeriae from a "fair percentage" of retail meat products that were approaching their expiration date and/or showing obvious signs of spoilage. Since *L. monocytogenes* apparently can grow in such meat products during refrigerated storage, these findings strongly support continuation of the policy of zero tolerance for the pathogen in ready-to-eat meat products.

While all studies discussed thus far have dealt with the incidence of listeriae in American-produced meats destined for human consumption, the reader is reminded that *L. monocytogenes* can seriously threaten the health and well-being of many domestic (i.e., cow, sheep, pig, goat, horse, rabbit) and wild animals (i.e., giraffe, leopard, moose, deer, marmoset) found in today's zoological parks. Consequently, Al-Sheddy and Richter (1) examined commercially prepared frozen zoo meat (mixture of chopped beef, beef byproducts, and chicken) for levels of *L. monocytogenes* and *Salmonella* as well as overall microbiological quality. Using an MPN procedure, 5 of 5 samples were positive for *L. monocytogenes* with a mean of 6.6 organisms/g, whereas 3 of 5 samples contained a mean of 5.3 salmonellae/g. Additional tests indicated that frozen zoo meat was similar to frozen ground beef destined for human consumption in terms of total aerobic plate ($\sim 10^6$ CFU/g) and fungal ($\sim 10^4$ CFU/g) counts; however, coliform counts were approximately 100-fold higher in frozen zoo meat ($\sim 10^4$ CFU/g) than in frozen ground beef. Subsequent experiments also demonstrated that thawing frozen zoo meat at <10°C largely prevented growth of *L. monocytogenes* as well as many other organisms. Therefore, proper handling of frozen zoo meat appears to be an important factor in controlling listeriosis and other foodborne illnesses among the many rare animals in today's zoological parks.

Incidence of *Listeria* spp. in Raw Meat Products Marketed Outside the United States

Canada

The incidence of listeriae in raw meat products also has received limited attention in Canada. While attempting to improve methodology for isolating listeriae from raw meat, Truscott and McNab (138) uncovered various *Listeria* spp. in 45 of 50 (90%) retail samples of raw ground beef by using a combination of eight different enrichment/isolation procedures. More important, *L. monocytogenes* was detected in 29 of 50 (58%) samples, which, like the American studies just discussed, indicates that contamination of raw ground beef with this pathogen is relatively common.

European Countries

As with raw milk, the potential for raw meat to transmit *L. monocytogenes* also was first recognized in 1944 by the Swedish worker Wramby (143), who isolated *Listeria* from raw meat that had been stored in 11% salt brine solution for up to 13 weeks. Subsequently European concerns about the possibility of contracting listeriosis through consumption of contaminated foods, as evidenced by several large listeriosis outbreaks that were likely associated with consumption of raw milk in post–World War II Germany, led to development of laws that now forbid the sale of meat from clinically infected animals (128). Despite the presumed health risks associated with consumption of *Listeria*-contaminated meat, the scientific literature contains relatively few pre-1980 studies that deal directly with incidence of listeriae in meat products.

In 1958, the Russian worker Slivko (133) isolated *L. monocytogenes* from brain, spleen, kidney, liver, and lymph node tissue from pigs and lambs that succumbed to natural listeric infections; however, the pathogen was never recovered from muscle tissue. Four years later, Kampelmacher (95) also was unable to identify *L. monocytogenes* in meat of cattle suffering from cerebral listeriosis. However, unlike the previous study, this is the first report in which the pathogen was identified in meat from similarly infected sheep. To our knowledge, *L. monocytogenes* was not conclusively identified in beef muscle until 1969, when Amtsberg (2) detected this pathogen in meat from 2 of 207 apparently healthy cows.

Ten years later, Elischerova et al. (73) detected *L. monocytogenes* in 12 of 63 (19%) and 6 of 35 (17%) samples of raw beef and pork, respectively, that were marketed in Czechoslovakia. In the only other pre-1980 study that was reported, Le Guilloux et al. (105), during 1978–1979, examined over 600 samples of French raw and/or processed meat for *L. monocytogenes*. Results of their effort will be discussed later in conjunction with other more recent Western European surveys of raw and processed meats.

Beginning in 1985, results from at least 20 primarily Western European surveys dealing with occurrence of *Listeria* spp. in raw meat products have found their way, both formally and informally, into the scientific literature (Table 11.4). While these surveys have provided the meat industry and public health officials with much-needed information, results from these studies, like those dealing with listeriae in cheese, need to be interpreted with some caution since sampling designs [i.e., number and size of sample, site of sample collection (slaughterhouse, processing facility, retail store), age of meat, portion of meat/meat product analyzed (carcass, ground meat, sausage meat, sausage with or without casing)] and methods for detection/identification of listeriae vary widely among the surveys.

In the only Austrian raw meat survey recorded to date, von Breuer and Prändl (59) examined 100 retail samples of raw ground pork and beef (~50 samples each) for listeriae. Overall, *Listeria* spp., *L. monocytogenes*, and *L. innocua* were detected in 65, 36, and 48% of the samples examined, respectively (Table 11.4). Using an MPN method, 30 (46%), 23 (35%), and 12 (18%) of the 65 positive samples were further shown to contain <12, 12–110, and >110 total *Listeria* CFU/g, respectively. These results, like those of other surveys to follow, indicate that *Listeria* contamination is a recurring problem in ground raw meat.

Working in Denmark, Skovgaard and Morgen (131) determined the incidence of listeriae in retail samples of raw ground beef. Overall, 45 of 67 (67%) and 19 of 67 (28%) ground beef samples collected from retail butcher shops and supermarkets contained *Listeria* spp. and *L. monocytogenes*, respectively (Table 11.4). As in the USDA-FSIS raw beef survey, these Danish researchers observed seasonal differences with listeriae being detected in 90% of summer samples but only in 57% of the winter samples. Presence of *L. monocytogenes* in about one-fourth of Danish ground beef samples was not unexpected since this organism also was present in 51% of fecal samples from cattle examined in this study. These findings indicate the potential for dissemination of *L. monocytogenes* along the slaughter line.

In a similar study, Skovgaard and Nørrung (132) determined the incidence of listeriae in raw ground pork. Overall, *Listeria* spp. were detected in 33 of 51 (64.7%) samples obtained from slaughterhouses or butcher shops with 12–51% of the samples positive for *L. monocytogenes* and *L. innocua*, respectively (Table 11.4). In contrast, *Listeria* spp. appeared in only 7 of 172 (4.1%) fecal samples from pigs, with only three such samples positive for *L. monocytogenes*. Nevertheless, fecal material remains the most likely vehicle through which *L. monocytogenes* enters slaughterhouses. Once established in the slaughterhouse environment, this pathogen can readily contaminate all types of animal carcasses during processing.

Interest in the incidence of listeriae in raw meat products marketed in France actually predates the emergence of *L. monocytogenes* as a bona fide foodborne pathogen. Le Guilloux et al. (105) failed to isolate *L. monocytogenes* from 62 beef carcasses that were examined between May 1978 and April 1979 (Table 11.4). While these researchers also failed to detect *L. monocytogenes* on the surface of pork carcasses, the pathogen was found in 14 of 30 (46%) samples of ground pork. These findings point directly to cutting, slicing, and/or grinding operations as major areas of concern in meat-processing facilities.

After more recent concerns about foodborne listeriosis, a series of surveys have been made to determine the incidence of listeriae in a variety of raw meat products marketed in France (Table 11.4). Overall, 4 of 82 (4.9%), 51 of 233 (21.2%), and 86 of 435 (19.8%) samples of beef carcasses, ground beef, and frozen ground beef, respectively, were positive for *L. monocytogenes* with isolates of serotype 1/2 predominating in at least three such studies (117,118,120). These results attest to the tenacity of *Listeria* in ground beef during frozen storage. As expected, *L. monocytogenes* also was detected more frequently in ground pork than on the surface of pork carcasses. These findings, along with results from Sweden (Table 11.4), show that, unlike ground beef and pork, complete animal carcasses are relatively free of *L. monocytogenes* shortly after slaughter. Hence, most contamination appears to occur when carcasses are cut into smaller pieces which are then reduced to ground meat.

Between February 1982 and June 1985, Luppi et al. (109) isolated organisms of the genus *Listeria* (including *L. monocytogenes* and *L. innocua*) from 1 of 19 (5.3%), 1 of 19 (5.3%), and 6 of 18 (33.3%) samples of raw veal, pork, and lamb, respectively, that were obtained from retail shops in the northern Italian province of Ferrara. Several years later, Cantoni et al. (63) also identified *L. monocytogenes* in 3 of 5 samples of both fresh and frozen meat (Table 11.4). While the number of samples examined in these two studies is small, these findings suggest that the incidence of listeriae in Italian meats is likely to be similar to that observed in other European countries.

Various *Listeria* spp. also have been uncovered in a substantial percentage of ground beef and pork samples from butcher shops and supermarkets in Switzerland. In 1989, Breer and Schopfer (58) isolated *Listeria* spp. from 6 of 18 (33%) and 14 of 31 (45%) samples of ground beef and pork, respectively (Table 11.4). Additional quantitative studies showed that 42 and 58% of the *Listeria*-positive samples contained <10 and 10–1000 listeriae CFU/g, respectively. Not surprisingly, these levels of contamination are similar to those observed earlier for ground beef and pork marketed in neighboring Austria.

German scientists also developed an interest in determining the extent to which West German meat products are contaminated with listeriae. In 1988, Karches and Teufel (97) found *Listeria* spp. in nearly half of the samples of ground beef and pork that were examined (Table 11.4). Using an MPN method, 24 of 50 (48%) positive samples were shown to contain <10 *Listeria* spp. CFU/g, with 17 (34%) and 9 (18%) samples harboring 10–99 and 100–1000 *Listeria* spp. CFU/g, respectively. More important, *L.*

Table 11.4 Incidence of Listeria spp. in Raw Beef, Beef/pork, Pork, Lamb, and Horse Meat Processed in Western Europe Between 1973 and 1989

Country of origin	Product	Number of samples analyzed	Number (%) of positive samples				Ref.
			L. monocytogenes	L. innocua	L. welshimeri	Other Listeria spp.	
Austria	Ground beef/pork	100	36 (36)	48 (48)	3 (3)	0	59
Denmark	Ground beef	67	19 (28)	36 (54)	NR[a]	16 (24)[b]	131
	Ground pork	51	6 (12)	26 (51)	0	1 (2)[c]	132
France	Beef	5	0	1 (20)	0	0	122
	Beef carcass	62	0	ND[d]	ND	ND	55
	Beef carcass-surface	20	4 (20)	0	0	0	115,117,118
	Ground beef	67	34 (51)	NR	NR	13 (19)[e]	55,120
	Ground beef	62	5 (8)	ND	ND	ND	105
	Ground beef	104	12 (11)	13 (12)	5 (5)	0	72
	Frozen ground beef	194	42 (22)	21 (11)	5 (3)	0	118
	Frozen ground beef	52	5 (10)	ND	ND	2 (4)[f]	115
	Frozen ground beef	149	39 (26)	18 (12)	4 (3)	0	116
	Pork	21	2 (9)	2 (9)	0	0	122
	Pork carcass-surface	20	1 (5)	0	0	0	115
	Ground pork	30	14 (47)	ND	ND	ND	105
	Lamb carcass-surface	20	0	0	0	0	115
	Lamb meat	7	1 (14)	0	0	0	115,118
	Ground horse meat	41	3 (7)	NR	NR	11 (27)[e]	55,120

Country	Product	n					Reference
Italy	Fresh meat	5	3 (60)	0	2 (40)	0	63
	Frozen meat	5	3 (60)	0	0	0	63
Sweden	Beef muscle-surface	45	0	ND	ND	ND	137
	Pork muscle-surface	45	0	ND	ND	ND	137
Switzerland	Ground meat	85	19 (22)	21 (25)	0	1 (1)[c]	57,58
	Ground beef	18	3 (17)	5 (28)	0	0	57,58
	Ground pork	31	4 (13)	13 (42)	0	0	57,58
West Germany	Ground meat	125	19 (15)	26 (21)	1 (1)	3 (2)[c]	119
	Beef	16	0	2 (12)	0	0	119
	Ground beef	21	11 (52)	8 (38)	NR	NR	141
	Ground beef	59	27 (46)	NR	NR	24 (41)	97
	Ground beef (lean)	50	15 (30)	23 (46)	ND	4 (8)[c]	127
	Ground beef/pork	50	8 (16)	7 (14)	ND	3 (16)[c]	127
	Ground beef/pork	48	10 (21)	NR	NR	NR	101
	Ground beef/pork/veal	19	3 (16)	NR	NR	NR	101
	Pork	10	0	1 (10)	1 (10)	0	119
	Ground pork	15	6 (40)	6 (40)	NR	NR	141
	Ground pork	90	15 (16)	NR	NR	NR	101
	Ground pork	30	24 (80)	14 (47)	9 (30)	1 (3)[c]	126
	Ground pork	58	23 (40)	NR	NR	21 (36)	97
	Lamb	7	1 (14)	0	0	0	119

[a] Not reported.
[b] Includes 7 samples with *L. grayi* and 9 other samples with *L. welshimeri*, *L. murrayi*, and/or *L. denitrificans*.
[c] Only *L. seeligeri*.
[d] Not determined.
[e] *L. innocua*, *L. welshimeri*, and *L. seeligeri*.
[f] Nonpathogenic *Listeria* spp.

monocytogenes was isolated from 13, 8, and 1 of the 50 positive samples at levels of <10, 10–100, and 270 CFU/g, respectively, thus indicating that slightly over half of the *Listeria*-positive samples contained more than one species of *Listeria*.

In addition to this study, Schmidt et al. (126) demonstrated that virtually all samples of ground pork purchased during the first half of 1988 for their West German study were contaminated with *L. monocytogenes, L. innocua, L. welshimeri,* and/or *L. seeligeri* (Table 11.4). While half of 16 selected samples contained <10 listeriae CFU/g, 7 of 16 (43.8%) and 1 of 16 (6.3%) samples had *Listeria* populations of 100–1000 and >1000/g, respectively. Additionally, 29 of 38 (80.6%) *L. monocytogenes* isolates available for serotyping were identified as serotype 1/2 with the remaining 7 (19.4%) as serotype 4b. A similar distribution of *L. monocytogenes* serotypes also is found among human listeriosis cases in West Germany, thus reinforcing the plausibility of meat as a possible infectious vehicle in at least some of these cases. However, the opposite situation appears to be true for France, England, and the United States (47).

Overall, data gathered from West Germany (Table 11.4) indicate that *L. monocytogenes* (strains of serotype 1/2 likely predominating) was present in 50 of 130 (38.4%) and 68 of 193 (35.2%) samples of ground beef and ground pork, respectively, with generally similar or slightly higher percentages of these samples harboring *L. innocua.* In addition to the West German findings in Table 11.4, Ozari and Stolle (119) identified *L. innocua* as the only *Listeria* contaminant in 1 of 18 (5.6%), 2 of 18 (11.1%), and 2 of 16 (12.5%) retail samples of beef liver, pork liver, and pork kidney, respectively. While 12 retail samples of beef kidney proved negative for listeriae, the overall findings suggest that organ meats also can serve as potential vehicles for listeric infections.

While recognizing some of the pitfalls in generalized data interpretation (i.e., different isolation/detection methods, missing and/or unreported data concerning the identity of all *Listeria* isolates), several important conclusions can be drawn from these European data (Table 11.4), which have been condensed and summarized in Table 11.5.

First, with the exception of one pork sample, *L. monocytogenes, L. innocua,* and *L. welshimeri* were absent from surfaces of both beef and pork carcasses. In contrast, approximately one-fourth of all ground beef samples were contaminated with *L.*

Table 11.5 Overall Incidence of *L. monocytogenes, L. innocua,* and *L. welshimeri* on Beef and Pork Carasses and in Ground Beef and Pork Produced in Western Europe

Product	Number of positive samples/Number of samples analyzed (%)		
	L. monocytogenes	*L. innocua*	*L. welshimeri*
Beef			
Carcasses	0/127 (0)	0/20 (0)	0/20 (0)
Ground	170/649 (26.2)	103/468 (22.0)	9/271 (3.3)
Pork			
Carcasses	1/65 (1.5)	0/20 (0)	0/20 (0)
Ground	78/275 (28.4)	59/127 (46.5)	9/112 (8.0)

monocytogenes and/or *L. innocua.* Similarly, approximately one-fourth and nearly one-half of all ground pork samples contained *L. monocytogenes* and *L. innocua,* respectively. From these findings, one can conclude that most *Listeria* contamination probably occurs during handling, cutting, and/or grinding of both beef and pork—long after the animals are slaughtered.

Second, as with raw milk (see Table 9.1), *L. innocua* was isolated from ground beef and pork with equal or somewhat greater frequencies than was *L. monocytogenes,* thus suggesting that both organisms may occupy similar niches in slaughterhouse and meat-processing/meat-packing environments. Therefore, presence of *L. innocua* in raw meat products should be indicative of possible contamination with *L. monocytogenes.*

Third, it is noteworthy that, as with raw milk, detectable levels of *L. welshimeri* occurred in a small percentage of both ground beef and ground pork samples examined in many of these European surveys. Although normally present in the external environment, *L. welshimeri* was isolated from feces of an asymptomatic human carrier in 1986, which, in turn, suggests that consumption of meat products may play a role in passive shedding of *L. welshimeri* in human feces. However, *L. welshimeri* is still regarded as nonpathogenic and is therefore of little public health concern when present in food.

Finally, according to results in Table 11.4, *L. seeligeri* was recovered from at least 10 samples of European-made ground beef and/or ground pork. While the non-pathogenicity of *L. seeligeri* has been recognized for many years, recent isolation of this organism in connection with a case of purulent meningitis in an immunocompetent adult (125) may raise new public health concerns about the sporadic occurrence of *L. seeligeri* in raw meat products.

Other Countries

As of July 1990, information regarding the incidence of listeriae in raw meats produced elsewhere was confined to two surveys completed in New Zealand and Japan. In the first of these investigations, Lowry and Tiong (108) identified *L. monocytogenes* in 5 of 25 (20%) and 9 of 15 (60%) boneless cuts of beef and lamb, respectively, that were obtained from a New Zealand slaughterhouse between January and May 1988. In contrast, only 3 of 10 (30%) swab samples from lamb carcasses were positive for the pathogen, which again suggests that listeriae most likely enter raw meats during cutting and processing operations. This mode of contamination is further supported by the isolation of *L. monocytogenes* from 27 to 73% of slaughterhouse work surfaces and 40% of the knives. Since *L. monocytogenes* also was detected in 23 of 25 (92%) and 17 of 25 (68%) corresponding samples of minced beef and pork cuts that were obtained from New Zealand supermarkets and butcher shops, the apparent higher incidence of listeriae in retail meats also points to cutting and processing operations as critical points for contamination. While few details concerning the incidence of listeriae in raw meats are available from other countries, the fact that 44 of 116 (37.9%) ground meat samples obtained from Japanese markets harbored *L. monocytogenes* (102) indicates that the problem of *Listeria*-contaminated meat is widespread and deserves the serious attention of industry in countries beyond the continental boundaries of Europe and North America.

Incidence of *Listeria* spp. in Sausage and Ready-to-Eat Meat Products Marketed Outside the United States

Two factors, namely development of proper methods to isolate *Listeria* from samples containing a diverse microflora and a heightened concern about foodborne listeriosis, have provided scientists worldwide with the "tools" and the incentive to examine sausage and other ready-to-eat meat products for listeriae. Consequently, numerous surveys have been made since 1985 to determine the incidence of listeriae in such products marketed outside the United States.

Canada

In 1988, Farber et al. (78) reported results from the first Canadian survey on occurrence of *L. monocytogenes* in ready-to-eat, dry-cured sausages such as Genoa and hard salami, both of which are generally prepared without cooking or smoking. Overall, 96 lots of fermented sausage manufactured by federally registered firms were examined for *L. monocytogenes* by two federal agencies. Overall, *L. monocytogenes* was detected in 15 of 96 (15.6%) sausages sampled immediately after fermentation, with 5 of 96 (5.2%) samples remaining positive after the drying period. In addition, *L. innocua* and *L. welshimeri*, respectively, were recovered from 12 of 96 (12.5%) and 7 of 96 (7.3%) sausages examined immediately after fermentation with four dried sausages also positive for *L. innocua*.

As was true for fermented dairy products, the apparent hardy nature of listeriae during manufacture and storage of fermented meats has prompted a government-sponsored monitoring program (similar to the USDA-FSIS program in the United States) to determine the incidence, source, and various means of controlling *Listeria* contamination in cooked/ready-to-eat meat products. In keeping with Canadian governmental policies, officials at Agriculture Canada's Food Production and Inspection Branch caused a Vancouver firm to issue a Class II recall for *L. monocytogenes*–contaminated frankfurters initially linked to listeriosis that caused the death of a woman whose refrigerator contained several other contaminated foods (44). However, subsequent testing revealed that the *L. monocytogenes* strains isolated from the patient and the incriminated frankfurters belonged to different serotypes, thus negating any role of the frankfurters in this isolated case of apparent foodborne listeriosis (47). USDA officials failed to recover this pathogen from sealed packages of frankfurters exported to the United States. Hence, even though a Class II recall was issued for this product in Canada, no further action was taken in the United States.

European Countries

Numerous studies have been made to determine the incidence of listeriae in cooked/ready-to-eat meat and sausage products produced in Western Europe (Table 11.6). In conjunction with the previously mentioned survey of ground pork and beef marketed in Austria, von Breuer and Prändel (59) determined incidence of listeriae in Austrian Mettwurst—a spreadable meat product (pH 4.75–5.50) that typically contains approximately 2.5% NaCl and 200 ppm sodium nitrite. Overall, 67 of 100 (67%) Mettwurst samples contained listeriae, with *L. monocytogenes* and *L. innocua* detected in 23 and 61 samples, respectively (Table 11.6). Thus incidence of listeriae in Mettwurst was similar to that observed for ground pork and beef (Table 11.4). However, unlike ground pork and beef, listeriae could not be quantitated in Mettwurst, which suggests that *Listeria* spp. failed to grow in this product, possibly as a result of low pH in combination with sodium chloride and sodium nitrite.

Beginning in 1987, Public Health Laboratory Service workers in England and Wales also made a series of surveys to determine the incidence of listeriae in various retail foods, including cooked/ready-to-eat meat products. According to several reports (79,124), *L. monocytogenes* was recovered from 49, 16, and 7% of retail samples of raw pork sausage, salami/continental sausage, and cooked, cured, or smoked meats, respectively (Table 11.6). While 21 of the 24 (87.5%) *L. monocytogenes* isolates were of serotype 1/2, nearly 80% of all clinical isolates from listeriosis victims during the same period were classified as serotype 4. A similar serotype distribution pattern among *L. monocytogenes* strains isolated from meat products and clinical cases of listeriosis also has been reported in France (118). Although not proven conclusively, a preliminary report (47) suggesting a possible relationship between virulence of *L. monocytogenes* and particular serotypes, with serotype 4 (reportedly dominant in dairy products) thought to be more virulent than strains of serotype 1/2 (reportedly dominant in meat products), may help explain some of the present difficulties in positively linking consumption of meat products to cases of human listeriosis.

As for raw beef and pork, several French investigators also have determined incidence of listeriae in French sausage and delicatessen products that are typically consumed either with or without heating (Table 11.6). In 1980, Le Guilloux et al. (105) found that 33 of 480 (6.9%) samples of ready-to-eat sausage spread and smoked sausage were contaminated with *L. monocytogenes*. While over half of the positive samples contained approximately 20 *L. monocytogenes* CFU/g, the pathogen was detected at levels as high as 2000 CFU/g in at least two sausages. Additional surveys of French ready-to-eat meat and delicatessen products (55,72,115,116) uncovered *L. monocytogenes* contamination rates of 12–27% (Table 11.6). Furthermore, 6 of 7 (85.7%) *L. monocytogenes* isolates from one of these surveys (116) were of serotype 1/2, thus indicating a serotype distribution pattern similar to that previously observed for un-cooked beef and pork (55).

Five recent surveys (55,106,115,116,122) also have uncovered *L. monocytogenes* and other *Listeria* spp. in 0–22% of French sausage and delicatessen products normally consumed after heating (Table 11.6). In one such study, Nicolas and Vidaud (116) classified 10 of 11 (91%) *L. monocytogenes* isolates as serotype 1/2, with the remaining strain being serotype 4a. Since dominance of *L. monocytogenes* serotype 1/2 in meat products normally consumed after cooking is again consistent with the serotype distribution pattern that was previously observed for this pathogen in raw and ready-to-eat meat and delicatessen products marketed in France, these data point to raw meat as the source of *L. monocytogenes* in meat-processing facilities.

In 1988, researchers in Hungary (123) recovered various strains of listeriae from 26 of 27 (96.3%), 27 of 46 (58.7%), and 2 of 3 (66.7%) samples of homemade raw, smoked, and flavored pork sausage, respectively, with four raw and two smoked sausages yielding corresponding MPN counts of 540 to >1600 and 6.8–540 *Listeria* CFU/g. Although none of the *Listeria* isolates was speciated biochemically, 26 of 40 (65%) positive sausages harbored virulent strains of listeriae (most likely *L. monocytogenes*) with isolates further

Table 11.6 Incidence of *Listeria* spp. in Western European Sausage, Ham, and Ready-to-Eat Meat Products Examined Between 1978 and 1989

Country of origin	Product	Number of samples analyzed	Number of positive samples (%)				Ref.
			L. monocytogenes	*L. innocua*	*L. welshimeri*	Other *Listeria* spp.	
Austria	Mettwurst	100	23 (23)	61 (61)	1 (1)	0	59
England	Salami and continental sausage	67	11 (16	NR[a]	NR	NR	79,124
Wales	Cooked, cured and smoked meat	29	2 (7)	NR	NR	NR	79,124
	Raw pork sausage	59	29 (49)	NR	NR	NR	124
France	Sausage	38	3 (8)	7 (8)	0	0	122
	Sliced cooked meat	10	0	2 (20)	0	0	122
	Sliced cured meat	15	0	1 (7)	0	0	122
	Fully matured raw ham	18	0	0	0	0	122
	Frankfurters	9	0	1	0	1 (11)[b]	106
	Delicatessen meats	72	9 (12)	2 (3)	2 (3)	0	72
	Sausage spread, smoked sausage	480	33 (7)	ND[c]	ND	ND	105
	Delicatessen meats normally consumed without heating (e.g. bologna)	33	9 (27)	NR	NR	14 (42)[d]	55
	Dry sausage	37	8 (22)	3 (8)	0	0	116,118
	Dry sausage	18	4 (22)	NR	NR	2 (11)[e]	115
	Fresh sausage and frozen pork for sausage-making	120	12 (10)	10 (8)	2 (2)	0	116,117
	Sausages normally consumed after heating (e.g. frankfurters, pork sausage)	98	4 (4)	NR	NR	12 (12)[e]	115
	Sausages normally consumed after heating	32	7 (22)	NR	NR	4 (12)[d]	55
Italy	Seasoned luncheon meat—casing	225	6 (3)	7 (3)	7 (3)	0	61
	—interior	225	0	0	0	0	61
	Sausage "paste"	15	2 (13)	1 (7)	0	1 (7)[f]	63
	Fresh sausage	10	2 (20)	1 (10)	0	0	63
	Aged raw salami	30	4 (13)	0	0	0	63
	Cold cuts, aged	243	0	0	0	0	63

Country	Product	No. of samples					Reference
Switzerland	Air-dried meat	44	4 (9)	3 (7)	0	0	57,58
	Uncooked ham	19	0	2 (10)	0	0	57,58
	Salami	63	4 (6)	7 (11)	0	2 (3)[b]	57,58
	Mettwurst	19	4 (21)	7 (37)	0	0	57,58
	Mettwurst	2	1 (50)	1 (50)	NR	NR	141
	Raw "country" sausage	59	3 (5)	5 (8)	0	1 (2)[b]	57,58
West Germany	Mettwurst	50	6 (12)	15 (30)	0	1 (2)[b]	127
	Mettwurst	30	17 (59)	24 (80)	7 (23)	1 (3)[b]	126
	Fresh onion Mettwurst	11	1 (9)	NR	NR	5 (45)	97
	Fresh spreadable fermented sausage	132	22 (17)	30 (23)	1 (1)	0	119
	Sliced raw sausage	126	2 (2)	17 (14)	1 (1)	0	119
	Raw ham	15	0	2 (13)	0	0	119
	Vacuum-packaged frankfurters	30	0	2 (7)	0	0	119
	Cooked liver sausage	22	0	0	0	0	119
	Pork sausage	50	3 (6)	1 (2)	0	0	127
Total (%)		2898	239 (8.35)	221 (10.67)	37 (1.79)	60 (2.65)	

[a]Not reported.
[b]*L. seeligeri* only.
[c]Not determined.
[d]*L. innocua*, *L. welshimeri*, and *L. seeligeri*.
[e]Nonpathogenic *Listeria* spp.
[f]*L. ivanovii*.
[g]Studies with ND and NR results omitted from calculations.

classified as serotypes 1/2, 4a, 4b, or 4ab (*L. monocytogenes* or *L. seeligeri*) as well as 6a and 6b (*L. innocua* or *L. welshimeri*).

Working in Italy, Cantoni et al. (61) investigated the extent to which seasoned cold cuts and luncheon meats are contaminated with listeriae. While these investigators failed to isolate *Listeria* spp. from the interior of such products, *L. monocytogenes*, *L. innocua*, and *L. welshimeri* were each detected on the surface and/or casings of 3% of the seasoned luncheon meat samples that were examined. Although these results suggest that *Listeria* spp., including *L. monocytogenes*, can be inactivated in sausage and luncheon meats during manufacture and aging, continued use of good manufacturing, cleaning, and sanitizing practices is essential to decrease chances for postprocessing contamination, which is implied by presence of listeriae on the surface of luncheon meats.

One year later, the same authors (63) found that 13–20% of sausage "paste," fresh sausage and aged raw salami were contaminated with detectable levels of *L. monocytogenes*, *L. innocua*, and/or *L. ivanovii* (Table 11.6). However, extensive testing failed to uncover any *Listeria* spp. in cold cuts that were aged >3 months.

A survey in Switzerland (57,58) also uncovered a substantial number of cooked, fermented, and/or otherwise processed meat products that contained listeriae. With the exception of air-dried meats that were contaminated both superficially and internally, *L. monocytogenes* and *L. innocua* could only be recovered from interior samples of sausage meat at levels of $\leq 10^3$ CFU/g. These results are in sharp contrast to those of Cantoni et al. (61), who reported isolating *L. monocytogenes* only from the outer casings of Italian cold cuts and luncheon meat. Overall, 12 of 15 (80%) *L. monocytogenes* isolates from air-dried meat, salami, Mettwurst, and raw "country" sausage produced in Switzerland were of serotype 1/2, with the remaining three strains classified as serotype 4b. Since most *L. monocytogenes* isolates from human listeriosis patients in Switzerland are of serotype 4b, these data, like those from England (79,124), France (117,118,120), and the United States (47), suggest that transmission of the pathogen via meat is relatively uncommon.

While the incidence of listeriae in cooked, fermented, and/or otherwise processed meat products made in West Germany (126) generally appears to be somewhat similar to that observed in other European countries (Table 11.6), Schmidt et al. (126) reported that 29 of 30 (97%) samples of fresh onion Mettwurst purchased in West Germany contained listeriae with 50 and 8% of these samples contaminated with two and three *Listeria* spp., respectively. Although 59 and 80% of these samples contained *L. monocytogenes* and *L. innocua*, respectively (Table 11.6), levels of *Listeria* spp. detected in Mettwurst were similar to those observed in other processed meats with 83 and 17% of the samples containing <10 and 100–1000 listeriae CFU/g, respectively. Results from serological testing reflected the distribution pattern identified in England, France, and Switzerland, with approximately 80 and 20% of all *L. monocytogenes* strains isolated from Mettwurst being identified as of serotypes 1/2 and 4, respectively.

Overall, results in Table 11.6 indicate that a substantial portion of European processed meats are contaminated with listeriae, including *L. monocytogenes* (8.3%), *L. innocua* (10.7%), and to a lesser extent *L. welshimeri* (1.8%). As was true for dairy products, presence of *Listeria* spp. other than *L. monocytogenes* in processed as well as raw meats may be indicative of possible contamination with *L. monocytogenes*. However, additional information concerning habitats, niches, and relative incidence of

Listeria spp. in all facets of the meat industry is needed before this can be confirmed definitively. Nevertheless, in the light of a recently reported case of human listeriosis that was linked to consumption of contaminated turkey frankfurters (53), it is now evident that presence of *L. monocytogenes* in processed meat products may pose a serious health hazard to certain individuals. Therefore, it is necessary to control all *Listeria* spp. in meat-processing facilities and to design procedures and/or treatments that will eliminate *L. monocytogenes* from ready-to-eat processed meat products.

BEHAVIOR OF *L. MONOCYTOGENES* IN MEAT PRODUCTS

Although *L. monocytogenes* was found during the 1950s in European meat products destined for human consumption, a general failure to positively link cases of human listeriosis to foods other than raw milk provided little incentive to examine behavior of listeriae in meat. This situation was further complicated by a lack of reliable and convenient methods to selectively isolate listeriae from heavily contaminated samples of animal origin, including organ as well as muscle tissue. Thus the first definitive studies on behavior of *L. monocytogenes* in raw meat were not begun until the 1970s. Even then, to accurately quantitate this organism in meat products during extended storage, it was generally deemed necessary to use specially treated "sterile" meat rather than raw meat products containing a normal microbial background flora.

Recent outbreaks of foodborne listeriosis linked to consumption of contaminated cheese prompted an almost immediate concern about the microbiological safety of raw and, particularly, ready-to-eat meat products marketed in North America and Europe. The outbreaks also demonstrated an urgent need for methods to rapidly and accurately detect listeriae in a wide range of foods. Subsequent development of the USDA procedure to detect listeriae in meat and poultry products provided researchers with a fairly accurate (albeit far from perfect) method by which to determine growth and survival of *L. monocytogenes* in raw and ready-to-eat products. Recent meat-oriented epidemiological studies along with a report implicating turkey frankfurters in a case of human listeriosis (53) suggest that behavior and control of *L. monocytogenes* in meat products is likely to remain an active area of research for some time to come. As in the previous section of this chapter, information concerning behavior of *L. monocytogenes* in raw meat will be presented first, followed by a discussion of the fate of this pathogen in processed meat products, with special emphasis on frankfurters and fermented sausage.

Listeric Infections in Domestic Livestock

As you will recall from Chapter 3, domestic farm animals such as cows, sheep, and pigs not only succumb to listeric infections, but also asymptomatically shed *L. monocytogenes* in their feces for many months. While virtually all meat from animals exhibiting obvious signs of listeriosis will be condemned and destroyed immediately after slaughter, meat from subclinically infected animals will likely be passed by inspectors as being fit for consumption. Since between 2 and 16% of all healthy cows, sheep, and pigs passively shed *L. monocytogenes* in their feces, there is ample opportunity for contamination of muscle tissue during slaughter, evisceration, and dressing of the animals.

In all likelihood, meat from domestic livestock will first be exposed to listeriae in the slaughterhouse environment. However, various organs from apparently healthy animals also can on occasion contain *L. monocytogenes*. In 1972, Höhne (86) reported that approximately 13% of the parotid glands from clinically healthy pigs contained *L. monocytogenes*. Five years later, Höhne et al. (87) detected *L. monocytogenes* in intestinal lymph nodes from eight apparently healthy slaughtered animals (5 small ruminants, 2 pigs, 1 cow) destined for human consumption. Subsequently, Cottin et al. (69) identified *L. monocytogenes* in 15 of 514 (3.1%) spleen and/or lung tissue samples obtained from apparently healthy cattle. According to Amtsberg et al. (2), *L. monocytogenes* was isolated from the spleen and muscle tissue of an apparently healthy animal. These findings suggest that *L. monocytogenes* might be transported to tissue via the bloodstream in animals suffering from symptomatic as well as asymptomatic septicemic listeric infections. Hence, to understand the behavior of *L. monocytogenes* in meat products, it is fitting to begin this section by first examining localization of *L. monocytogenes* in organ and particularly muscle tissue from infected animals.

Localization in Tissue

In 1988, Johnson et al. (93) reported results from a study in which samples of muscle, organ, and lymphoid tissue as well as feces and blood from several Holstein cows previously inoculated intravenously with 10^{10}–10^{11} *L. monocytogenes* cells were examined for the pathogen 2, 6, or 54 days after inoculation using a combination of direct plating and cold enrichment. As expected, recovery of listeriae varied among animals and was strongly influenced by the time that elapsed between inoculation and slaughter (Table 11.7). Overall, 94% of all samples obtained from cows slaughtered 2 days after inoculation contained *L. monocytogenes* with 23 of 32 (72%) samples positive by direct plating. More important, the pathogen was routinely detected in muscle tissue from the same animals, frequently at levels of 120–280 CFU/g. Despite a marked decrease in recovery of *L. monocytogenes* from animals examined 6 and 54 days postinoculation, the pathogen was still present at levels of ~140–675 CFU/g in kidney tissue as well as in mesenteric and mammary lymph nodes, with populations about two orders of magnitude lower in liver and spleen tissue. Following 2 weeks of cold enrichment, the pathogen also was detected in plate-flank tissue taken from an animal 6 days after slaughter. These findings suggest that consumption of animal organs may constitute a greater health hazard than muscle tissue and also readily explain how evisceration of domestic animals can lead to surface contamination of muscle tissue.

Assuming that most contamination occurs during handling of carcasses after slaughter, Chung et al. (66) investigated the ability of *L. monocytogenes* to attach to (or become entrapped) and proliferate on muscle and fat tissue both alone and in the presence of *Pseudomonas aeruginosa*. Immersion of lean muscle and fat tissue in broth cultures containing 10^5 or 10^8 *L. monocytogenes* CFU/ml for various times followed by thorough rinsing resulted in large numbers of listeriae being attached to (or entrapped in) both types of samples within the first 10 minutes (Fig. 11.4). Despite large differences in

Table 11.7 Levels of *L. monocytogenes* in Feces, Blood, and Tissues from Four Intravenously Inoculated Cows

Sample	Days postinoculation after which cows were slaughtered and examined		
	2[a]	6	54
Feces	+[b]/−[c]	−	+
Blood	2.79[d]	−	−
Brain	+/−	−	+
Spinal cord	+/+	−	−
Mammary gland	3.27	+	+
Mesenteric lymph node	2.03	−	2.83
Mammary lymph node	3.06	2.15	+
Spleen	4.74	−	+
Kidney	3.12	−	2.56
Tongue	2.38/+	−	−
Heart	2.23	−	+
Liver	4.39	−	+
Chuck-rib	2.09	−	−
Loin	2.25/+	−	−
Plate-flank	2.26	+	−
Round	2.45/+	−	−
Total recovery (%)	94	19	56

[a]Average of two trials.
[b]*L. monocytogenes* detected during 8 weeks of cold enrichment.
[c]*L. monocytogenes* not detected during 8 weeks of cold enrichment.
[d]Log_{10} CFU/g.
Source: Adapted from Ref. 93.

hydrophobicity, pliability, and surface qualities, *L. monocytogenes* adhered (entrapped) equally well to lean muscle and fat tissue during 50–60 minutes of incubation at ambient temperature. [According to an earlier report by Herald and Zottola (85), attachment of *L. monocytogenes* to stainless steel and presumably meat surfaces is related to flagellae, fibrils, and exopolymeric substances (i.e., polysaccharides), all of which are readily produced by *Listeria* during extended incubation at room temperature.] However, lean muscle tissue supported faster growth of the pathogen than fat tissue when samples were stored 1 day at ambient followed by 7 days at refrigeration temperature. Following attachment (and/or entrapment) of ~10^6 *L. monocytogenes* and *P. aeruginosa* CFU/4 cm^2 to lean meat, *Listeria* populations increased approximately 100-fold during 24 hours of incubation at room temperature and remained at this level during 7 days of refrigerated storage, regardless of presence or absence of *P. aeruginosa*. In contrast, populations of *P. aeruginosa* on lean meat increased >100-fold during initial storage at room temper-

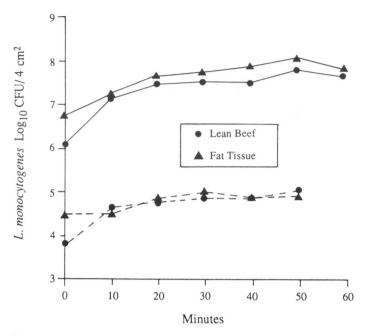

Figure 11.4 Effect of holding time on attachment of *L. monocytogenes* to lean beef and fat tissue when samples were immersed in a medium containing 10^8 (———) and 10^6 (– – –) *L. monocytogenes* CFU/ml. (Adapted from Ref. 66.)

ature, but then decreased with levels frequently 10 times lower than the *Listeria* population following 7 days of refrigerated storage.

Dickson (71) simulated contamination of raw beef during processing, handling, and storage by placing surfaces of heavily inoculated lean and fat beef tissue (~2 × 10^6 *L. monocytogenes* CFU/cm^2) in direct contact with uninoculated tissue. Overall, transfer of listeriae was largely dependent on the type of tissue with minimum and maximum transfer observed from fat-to-fat and lean-to-fat tissue, respectively. However, bacterial transfer also was influenced by adsorption time of the original inoculum and contact time with uninoculated tissue. Adsorption times of <60 minutes generally led to highest *Listeria* transfer rates, particularly between inoculated and uninoculated lean beef tissue. These findings are readily explained when one considers that most listeriae are likely to be freely suspended (unattached) in water films on tissue surfaces shortly after inoculation. Following an adsorption time of 30 minutes, approximately 30 and 50% of the original *Listeria* inoculum migrated from lean and fat tissue, respectively, to lean tissue after 5 minutes of direct contact at ambient temperature. When contamination between fat and lean tissue was simulated using shorter contact times of 15–60 seconds, a greater percentage of listeriae migrated from inoculated fat to uninoculated lean tissue, which, in turn, likely reflects the transfer of cells in unadsorbed water from hydrophobic fat to hydrophilic lean tissue. More important, the fact that bacterial transfer also occurred at 5°C with 0.6–9.5% of the original *Listeria* population migrating from inoculated to uninoculated lean and/or fat tissue after an 18-hour adsorption period provides a reasonable means for spread of this pathogen to *Listeria*-free meat during storage in walk-in coolers.

These findings attest to the hardy nature of *L. monocytogenes* on the surface of raw meats and to the need for effective means of reducing surface contamination on carcasses. Regarding the latter, Chung et al. (67) reported that wash solutions containing nisin effectively delayed growth of *L. monocytogenes* on surfaces of raw meats, particularly when such products were incubated at refrigeration rather than ambient temperatures. Although nisin-producing bacterial starter cultures have been used in the dairy industry for many years, with the exception of certain types of cheese spread, present laws in the United States still prevent direct addition of nisin to most foods, including raw meat.

Populations of enteric pathogens (i.e., *Salmonella* spp., enteropathogenic *Escherichia coli*, and *Yersinia* spp.) on raw meats can be sharply reduced by exposing the water phase of meat surfaces to 0.2 M lactic acid (pH 2.5) at 21°C (114). While *L. monocytogenes* is generally recognized as being more acid-tolerant than the previously mentioned enteric pathogens, this organism is nevertheless inactivated at pH values < 4.0. Hence, provided that *L. monocytogenes* is exposed to lactic acid for sufficient time, acid washes may be somewhat helpful in decreasing *Listeria* populations on the surface of animal carcasses.

As noted by Johnson et al. (93), *L. monocytogenes* was routinely detected in muscle tissue from cows that were killed 2 days after being inoculated intravenously with the pathogen. While some contamination of muscle tissue might have occurred during sampling, results from this study suggest that *L. monocytogenes* can enter muscle tissue via the bloodstream.

To further investigate this hypothesis, Johnson et al. (92) examined muscle, liver, and spleen tissue from two lambs and one calf that had been inoculated intravenously with *L. monocytogenes*. Microscopic examination of tissues stained with immunoperoxidase or Azure A revealed *L. monocytogenes* cells at levels of 10^3–10^4 CFU/g in muscle tissue and 10^3–10^6 CFU/g in both liver and spleen tissue. While *L. monocytogenes* appeared to be associated with phagocytes in liver and spleen tissue, the pathogen was observed in loose connective tissue between muscle fibers and also within muscle fibers themselves.

Using the USDA enrichment method, Johnson et al. (91) subsequently detected *L. monocytogenes* serotype 1a at ≤10 CFU/g in aseptically removed interior samples from 2 of 50 (4%) and 3 of 50 (6%) retail whole muscle beef and pork roasts, respectively. One beef sample also was positive for *L. innocua* and *L. welshimeri*. Although presence of these two nonpathogenic (i.e., noninvasive) *Listeria* spp. within a whole muscle roast suggests possible contamination during sampling, other results from Johnson et al. (91–93) strongly support at least limited transmission of *L. monocytogenes* from the bloodstream into muscle tissue. If this proves to be true, the meat industry, and particularly veterinarians, will be faced with a far greater challenge in that even complete elimination of *L. monocytogenes* from the slaughterhouse environment, probably an unobtainable goal, may still not lead to raw meats that are consistently free of *L. monocytogenes*.

Raw Beef

Growth and Survival

Interest in behavior of *Listeria* in raw meat products dates back to at least 1966 when Sielaff (130) inoculated beef, pork, and rabbit with *L. monocytogenes* immediately after slaughter and examined these samples for listeriae during extended storage at 3–4°C. Under these conditions, the pathogen survived at least 15 days in all three products.

While this study was among the first to examine the ability of *L. monocytogenes* to survive in raw beef, information concerning actual growth of this pathogen in raw beef was not available until 1978. In that year Gouet et al. (82) reported results from a study which examined multiplication of *L. monocytogenes* in "sterile" minced beef alone and in combination with a defined microflora. *Listeria monocytogenes* failed to grow alone in minced beef (pH 5.8) stored at 8°C, and populations decreased ≤10-fold during 17 days of incubation. In contrast, numbers of listeriae decreased approximately 100-fold in samples of minced beef (pH 5.8) that were simultaneously inoculated with *Lactobacillus plantarum* and held at 8°C for 17 days (Fig. 11.5). These researchers also found that higher concentrations of *L. monocytogenes* (10^6 CFU/g) enhanced growth of *L. plantarum*. When samples of minced beef were simultaneously inoculated to contain equal numbers of *L. monocytogenes*, *Pseudomonas fluorescens*, and *Escherichia coli*, *Listeria* populations decreased approximately 10-fold after 24 hours of incubation at 8°C, with numbers rapidly increasing after day 7 (Fig. 11.6). Rapid growth of listeriae during the latter half of incubation was likely prompted by proteolysis of meat proteins by *P. fluorescens*, which, in turn, led to a gradual increase in pH of the meat from 5.8 to 6.8. With a complex microflora consisting of ~10^3 CFU/g each of *L. plantarum*, *P. fluorescens*, *E. coli*, *Micrococcus sp.*, *Clostridium perfringens*, and *Streptococcus*

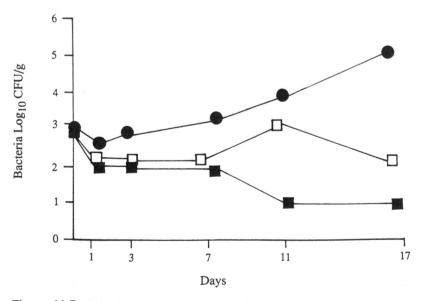

Figure 11.5   Behavior of *L. monocytogenes* alone (□) and in combination (■) with *Lactobacillus plantarum* (●) in minced beef stored at 8°C. (Adapted from Ref. 82.)

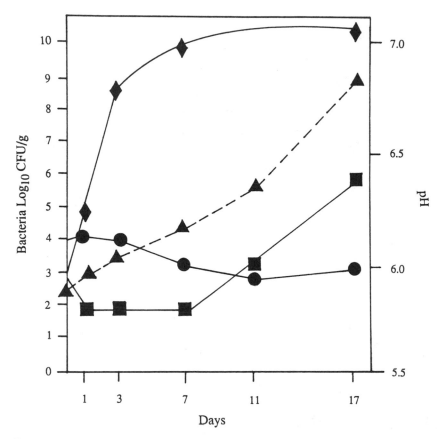

Figure 11.6 Behavior of *L. monocytogenes* alone (■) and in combination with *Escherichia coli* (▲) and *Pseudomonas fluorescens* (◆) in minced beef stored at 8°C. Dashed line (▲ – – –) designates the change in pH during storage. (Adapted from Ref. 82.)

faecalis, behavior of *L. monocytogenes* was similar to that previously observed for the pathogen in the presence of *P. fluorescens* and *E. coli*, with listeriae populations reaching approximately 6×10^5 CFU/g in minced beef following 17 days at 8°C (Fig. 11.7). A rapid increase in numbers of *P. fluorescens* before growth of *L. plantarum* again appeared instrumental in raising the pH from 5.8 to 7.2, which, in turn, stimulated growth of listeriae. Hence results from this early study suggest that *L. monocytogenes* can grow in temperature-abused retail ground beef since the microbial composition of this product is fairly similar to that found in ground beef inoculated with seven different organisms used in this study.

In a similar investigation completed 11 years later, Kaya and Schmidt (98) also found that growth of *L. monocytogenes* in artificially contaminated sterile minced meat during extended incubation at 8–20°C was suppressed by addition of 10^6 *Lactobacillus* CFU/g but was unhindered in the presence of 10^6 *Pseudomonas* sp. CFU/g. However, unlike in the previous study by Gouet et al. (82), this strain of *L. monocytogenes* readily grew in the absence of other microorganisms with populations increasing approximately 2 and ≥ 4 orders of magnitude in sterile minced meat after 10 and 1–5 days of storage at 4 and 8–20°C, respectively. Thus, in this particular instance, proteolysis of meat proteins

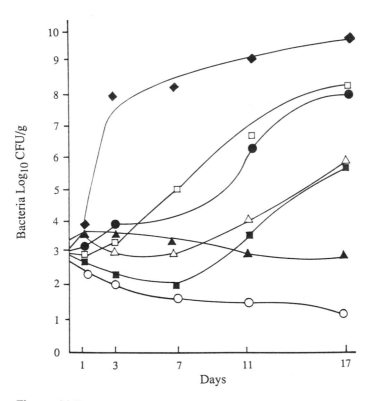

Figure 11.7 Behavior of *L. monocytogenes* alone (■) and in combination with *Lactobacillus plantarum* (●), *Pseudomonas fluorescens* (♦), *Escherichia coli* (▲), *Micrococcus* sp. (△), *Clostridium perfringens* (○), and *Streptococcus faecalis* (□) in minced beef stored at 8°C. (Adapted from Ref. 82.)

by pseudomonads apparently was not a prerequisite for growth of *L. monocytogenes* in sterile minced meat with an initial pH value of 5.8–6.0.

During 1988 and 1989, three additional studies were made to determine the behavior of listeriae in ground beef; however, unlike previous investigations, the meat was not pretreated to eliminate the normal background flora. When ground beef at pH 5.6–5.9 was inoculated to contain 10^5 and 10^6 *L. monocytogenes* strain Scott A or V7 CFU/g, packaged in oxygen-permeable or -impermeable film and examined for numbers of listeriae during extended storage at 4°C, Johnson et al. (90) found that the numbers and pH remained relatively constant in both products during 14 days of incubation, regardless of the film's degree of permeability. Unlike the previous study by Gouet et al. (82) in which the pH of minced beef containing a complex microflora increased from 5.8 to 7.2 during extended incubation at 8°C, the pH of all packaged ground beef samples in this study remained in the range of pH 5.6–5.9 throughout storage. Thus the lower pH of the meat in this study, along with a lower incubation temperature (4 vs. 8°C) are likely to have been at least partly responsible for inhibiting growth of listeriae in packaged samples of "retail-like" ground beef.

In keeping with these findings, Shelef (129) also reported that *L. monocytogenes* failed to grow in artificially contaminated ground beef or ground liver during 1 and 40 days of incubation at 25 and 4°C, respectively. However, in contrast to results of the previous study by Johnson et al. (90), the pathogen failed to grow in ground beef despite a final pH value of 7.8. While the reason(s) for this behavior remain(s) obscure, inability of *L. monocytogenes* to multiply in ground beef under these conditions is likely related to the type and load of inherent microflora in the product.

This hypothesis is supported by a West German study in which Kaya and Schmidt (98) showed that an increase in the natural bacterial flora of ground beef from 10^5 to 10^7 CFU/g led to increased inhibition of *L. monocytogenes* in artificially contaminated meat. When ground beef was inoculated to contain ~10^5 *L. monocytogenes* CFU/g, the pathogen grew after 1–5 days at 7–20°C in samples harboring ~10^5 non-*Listeria* contaminants/g but failed to multiply in corresponding samples containing higher levels of naturally occurring organisms. Although a similar growth pattern was observed for samples naturally contaminated with 10^2 *Listeria* CFU/g and 10^5 non-*Listeria* CFU/g, growth was markedly hindered in naturally rather than artificially contaminated samples with *Listeria* populations remaining constant in the former during 14 days at 8°C. However, behavioral differences were no longer observed at lower temperatures with the organism failing to grow during 14 days of incubation at 4°C in both artificially and naturally contaminated ground beef containing similar background populations. While these findings attest to the hardy nature of listeriae in fresh ground beef, *L. monocytogenes* also was equally tenacious in artificially contaminated frozen ground beef, with populations remaining unchanged at ~10^5 CFU/g during 6 months of storage at –18°C.

Listeria monocytogenes may well behave similarly on the surface of fresh intact beef muscle; however, little information is currently available to support this hypothesis. In two such studies conducted shortly before *L. monocytogenes* emerged as a serious foodborne pathogen, Lee et al. (103,104) dealt indirectly with the incidence and subsequent behavior of *Listeria* spp. along with many other psychrotrophic as well as mesophilic organisms present on the surface of hot-boned and conventionally boned beef. In this study, hot-boned beef was obtained from five steers 2 hours after slaughter, vacuum-packaged, and cooled from 32 to 21°C. In contrast, conventionally processed beef was obtained from carcasses that were hung in a cold room at 2°C for 2 days after slaughter. Both types of beef were then examined for mesophilic and psychrotrophic organisms at day 0 when the surface temperature had decreased to 21°C (<1 hour for conventionally processed beef) and again following 14 days of storage at 2°C. Nearly 1250 bacterial isolates were subsequently identified by feeding results from 116 miniaturized tests/isolate into a computer. Although *Listeria* spp. were never isolated from slow or moderately chilled, hot-boned beef at day 0, 9.1–13.5% of all microorganisms present on the surface of such beef after 14 days were identified as *Listeria* spp., some isolates of which were likely *L. monocytogenes* (Table 11.8). Overall, only one isolate from conventionally processed beef was identified as in the genus *Listeria*. From these data one can infer that *Listeria* can grow on the surface of vacuum-packaged hot-boned beef but not on the surface of unpackaged conventionally processed beef during 2 weeks of storage at 2°C. Since the high water-binding properties of hot-boned beef make this product particularly well suited for sausage-making, widespread use of hot-boned beef by the processed meat industry may be partially related to the relatively high incidence of listeriae in ready-to-eat meat products. If this is true, additional efforts may be needed to improve the microbiological safety of hot-boned meats.

In a more definitive Australian study reported in 1988, Grau and Vanderlinde (83) specifically examined the ability of *L. monocytogenes* to grow on the surface of artificially contaminated (10^2–10^3 CFU/cm^2) vacuum-packaged, nonsterile beef striploin during extended incubation at 0 and 5.3°C. While *L. monocytogenes* populations increased in all samples (and product exudates that developed in packages) during storage, the extent of *Listeria* growth was markedly influenced by incubation temperature, pH of the sample (5.6 vs. 6.0), and type of tissue (lean vs. fat). Overall, higher

Table 11.8 Fate of *Listeria* spp. on the Surface of Hot-Boned (HB) and Conventionally Processed (CP) Beef After Both Products Were Cooled at 21°C (day 0) and Stored at 2°C for 14 Days

Bacterial group	HB chilling rate	Time (days)	Processing method HB	CP
	Slow	0	0/83[a]	1/89
Mesophiles	Slow	14	0/99	0/77
Psychrotrophs	Slow	0	0/84	0/36
	Slow	14	1/100	0/58
Mesophiles	Moderate	0	0/96	0/81
	Moderate	14	9/99 (9.1)	0/89
Psychrotrophs	Moderate	0	0/66	0/25
	Moderate	14	13/96 (13.5)	0/71

[a]Number of isolates identified as *Listeria* spp./Total number of isolates identified as non-*Listeria* spp. (%).
Source: Adapted from Ref. 104.

Listeria populations consistently developed on fat tissue, with growth also more rapid at the higher of the two incubation temperatures and pH values. Numbers of listeriae on fat tissue of pH 5.6 increased from 5×10^3 to 3×10^7 CFU/cm^2 during 16 days of incubation, whereas the pathogen was just beginning to grow on corresponding samples after 7–14 days of storage at 0°C. These researchers also noted that *Listeria* populations increased <10- and ~1000-fold on vacuum-packaged meats of pH 5.6 and 6.0, respectively, after 10–11 weeks of storage at 0°C. Thus it appears that two conditions, (a) a storage temperature of 0°C and (b) a product pH value of 5.6, must be met simultaneously to prevent significant growth of *L. monocytogenes* in vacuum-packaged raw meats destined for export.

Thermal Inactivation

Interest in heat resistance of listeriae in raw meat products dates back to at least 1980 when Karaioannoglou and Xenos (96) reported on survival of *Listeria* in grilled meatballs. In their experiments, minced beef was inoculated to contain 10^2, 10^3, 10^4, or 10^5 *L. monocytogenes* CFU/g, was then combined with eggs, bread, onion, garlic, salt, and spices, and was fashioned into meatballs weighing 35–40 g each. Meatballs were then placed on a coal-fired grill at 110 to 120°C and cooked for 15 minutes until they attained an internal temperature of 78 to 85°C. After grilling, *L. monocytogenes* was isolated from all meatballs that originally contained 10^4–10^5 listeriae/g. However, the pathogen was discovered in only 1 of 4 meatballs inoculated to contain 10^3 listeriae/g and was absent from meatballs that originally contained 10^2 listeriae/g. Since data from the European surveys discussed earlier indicate that retail raw beef occasionally may contain up to 10^3 *Listeria* CFU/g (some of which are likely to be *L. monocytogenes*), thorough cooking of raw meat is presently advised to eliminate *L. monocytogenes* as well as salmonellae, *Campylobacter* spp., pathogenic strains of *E. coli*, and other organisms that have been associated with foodborne illness.

Recent concern about possible resistance of *L. monocytogenes* to pasteurization of milk, along with detection of this pathogen in cooked meats, prompted renewed interest in the possibility of *L. monocytogenes* surviving thermal processing steps commonly used to convert raw meat into ready-to-eat products. Consequently, Boyle et al. (56) investigated thermal destruction of *L. monocytogenes* strain Scott A in ground beef (~20% fat) by submerging sealed tubes containing ground beef with 10^8 listeriae/g in a water bath at 75°C until the internal temperature of samples was 50, 60, 65, or 70°C. Samples then were examined for listeriae by direct plating and selective and cold enrichment. According to these researchers, *Listeria* populations failed to decrease in samples heated to an internal temperature of 50°C over 6.2 minutes. Numbers of listeriae decreased 4.4–6.1 orders of magnitude in samples of ground beef during 8.4 and 10.6 minutes of heating to 60 and 65°C, respectively; similar results also were reported in 1988 by Farber et al. (77). However, healthy listeriae cells could still be readily quantitated by direct plating of appropriate dilutions on a selective medium. Similar results also were obtained when inoculated samples of ground beef were stored at 4°C before being heated to internal temperatures of 50, 60, or 65°C. Although *L. monocytogenes* was not detected by directly plating samples heated to an internal temperature of 70°C, the pathogen was recovered from 8 of 9 samples following selective and/or cold enrichment. These findings together with those of another recent report (110) in which

L. monocytogenes exhibited D-values of approximately 4.5, 0.65, and 0.15 minute in raw beef heated to 60, 65, and 70°C, respectively, suggest this pathogen is more heat resistant in meat than in fluid dairy products. Increased thermal resistance in the former probably is related to lower a_w values (136) as well as to possible protective effects from fat and drying during heating (110).

Subsequently, Farber and Brown (76) examined the effect of prior heat shock on heat resistance of *Listeria* in ground beef. Following irradiation to reduce background flora, samples of ground beef were inoculated to contain ~10^7 *L. monocytogenes* CFU/g and held at 48°C for 30, 60, or 120 minutes before being heated to internal temperatures of 62 to 64°C. Surprisingly, recovery of the pathogen increased by 1.2–2.7 orders of magnitude for preheated than for nonpreheated samples. Furthermore, when inoculated samples were preheated at 48°C for 60 minutes and refrigerated for 24 hours before being heated to an internal temperature of 64°C, heat-shocked cells of *L. monocytogenes* within the meat retained their increased heat resistance as compared to that of control cells that were not heat-shocked. Unlike results from other studies reported thus far, these findings demonstrate an apparent ability of *L. monocytogenes* to become more heat-tolerant under certain conditions. Furthermore, these results emphasize the importance of thoroughly reheating refrigerated leftover meats, particularly if such items were prepared in cafeterias or food service establishments and kept warm (via steam table or heat lamp) for extended times.

These concerns about thoroughly reheating leftover meat products are further supported by preliminary results from a recent study indicating that *L. monocytogenes* is more heat-tolerant than *Salmonella* spp. in fatty ground beef (30.5% fat), with *L. monocytogenes* exhibiting D-values of 90.1, 6.6, and 1.2 minutes at 51.7, 57.2, and 62.8°C, respectively (23). In contrast, *Salmonella* exhibited a D-value of only 63–64 minutes at 51.7°C and was no longer detected in samples of ground beef held at the two higher temperatures. These researchers further demonstrated that *L. monocytogenes* was slightly more heat resistant in ground beef containing 2% rather than 30.5% fat.

Resistance to Gamma Irradiation

Recent trends toward extending both shelf life and safety of many foods by use of ionizing radiation prompted El-Shenawy et al. (74) to examine the ability of gamma irradiation to destroy and/or injure *L. monocytogenes* in raw meat. In their study, retail samples of ground beef were inoculated to contain ~10^8 *L. monocytogenes* strain Scott A, V7, or CA/g and irradiated with doses of gamma irradiation between 0.75 and 4.50 kGy. Samples of irradiated meat were then plated on permissive and nonpermissive agar to determine the extent of *Listeria* cell death and injury, respectively. According to these researchers, strain V7 was most resistant to gamma irradiation in ground beef (average D-value of 1.0 kGy) followed by strains CA and Scott A with average D-values of 0.58 and 0.51 kGy at room temperature, respectively. Since Stegeman (134) also reported D-values of 0.38 and 1.06 kGy for *L. monocytogenes* strain Scott A in minced meat irradiated at 4 and –18°C, respectively, it appears that this organism is equally or slightly more resistant to gamma irradiation in ground beef than are other non–spore-forming foodborne pathogens such as *Salmonella typhimurium*, *Staphylococcus aureus* (140), *Yersinia enterocolitica* (75), and *Campylobacter jejuni* (140). While El-Shenawy et al. (74) found that exposure to gamma irradiation led to limited dose-dependent injury of all three *Listeria* strains, these authors concluded that relatively mild doses of gamma irradiation can be used to effectively kill large populations of *L. monocytogenes* in artificially and probably naturally contaminated ground beef.

Raw Lamb and Pork

Most investigations have focused almost exclusively on behavior of *Listeria* in raw beef; however, several reports on fate of this pathogen in raw lamb and pork are in the scientific literature. As early as 1973, Khan et al. (99) published results from a study in which aseptically obtained "sterile" raw lamb meat was inoculated to contain ~10^5 *L. monocytogenes* CFU/g; packaged in gas-permeable or gas-impermeable film, and examined for numbers of listeriae during extended storage at 0 and 8°C. Although *Listeria* populations remained relatively constant in lamb meat packaged in gas-permeable film during 20 days at 0°C, numbers of listeriae decreased approximately 10-fold in corresponding samples that were packaged in a gas-impermeable film. These results are similar to those obtained by Johnson et al. (90), who concluded that *L. monocytogenes* also was unable to grow in refrigerated ground beef that was packaged in gas-permeable or -impermeable film. Following 12 days of storage at 8 rather than 0°C, populations of listeriae in lamb increased >1000-fold; however, unlike meat packaged in gas-permeable film, the pathogen exhibited a 2-day lag period and grew markedly slower in gas-impermeable packages (Fig. 11.8). Various physical differences of the meat, combined with an increased concentration of CO_2 (and presumably a lower pH) in gas-impermeable packages, may be largely responsible for partially inactivating the pathogen at 0°C and delaying onset of growth at 8°C.

Two years later, Khan et al. (100) examined behavior of *L. monocytogenes* in preparations of sarcoplasmic pork, beef, and lamb protein that were inoculated to contain ~10^4 *L. monocytogenes* CFU/ml and then held at 4°C. According to these investigators, the pathogen grew readily in preparations of pork and beef protein, reaching levels of approximately 10^5 and 10^7/ml, respectively, after 12 days of refrigerated storage. Although *Listeria* populations remained relatively constant in corresponding preparations of lamb protein held at 4°C, the pathogen grew readily in lamb meat stored at 8°C. Hence, it appears that raw pork, beef, and lamb can support rapid growth of listeriae, particularly when these products have undergone temperature abuse, as frequently occurs at the retail level.

These early observations were recently confirmed by Lovett et al. (107), who found that *L. monocytogenes* reached levels of at least 10^8 CFU/g in inoculated samples of retail lamb, pork, and beef after 14 days at 7°C (Fig. 11.9). *Listeria monocytogenes* exhibited both a 2-day lag period and a slower rate of growth in beef and pork than lamb. Such variations in growth rate might be related to differences in concentrations of various amino acids (particularly lysine, serine, and valine, which are reportedly essential for growth of *L. monocytogenes*), as first suggested by Khan et al. (99) in 1973.

As previously discussed, retail samples of raw lamb, pork, and beef can occasionally contain low to moderate levels of *L. monocytogenes*, particularly if such products have undergone temperature abuse. Moreover, a recent government survey led to respective discovery of *L. monocytogenes* and catalase activity (an indication of gross underprocessing) in 4 of 64 and 15 of 64 precooked meat patties (51). Consequently, in an

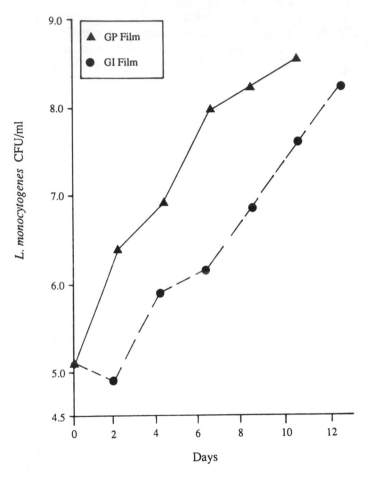

Figure 11.8 Effect of gas-permeable (GP) and gas-impermeable (GI) films on growth of *L. monocytogenes* in sterile lamb meat during storage at 8°C. (Adapted from Ref. 99.)

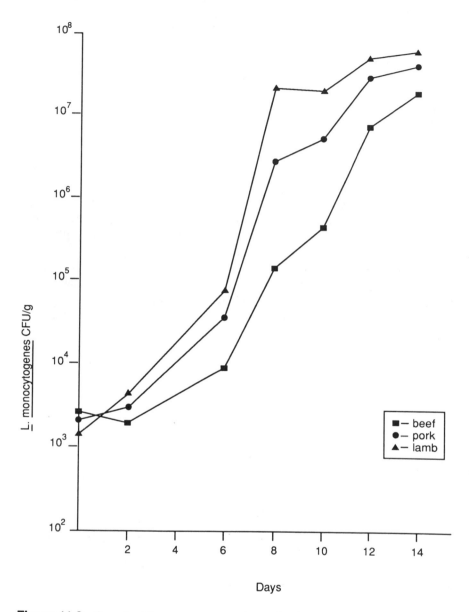

Figure 11.9 Growth of *L. monocytogenes* in raw beef, pork, and lamb during extended storage at 7°C. (Adapted from Ref. 107.)

effort to safeguard public health, USDA-FSIS officials announced new time-temperature guidelines for cooking and storing all perishable meat products (17). In June 1990, USDA officials proposed a minimum 5-D kill of *L. monocytogenes* during commercial manufacture of precooked hamburgers and other meat patties (51). Such reductions in numbers of listeriae could be accomplished by holding a product at an internal temperature of 66.1°C for 51 seconds or at slightly higher temperatures for less time. The agency now requires that cooked meat products (other than roast beef, cooked corned beef, shelf-stable meats, and "hot-shipped" products, which must at all times be maintained at ≥60°C or discarded) be cooled from 54.4 to 26.7°C within 1.5 hours and from 16.7 to 4.4°C within 5 hours. However, another proposal was made in June 1990 which would require that the temperature of such products be reduced to 4.4°C within only 2 hours after cooking (51). Additionally, all meat products to be stored longer than 7 days must now be held at a maximum of 1.7 rather than 4.4°C as was previously required. (Currently, FDA officials require that all perishable foods under their jurisdiction be stored at ≤7.2°C by retail establishments.) While ingestion of pork products, which are normally well cooked before consumption, should pose a very low risk of listeric infection, one would expect far more cases of listeriosis to be linked to consumption of beef and lamb since both products are frequently consumed after only partial cooking. Therefore, storing all raw meat at ≤1.7°C should be useful in preventing extensive growth of *L. monocytogenes* and most other foodborne pathogens, extending the shelf life of these foods, and reducing involvement of meat products in foodborne illness.

Cooked and Ready-to-Eat Meats

Cured Ham

Investigators in Europe and the United States also have determined the behavior of *L. monocytogenes* in ham during processing and extended storage. Working in The Netherlands, Stegeman et al. (135) examined thermal resistance of listeriae in experimentally produced hams to which 2 or 3% NaCl and 120 or 180 ppm sodium nitrite were added during manufacture. After inoculating the product to contain ~10^4 *L. monocytogenes* CFU/g, all hams were canned, heated to internal temperature of 68.9–71.0 (or 64.0°C) within 5 hours to simulate normal and underprocessing, respectively, cooled, and sampled after 5 days of storage of 4°C. According to these authors, three different enrichment procedures failed to recover viable listeriae from any samples.

Results from the study just described indicate that standard thermal treatments are more than sufficient for producing *Listeria*-free ham. However, once removed from protective packaging, all cooked/ready-to-eat meats can become contaminated with listeriae during slicing and further handling, as suggested by recent surveys. To simulate postprocessing contamination, Glass and Doyle (80) inoculated the surface of commercially produced ham slices and five other meat products (to be discussed shortly) to contain approximately 0.2 or 500 *L. monocytogenes* CFU/g. All samples were then vacuum-packaged and periodically examined for numbers of listeriae during prolonged incubation at 4.4°C. Regardless of the original inoculum, *L. monocytogenes* attained populations of 10^5–10^6 CFU/g on organoleptically acceptable ham (pH 6.3–6.5) after 4 weeks of refrigerated storage, thus indicating that manufacturers cannot rely on the combination of vacuum-packaging and refrigeration for control of listeriae on ham.

Cooked Roast Beef

Glass and Doyle (80) also used the procedure just described to evaluate the potential for *L. monocytogenes* to grow on the surface of vacuum-packaged samples of cooked roast beef having initial pH values of ~5.90. Unlike sliced ham, cooked roast beef supported far less growth of listeriae, with populations increasing ≤2 orders of magnitude on organoleptically acceptable product after 4 weeks of refrigerated storage. Slower growth of the pathogen on precooked roast beef correlated well with a decrease in product pH to values ≤ 5.15 in 4-week-old samples.

Unfermented Sausage

Even though potentially contaminated raw meats find their way into enormous quantities of sausage products, with over 200 varieties manufactured in the United States alone, no information pertaining to behavior of *L. monocytogenes* during manufacture and storage of these popular meat products appeared in the scientific literature before 1988. While the California listeriosis outbreak of 1985 eventually led to the aforementioned surveys in which *Listeria* was detected in raw and processed meats, including sausage, the general consensus, until recently, was that consumption of such products did not pose a serious threat of contracting listeriosis as shown by a lack of any confirmed cases of meatborne listeriosis. However, this situation changed in December 1988 following the report of a breast cancer patient who developed listeric meningitis and eventually died after consuming turkey frankfurters that were contaminated with *L. monocytogenes*. Although current research findings will now be presented on behavior of *L. monocytogenes* during manufacture and storage of various sausage products, the reader should keep in mind that results of additional investigations prompted by the recent listeriosis case linked to consumption of *Listeria*-contaminated turkey frankfurters will be available in the future.

Unfermented sausages are best classified according to the following five categories, which are based on the method of manufacture: (a) fresh sausage (e.g., fresh pork sausage, bratwurst), (b) cooked sausage (e.g., liver sausage, Braunschweiger), (c) cooked smoked sausage (e.g., frankfurters, bologna), (d) uncooked smoked sausage (e.g., Mettwurst, smoked country-style pork sausage, Kielbasa), and (e) cooked meat specialty items (e.g., head cheese). Current research efforts have dealt primarily with behavior of *Listeria* in sausages belonging to three of these five categories, with little if any information presently available on cooked sausage and cooked meat specialty items.

Fresh Sausage

While fresh pork sausage is by far the most widely manufactured fresh sausage, this category also includes other well-known varieties such as fresh Italian, breakfast, and beef sausage as well as fresh bratwurst, Thuringer, and bockwurst. The last two are most popular in Germany. All varieties of fresh sausage are normally prepared from coarse or finely comminuted pork, beef, or veal to which water is added along with an array of spices which varies with the type of sausage to be produced. In the United States, certain varieties of fresh sausage also may contain binders and/or extenders (e.g., cereal, vegetable starch, nonfat dry milk, dried whey) at levels not exceeding 3.5% by weight. After being stuffed into natural or artificial casings, the product is twisted and cut to form individual sausage links which are cooled rapidly to preserve freshness and flavor. Unlike cooked and fermented sausages, fresh sausages have a short shelf life and must be constantly refrigerated to prevent growth of spoilage organisms, including lactic acid bacteria and micrococci.

Thus far efforts to define the behavior of *L. monocytogenes* in fresh sausage have been limited to two 1989 studies involving artificially contaminated bratwurst. When commercially prepared fresh bratwursts were surface-inoculated to contain approximately 0.1 or 600 *L. monocytogenes* CFU/g, vacuum-packaged, and stored at 4.4°C, Glass and Doyle (80) found that the pathogen attained populations of 10^6 CFU/g on organoleptically acceptable 4-week-old bratwursts, regardless of the initial inoculum. As with ham, profuse growth of listeriae on fresh bratwurst was attributed to a pH value > 6.0 was maintained by the product throughout the first 4 weeks of refrigerated storage.

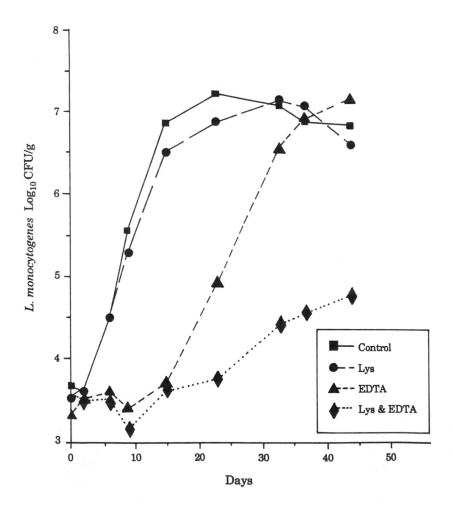

Figure 11.10 Effect of lysozyme (Lys) and EDTA on growth of *L. monocytogenes* in fresh bratwurst. (Adapted from Ref. 89.)

In the only other reported study involving fresh sausage, Hughey et al. (89) investigated the ability of lysozyme to prevent growth of *L. monocytogenes* in bratwurst prepared from coarsely ground pork. After addition of commercial bratwurst spice, distilled water was added with or without 100 ppm lysozyme and 5 mM EDTA—a generally recognized as safe chelating agent that enhances antibacterial activity of lysozyme. This meat mixture was then inoculated to contain ~4 × 10³ *L. monocytogenes* CFU/g and stuffed into natural hog casings which were subsequently linked, separated, vacuum-packaged, and stored at 5°C for 45 days.

As expected from the previous study, *Listeria* populations increased rapidly in fresh bratwurst (pH ≅ 6.0) without added lysozyme or EDTA, reaching levels of >10⁶ CFU/g following 10 days of refrigerated storage (Fig. 11.10). *Listeria monocytogenes* also behaved similarly in bratwurst containing lysozyme alone; however, presence of EDTA alone resulted in a 15-day lag period, thus preventing the pathogen from reaching populations of 10⁶ CFU/g until nearly 30 days of storage. In contrast, lysozyme and EDTA acted synergistically to retard growth of *L. monocytogenes* in fresh bratwurst. Under these conditions, the pathogen exhibited a lag period of nearly 21 days, i.e., approximately 7 days beyond the normal shelf life of the product, and reached populations of <10⁵ CFU/g following 44 days of refrigerated storage. While only listeriostatic, the combined use of lysozyme and EDTA appears to be an effective means of controlling *Listeria* growth during the normal shelf life of fresh bratwurst. Furthermore, once growth is prevented, low levels of *L. monocytogenes* that occasionally appear in fresh bratwurst (<10³ CFU/g) should be readily eliminated by proper cooking.

Cooked Smoked Sausage

This group of sausages, which includes the ever-popular frankfurter (hot dog) as well as bologna and various luncheon meats, is prepared from mixtures of comminuted beef and/or pork to which salt, sugar, sodium nitrite, and spices are normally added. When making frankfurters, this meat/ingredient mixture, commonly referred to as the sausage emulsion, is stuffed into natural or artificial casings, which are then twisted to form sausage links. This string of frankfurter links is cooked to an internal temperature of ~71.1°C (160°F) to (a) coagulate protein, (b) fix the color, and (c) pasteurize the product. Although not absolutely required, frankfurters and other similar sausages are frequently hung in smoking rooms either before or after cooking. Alternatively, commercially available liquid smoke products can be added to the sausage emulsion or applied directly to the surface of frankfurters before or during heating. In either event, beside imparting a pleasant smoked flavor to the finished product, some smoke components (i.e., formaldehyde, acetic acid, creosote, and phenols with high boiling points) are bacteriostatic and/or bactericidal toward many microbial contaminants. After cooking, frankfurters are carefully cooled, packaged, and refrigerated during shipment to wholesale and retail markets. Skinless frankfurters, which are very popular, are produced in a similar manner except the casing is mechanically peeled from the sausage after cooking or smoking.

Although still controversial, recent epidemiological data from the CDC showing an apparent association between listeriosis and undercooked frankfurters has prompted several studies to examine the thermal resistance of *L. monocytogenes* in this sausage. Zaika et al. (144) prepared frankfurters from a sausage emulsion inoculated to contain ~10⁸ *L. monocytogenes* CFU/g. After stuffing, all frankfurters were thermally processed (without smoke) according to a standard commercial heating schedule. These USDA officials found that *L. monocytogenes* populations decreased approximately 1000-fold in frankfurters that were heated to an internal temperature of 71.1°C (160°F). [Preliminary results also suggest that *L. monocytogenes* is eliminated faster from liver sausage than frankfurters (18), probably because of longer processing times required for large-diameter liver sausage.] Hence, based on these data, cooking frankfurters to an internal temperature of 71.1°C should eliminate maximum levels of *L. monocytogenes* ($<10^3$ CFU/g) that could conceivably occur in raw frankfurter emulsions.

Data gathered by the American Meat Institute in 1988 have pointed to frankfurters as being among the most likely carriers of *L. monocytogenes* and also have suggested that poor environmental conditions before packaging may play a major role in contaminating the finished product (16). Moreover, Glass and Doyle (80) reported that this pathogen can proliferate on vacuum-packaged, artificially contaminated (~0.01 *L. monocytogenes* CFU/g) retail frankfurters during incubation at 4.4°C with populations two to five orders of magnitude higher on organoleptically acceptable samples after 4 weeks of refrigerated storage. Prevention of *Listeria* contamination and impending growth is further complicated by present consumer demands for reduced amounts of salt and preservatives along with longer shelf life, smaller packages, and greater convenience, all of which will require the processed meat industry to develop even stricter requirements for processing, cooking, handling, packaging, and refrigeration of products.

Several studies were initiated by the food industry to examine the feasibility of using heat to eliminate *L. monocytogenes* from the surface of finished frankfurters. In one such study (19), frankfurters were dipped in a broth culture of *L. monocytogenes* (10^6–10^8 CFU/ml) to simulate postprocessing contamination. Unfortunately, *Listeria* populations on the surface of the frankfurters decreased only 100-fold after 8 minutes of heating at 86.1–87.8°C (187–190°F). Furthermore, this heat treatment rendered the sausages organoleptically unacceptable for most consumers. Hence "postprocess pasteurization" does not appear to be a viable means for eliminating *L. monocytogenes* from the surface of frankfurters that have been contaminated after manufacture.

Additional efforts to control *Listeria* contamination on the surface of frankfurters have focused on the bactericidal properties of commercially available liquid smoke products. In one study (112), beef frankfurters were immersed in a culture containing 1×10^3 *L. monocytogenes* CFU/ml, removed, thoroughly air-dried, and then dipped in full-strength commercially available liquid smoke solution (CharSol C-10). Although *Listeria* populations were unchanged in control frankfurters that were dipped in phosphate buffer, vacuum-packaged, and analyzed after 72 hours at 4°C, numbers of listeriae had decreased 60 to ≥99.9% 15 minutes after the frankfurters were treated with liquid smoke. Furthermore, the pathogen was never detected in smoke-treated sausage following 72 hours of refrigerated storage. Hence, while dipping frankfurters in full-strength liquid smoke eliminated *L. monocytogenes*, this treatment produces an extremely intense smokey-flavored product that is no longer organoleptically acceptable to consumer.

Preliminary results from several additional experiments dealing with antilisterial effects of less concentrated liquid smoke solutions were reported by Wendorff (142). Initially, beef frankfurters were dipped into a concentrated broth culture of *L. monocytogenes*, removed, thoroughly dried, dipped into aqueous liquid smoke solutions containing 10–40% CharSol C-10 or Poly-10 (concentrations normally used in frankfurter production) and then analyzed for listeriae after 72 hours of refrigerated storage, using the Gene-Trak DNA hybridization assay. Although *L. monocytogenes* was eliminated from the surface of frankfurters dipped in 40% solutions of CharSol C-10 or Poly-10, the pathogen was still detected on frankfurters treated with 10 and 25% solutions of CharSol C-10.

After demonstrating that these liquid smoke compounds lost their activity against *Listeria* on the surface of frankfurters when added directly to sausage emulsion before stuffing, Wendorf (142) examined the ability of liquid smoke compounds to inactivate listeriae on surface-inoculated skinless frankfurters that were sprayed with five levels of CharSol Poly-10 and CharSol Supreme (twice the strength of CharSol C-10) just before vacuum packaging (Table 11.9). When used at organoleptically acceptable concentrations, CharSol Supreme was more effective than CharSol Poly-10, with *Listeria* populations on the surface of frankfurters decreasing >40% following 72 hours of refrigerated storage. When this study was repeated with a more realistic *L. monocytogenes* inoculum level (~10^3 CFU/g), approximately 89% of the *Listeria* population was inactivated on frankfurters treated with CharSol or CharSol Poly-10 at levels of 2.0 and 4.0 oz./100 lb. of frankfurters, thus indicating that none of these treatments can guarantee a *Listeria*-free product. Hence, to avoid contamination of finished product, efforts must be made to develop microbial monitoring, sampling, and HACCP programs that can effectively address problems pertaining to lack of separation between raw and finished processing areas as well as procedures used to clean and sanitize the factory environment and equipment such as grinders, mixers, and particularly sausage peelers.

Table 11.9 Fate of *L. monocytogenes* on the Surface of Beef Frankfurters Sprayed with CharSol Poly-10 or CharSol Supreme Liquid Smoke and Stored at 4°C for 72 Hours

Treatment	Level (oz./100 lb. frankfurters)	*L. monocytogenes* Initial inoculum (CFU/g)	Inactivation after 72 h (%)
Control	0	5.28	0
CharSol Poly-10	1.7[a]	5.30	Growth
	3.4[a]	5.28	0
	5.1[a]	5.16	23.6
	8.5	4.84	63.1
	12.0	4.67	75.2
CharSol Supreme	1.8[a]	5.02	44.7
	3.6[a]	5.04	42.1
	5.4	4.73	71.5
	9.0	4.41	86.3
	12.6	4.30	89.5

[a]Organoleptically acceptable concentration of liquid smoke.
Source: Adapted from Ref. 142.

In the only other reported study involving cooked smoked sausage, Glass and Doyle (80) examined the behavior of *L. monocytogenes* on vacuum-packaged, artificially contaminated slices of commercially produced bologna. As was true for ham and bratwurst, the pathogen also grew well on bologna (pH 6.1–6.4) with populations generally three to four orders of magnitude higher than initially on organoleptically acceptable samples held 4 weeks at 4.4°C. These findings again stress the importance of following good manufacturing practices, which will, in turn, greatly reduce the possibility of listeriae contaminating ready-to-eat meats during slicing and packaging.

Uncooked Smoked Sausage

According to incidence data in Table 11.6, one variety of Western European uncooked smoked sausage, namely Mettwurst, appears to be particularly prone to contamination with *Listeria* spp., including *L. monocytogenes*. These observations prompted a 1989 study by Trüssel and Jemmi (139) in which an experimentally produced Mettwurst emulsin (pH 5.3) containing ~2.6% NaCl and 100 ppm sodium nitrate was artificially contaminated with *L. monocytogenes* at levels of 10^3 or 10^7 CFU/g and examined for numbers of listeriae during manufacture, after 7 days of ripening at 14°C, and after 3 weeks of subsequent storage of 4°C. Overall, *Listeria* populations remained relatively constant during manufacture and ripening, which, in turn, reflects the apparent inability of this organism to multiply in ready-to-eat meat products having pH values < 5.5. As expected from the results of European surveys, this pathogen also survived well in Mettwurst during the product's entire refrigerated shelf life with 4-week-old samples still containing approximately 10^2 and 10^6 *L. monocytogenes* CFU/g. Given these findings, it would be prudent for Mettwurst producers to review their manufacturing practices and develop procedures for decreasing *Listeria* contamination during all facets of production. Such efforts would go a long way toward averting any potential public health problems with Mettwurst.

Fermented Sausage

Sausages classified as fermented undergo a controlled lactic acid–type fermentation usually through action of a commercially produced starter culture added to the comminuted meat. While all fermented sausages can be further classified according to moisture content as either semi-dry or dry, manufacturing procedures for both types are generally similar until the point of drying. Fermented sausages are normally prepared from comminuted beef and/or pork to which sugar and various spices are added along with sodium or potassium nitrate and/or nitrite. This meat preparation, known as a mix rather than an emulsion, is inoculated with a commercial mixture of lactic acid bacteria, which frequently includes species of *Pediococcus* (particularly *P. cerevisiae* and *P. acidilactici*), *Lactobacillus*, and *Leuconostoc*. After stuffing the inoculated sausage mix into natural or artificial casings, the strings of sausage links are hung in ripening or "green-rooms" at 27–40°C/80 to 90% R.H. Within 2–3 days, sugar added to the mix is fermented to lactic acid by the starter culture, which, in turn, decreases the pH to ~5.1 and produces the characteristic tangy flavor found in fermented sausages. As in cheesemaking, controlled lowering of the sausage pH to levels near the isoelectric point of meat protein also is important for proper removal of water during later stages of sausage manufacture.

Following fermentation, sausages destined to become semi-dry varieties containing ~50% moisture (e.g., Cervelat-type sausages and Lebanon bologna) are normally placed in smokehouses where they are smoked and cooked to internal temperatures of 60–68°C. In contrast, dry sausages which will ultimately contain ~35% moisture (e.g., pepperoni, Genoa, and Milano salamis) are moved to drying rooms (10–17°C/65–80% R.H.) where they remain for various times, depending on the type and size of sausage. Some varieties also may be exposed to cool smoke before drying; however, unlike semi-dry varieties, dry sausages are never cooked. Although fermented sausages keep well because of their relatively high salt content, low pH, and low moisture (a_w) content, both varieties, and particularly semi-dry sausages, should be refrigerated.

Semi-dry Fermented Sausage

The relatively severe heat treatment that semi-dry sausages receive during manufacture generally has been regarded as sufficient to eliminate most commonly encountered non–spore-forming foodborne pathogens. Hence, despite concerns regarding presence of listeriae in meat products, behavior of *L. monocytogenes* during manufacture and storage of semi-dry fermented sausage has received relatively little attention.

A report indicating that a bacteriocin-producing strain of *Pediococcus acidilactici* inactivated *L. monocytogenes* in experimentally produced fermented dairy products (121) prompted Berry et al. (54) to examine the possibility of using a similar starter culture to inhibit growth of *L. monocytogenes* during manufacture of fermented summer sausage. According to these authors, a commercial summer sausage mix was inoculated to contain ~10^6 *L. monocytogenes* CFU/g and fermented with either bacteriocin-producing or non–bacteriocin-producing strains of *P. acidilactici*. Following 12–14 hours of fermentation at 37.8°C, populations of listeriae decreased approximately 100-fold and 10-fold in summer sausage fermented with bacteriocin-producing and non-bacteriocin-producing strains of *P. acidilactici*, respectively. The pathogen also was inactivated in sausages with slower acid production (pH > 5.5), which suggests that bacteriocin production occurred independent of carbohydrate fermentation. However, *L. monocytogenes* was still detected in 9 of 90 (10.0%) sausage samples that had been heated to an internal temperature of 64°C and then refrigerated for up to 2 weeks. Thus, while use of this bacteriocin-producing starter culture led to a dramatic decrease in numbers of viable listeriae in summer sausage, it did not completely inactivate the pathogen in finished product prepared from sausage mix containing 10^6 *L. monocytogenes* CFU/g. However, since the presence of >10^3 *L. monocytogenes* CFU/g in commercially prepared sausage mix is highly unlikely, it appears that current heat treatments are adequate to produce *Listeria*-free semi-dry sausage.

While *L. monocytogenes* is unlikely to survive during manufacture of semi-dry sausage, ample opportunity exists for this pathogen to contaminate the finished product during slicing and packaging. Hence, to simulate postprocessing contamination, Glass and Doyle (80) inoculated slices of commercially produced, fermented semi-dry sausage to contain approximately 0.01 or 100 *L. monocytogenes* CFU/g, after which all samples were vacuum-packaged and quantitatively examined for listeriae during prolonged incubation at 4.4°C. Unlike ham, bologna, and frankfurters, the pathogen failed to grow on fermented semi-dry sausage of pH 4.8–5.2, with populations generally decreasing ≤10-fold on organoleptically acceptable samples after 6–12 weeks of refrigerated storage.

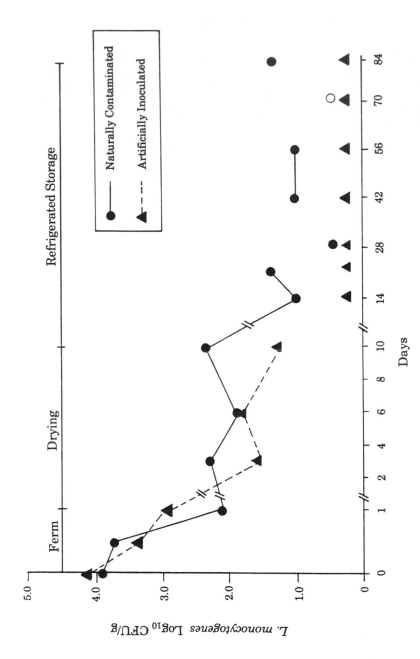

Figure 11.11   Behavior of *L. monocytogenes* during fermentation (Ferm), drying, and storage of hard salami prepared from naturally contaminated and artificially inoculated ground beef. Solid (●, ▲) and open (○) symbols at <1.0 $\log_{10}$ CFU/g represent positive and negative results, respectively, after 8 weeks of cold enrichment. (Adapted from Ref. 93.)

Recognizing the likelihood of listeriae being introduced into semi-dry sausage during slicing/packaging and surviving throughout the normal shelf life of the product, Cirigliano et al. (68) investigated the possibility of eliminating *L. monocytogenes* from inoculated slices of German- and Polish-type beef sausage (10^4–10^5 *L. monocytogenes* strain Scott A or V7 CFU/g) by exposing vacuum-packaged product to temperatures of 32.2–51.7°C (90–125°F) for up to 72 hours. According to the authors, *L. monocytogenes* populations failed to change in product held at 32.2°C (90°F); however, numbers of both *Listeria* strains decreased approximately 100-fold after product was held at 37.8°C (100°F) for 72 hours, with a slightly faster rate of inactivation observed in Polish- than German-type sausage. Although increasing the temperature to 43.3°C (110°F) led to elimination of strain V7 from Polish- and German-type sausage after 8 and 48 hours, respectively, strain Scott A was not eliminated from either product until completion of a 72-hour heat treatment. When exposed to 48.9 and 51.7°C (120 and 125°F), strain V7 was inactivated in Polish- and German-type sausages within 4 and 24 hours, respectively. While somewhat more heat resistant, strain Scott A was eliminated from both products after 24 hours at 51.7°C (125°F). In some instances, objectionable fat losses were observed for both product types; however, the authors concluded that mild heat treatments can be used to salvage *Listeria*-contaminated German- and Polish-type sausage without seriously affecting product quality.

Dry Fermented Sausage

Unlike semi-dry varieties, dry fermented sausages are never exposed to temperatures that would be expected to inactivate even small numbers of listeriae. Consequently, dry sausages have attracted more attention, as shown by several recent studies that examined the fate of *L. monocytogenes* during fermentation, drying, and storage of hard salami, pepperoni, and dry Finnish sausage.

In the first such study, Johnson et al. (93) prepared hard salami from naturally contaminated (i.e., meat from cows inoculated intravenously with *L. monocytogenes*) as well as artificially inoculated ground beef, both of which contained ~10^4 *L. monocytogenes* CFU/g. Glucose, spices, sodium nitrite, and salt were added to the ground beef along with a glucose-fermenting strain of *Pediococcus acidilactici*. After stuffing the mix into casings, all sausages were fermented at 40°C for 24 hours, dried at 13°C for 9 days, vacuum-packaged in gas-impermeable film, and stored at 4°C for 12 weeks. As shown by data in Fig. 11.11, *Listeria* populations decreased approximately 10- and 100-fold during fermentation (40°C/24 hours) of hard salami prepared from naturally contaminated and artificially inoculated ground beef, respectively. As will be seen shortly, inactivation of listeriae during the fermentation appears to be primarily attributable to production of lactic acid (or other metabolites) by the starter culture, with pH values decreasing from approximately 5.7 to 4.4 by the end of fermentation. Although numbers of listeriae remained relatively constant in naturally contaminated hard salami following 9 days of drying (13°C/65% R.H.), *Listeria* populations decreased nearly 100-fold during drying of product prepared from artificially inoculated ground beef. *Listeria monocytogenes* was detected in both products during 8 weeks of refrigerated storage; however, higher levels of listeriae were recovered from naturally contaminated rather than artificially inoculated hard salami, thus suggesting that behavior of this pathogen is best studied using sausage prepared from naturally contaminated rather than artificially inoculated ground beef. Compositionally, both products were very dry, having a_w values of 0.79–0.81 as compared to ~0.91 for commercially produced hard salami. Although *L. monocytogenes* might be expected to survive more readily in higher moisture commercial products, growth of the pathogen in retail hard salami appears unlikely given the presence of 5–7% NaCl and 100–150 ppm sodium nitrite combined with a pH of 4.3–4.5 and a relatively low storage temperature.

In contrast to the study just described, Truüssel and Jemmi (139) reported that *L. monocytogenes* populations in salami prepared from a mix inoculated to contain approximately 10^3 or 10^7 *L. monocytogenes* CFU/g decreased ≤10-fold in product of pH ≤5.6 during 7 days of ripening at 12–22°C/82–95% R.H. After 8 weeks of drying at 10–17°C/78–82% R.H., numbers of listeriae in salami of pH 5.4–5.7 decreased to <10 CFU/g, regardless of the initial inoculum. However, when an enrichment procedure was used, the pathogen still could be detected in these sausages after an additional 6–11 weeks of drying at 10–17°C/35–50% R.H. to a_w values of 0.68–0.69. Thus, as was true for certain fermented dairy products discussed in Chapter 10, small numbers of *L. monocytogenes* cells also can persist in fermented dry sausages for at least 14–19 weeks.

After recognizing that *L. monocytogenes* may survive the typical process used to manufacture hard salami, Glass and Doyle (81) attempted to identify various heat treatments that could be used to inactivate *L. monocytogenes* during manufacture of dry fermented sausage. Work with "beaker sausage" prepared from ground beef/pork containing 3.5% salt, 103 ppm sodium nitrite, and approximately 5×10^3 *L. monocytogenes* CFU/g indicated that numbers of listeriae decreased >10-fold following an active fermentation (32.2°C/16 h) with *P. acidilactici* during which the pH decreased from approximately 6.3 to 4.8. Prolific growth of *L. monocytogenes* in a similar lot of "beaker sausage" prepared without *P. acidilactici* confirms the importance of an active starter culture in preventing growth of listeriae in fermented sausage. Furthermore, these findings suggest that 3.5% salt and 103 ppm sodium nitrite are of virtually no value in preventing growth of listeriae in sausage mix. Subsequent holding of fermented "beaker sausage" at 46.1°C for 8 hours or heating to an internal temperature of 51.7 or 57.2°C failed to eliminate listeriae, with the pathogen still present in all samples examined according to the USDA enrichment method. While holding samples at 51.7°C for 8 hours or 57.2°C for 4 hours reduced *Listeria* populations >100-fold, enrichment results showed the pathogen was still present in one of two samples that received each of the two heat treatments. Only after heating "beaker sausage" to an internal temperature of 62.8°C was the pathogen no longer detected either by direct plating or enrichment.

Subsequently, Glass and Doyle (81) investigated the fate of *L. monocytogenes* in pepperoni during normal processing and storage and during heating to an internal temperature of 51.7°C for 4 hours immediately after fermentation or drying. After inoculating commercially prepared pepperoni mix to contain 10^4 *L. monocytogenes* CFU/g, populations of listeriae decreased approximately 100-fold following fermentation (35.6°C/12 h) by *P. acidilactici* which caused the pH to decrease from 6.0 to 4.7. These findings are similar to those of Johnson et al. (93) (Fig. 11.11), who found *Listeria* populations decreased 10- to 100-fold during fermentation of hard salami. Following 5 days of drying at 12.8°C, numbers of listeriae decreased to <10 CFU/g in normally processed pepperoni; however, with the USDA enrichment procedure, *L. monocytogenes* could still be detected in 82-day-old refrigerated samples of vacuum-packaged pepperoni. Heating the same pepperoni to an internal temperature of 51.7°C between fermentation and drying had relatively little effect on *L. monocytogenes*, with viable populations decreasing only about 10-fold. Although holding pepperoni for 4 hours at 51.7°C reduced *Listeria* populations to undetectable levels, as determined by direct plating and enrichment, the pathogen was sporadically recovered with the USDA enrichment procedure from 5- to 22-day-old sausage. Subsequent holding of the same pepperoni (pH 4.6) at an internal temperature of 51.7°C for 4 hours immediately after 26 days of drying at 12.8°C led to complete demise of the pathogen as determined by direct plating and enrichment procedures. Additional experiments conducted on pepperoni containing 5.3×10^3 *L. monocytogenes* CFU/g after 19 days of drying verified that a minimum heat treatment of 4 hours at 51.7°C was required to obtain a *Listeria*-free product. Thus, while normal processes used to manufacture pepperoni are not sufficient to eliminate *L. monocytogenes* from heavily contaminated product, holding pepperoni and possibly other dry sausages at an internal temperature of 51.7°C for at least 4 hours may prove to be a viable means of salvaging contaminated product.

Although the antibotulinal properties of nitrate and particularly nitrite have been recognized for years, present scientific literature contains relatively little information concerning the effect of these preservatives on *Listeria* behavior in dry fermented sausage. As of July 1990, only one such study was reported in which Junttila et al. (94) examined the ability of *L. monocytogenes* to survive in dry Finnish sausage containing various levels of potassium nitrate, sodium nitrite, and salt. All sausage was prepared from a mixture of ground beef and pork to which sugar, spices, and 3 or 3.5% salt were added along with 50–1000 ppm potassium nitrate and/or sodium nitrite. After inoculation to contain ~10^5 *L. monocytogenes* CFU/g and a starter culture consisting of *Staphylococcus carnosus* and *Lactobacillus plantarum*, the sausage mix was stuffed into casings. All sausage links were fermented 2 days at 23°C, smoked 5 days at 20–22°C and dried 1 week each at 18 and 10°C. *Listeria monocytogenes* populations in sausage containing commonly used levels of salt (3.0%) and sodium nitrite (120 ppm) decreased 1.14 orders of magnitude over 21 days (Fig. 11.12). Similar findings also were reported when 3.5 rather than 3.0% salt was used. Increasing levels of sodium nitrite (200 ppm) and potassium nitrate (330 ppm) to those commonly used 30 years ago led to somewhat faster demise of listeriae in dry fermented sausage, with inactivation again most pronounced during the later stage of drying. Over the same 21-day period, *Listeria* populations decreased approximately 3.3 orders of magnitude in sausage containing 3.5% salt and 1000 ppm potassium nitrate; however, this concentration of potassium nitrate is no longer permitted in dry fermented sausage. Growth of *L. monocytogenes* in this product apparently was suppressed by the combination of salt, sodium nitrite, and a pH of 4.7; however, given the pathogen's known tolerance to salt, acid, and low temperatures, addition of commonly used levels of sodium nitrite to fermented sausage was only marginally effective in inactivating listeriae. Thus, while this and other studies have provided valuable information concerning behavior of *L. monocytogenes* in sausage products, an understanding of interactions between various factors such as starter cultures, food additives, and various heat treatments is still needed to develop suitable methods to eliminate *L. monocytogenes* from fermented sausage and other processed meat products.

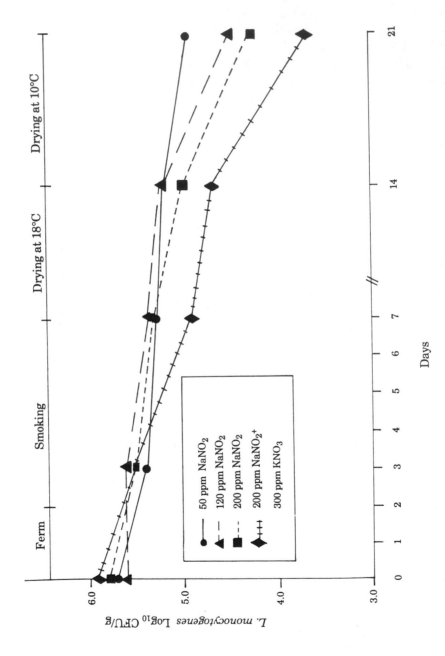

Figure 11.12 Fate of *L. monocytogenes* during fermentation (Ferm), smoking, and drying of Finnish sausage prepared from ground beef/pork containing 3% NaCl and various concentrations of $NaNO_2$ and/or KNO_3. (Adapted from Ref. 94.)

REFERENCES

1. Al-Sheddy, I., and E. R. Richter. 1989. Microbiological quality/safety of zoo food. Ann. Mtg., Inst. Food Technol., Chicago, IL, June 26–29, Abstr. 476.
2. Amtsberg, G. von, A. Elsner, H. A. Gabbar, and W. Winkenwerder. 1969. Die epidemiologische und lebensmittelhygienische Bedeutung der Listerieninfektion des Rindes. *Dtsch. tierärztl. Wschr.* 76:497–536.
3. Anonymous. 1985. FSIS to expand *Listeria, Salmonella* control efforts. *Food Chem. News* 27(42):20–22.
4. Anonymous. 1987. FSIS to give firms 5 days for clean-up before resampling for *Listeria. Food Chem. News* 29(32):7–9.
5. Anonymous. 1987. Ice cream industry seeks parity with meat industry on *Listeria* policy. *Food Chem. News* 29(23):15.
6. Anonymous. 1987. *Listeria* confirmed by FSIS in Florida plant's corned beef. *Food Chem. News* 29(40):32–33.
7. Anonymous. 1987. USDA *Listeria* policy allows chance for cleanup before recall. *Food Chem. News* 29(24):50–54.
8. Anonymous. 1987. USDA *Listeria* policy to consider control problems, Houston indicates. *Food Chem. News* 29(15):32.
9. Anonymous. 1987. *Listeria* proposed plan would permit sale of contaminated products. *Food Chem. News* 29(19):3–6.
10. Anonymous. 1987. *Listeria* sampling of sliced lunch meats, jerky expected by year-end. *Food Chem. News* 29(27):28–29.
11. Anonymous. 1987. Microbiological criteria group should consider *Listeria* issue: NFPA. *Food Chem. News* 29(8):44–45.
12. Anonymous. 1987. USDA *Listeria* recalls to be restricted to single items. *Food Chem. News* 29(25):9.
13. Anonymous. 1987. USDA to delay *Listeria* testing of meat, poultry. *Food Chem. News* 29(5):3.
14. Anonymous. 1987. USDA to limit *Listeria* recalls to sampled production lot. *Food Chem. News* 29(31):30.
15. Anonymous. 1987. Zero *Listeria* tolerance in meat, poultry may be recommended. *Food Chem. News* 29(11):31–32.
16. Anonymous. 1988. AMI data show frankfurters most likely *Listeria* carrier in meat. *Food Chem. News* 30(16):37–39.
17. Anonymous. 1988. FSIS recommends 35°F for long-term storage of meat, poultry. *Food Chem. News* 30(12):25–28.
18. Anonymous. 1988. Hot dog processing "borderline" for *Listeria* destruction: ARS. *Food Chem. News* 30(41):46.
19. Anonymous. 1988. *Listeria* destruction in cooked meat products ineffective: Hormel. *Food Chem. News* 30(15):32–34.
20. Anonymous. 1988. *Listeria*-in-meat monitoring results reported by USDA. *Food Chem. News* 30(10):36–37.
21. Anonymous. 1988. Wisconsin agrees to delay *Listeria* testing of meat products. *Food Chem. News* 30(14):32–33.
22. Anonymous. 1988. Wisconsin *Listeria* testing program for processed meat set. *Food Chem. News* 30(40):52.
23. Anonymous. 1989. Current meat processing may not kill *Listeria*, study shows. *Food Chem. News* 30(52):57–58.
24. Anonymous. 1989. FDA to survey prepared sandwiches for *Listeria, Salmonella. Food Chem. News* 31(25):25–26.
25. Anonymous. 1989. Frozen heat and serve chili dog, chili and cheese dog sandwiches recalled. FDA Enforcement Report, Nov. 29.
26. Anonymous. 1989. FSIS asserts jurisdiction in Wisconsin *Listeria*-in-meat program. *Food Chem. News* 30(49):42–44.

27. Anonymous. 1989. FSIS issues directive outlining *Listeria* program. *Food Chem. News* *30*(52):58.
28. Anonymous. 1989. *Listeria* found by FSIS in small number but wide range of products. *Food Chem. News 31*(30):47–48.
29. Anonymous. 1989. *Listeria* recalls can be avoided, USDA tells meat processors. *Food Chem. News 31*(17):3–5.
30. Anonymous. 1989. *Listeria* tolerances asked by meat, poultry group. *Food Chem. News 31*(14):46–48.
31. Anonymous. 1989. *Listeria* zero tolerance is warranted, USDA says. *Food Chem. News 31*(19):47–48.
32. Anonymous. 1989. Prepared meat and cheese sandwiches recalled. FDA Enforcement Report, Oct. 11.
33. Anonymous. 1989. Prepared sandwiches recalled because of *Listeria*. *Food Chem. News 31*(16):23.
34. Anonymous. 1989. Refrigerated fresh and frozen sandwiches recalled. FDA Enforcement Report, Dec. 20.
35. Anonymous. 1989. Sausage and egg biscuit sandwiches recalled. FDA Enforcement Report, Dec. 13.
36. Anonymous. 1989. Sausage recalled in Rhode Island, Massachusetts because of *Listeria*. *Food Chem. News 31*(38):33.
37. Anonymous. 1989. Smaller *Listeria* test sample decreases sensitivity, study shows. *Food Chem. News 31*(11):47.
38. Anonymous. 1989. USDA announces first *Listeria* recall under amended policy. *Food Chem. News 31*(24):20.
39. Anonymous. 1989. USDA to increase *Listeria* sample size, demand recalls of positives. *Food Chem. News 31*(11):65–67.
40. Anonymous. 1989. USDA to toughen regulatory policy on *Listeria* in meat, poultry. *Food Chem. News 31*(8):52–53.
41. Anonymous. 1989. Various prepared sandwiches recalled. FDA Enforcement Report, June 14.
42. Anonymous. 1990. CDC links Cajun pork sausage to listeriosis case: Product recalled. *Food Chem. News 31*(44):35.
43. Anonymous. 1990. Class I recall made of sandwiches because of *Listeria*. *Food Chem. News 31*(49):52–53.
44. Anonymous. 1990. Food-borne *Listeria* implicated in 1989 death of Canadian woman. *Food Chem. News 32*(13):61.
45. Anonymous. 1990. FSIS blocklists cooked beef from Argentine plant due to *Listeria*. *Food Chem. News 32*(9):62–63.
46. Anonymous. 1990. FSIS plans adjustments to *Listeria* regulatory program. *Food Chem. News 31*(27):49–50.
47. Anonymous. 1990. Investigators unable to pinpoint *Listeria* source in Canadian death. *Food Chem. News 32*(14):48–49.
48. Anonymous. 1990. *Listeria monocytogenes* contamination of sandwiches uncovered by FDA at Stewart Sandwiches, Inc., Norfolk, VA. *Food Chem. News 32*(14):2.
49. Anonymous. 1990. Prepared sandwiches recalled. FDA Enforcement Report, Jan. 31.
50. Anonymous. 1990. Stewart sandwiches injunction would close plant. *Food Chem. News 32*(15):17–19.
51. Anonymous. 1990. USDA meat patty reproposal cites *Listeria* concern, drops micro tests. *Food Chem. News 32*(15):26–30.
52. Anonymous. 1990. USDA monitoring finds *Listeria* in ready-to-eat products at 78 plants. *Food Chem. News 32*(7):71–73.
53. Barnes, R., P. Archer, J. Stack, and G. R. Istre. 1989. Listeriosis associated with consumption of turkey franks. *Morbid. Mortal. Weekly Report 38*:267–168.

54. Berry, E. D., M. B. Liewen, R. W. Mandigo, and R. W. Hutkins. 1990. Inhibition of *Listeria monocytogenes* by bacteriocin-producing *Pediococcus* during the manufacture of fermented semidry sausage. *J. Food Prot.* 53:194–197.
55. Bind, J.-L. 1988. Review of latest information concerning data about repartition of *Listeria* in France. WHO Working Group on Foodborne Listeriosis, Geneva, Switzerland, February 15–19.
56. Boyle, D. L., J. N. Sofos, and G. R. Schmidt. 1989. Thermal destruction of *Listeria monocytogenes* in a meat slurry and in ground beef. *J. Food Sci.* 55:327–329.
57. Breer, C., and G. Breer. 1988. The isolation of *Listeria* spp. in meat and meat products. In *Proc. 34th Int. Congress Meat Sci. Technol.*, Brisbane, Australia, Part B, pp. 520–521.
58. Breer, C., and K. Schopfer. 1989. Listerien in Nahrungsmitteln. *Schweiz. med. Wschr. 119*:306–311.
59. Breuer, J. von, and O. Prändl. 1988. Nachweis von Listerien und deren Vorkommen in Hackfleisch und Mettwürsten in Österreich. *Arch. Lebensmittelhyg. 39*:28–30.
60. Buchanan, R. L., H. G. Stahl, M. M. Bencivengo, and F. del Corral. 1989. Comparison of lithium chloride-phenylethanol-moxalactam and modified Vogel-Johnson agars for detection of *Listeria* spp. in retail-level meats, poultry and seafood. *Appl. Environ. Microbiol.* 55:599–603.
61. Cantoni, C., M. Valenti, and G. Comi. 1988. *Listeria* in formaggi e in salumi. *Ind. Aliment.* 27:859–861.
62. Cantoni, C., C. Balzaretti, and M. Valenti. 1989. A case of *Listeria monocytogenes* human infection associated with consumption of "Testa in Cascetta" (cooked meat pork product). *Arch. Vet. Ital. 40*:141–142.
63. Cantoni, C., M. Valenti, and G. Comi. 1989. *L. monocytogenes* nei salumifici e nei prodotti di salumeria. *Ind. Aliment. 28*:605–607, 610.
64. Carosella, J. M. 1988. Occurrence of *Listeria monocytogenes* in meat and poultry. Society for Industrial Microbiology—Comprehensive Conference on *Listeria monocytogenes*, Rohnert Park, CA, Oct. 2–5, Abstr. I-23.
65. Carosella, J. M. 1989. Personal communication.
66. Chung, K.-T., J. S. Dickson, and J. D. Crouse. 1989. Attachment and proliferation of bacteria on meat. *J. Food Prot. 52*:173–177.
67. Chung, K.-T., J. S. Dickson, and J. D. Crouse. 1989. Effects of nisin on growth of *Listeria monocytogenes* on meat. Ann. Mtg., Amer. Soc. Microbiol., New Orleans, LA, May 14–18, Abstr. P-11.
68. Cirigliano, M. C., R. M. Ehioba, and R. T. McKenna. 1989. Unpublished data.
69. Cottin, J., H. Genthon, C. Bizon, and B. Carbonnelle. 1985. Recherche de *Listeria monocytogenes* dans des viandes prélevées sur 514 bovins. *Sci. Aliment. 5*:145–149.
70. Crawford, L. M. 1989. Food Safety and Inspection Service—revised policy for controlling *Listeria monocytogenes*. Fed. Reg. 54:22345–22346.
71. Dickson, J. S. 1990. Transfer of *Listeria monocytogenes* and *Salmonella typhimurium* between beef tissue surfaces. *J. Food Prot. 53*:51–55.
72. Dumur, P., J.-L. Bind, and A. Audurier. Ecologie des *Listeria* dans les aliments autres que les produits laitiers. *Sci. Aliment. 9*:97–102.
73. Elischerova, K., S. Stupalova, and J. Stepanek. 1979. Some ecological aspects of *Listeria monocytogenes* in the meat industry. In I. Ivanov (ed.), *Problems of Listeriosis. Proc. 7th Int. Symp. National Agroindustrial Union*, Center for Scientific Information, Sofia, pp. 148–155.
74. El-Shenawy, M. A., A. E. Yousef, and E. H. Marth. 1989. Radiation sensitivity of *Listeria monocytogenes* in broth or in raw ground beef. *Lebensm. Wiss. Technol. 22*:387–390.
75. El-Zawahry, Y. A., and D. B. Rowley. 1979. Radiation resistance and injury of *Yersinia enterocolitica*. *Appl. Environ. Microbiol. 37*:50–54.
76. Farber, J. M., and B. E. Brown. 1989. The effect of prior heat shock on the heat resistance of *Listeria monocytogenes* in meat. *J. Food Prot. 52*:750. (Abstr.)
77. Farber, J. M., A. Hughes, and R. Holley. 1988. Thermal resistance of *Listeria monocytogenes* in sausage meat. Tenth Int. Symposium on Listeriosis, Pecs, Hungary, Aug. 22–26, Abstr. 51.

78. Farber, J. M., F. Tittiger, and L. Gour. 1988. Surveillance of raw-fermented (dry-cured) sausages for the presence of *Listeria* spp. *Can. Inst. Food Sci. Technol. J. 21*:430–434.
79. Gilbert, R. J., S. M. Hall, and A. G. Taylor. 1989. Listeriosis update. *Public Health Laboratory Service Digest 6*:33–37.
80. Glass, K. A., and M. P. Doyle. 1989. Fate of *Listeria monocytogenes* in processed meat products during refrigerated storage. *Appl. Environ. Microbiol. 55*:1565–1569.
81. Glass, K. A., and M. P. Doyle. 1989. Fate and thermal inactivation of *Listeria monocytogenes* in beaker sausage and pepperoni. *J. Food Prot. 52*:226–231, 235.
82. Gouet, Ph., J. Labadie, and C. Serratore. 1978. Development of *Listeria monocytogenes* in monoxenic and polyxenic beef minces. *Zbl. Bakteriol. Hyg., I Abt. Orig. B 166*:87–94.
83. Grau, F. H., and P. B. Vanderlinde. 1988. Growth of *Listeria monocytogenes* on vacuum packaged beef. In *Proc. Int. Congress Meat Sci. Technol.*, Brisbane, Australia, Part B, pp. 518–519.
84. Green, S. 1990. Personal communication.
85. Herald, P. J., and E. A. Zottola. 1988. Attachment of *Listeria monocytogenes* to stainless steel surfaces at various temperatures and pH values. *J. Food Sci. 53*:1549–1552, 1562.
86. Höhne, K. 1972. Über die Entwicklung eines neuen selecktiven Kombinations-Medium zum Nachweis von *Listeria monocytogenes* mit einem Hinweis auf den Listeriabefall des Schlachtschweines. Inaug. Diss., Univ. Würzburg. In Höhne, K., B. Loose, and H. P. R. Seeliger. 1975. Isolation of *Listeria monocytogenes* in slaughter animals and bats of Togo (West Africa). *Ann. Inst. Pasteur Microbiol. 126A*:501–507.
87. Höhne, K., B. Loose, and H. P. R. Seeliger. 1975. Isolation of *Listeria monocytogenes* in slaughter animals and bats of Togo (West Africa). *Ann. Inst. Pasteur Microbiol. 126A*:501–507.
88. Houston, D. L. 1987. Food Safety and Inspection Service—testing for *Listeria monocytogenes*. *Fed. Reg. 52*:7464–7465.
89. Hughey, V. L., P. A. Wilger, and E. A. Johnson. 1989. Antibacterial activity of hen egg white lysozyme against *Listeria monocytogenes* Scott A in foods. *Appl. Environ. Microbiol. 55*:631–638.
90. Johnson, J. L., M. P. Doyle, and R. G. Cassens. 1988. Survival of *Listeria monocytogenes* in ground beef. *Int. J. Food Microbiol. 6*:243–247.
91. Johnson, J. L., M. P. Doyle, and R. G. Cassens. 1990. Incidence of *Listeria* spp. in retail meat roasts. *J. Food Sci. 55*:572–574.
92. Johnson, J. L., R. G. Cassens, M. P. Doyle, and J. T. Beery. 1988. Microbiological and histochemical examination of muscle for *Listeria monocytogenes*. Ann. Mtg., Inst. Food Technol., New Orleans, LA, June 19–22, Abstr. 324.
93. Johnson, J. L., M. P. Doyle, R. G. Cassens, and J. L. Schoeni. 1988. Fate of *Listeria monocytogenes* in tissues of experimentally infected cattle and in hard salami. *Appl. Environ. Microbiol. 54*:497–501.
94. Junttila, J., J. Hirn, P. Hill, and E. Nurmi. 1989. Effect of different levels of nitrite and nitrate on the survival of *Listeria monocytogenes* during the manufacture of fermented sausage. *J. Food Prot. 52*:158–161.
95. Kampelmacher, E. H. 1962. Animal products as a source of listeric infection in man. In M. L. Gray (ed.), Second symposium on listeric infection, Montana State College, Bozeman, MT, pp. 146–156.
96. Karaioannoglou, P. G., and G. C. Xenos. 1980. Survival of *Listeria monocytogenes* in meatballs. *Hell. Vet. Med. 23*:111–117.
97. Karches, H., and P. Teufel. 1988. *Listeria monocytogenes* Vorkommen in Hackfleisch und Verhalten in frischer Zwiebelmettwurst. *Fleischwirtschaft 68*:1388–1392.
98. Kaya, M., and U. Schmidt. 1989. Verhalten von *Listeria monocytogenes* im Hackfleisch bei Kühl- und Gefrierlagerung. *Fleischwirtschaft 69*:617–620.
99. Khan, M. A., C. V. Palmas, A. Seaman, and M. Woodbine. 1973. Survival versus growth of a facultative psychrotroph in meat and products of meat. *Zbl. Bakteriol. Hyg., I Abt. Orig. B 157*:277–282.

100. Khan, M. A., I. A. Newton, A. Seaman, and M. Woodbine. 1975. Survival of *Listeria monocytogenes* inside and outside its host. In M. Woodbine (ed.), *Problems of Listeriosis.* Leicester University Press, Surrey, England, pp. 75–83.

101. Kleinlein, N., F. Untermann, and H. Beissner. 1989. Zum Vorkommen von *Salmonella* und *Yersinia*—Spezies sowie *Listeria monocytogenes* in Hackfleisch. *Fleischwirtschaft 69*:1474–1476.

102. Kokubo, Y., I. Takashi, S. Kaneko, and T. Maruyama. 1990. Evaluation of enrichment and plating media for isolating *Listeria monocytogenes* from raw meat. *Shokuhin Eiseigaku Zusshi 31*:51–56.

103. Lee, C. Y., D. Y. C. Fung, and C. L. Kastner. 1982. Computer-assisted identification of bacteria on hot-boned and conventionally processed beef. *J. Food Sci. 47*:363–367, 373.

104. Lee, C. Y., D. Y. C. Fung, and C. L. Kastner. 1985. Computer-assisted identification of microflora on hot-boned and conventionally processed beef: Effect of moderate and slow chilling rate. *J. Food Sci. 50*:553–567.

105. Le Guilloux, M., Cl. Dollinger, and G. Freyburger. 1980. *Listeria monocytogenes*—Sa fréquence dans les produits de charcuterie. *Bull. Soc. Vet. Prat. France 64*(1):45–53.

106. Lieval, F., J. Tache, and M. Poumeyrol. 1989. Qualité microbiologique et *Listeria* sp. dans les produits de la restauration rapide. *Sci. Aliment. 9*:111–115.

107. Lovett, J., D. W. Francis, and J. G. Bradshaw. 1988. Outgrowth of *Listeria monocytogenes* in foods. Society for Industrial Microbiology—Comprehensive Conference on *Listeria monocytogenes*, Rohnert Park, CA, Oct. 2–5, Abstr. I-26.

108. Lowry, P. D., and I. Tiong. 1988. The incidence of *Listeria monocytogenes* in meat and meat products: Factors affecting distribution. In *Proc. 34th Int. Congress Meat Sci. Technol.*, Brisbane, Australia, Part B, pp. 528–530.

109. Luppi, A., G. Bucci, P. Maini, and J. Rocourt. 1988. Ecological survey of *Listeria* in the Ferrara area (Northern Italy). *Zbl. Bakteriol. Hyg. A 269*:266–275.

110. Mackey, B. M., and N. Bratchell. 1989. A review—The heat resistance of *Listeria monocytogenes. Lett. Appl. Microbiol. 9*:89–94.

111. McClain, D., and W. H. Lee. 1988. Development of USDA-FSIS method for isolation of *Listeria monocytogenes* from raw meat and poultry. *J. Assoc. Off. Anal. Chem. 71*:660–664.

112. Messina, M. C., H. A. Ahmad, J. A. Marchello, C. P. Gerba, and M. W. Paquette. 1988. The effect of liquid smoke on *Listeria monocytogenes. J. Food Prot. 51*:629–631, 638.

113. Montgomery, E. 1990. Personal communication.

114. Netten, P. van, and D. A. A. Mossel. 1981. The ecological consequences of decontaminating raw meat surfaces with lactic acid. *Arch. Lebensmittelhyg. 33*:190–191.

115. Nicolas, J.-A. 1985. Contamination des viandes et des produits de charcuterie par *Listeria monocytogenes* en Haute-Vienne. *Sci. Aliment. 5*:175–180.

116. Nicolas, J.-A., and N. Vidaud. 1987. Contribution à l'étude des *Listeria* présentes dans les denrées d'origine animale destinées à la consommation humaine. *Recueil de Medecine Veterinaire 163*:283–285.

117. Nicolas, J.-A., M. J. Cornuejols, N. Hangard-Vidaud, C. Boisgiraud, and A. Menudier. 1989. Etude de la virulence de *Listeria monocytogenes* isolées des aliments. *Sci. Aliment. 9*:31–37.

118. Nicolas, J.-A., E.-C. Espaze, B. Catimel, N. Vidaud, J. Rocourt, and A.-L. Courtieu. 1989. Isolation of *Listeria* from French meat products. *Zbl. Bakteriol. 272*:242–247.

119. Ozari, R. von, and F. A. Stolle. 1990. Zum Vorkommen von *Listeria monocytogenes* in Fleisch und Fleisch-Erzeugnissen einschliesslich Geflügelfleisch des Handels. *Arch. Lebensmittelhyg. 41*:47–50.

120. Poumeyrol, M. 1988. Bactéries "nouvelles" dans les viandes. *Viandes Produits Carnés 9*:135–141.

121. Pucci, M. J., E. R. Vedamuthu, B. S. Kunka, and P. A. Vandebergh. 1988. Inhibition of *Listeria monocytogenes* by using bacteriocin PA-1 produced by *Pediococcus acidilactici* PAC 1.0. *Appl. Environ. Microbiol. 54*:2349–2353.

122. Quintavalla, S., and S. Barbuti. 1989. Caractérisation microbiologique et résistance thermique de *Listeria* isolée de produits de viande. *Sci. Aliment.* 9:125–128.
123. Ralovich, B., and A. Proksza. 1988. Presence of *Listeria*—strains in home-made sausage. Tenth Int. Symposium on Listeriosis, Pecs, Hungary, Aug. 22–26, Abstr. P58.
124. Richmond, M. 1990. Report of the Committee on the Microbiological Safety of Food, HMSO, pp. 133–137.
125. Rocourt, J., H. Hoff, A. Schrettenbrunner, R. Malinverni, and J. Bille. 1986. Méningite purulente aiguë à *Listeria seeligeri* chez un adulte immunocompétent. *Schweiz med. Wschr.* 116:248–251.
126. Schmidt, V., H. P. R. Seeliger, E. Glenn, B. Langer, and L. Leistner. 1988. *Listeria* findings in raw meat products. *Fleischwirtschaft* 68:1313–1316.
127. Schoen, R., and G. Terplan. Personal communication.
128. Seeliger, H. P. R. 1961. *Listeriosis*, Hafner Publishing Co., New York.
129. Shelef, L. A. 1989. Survival of *Listeria monocytogenes* in ground beef or liver during storage at 4 and 25°C. *J. Food Prot.* 52:379–383.
130. Sielaff, H. 1966. Die lebensmittelhygienische Bedeutung der Listeriose. *Monatsh. Veterinarmed.* 21:750–758.
131. Skovgaard, N., and C.-A. Morgen. 1988. Detection of *Listeria* spp. in faeces from animals, in feeds, and in raw foods of animal origin. *Int. J. Food Microbiol.* 6:229–242.
132. Skovgaard, N., and B. Nørrung. 1989. The incidence of *Listeria* spp. in faeces of Danish pigs and in minced pork meat. *Int. J. Food Microbiol.* 8:59–63.
133. Slivko, V. V. 1958. Survival of *Listeria* in meat. *Vet. Bull.* 29:168.
134. Stegeman, H. 1988. Radiation resistance of *Listeria monocytogenes*. Tenth Int. Symposium on Listeriosis, Pecs, Hungary, Aug. 22–26, Abstr. P56.
135. Stegeman, H., B. J. Hartog, F. K. Stekelenburg, and J. P. M. den Hartog. 1988. The effect of heat pasteurization on *Listeria monocytogenes* in canned cured ham. Tenth Int. Symposium on Listeriosis, Pecs, Hungary, Aug. 22–26, Abstr. P55.
136. Sumner, S. S., T. M. Sandros, M. Harmon, V. N. Scott, and D. T. Bernard. 1989. Effect of water activity on the heat resistance of *Salmonella* and *Listeria*. Ann. Mtg., Inst. Food Technol., Chicago, IL, June 25–29, Abstr. 465.
137. Ternström, A., and G. Molin. 1987. Incidence of potential pathogens on raw pork, beef and chicken in Sweden, with special reference to *Erysipelothrix rhusiopathiae*. *J. Food Prot.* 50:141–146, 149.
138. Truscott, R. B., and W. B. McNab. 1988. Comparison of media and procedures for the isolation of *Listeria monocytogenes* from ground beef. *J. Food Prot.* 51:626–628, 638.
139. Trüssel, M., and T. Jemmi. 1989. The behavior of *Listeria monocytogenes* during the ripening and storage of artificially contaminated salami and Mettwurst. *Fleischwirtschaft* 69:1586–1593.
140. Urbain, W. M. 1986. *Food Irradiation*, Academic Press, New York.
141. Weis, J. 1989. Vorkommen von Listerien in Hackfleisch. *Tierärztl. Umschau* 44:370–375.
142. Wendorff, W. L. 1989. Effect of smoke flavorings on *Listeria monocytogenes* in skinless franks. Seminar presentation, Department of Food Science, University of Wisconsin-Madison, Jan. 13.
143. Wramby, G. O. 1944. Unpublished data. In Bojsen-Møller, J. 1972. Human listeriosis—Diagnostic, epidemiological and clinical studies. *Acta Pathol. Microbiol. Scand. B* 229:39.
144. Zaika, L. L., S. A. Palumbo, J. L. Smith, F. del Corral, S. Bhaduri, C. O. Jones, and A. H. Kim. 1990. Destruction of *Listeria monocytogenes* during frankfurter processing. *J. Food Prot.* 53:18–21.

12

Incidence and Behavior of *Listeria monocytogenes* in Poultry and Egg Products

INTRODUCTION

Avian listeriosis was first recognized in 1932 when TenBroeck isolated *L. monocytogenes* (then *Bacterium monocytogenes*) from diseased chickens (76). While chickens have remained the most common avian host for *L. monocytogenes*, during the nearly 60 years since avian listeriosis was recognized (40), listeriosis also has been observed in at least 22 other avian species, including such frequently consumed fowl as turkeys (22,44,64), ducks (40,77), geese (40,77), and pheasants (40). Large outbreaks of listeriosis in domestic fowl are relatively rare (63); however, sporadic cases occur much more frequently and are often accompanied by asymptomatic shedding of *L. monocytogenes* in feces. Hence, as was true for beef, pork, and lamb, poultry meat destined for human consumption also is at risk of becoming contaminated with *L. monocytogenes*, particularly when birds are slaughtered, defeathered, and eviscerated. Several early studies suggested that poultry- and egg-processing workers can contract listeric infections by handling contaminated birds (30,52). Additionally, several reports from England during the 1970s indicated that *L. monocytogenes* could be isolated with some frequency from raw chicken as well as turkey, duck, and pheasant. Nevertheless, consumption of poultry products has only recently been linked to human cases of listeriosis. An added concern with poultry relates to eggs that might become contaminated with this pathogen during collecting and processing.

The emergence of *L. monocytogenes* as a bona fide foodborne pathogen following the Mexican-style cheese outbreak of 1985 prompted immediate concern about presence of listeriae in dairy products and also generated a parallel interest in the incidence and behavior of *L. monocytogenes* in meat and poultry products; the latter is the topic of this chapter. Interest in this area has increased as a result of several listeriosis cases that were directly linked to consumption of turkey frankfurters and ready-to-eat/cook-chill poultry products in the United States and England, respectively.

In the same format used in Chapter 11, the position of the USDA-FSIS regarding presence of listeriae in raw and processed poultry products will be reviewed first before discussing results from surveys done to establish the incidence of *L. monocytogenes* in raw and processed poultry products manufactured in the United States and Western Europe. This information will be followed by findings that pertain to growth and survival as well as thermal and irradiation resistance of *L. monocytogenes* in poultry products. A

463

discussion of the incidence and behavior of *L. monocytogenes* in egg products appears on the final pages of this chapter.

USDA-FSIS *LISTERIA*-MONITORING/VERIFICATION PROGRAM FOR COOKED/READY-TO-EAT POULTRY PRODUCTS

Public health concerns about *Listeria*-contaminated raw and, particularly, processed ready-to-eat poultry products sold in the United States also stem directly from the 1985 listeriosis outbreak in California associated with consumption of Mexican-style cheese. Consequently, as mentioned in the previous chapter, it is not surprising that USDA-FSIS officials soon thereafter announced their intentions to develop *Listeria*-monitoring/verification programs for cooked and ready-to-eat meat as well as poultry products. Since these *Listeria*-monitoring/verification programs for meat and poultry products developed in parallel and were both similar in terms of sampling scheme, methodology, and action taken upon finding *L. monocytogenes* in a product, the following discussion will focus on the various products tested and pertinent results rather than on an in-depth analysis of this program. Such an analysis can be found in Chapter 11 and deals with the program as it pertains to cooked/ready-to-eat meat products.

A *Listeria*-monitoring/verification program for cooked/ready-to-eat poultry was first suggested in December 1985 and was to cover all such products prepared in federally inspected establishments as well as those produced by certified foreign manufacturers (45). However, actual testing of poultry sausage, i.e., the first category of ready-to-eat poultry products examined, did not begin until September 1988, one year after the *Listeria* monitoring/verification program was first instituted for cooked beef, roast beef, and cooked corned beef.

Before April 1989, USDA's *Listeria* policy, which gave firms the opportunity to clean up their facility before additional verification samples were analyzed under hold-test procedures, was consistent with the fact that listeriosis had not yet been linked to consumption of poultry products. However, the official USDA-FSIS position regarding presence of *L. monocytogenes* in cooked and ready-to-eat poultry products changed radically on April 14, 1989, when CDC investigators directly linked consumption of contaminated turkey frankfurters to a case of listeric meningitis in a breast cancer patient in Oklahoma (14). After isolating *L. monocytogenes* serotype 1/2a of the same electrophoretic enzyme type from the woman and opened as well as unopened retail packages of turkey frankfurters, USDA-FSIS officials requested that the manufacturer issue an immediate Class I recall for approximately 600,000 pounds of Texas-produced turkey frankfurters that were marketed by retail and institutional establishments in Alaska, Arizona, Arkansas, California, Florida, Georgia, Idaho, Illinois, Indiana, Kentucky, Louisiana, Mississippi, Missouri, New Jersey, New York, Ohio, Oklahoma, Pennsylvania, Tennessee, Texas, Utah, and Washington. As expected, this recall immediately prompted an intensified monitoring/verification program to determine the extent of *Listeria* contamination in a far wider range of cooked/ready-to-eat poultry products marketed in the United States.

Despite pleas by the National Turkey Association to adopt tolerance levels for *L. monocytogenes* in cooked and ready-to-eat poultry products (9), USDA-FSIS officials rightly maintained that since an "acceptable level" of *L. monocytogenes* in such products cannot be determined from present knowledge of foodborne listeriosis, the only acceptable alternative is to adopt a policy of "zero tolerance" for this pathogen in cooked/ready-to-eat poultry and meat products (10). Consequently, under the new program (29) which is identical to that developed for cooked and ready-to-eat red meat products, USDA-FSIS officials will request firms to issue a Class I recall for all lots of cooked and ready-to-eat poultry products in which *L. monocytogenes* is detected in monitoring samples taken from intact packages of product. However, *Listeria*-positive lots that are still under direct control of the manufacturer can be recalled internally, thus avoiding adverse publicity. If the pathogen is initially detected in monitoring samples from unpackaged products, USDA-FSIS officials will not request firms to immediately recall the sampled lot. Instead, government officials will analyze subsequent lots and, if necessary, initiate further steps (i.e., hold-test programs) to prevent production of contaminated products.

Our knowledge concerning the incidence of listeriae in cooked/ready-to-eat poultry products marketed in the United States is currently limited to data gathered from the USDA-FSIS *Listeria*-monitoring/verification programs with present results indicating that ~1.5–2.0% of all such products are contaminated with *L. monocytogenes* (7,18,26). During the 12-month period beginning in April 1989, 12 poultry processors were cited for producing various cooked/ready-to-eat poultry products that contained *L. monocytogenes*. Included were chicken patties (7), chicken thighs (7), chicken salad (7), diced poultry (7), poultry salad (18), poultry spread (18), poultry frankfurters (7), poultry bologna (7), and turkey sausage (7). In all likelihood, the pathogen entered these products during the later stages of manufacture and/or packaging. Since most manufacturers retained all product lots that were sampled until results of *Listeria* testing became known, formal Class I recalls for such products thus far appear to be limited to the aforementioned recall of turkey frankfurters (14), two recalls of chicken salad (4,6), and one additional incident involving 13,000 pounds of chicken spread produced by a Virginia-based firm (15). However, numerous Class I recalls have been issued for prepared delicatessen-type sandwiches (see Table 11.2), with at least two of these recalls (11,17) involving items that also contained processed chicken and/or turkey.

INCIDENCE OF *LISTERIA* SPP. IN RAW POULTRY MARKETED IN THE UNITED STATES

Immediately after the 1985 listeriosis outbreak in California was announced, public concerns were raised about safety of dairy products and other potentially contaminated foods, including meat and poultry products. Interest in the safety of raw poultry soon escalated following a nationwide telecast which informed the general public that ~50% of all raw chicken marketed in the United States was contaminated with *Salmonella*. Consequently, several surveys were initiated to determine the extent to which raw chicken and turkey meat are contaminated with *Listeria* and *Salmonella*.

Chicken

The aforementioned concerns prompted USDA-FSIS officials to initiate a poultry back/neck testing program for *L. monocytogenes*, *Salmonella*, and *Escherichia coli*

Table 12.1 Incidence of *Listeria* spp. on Fresh and/or Semi-Frozen Chicken and Turkey Parts Purchased from Three California Supermarkets Between June 1988 and May 1989

Type and part of poultry		Number of parts examined	Number (%) of positive parts			
			L. monocytogenes	*L. innocua*	*L. welshimeri*	Total *Listeria* spp.
Chicken						
Wings	fresh	40	5 (12.5)	14 (35.0)	1 (2.5)	17[a] (42.5)
	semi-frozen	10	0	1 (10.0)	0	1(10.0)
Legs	fresh	50	8 (16.0)	19 (38.0)	0	27 (54.0)
	semi-frozen	10	1 (10.0)	0	0	1 (10.0)
Livers	fresh	40	6 (15.0)	8 (20.0)	1 (2.5)	13[a] (32.5)
	semi-frozen	10	1 (10.0)	0	0	1 (10.0)
Turkey						
Wings	fresh	60	12 (20.0)	3 (5.0)	12 (20.0)	27 (45.0)
Legs	fresh	60	8 (13.3)	0	9 (15.0)	17 (28.3)
Tails	fresh	60	7 (11.7)	0	7 (11.7)	14 (23.2)

[a]Some chicken parts contained both *L. monocytogenes* and *L. innocua* or *L. innocua* and *L. welshimeri*.
Source: Adapted from Refs. 33, 34.

serotype O157:H7 in January of 1989. As of February 1990, *L. monocytogenes* and *Salmonella* were detected in 508 of 2686 (18.9%) and 792 of 2739 (28.9%) samples, respectively, with *E. coli* serotype O157:H7 reported absent from 2696 samples (18). While no additional governmental surveys have thus far been reported, several researchers have independently investigated the incidence of listeriae in poultry processed in the southeastern United States and California.

In the first of these independent surveys, Bailey et al. (19) determined the incidence of *L. monocytogenes* and other *Listeria* spp. on the surface of broiler carcasses processed in the southeastern United States. They also compared *L. monocytogenes* serotypes isolated from raw chicken to those that are commonly associated with human cases of listeriosis. Using an enrichment procedure together with three selective plating media, *Listeria* spp. were detected in rinse samples from 34 of 90 (37.8%) chicken carcasses; however, recovery of listeriae varied widely with three lots of 10 birds each being reported as negative. More important, 21 of 90 (23.3%) carcasses contained *L. monocytogenes* with 64, 18, 6, and 12% of the isolates identified as serotypes 1/2b, 1/2c, 3b, and nontypable strains, respectively. While only 7 of 115 (6.1%) *L. monocytogenes* isolates from recent listeriosis victims in the United States have been of serotype 1/2b or 1/2c, the fact that most strains of *L. monocytogenes* isolated from chickens were pathogenic to mice suggests chicken meat as a possible vehicle in human cases of listeriosis.

Between June 1988 and May 1989, Genigeorgis et al. (33,34) conducted two large surveys which examined the incidence of *Listeria* spp. on fresh and/or semi-frozen chicken and turkey parts obtained from retail and slaughterhouse sources. According to their results for chicken, 12.5% of fresh wings, 16.0% of fresh legs, and 15.0% of fresh livers purchased at three supermarkets in northern California contained detectable levels of *L. monocytogenes* (Table 12.1). Furthermore, with the exception of fresh chicken liver, *L. innocua* was generally two to three times more prevalent in the remaining samples than was *L. monocytogenes*. Overall, the highest incidence of *Listeria* spp. was observed for fresh legs (54.0%) followed by fresh wings (42.5%) and fresh livers (32.5%). In contrast to fresh products, only 10% of semi-frozen chicken wings, legs, and livers contained *Listeria* spp. However, finding *L. monocytogenes* alone in 1 of 10 semi-frozen legs and livers points to the ability of this pathogen to survive in semi-frozen raw chicken and turkey, as also was observed by Palumbo and Williams (67).

In addition to these efforts, Genigeorgis et al. (33) also attempted to trace the route of *Listeria* contamination on fresh chicken wings, legs, and livers by examining samples at various stages of production and storage. While all chicken parts from the beginning of the production line were free of *L. monocytogenes*, results in Table 12.2 indicate that most contamination occurred during the latter stages of production when carcasses came in direct contact with *Listeria*-laden fecal material since at the time of packaging, 70, 30, and 33% of chicken wings, legs, and livers contained *L. monocytogenes*, respectively. Not surprisingly, *L. innocua*, which was virtually absent from chicken parts at the beginning of production, also was routinely isolated from wings, livers, and particularly legs at the end of production. Despite these relatively high contamination rates, both *Listeria* spp. failed to grow on all three packaged products during the first 4 days of refrigerated storage. Wimpfheimer et al. (89) observed a 3- to 4-day lag phase for *L. monocytogenes* when inoculated samples of raw minced chicken were held at 4°C. Given

Table 12.2 Incidence of *Listeria* spp. on Commercially Produced Fresh Chicken and Turkey Parts Before and After Being Packaged and/or Stored at 4°C

| Type and part of poultry | *Listeria* sp. | Production line | | 4-Day-old packaged product stored at 4°C |
		Beginning	End	
Chicken				
Wings	*L. monocytogenes*	0/20[a]	21/30 (70)	18/25 (72)
	L. innocua	0/20	6/30 (20)	4/25 (16)
Legs	*L. monocytogenes*	0/20	11/30 (37)	13/25 (52)
	L. innocua	0/20	19/30[c] (67)	17/25 (68)
Livers	*L. monocytogenes*	0/31	5/15 (33)	6/15 (40)
Turkey	*L. innocua*	2/31 (6.5)[b]	4/15 (27)	4/15 (27)
Wings	*L. monocytogenes*	1/30 (3.3)	0/30	ND[d]
	L. welshimeri	1/30 (3.3)	4/30 (13.3)	ND
Legs	*L. monocytogenes*	0/30	2/30 (6.7)	ND
	L. welshimeri	1/30 (3.3)	1/30 (3.3)	ND
Livers	*L. monocytogenes*	0/30	0/30	ND
	L. welshimeri	1/30 (3.3)	5/30 (16.7)	ND

[a]Number of positive parts/number of parts examined.
[b]Percent positive.
[c]Strain of *L. welshimeri* also detected.
[d]Not determined.
Source: Adapted from Refs. 33, 34.

this information, the failure of Genigeorgis et al. (33) to detect growth of *L. monocytogenes* and *L. innocua* on naturally contaminated packaged chicken parts is not surprising.

It is important to remember that like meats, poultry products also can be used for purposes other than human consumption. In Chapter 11 we mentioned that Al-Sheddy and Richter (1) determined the incidence of *L. monocytogenes* in frozen ground meat that contained raw chicken together with chopped beef byproducts. While not conclusive, the finding of *L. monocytogenes* in all five samples examined and the fact that this pathogen is more commonly found in chicken rather than beef products leads one to conclude that raw chicken was the most likely source of contamination. Hence, considering the high incidence of *L. monocytogenes* in raw chicken, it may be prudent to eliminate raw poultry products from the diet of zoo animals to curb the number of listeriosis cases occurring in zoological parks.

Turkey

Since there are many similarities between processing of chickens and other types of domesticated fowl, one would expect various *Listeria* spp., including *L. monocytogenes*, to superficially contaminate other raw poultry products, including turkeys, ducks, and pheasants. After completing the aforementioned survey of California chicken parts for listeriae (33), Genigeorgis et al. (34) initiated a similar study to determine the prevalence of various *Listeria* spp. on fresh turkey parts obtained from retail and slaughterhouse sources.

Listeria contamination rates were generally similar to those previously observed for fresh chicken, with 45.0% of fresh turkey wings, 28.3% of fresh legs, and 23.3% of fresh tails obtained from three local northern California supermarkets harboring various *Listeria* spp. (Table 12.1). While their findings further demonstrate that *L. monocytogenes* is equally common on fresh chicken and turkey parts, with isolation rates of 10.0–16.0% and 11.7–20.0%, respectively, the same cannot be said for *L. innocua* and *L. welshimeri*. In fact, *L. innocua*, the *Listeria* sp. most commonly detected on fresh chicken, was recovered from only 3 of 180 (1.7%) fresh turkey parts. Similarly, *L. welshimeri*, the dominant *Listeria* sp. on fresh turkey, was only rarely observed on fresh chicken. Although both surveys were confined to fresh chicken and poultry parts available from three local supermarkets, nevertheless these findings suggest the interesting possibility that chickens and turkeys may be preferential hosts for *L. innocua* and *L. welshimeri*, respectively. However, additional data need to be gathered from other parts of the country to prove or disprove this theory.

As was true for fresh chicken, additional testing at a local slaughterhouse once again demonstrated that fresh turkey parts are most likely to become contaminated with listeriae during later stages of processing (Table 12.2). This scheme, mentioned earlier as the way fresh poultry becomes contaminated, was further confirmed by identification of various *Listeria* spp., including *L. monocytogenes*, in 4 of 15 (26.7%) samples of mechanically deboned raw turkey meat obtained from the same slaughterhouse. Detailed information regarding the incidence and control of listeriae in poultry-processing facilities appears in Chapter 15.

INCIDENCE OF *LISTERIA* SPP. IN POULTRY PRODUCTS MARKETED IN WESTERN EUROPE

Raw Poultry

European scientists have been aware of the possible relationship between listeriosis in fowl and humans for nearly 40 years as evidenced by several reports in which infected poultry was found in the immediate vicinity of human cases. Considering the relatively high fecal carriage rate for *L. monocytogenes* in domestic and wild fowl as well as the mechanized slaughtering practices that result in heavy fecal contamination of carcasses during defeathering, evisceration, and subsequent chilling in "spin-chillers," it is not surprising that interest in the incidence of listeriae in poultry has escalated. However, since the first European case of avian listeriosis was diagnosed in England during 1936 (68) and no additional cases were recorded in England over the next 22 years (40), one would probably not expect to learn that our present-day knowledge concerning the incidence of *Listeria* in European raw poultry products originates from surveys made in England and Wales during the 1970s.

After identifying *L. monocytogenes* in human stool samples from 32 of 5100 (0.6%) asymptomatic individuals that resided in an area of Wales in which clinical cases of listeriosis had not been identified for 15 years, Kwantes and Isaac (54) postulated that the fecal carriage rate may be related to food consumption and began surveying both fresh and frozen chicken for *L. monocytogenes*. Following a 1971 preliminary report (54), Kwantes and Isaac (55) published final results of their study in 1975 when they reported detecting *L. monocytogenes* on the internal/external surfaces of 27 of 51 (52.9%) raw chickens obtained from a local processor (Table 12.3), with 23 (85.2%) and 4 (14.8%) *L. monocytogenes* isolates identified as serotype 1 and 4b, respectively. To determine the public's actual exposure to contaminated poultry, these investigators went to homes of poultry consumers in Wales and swabbed the external/internal surfaces of fresh and frozen carcasses of chickens, turkeys, ducks, and pheasants that were purchased from local stores.

Overall, *L. monocytogenes* was isolated from 50% of the fresh chickens sampled from home refrigerators, and also from 64% of the frozen chickens stored in home freezers, thus demonstrating the ability of this pathogen to readily survive in frozen foods. However, unlike chickens obtained directly from the processor, *L. monocytogenes*

Table 12.3 Incidence of *L. monocytogenes* in or on Raw Poultry Carcasses Marketed in Western Europe Between 1971 and 1989

Origin	Type of poultry	Number of carcasses examined	Number (%) of positive carcasses	Ref.
Denmark	Fresh chicken	17	8 (47.1)	82
England/Wales	Fresh chicken	51	27 (52.9)	55
	Fresh chicken	38	19 (50.0)	55
	Fresh chicken	50	33 (66.0)	71,72
	Fresh chicken	6	2 (33.3)	38
	Fresh chicken	100	60 (60.0)	36,73
	Fresh chicken	30	15 (50.0)	47
	Fresh chicken	16	10 (62.5)	60
	Frozen chicken	64	41 (64.0)	55
	Frozen chicken	50	27 (54.0)	71,72
	Frozen chicken	56	7 (12.5)	38
	Turkey	4	1 (25.0)	55
	Fresh turkey	1	0	38
	Frozen turkey	3	0	38
	Duck	3	3 (100.0)	55
	Frozen duck	2	1 (50.0)	38
	Wild pheasant	2	1 (50.0)	55
Italy	Fresh chicken	~200	0	28
Sweden	Fresh chicken	45	0	85
Switzerland	Fresh chicken	24	5 (20.8)	24
West Germany	Fresh/Frozen chicken	100	85 (85.0)	75,83
	Unspecified poultry	30	6 (20.0)	66
	Unspecified poultry	11	3 (27.3)	83

isolates belonging to serotype 4b outnumbered those belonging to serotype 1 on fresh and, particularly, on frozen chickens obtained from consumers' homes. Although relatively few samples were examined, isolation of *L. monocytogenes* from the internal/external surface of one turkey, three ducks, and one wild pheasant (Table 12.3) indicates that improperly handled poultry products other than chicken also may pose a potential threat to consumers.

One year later, Gitter (38) published results from a similar study which examined incidence of *L. monocytogenes* on surfaces of various "oven-ready" poultry products purchased at 26 different shops and supermarkets in southern England. Using a combination of direct plating and cold enrichment, he discovered *L. monocytogenes* on 7 of 56 (12.5%) frozen and 2 of 6 (33.3%) fresh chickens as well as on 1 of 2 frozen ducks (Table 12.3). While the incidence of *L. monocytogenes* on raw poultry products was markedly lower than that previously found by Kwantes and Isaac (55), *L. monocytogenes* isolates identified as serotype 4 again outnumbered those identified as serotype 1/2.

Following emergence of *L. monocytogenes* as a serious foodborne pathogen in June 1985, Pini and Gilbert (72) investigated prevalence of the pathogen in uncooked fresh and frozen chickens obtained from retail outlets throughout metropolitan London. Unlike previous studies, which relied on swab samples from carcasses, these researchers examined two different samples from each chicken carcass whenever possible—one sample consisting of edible offal (trimmings and/or viscera) and the other a composite sample of skin and carcass remnants. Use of cold enrichment in conjunction with the FDA procedure resulted in isolation of *L. monocytogenes* from 33 of 50 (66%) fresh and 27 of 50 (54%) frozen chickens. These results also compare favorably to those obtained from two additional 1987–1989 surveys (36,47,60,73) in which *L. monocytogenes* was detected on 10 of 16 (62.5%), 15 of 30 (50%), and 60 of 100 (60%) fresh chicken carcasses marketed in England and Wales (Table 12.3). According to a second report by Pini and Gilbert (71), other *Listeria* spp., including *L. innocua*, *L. seeligeri*, and *L. welshimeri*, also were detected either alone or together with *L. monocytogenes* in 26 and 30% of the fresh and frozen chicken samples tested, respectively. Overall, 74 *L. monocytogenes* strains representing serotypes 1/2, 3a, 3b, 3c, 4b, 4d, and two nontypable strains, with serotype 1/2 predominating, were isolated from 160 samples consisting of 60 edible offal and 100 composite samples. Composite samples yielded more isolates of *L. monocytogenes* (57%) than did edible offal samples (22%) and also a higher percentage of other *Listeria* spp. (23%) than did the edible offal samples (15%). Although there were differences in methodologies and types of samples analyzed in the above-mentioned studies, averaging the results in Table 12.3 indicates that 166 of 291 (57.0%) fresh chickens and 75 of 170 (44.1%) frozen chickens marketed in England and Wales between 1971 and 1989 were contaminated with *L. monocytogenes*. That the 1986 findings of Pini and Gilbert (71,72) are similar to those obtained in both American and European surveys as far back as the mid-1970s underscores the continuing importance of proper kitchen hygiene and cooking of raw poultry products and also the need for continuous inspection of carcasses (e.g., identification of liver and heart lesions), along with use of good manufacturing and sanitizing practices in poultry-processing facilities. Since 152 of 214 (71%) clinical *L. monocytogenes* isolates obtained from British patients between November 1986 and 1987 (59) were identified as being of serotype 4b, poultry products, in which *L. monocytogenes* serotype 1/2 predominates, may be a less common vehicle for listeriosis than other foods. However, as will soon be evident, patés, which are in essence poultry spreads prepared from chicken or goose liver, may be an exception.

European concern about the incidence of *L. monocytogenes* in raw poultry products consumed outside of England/Wales dates back to at least 1982 when two Swedish workers, Ternström and Molin (85), examined 45 chickens obtained from two local slaughterhouses (Table 12.3). Although these researchers failed to isolate *L. monocytogenes* from any of the chickens examined, it appears that the *Listeria* isolation/detection methods used in this study were primarily responsible for their lack of success since listeriosis in Swedish poultry is relatively common with 112 cases diagnosed in the 10-year period between 1948 and 1957 (64). In view of the high incidence of *L. monocytogenes* in raw poultry marketed in the United States and England, inadequate isolation/detection methods also are likely responsible for the inability of Comi and Cantoni (28) to isolate this pathogen from approximately 200 chicken samples (i.e., carcass, skin, entrails) obtained from slaughterhouses in northern Italy during the early 1980s.

After the 1985 cheeseborne listeriosis outbreak in California, other Western European scientists began to determine the incidence of listeriae in a wide range of foods, including fresh poultry products. In the first of these studies, which was published in 1988, Skovgaard and Morgen (82) visited two large Danish poultry slaughterhouses and examined chilled chicken carcasses for evidence of *Listeria* contamination. According to these authors, *Listeria* spp. were detected in neck-skin samples from 16 of 17 (94.1%) chicken carcasses, with *L. innocua* identified in all but two *Listeria*-positive samples. While most of the poultry processed at these two facilities was heavily contaminated with *L. innocua*, 8 of 17 (47.1%), 1 of 17 (5.9%), and 2 of 17 (11.8%) carcasses also contained detectable levels of *L. monocytogenes* (Table 12.3), *L. innocua*, and other *Listeria* spp. (*L. welshimeri, L. murrayi,* and/or *L. denitrificans*), respectively. Thus the *L. monocytogenes* contamination rate for chickens processed in Denmark is only slightly lower than the average we have calculated (56.7%) for fresh chicken carcasses marketed in England and Wales. These Danish researchers also identified *Listeria* spp., including *L. monocytogenes*, in chicken feces and transport cage material; this further supports the widespread belief that poultry carcasses most likely become contaminated with listeriae during evisceration and subsequent handling, as also was suggested by Genigeorgis et al. (33,34) based on results of two recent surveys of poultry-processing facilities in California.

Interest in the incidence of listeriae in European fresh poultry again intensified following reports that 34 individuals in Switzerland died after consuming contaminated Vacherin Mont d'Or soft-ripened cheese. While results from most of these surveys (Table 12.3) have not yet been formally published, Breer (24) isolated *L. monocytogenes*, *L. innocua*, and *L. seeligeri* from 5 of 24 (20.8%), 6 of 24 (25.0%), and 1 of 24 (4.2%) raw chickens purchased in Switzerland, respectively. West German researchers (75,83), using a modified version of the FDA procedure, found *Listeria* spp. and *L. monocytogenes* in 94 of 100 (94%) and 85 of 100 (85%) chicken carcasses, respectively. However, results from two smaller surveys of West German poultry (66,83) suggested far lower *L. monocytogenes* contamination rates, with only 20.0–27.3% of unspecified fresh poultry carcasses (presumably chicken) containing this pathogen (Table 12.3). Present information also indicates that *L. monocytogenes* has been detected in raw poultry produced in

France (23). While detailed findings from this survey as well as several others will likely be available in the future, current data suggest that *L. monocytogenes* as well as other *Listeria* spp. will likely be detected in large numbers of poultry carcasses marketed throughout Western Europe.

Cooked/Ready-to-Eat Poultry

The association between consumption of cooked/cooked-chilled/ready-to-eat poultry products and several previously described cases of listeriosis in England (see Chapter 8) prompted interest in the incidence of *L. monocytogenes* in products which are cooked, rapidly chilled, and frequently held refrigerated for at least 5 days before being consumed without further heating. Preliminary findings from one survey conducted by the Public Health Laboratory Service in London (36,37,73) indicate that *L. monocytogenes* was present in 63 of 527 (12.0%) precooked, ready-to-eat poultry products collected from London-area retail establishments between mid-November 1988 and mid-January 1989. Little information is available concerning actual numbers of *L. monocytogenes* present in cooked poultry products; however, 14 samples that were examined quantitatively contained <100 CFU/g. In addition, *L. monocytogenes* was isolated from 13 of 74 (18%) retail chilled meals, most of which were poultry products given to hospital patients. The pathogen also was discovered in 6 of 24 (25%) cook-chilled poultry products (13), seven cook-chilled poultry dishes at levels up to 700 *L. monocytogenes* CFU/g, and two cooked chicken products labeled "ready-to-eat," one of which contained 400 *L. monocytogenes* CFU/g. Although the chilled meals mentioned earlier carried reheating instructions, current evidence indicates that ready-to-eat and inadequately reheated chilled foods may constitute a potential public health risk if consumed by pregnant women, immunocompromised adults, and the elderly, all of whom are at great risk of contracting listeriosis. Since there is a recent account in which *L. monocytogenes* populations increased approximately 100-fold in an inoculated chicken casserole during 5 days of storage at 6°C (a temperature not uncommon in many home refrigerators), consumption of such food after extended refrigeration appears to be particularly hazardous.

Working at the Cardiff Public Health Laboratory Service in Wales, Morris and Ribeiro (61) also initiated a survey in July 1989 to determine the potential *Listeria*-related risks associated with consumption of paté, an appetizer-type poultry spread that is typically prepared from chicken or goose liver. According to their report, 14 varieties of patés (primarily imported, many from Belgium) were obtained in bulk from area delicatessen counters or in unopened packages from supermarket refrigerators and examined for *L. monocytogenes* using established methods. Overall, this pathogen was isolated from 37 of 73 (50.4%) patés with 28 (75.7%) and 9 (24.3%) of these positive samples originating from delicatessens and supermarket refrigerators, respectively. These patés were subsequently withdrawn from the market after officials discovered dangerously high *L. monocytogenes* populations of 10^4–$\geq 10^5$ CFU/g in seven samples (8). It is noteworthy that *L. monocytogenes* strains of serotype 4b, the serotype responsible for ~80% of all human listeriosis cases in England and Wales, were isolated from 36 of 37 (97.3%) positive samples with one strain of *L. monocytogenes* serotype 4b matching clinical isolates from a 1987 cluster of listeriosis cases in which the exact origin of illness could never be determined.

These findings prompted Public Health Laboratory officials to greatly expand their survey of paté. As of March 1990 (35,73), government officials at 48 of 53 (90.6%) participating laboratories in England and Wales isolated *L. monocytogenes* from 187 of 1834 (10.2%) samples of imported and domestic paté. As in the previous survey, ~10% of all positive samples contained 10^4–$>10^6$ *L. monocytogenes* CFU/g, with over half of all isolates being of serotype 4. As of spring 1990, the number of listeriosis cases reported in England and Wales has decreased to approximately half the level reported in 1988, with further decreases expected for 1990 (35,73). Although pregnant women and other susceptible individuals were warned against consuming paté, which provides a tentative explanation for the decreasing incidence of listeriosis in England and Wales, it is still difficult to surmise how such a specialty product consumed by relatively few people could have such a dramatic impact. Since paté has not yet been positively linked to any listeriosis cases in England or elsewhere, further epidemiological and laboratory work is needed to clarify the relationship, if any, between consumption of tainted paté and human listeriosis.

In the only other European survey of cooked/ready-to-eat poultry products thus far reported, Lieval et al. (57) isolated *L. monocytogenes*, *L. seeligeri*, and *L. innocua* from 1 of 9, 2 of 9, and 1 of 9 chicken sandwiches obtained from cafes in and around Paris. While identical efforts to recover listeriae from 20 fast-food fried chicken items ended in failure, the ability of such foods to harbor listeriae, including *L. monocytogenes*, has been well established by the previously discussed surveys in England. In view of such evidence, the problem of *Listeria*-contaminated cooked/ready-to-eat poultry products is likely to become more widespread as researchers and public health officials look for *L. monocytogenes* and *Listeria* spp. in foods that have been previously ignored.

BEHAVIOR OF *L. MONOCYTOGENES* IN RAW AND COOKED POULTRY PRODUCTS

Although *L. monocytogenes* was first detected on European raw chicken nearly 20 years ago, behavior of *Listeria* in raw and processed poultry products received no attention until this organism was recognized as a bona fide foodborne pathogen in the mid-1980s. Recent research efforts, primarily in the United States, have provided the poultry industry with valuable information concerning growth of *L. monocytogenes* in raw and cooked chicken products, including the levels of heat and microwave and gamma irradiation needed to destroy this organism in raw chicken. However, our present-day knowledge about behavior of listeriae in raw and processed chicken products is still only rudimentary. While results from these efforts will now be summarized, several recently reported cases of listeriosis that were positively linked to consumption of processed poultry products in the United States and England have already prompted additional work in this area. Results from these studies should add much to our knowledge about behavior of listeriae in poultry products and aid in development of processing methods that might decrease the incidence of this pathogen in raw and cooked-chilled poultry products.

Growth-Raw Chicken

Despite the long-time recognition of *L. monocytogenes* as a contaminant of raw poultry products, Wimpfheimer and Hotchkiss (89) are, to date, the only investigators who have examined in some detail the behavior of *L. monocytogenes* in raw chicken. In their study, raw minced chicken meat was inoculated to contain 10^2 *L. monocytogenes* CFU/g, packaged anaerobically (75% CO_2:25% N_2), microaerobically (72.5% CO_2:22.5% N_2:5% O_2), or aerobically (air), and examined for numbers of *L. monocytogenes* as well as aerobic spoilage organisms during storage at 4, 10, or 27°C. As expected, neither *L. monocytogenes* nor aerobic spoilage organisms grew in anaerobically packaged raw chicken during extended storage at any of the three temperatures, with both populations decreasing to <10 CFU/g after 6 days of storage at 4°C (Fig. 12.1). When packaged microaerobically under conditions that more closely duplicate commercial practices, numbers of *L. monocytogenes* in raw chicken increased rapidly during extended storage at 4°C while growth of aerobic spoilage organisms was strongly inhibited (Fig. 12.1). Hence, under these conditions, a potentially serious situation may develop in which *L. monocytogenes* can rapidly proliferate in seemingly normal, unspoiled raw chicken during what would be considered excellent refrigerated storage. While the ability of *L. monocytogenes* to grow in microaerobically packaged raw chicken was not affected by the initial level of *Listeria* (<10^1 or 10^2 CFU/g) or aerobic spoilage organisms (10^4 or 10^8 CFU/g), the ratio of listeriae to spoilage organisms was strongly temperature-dependent with both organisms reaching populations of 10^7–10^8 and 10^9–10^{10} CFU/g in

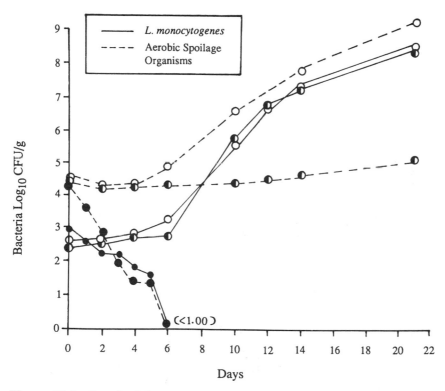

Figure 12.1   Growth of *L. monocytogenes* and aerobic spoilage organisms in aerobically (O), microaerobically (◑), and anaerobically (●) packaged raw chicken during incubation at 4°C. (Adapted from Ref. 89.)

Table 12.4 Populations of *L. monocytogenes* (log$_{10}$ CFU/g) in Artificially Contaminated Cooked/Ready-to-Eat Poultry Products of Acceptable Organoleptic Quality During Extended Refrigerated Storage

Product	Incubation temp. (°C)	Initial inoculum	Length of incubation (days)							Ref.
			3	6	8	10	14	20	28	
Sliced chicken[a]	4.4	2.79	—[b]	—	—	—	6.94	—	—	39
	4.4	0[c]	—	—	—	—	5.90	—	—	
Sliced turkey (Brand A)[a]	4.4	3.04	—	—	—	—	5.04	—	6.15	39
	4.4	−1.30	—	—	—	—	2.38	—	3.73	
Sliced turkey (Brand B)[a]	4.4	2.87	—	—	—	—	6.70	—	—	39
	4.4	−1.70	—	—	—	—	4.79	—	7.70	
Chicken homogenate	4	6.7	—	—	—	—	—	9.4	—	81
	4	2.7	—	—	—	—	—	7.9	—	
Breaded chicken fillets	5	2.7	—	3.6	—	—	—	—	—	80
	5	1.7	—	3.6	—	—	—	—	—	
Chicken casserole	3	2.7	2.9	3.5	3.3	3.6	—	—	—	36
	6	2.7	3.6	5.3	6.3	7.5	—	—	—	

[a]Vacuum packaged.
[b]Not tested.
[c]1 CFU/g.

microaerobically packaged chicken following <2 and 8 days of storage at 10 and 27°C, respectively. Not surprisingly, neither *L. monocytogenes* nor aerobic spoilage organisms were inhibited in aerobically packaged raw chicken, with listeriae and spoilage organisms attaining populations in excess of 10^7 and 10^9 CFU/g, respectively, in products stored at 4, 10, or 27°C. Thus, with exception of the microaerobically packaged product, raw chicken would likely become overtly spoiled before *L. monocytogenes* could proliferate to the point where the pathogen might be detectable in minimally cooked chicken. (Thermal inactivation of *L. monocytogenes* in poultry will be discussed shortly.) Nevertheless, it is important to remember that consumers must take special precautions to prevent cross-contamination between raw chicken that may contain *L. monocytogenes* and/or *Salmonella* spp. and ready-to-eat products including cooked chicken.

Growth-Cooked/Ready-to-Eat Poultry Products

Confirmation of cooked-chilled chicken and turkey frankfurters as vehicles of *Listeria* infection in England and the United States during 1988 and 1989 prompted immediate international efforts to assess the potential hazards associated with growth of *L. monocytogenes* in a wide range of retail cooked/ready-to-eat poultry products. A June 1990 search of the scientific literature has uncovered results from at least seven such studies, four of which have been briefly summarized in Table 12.4. Since all of these studies differ in experimental design, sampling times, and initial inoculum levels of *L. monocytogenes*, these findings cannot be compared directly. However, it is evident that numbers of listeriae increased 1–6 orders of magnitude in all six artificially contaminated products after 6–28 days of storage at 3–6°C. Equally important, organoleptic acceptability of these products was not altered by growth of this pathogen. Overall, *L. monocytogenes* grew most abundantly in vacuum-packaged sliced chicken and one brand of sliced turkey, both of which were similar in pH (6.3, 6.4), and in contents of moisture (71.3, 74.0%), protein (18.9, 22.6%), carbohydrate (1.3, 0.9%), and salt (1.7, 1.4%). These authors attributed decreased growth of the pathogen in a second brand of sliced turkey to higher levels of salt (2.7%) and carbohydrate (1.7%); the latter was largely responsible for the eventual decrease in pH of this product to 4.97.

As mentioned in the preceding paragraph, results from three additional studies dealing with behavior of listeriae in cooked poultry products also have been made available to the scientific community. In the first of these reports (49), cooked/sterilized chicken loaf was inoculated to contain 10^3 *L. monocytogenes* and 10^3 *Pseudomonas fragi* CFU/g, packaged aerobically (air), microaerobically (10% O_2), or anaerobically, and examined for both organisms during 6 days of incubation at 3, 7, and 11°C. Regardless of incubation temperature, *P. fragi* attained maximum populations of approximately 4 × 10^9 CFU/g in all aerobic samples after 6 days of storage (Fig. 12.2). However, growth of listeriae was partially suppressed with population differences as great as 3.4 orders of magnitude observed in samples after 6 days of incubation at 3°C. While both organisms attained lower maximum populations in cooked chicken loaf following 6 days of microaerobic or anaerobic incubation at all three temperatures, these conditions led to *Listeria* populations that were 1–2 orders of magnitude higher than those attained by *P. fragi*. Thus, as was true for raw poultry (Fig. 12.1), microaerobic and anaerobic refrigerated storage both appear to selectively favor growth of *L. monocytogenes* over

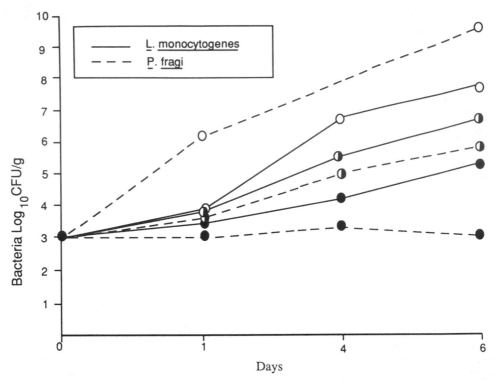

Figure 12.2 Growth of *L. monocytogenes* and *Pseudomonas fragi* in aerobically (○), microaerobically (◑), and anaerobically (●) packaged cooked chicken loaf during incubation at 7°C. (Adapted from Ref. 49.)

P. fragi and possibly other spoilage organisms which, in turn, could potentially yield an organoleptically acceptable product with dangerously high numbers of listeriae.

Finally, two additional investigations also have assessed behavior of listeriae in inoculated samples of chicken gravy and chicken broth during cooling and/or refrigerated storage. According to Huang et al. (46), *L. monocytogenes* populations in individual 1000-g samples of artificially contaminated chicken gravy (prepared from poultry stock, spices, waxy maize wash, and chicken base) increased by two orders of magnitude as the product cooled from 40 to 9°C during 24 hours of storage in a refrigerator at 7°C (Fig. 12.3). After the chicken gravy stabilized at 7°C, generation times for *L. monocytogenes* approximately doubled. However, the pathogen still attained a maximum population of 10^9 CFU/g in 8-day-old gravy. Of perhaps greater importance is a 1990 study by Walker et al. (88) that demonstrated the ability of three *L. monocytogenes* strains to multiply in artificially contaminated sterile chicken broth (pH ≅ 6.4) held at even lower temperatures, with *Listeria* populations in this product increasing 100-fold during extended incubation at 0.8°C (Fig. 12.4). In fact, growth of this pathogen also was evident in samples of chicken broth that were held at temperatures as low as –0.4°C, below which the broth could no longer be sampled because it was frozen.

Results from these two investigations stress the importance of cooling foods as

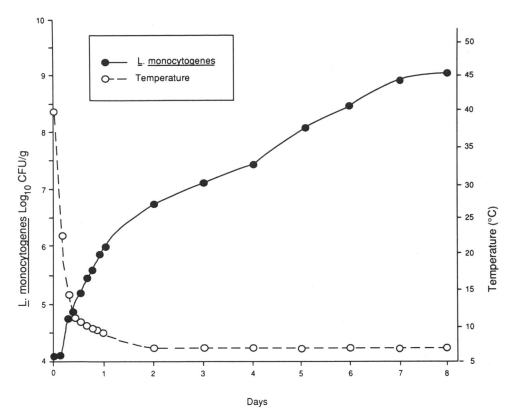

Figure 12.3 Behavior of *L. monocytogenes* in chicken gravy during cooling to 7°C and extended storage. (Adapted from Ref. 46.)

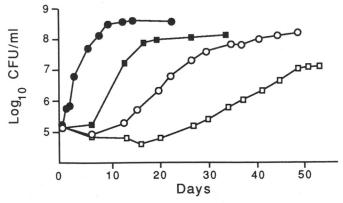

Figure 12.4 Growth of *L. monocytogenes* in sterile chicken broth during extended incubation at 8.7 (●), 3.5 (■), 1.5 (○), and 0.8°C (□). (Adapted from Ref. 88.)

rapidly as possible and show that hazardous situations can easily develop if refrigerated foods are subjected to mild temperature abuse, i.e., holding at temperatures above 4.4°C. In an effort to increase the safety of cooked, cooked-chilled, and ready-to-eat poultry, USDA officials recently lowered the recommended long-term storage temperature for such products from 4.4 (40°F) to 1.7°C (35°F) and also have developed stricter guidelines that require faster (than recommended previously) cooling of warm products at the end of manufacture (3). Continued attention to rapid cooling of finished products and avoidance of postprocessing contamination are both essential to decrease the incidence of this psychrotrophic pathogen in cooked/ready-to-eat poultry products.

Thermal Inactivation

The most obvious means of destroying *L. monocytogenes* and other foodborne pathogens in any raw food, including poultry, is by use of heat. However, numerous reports attesting to unusual thermal tolerance of *L. monocytogenes* in various foods, coupled with discovery of *L. monocytogenes* in several cooked poultry products that were directly linked to cases of listeriosis, have raised questions about the exact thermal processing times and temperatures required to completely eliminate this pathogen from raw poultry products. In response to these concerns, Carpenter and Harrison conducted three studies in which raw chicken breasts were surface-inoculated to contain ~10^5–10^7 *L. monocytogenes* CFU/g and cooked to internal temperatures of 65.6, 71.1, 73.9, 76.7, or 82.2°C using dry heat (27), moist heat (42), and microwave radiation (43). All cooked chicken breasts were then vacuum-packaged or wrapped in oxygen-permeable film and analyzed for numbers of listeriae during 4 weeks of storage at 4 and 10°C.

Overall, *L. monocytogenes* was recovered from chicken breasts cooked to all five internal temperatures, using dry heat, moist heat, and microwave radiation. As expected, the magnitude of lethality was directly related to cooking temperature. Since chicken breasts contained somewhat different levels of *L. monocytogenes* before heating, one cannot directly compare the effectiveness of the three cooking methods used in these studies. However, if one assumes that *L. monocytogenes* populations decreased linearly during most of the time that chicken breasts were heat-treated (admittedly, some "tailing" of the survivor curve likely occurred at the three highest temperatures using dry, moist heat, and microwave irradiation), then it is possible to estimate the number of survivors in chicken breasts that contained any initial inoculum. Thus, if Carpenter and Harrison had used an initial population of 1.0×10^6 *L. monocytogenes* CFU/g in all three studies, one would expect their results to have been similar to the estimated number of survivors shown in Table 12.5. Considering these approximations, it appears that *L. monocytogenes* was generally more tolerant of microwave radiation than dry or moist heat, with numbers of listeriae decreasing less than four orders of magnitude on chicken cooked to an internal temperature of 82.2°C. Of greater importance is the fact that *Listeria* populations decreased ≤2 orders of magnitude on chicken breasts cooked to an internal temperature of 71.1°C, the minimum internal temperature to which poultry must be heated to designate the product as fully cooked in the United States (2). Although populations of listeriae generally decreased approximately five orders of magnitude when chicken was cooked to higher internal temperatures using either dry or moist heat, these authors (41) later demonstrated that moist heating of surface-inoculated chicken

Table 12.5 Estimated Decrease in Numbers of *L. monocytogenes* on the Surface of Chicken Breasts Inoculated to Contain 6.00 $\log_{10}$ CFU/g and Cooked to Various Internal Temperatures Using Dry Heat, Moist Heat, or Microwave Radiation

Cooking method	No.[a] of *L. monocytogenes* ($\log_{10}$ CFU/g) decrease after cooking to internal temp. of				
	65.6°C	71.1°C	73.9°C	76.7°C	82.2°C
Dry heat	2.42	2.00	5.05	5.24	5.04
Moist heat	2.08	1.83	3.46	5.08	4.96
Microwave radiation	0.82	1.95	2.50	3.77	3.26

[a]Initial inoculum of 6.00 $\log_{10}$ *L. monocytogenes* CFU/ml.
Source: Adapted from Refs. 27, 42, 43.

breasts to an internal temperature of 73.9°C also failed to completely inactivate more realistic *L. monocytogenes* populations of 10^2–10^4 CFU/g. Overall, microwave heating was less effective than either dry or moist heating, with *Listeria* populations decreasing less than four orders of magnitude on chicken breasts cooked to an internal temperature of 82.2°C (Table 12.5). In 1989, researchers in England (58) also reported that microwave heating was less effective than other forms of cooking for eliminating *L. monocytogenes* from the surface and interior (stuffing) of whole stuffed chickens (~1.7 kg each) inoculated to contain 10^6 and 10^7 *Listeria* CFU/g of skin and stuffing, respectively. Uneven heating, which is an inherent problem in microwave cooking, accounted for the 20 minutes of additional standing time that was required after 38 minutes of cooking (final skin temperature of 80–99°C) to completely inactivate the pathogen on the surface of whole chickens. However, low levels of *L. monocytogenes* (<10 CFU/g) were still detected in stuffing samples from one of two similarly treated whole chickens that attained temperatures of 72–85°C after 20 minutes of standing. Thus these findings serve as a warning to persons who regularly cook large stuffed birds (particularly turkeys) in microwave ovens and they also stress the importance of postcooking standing time for further inactivation of listeriae and other foodborne pathogens in poultry products after microwave cooking.

Not surprisingly, follow-up work by Carpenter and Harrison (27,42,43) demonstrated that *L. monocytogenes* survivors (likely sublethally injured during heating) can persist and multiply on both oxygen-permeable film-wrapped and vacuum-packaged cooked chicken during extended storage at 4 and 10°C. As shown in Figure 12.5, growth of listeriae on chicken breasts packaged in oxygen-permeable film was most evident after 2 weeks of refrigerated storage with larger populations generally developing on products that were cooked using microwave radiation, followed by those given moist or dry heat. Most important, *L. monocytogenes* was recovered via direct plating from all 4-week-old aerobically packaged chicken breasts except those that were cooked to an internal temperature of 82.2°C using moist heat. In addition, higher numbers of listeriae also developed on aerobically packaged chicken breasts that were exposed to less severe heat treatments. As expected, increasing the incubation temperature also led to much faster growth of *Listeria*, with the pathogen generally attaining populations of 10^6–10^7 CFU/g on aerobically packaged chicken breasts after only 7 days at 10°C.

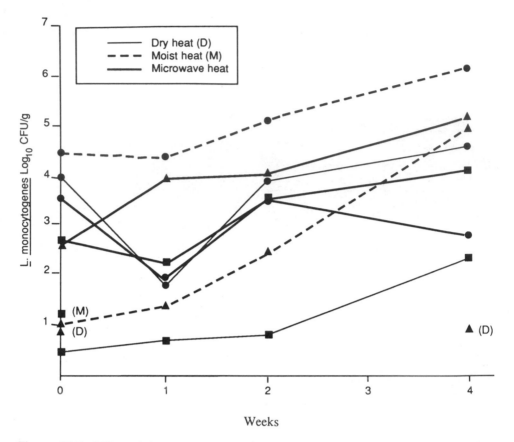

Figure 12.5 Effect of three different heating methods on behavior of *L. monocytogenes* on incubated chicken breasts that were cooked to internal temperatures of 71.1 (●), 76.7 (▲), or 82.2°C (■), packaged in oxygen-permeable film, and stored at 4°C. (Adapted from Refs. 27, 42, 43.)

Behavior of *L. monocytogenes* on chicken breasts was influenced by the heating method/treatment, temperature at which the cooked product was ultimately stored, and type of packaging material. According to these authors, *Listeria* populations were generally one to two orders of magnitude lower in vacuum-packaged than in aerobically wrapped product following 4 weeks of storage at 4°C; however, the pathogen was present in all 4-week-old samples except those that were originally cooked to an internal temperature of 82.2°C using moist or dry heat (Fig. 12.6). While numbers of listeriae were again generally one to two orders of magnitude lower in vacuum-packaged than in aerobically wrapped chicken breasts following 1 week at 10°C, populations were as much as five orders of magnitude lower in vacuum-packaged chicken breasts that were cooked to an internal temperature of 82.2°C using moist heat.

Since raw chicken normally contains ≤1000 *L. monocytogenes* CFU/g (60) and *Listeria* populations generally decrease approximately three to five orders of magnitude in fully cooked poultry heated to an internal temperature of 63.9°C, as specified in the United States Code of Federal Regulations, it appears that present cooking temperatures are at best only marginally adequate to eliminate this pathogen from raw poultry products. In fact, Harrison and Carpenter (41) reported that moist heating of inoculated chicken breasts to an internal temperature of 73.9°C failed to completely inactivate *L. monocytogenes* surface populations of 10^2–10^4 CFU/g, with the pathogen reestablishing itself at levels equal to or above the original inoculum level after 4 weeks at 4°C. Nonetheless, the adequacy of current poultry-processing methods was maintained by another recent report (5) which indicated that a turkey meat emulsion (containing salt, sodium tripolyphosphate, carrageenan, and water) inoculated to contain 5.78 *L. monocytogenes* $\log_{10}$ CFU/g was free of the pathogen after holding the product at 71.1°C for 2 minutes (est. $D_{71.1°C}$ = 0.28 minute). However, in view of at least three human listeriosis cases linked to cooked-chilled chicken meat and turkey frankfurters (the latter was reportedly warmed 45–60 seconds in a microwave oven before consumption) and that small numbers of *L. monocytogenes* survived a wide range of heat treatments given to chicken breasts and frequently grew in these products during refrigeration, it is prudent for poultry processors to cook their products to somewhat higher internal temperatures (76.7–82.2°C) than is now routinely practiced until the adequacy of the current minimum

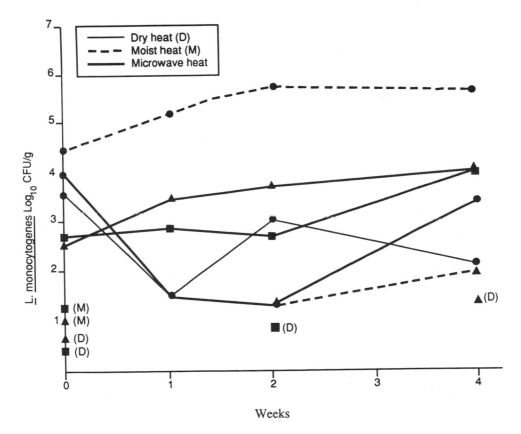

Figure 12.6 Effect of three different heating methods on behavior of *L. monocytogenes* on incubated chicken breasts cooked to internal temperatures of 71.1 (●), 76.7 (▲), or 82.2°C (■), vacuum-packaged, and stored at 4°C. (Adapted from Refs. 27, 42, 43.)

heat treatment can be firmly established. Future studies should give attention to the effect of processed poultry ingredients (i.e., salt, preservatives) on thermal resistance of listeriae during conventional as well as microwave heating since Harrison and Carpenter (43) found that the latter cooking method was less successful in eliminating *L. monocytogenes* from the surface of chicken breasts than either dry or moist heating.

Susceptibility to Gamma Radiation

Results from recent surveys indicate that up to ~60% of all raw poultry products sold in retail stores may be contaminated with *L. monocytogenes* and *Salmonella* spp. Such statistics have prompted development of various processes to eliminate hazardous pathogens from raw poultry. Of these, exposure to the bactericidal effects of gamma radiation appears to be among the most effective means of reducing populations of both pathogenic and spoilage organisms. While presently allowable gamma radiation doses of 2.5–7.0 kGy in England (147) and ≤3.0 kGy in the United States (16) are generally regarded as sufficient for eliminating these organisms from raw poultry, readers should be aware that exposing cooked poultry to levels >2.5 kGy may adversely affect product odor, color, and flavor (60).

In 1989, Patterson (70) examined sensitivity of *Listeria* to gamma radiation using radiation-sterilized raw minced chicken meat that was inoculated to contain ~10^6 *L. monocytogenes* CFU/g. After exposing the product to gamma radiation doses of 0, 0.5, 1.0, 1.5, 2.0, and 2.5 kGy, *L. monocytogenes* exhibited a D_{10}-value (i.e., radiation dose required to decrease the population 10-fold) of 0.4177–0.553 kGy, depending on the bacterial strain and the type of plating medium used to quantitate the pathogen in minced poultry following irradiation. In support of these findings, Huhtanen et al. (48) also reported that a gamma radiation dose of 2 kGy was sufficient to inactivate an *L. monocytogenes* population of ~10^4 CFU/g (average D_{10}-value of 0.45 kGy) in artificially contaminated, mechanically deboned chicken. Similar D_{10}-values also have been published for *Salmonella* spp. in fresh poultry (62).

While all of the studies discussed thus far support the use of 2.5 kGy of gamma radiation to eliminate <10^4 *L. monocytogenes* CFU/g from raw poultry meat, researchers in England (60) subsequently recovered this pathogen from 1 of 12 (8.3%) fresh chicken carcasses that had been surface-inoculated to contain approximately 10^2 or 10^4 *L. monocytogenes* CFU/cm^2 and exposed to 2.5 kGy of gamma radiation. More important, after extended storage at 5–10°C, the pathogen was recovered from 1 of 18 (5.6%) and 7 of 18 (38.8%) irradiated carcasses that originally contained low and high *Listeria* inocula, respectively. Hence, unlike previous studies, these findings suggest that small numbers of listeriae either escaped sublethal injury or underwent repair and grew on these carcasses during refrigerated storage.

From this information it appears that a gamma radiation dose of 2.5 kGy may be only marginally sufficient to inactivate levels of listeriae that one might reasonably expect to find on naturally contaminated raw poultry. Nevertheless, provided that irradiated poultry products are properly packaged to prevent recontamination (and subsequent growth) with listeriae and other foodborne pathogens, this procedure should markedly decrease the risk of contaminating ready-to-eat foods (e.g., salads, raw vegetables) when raw poultry is prepared by the consumer. Unfortunately, while the scientific community generally contends that foods exposed to such low levels of radiation are safe for human consumption, irradiated foods have not yet gained widespread acceptance by most consumers. Perhaps the continued outpouring of scientific evidence will eventually curb the unfounded fear of irradiated foods in the mind of the general public.

EGG PRODUCTS

Listeria monocytogenes is most frequently isolated from heart, liver, and spleen tissue of poultry suffering from listeriosis; however, according to the early scientific literature, this pathogen also has been detected in necrotic oviduct lesions of several infected hens (40) and in follicles of one artificially infected chicken (51). These observations prompted a large-scale survey in 1958 (5) in which *L. monocytogenes* was not isolated from 600 intact hen's eggs. In keeping with these findings, consumption of eggs and egg products also has not yet been linked to a single case of listeriosis. However, the possible presence of *L. monocytogenes* on egg shells which may contain minute cracks and the ability of this pathogen to survive 90 days on eggs stored at 5°C (21) and grow in artificially contaminated eggs stored at refrigeration and ambient temperatures suggests that eggs cannot be ignored as a possible source of listeric infection in humans. Hence, it is not surprising that recent concerns about contaminated poultry products also have prompted efforts to define both the incidence and behavior of *L. monocytogenes* in eggs and egg products, including pasteurized liquid and dried egg.

Incidence

As mentioned in the preceding paragraph, isolation of *L. monocytogenes* from intact whole eggs has not yet been documented; however, the same is not true for broken eggs. According to Leasor and Foegeding (56), *Listeria* spp. were isolated from 15 of 42 (36%) previously frozen samples of raw, commercially broken, solids-adjusted liquid whole egg (21 samples), natural-proportion liquid whole egg (20 samples), and yolk (1 sample) obtained on several occasions from 6 of 11 (54%) commercial manufacturers located throughout the United States. Upon closer examination of the data, it is evident that *L. innocua* and *L. monocytogenes* were identified in 15 of 15 (100%) and 2 of 15 (13.3%) positive samples, respectively. Twelve of 15 (80%) and 3 of 15 (20%) positive samples, including one sample each with *L. monocytogenes*, were classified as solids-adjusted and natural-proportion liquid whole egg, respectively. Increased handling during manufacture and, as suggested by the authors, a higher solids content which may enhance growth and survival of listeriae are just two of many possible reasons why a higher incidence of listeriae was observed in solids-adjusted rather than natural-proportion liquid whole egg. While results from direct plating indicated that the two *L. monocytogenes*-positive samples contained approximately 1 and 8 *L. monocytogenes* CFU/g at the time of analysis, the fact that these samples were held frozen for up to 4.5 months and subjected to two freeze-thaw cycles suggests that numbers of listeriae likely decreased by at least 50% during storage (see Chapter 5). Hence, both samples probably contained <100 *L. monocytogenes* CFU/g before being frozen. Nonetheless, the 2-week and 6-month refrigerated shelf life of pasteurized and ultrapasteurized liquid whole egg products, respectively, is more than ample to allow this pathogen to increase from very low to very high numbers, as is evident from the following discussion.

Growth

The ability of *Listeria* to grow in hen's eggs was first recognized in 1940 when Paterson (69) inoculated a laboratory culture of *L. monocytogenes* into the chorioallantoic membrane of a chicken embryo. This procedure is still useful in determining virulence of particular *L. monocytogenes* strains (84). Information concerning growth of this pathogen in nonfertile eggs and egg products is limited.

A search of the scientific literature has uncovered only two studies pertaining to growth of *L. monocytogenes* in raw whole eggs or egg components. According to results from the first such paper published in 1955, Urbach and Schabinski (86) found that populations of *L. monocytogenes* in intact experimentally infected nonfertile eggs increased nearly six orders of magnitude during 10 days of storage at ambient temperature. Following this study, 20 years passed until viability of *L. monocytogenes* was again examined in artificially contaminated raw as well as cooked (121°C/15 min) whole egg, albumen, and egg yolk during extended storage at 5 and 20°C (53). Results for raw whole and separated egg showed that growth of *L. monocytogenes* was primarily confined to egg yolk (Fig. 12.7), with the pathogen exhibiting respective generation times of 1.7 days and 2.4 hours at 5 and 20°C. Overall, *Listeria* populations in raw whole egg generally varied less than one order of magnitude from the original inoculum during extended storage at either temperature; however, numbers of listeriae in raw albumen (pH 8.9) decreased three and five orders of magnitude during prolonged incubation at 5 and 20°C, respectively. Despite the reported ability of *L. monocytogenes* to grow in laboratory media having pH values as high as 10.0 (78), loss of viability by *Listeria* in raw albumen was pH-related, with numbers of listeriae decreasing less than two orders

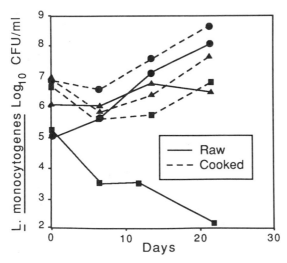

Figure 12.7 Behavior of *L. monocytogenes* in raw and cooked whole egg (▲), albumen (■), and egg yolk (●) during extended incubation at 5°C. (Adapted from Ref. 53.)

of magnitude in samples that were preadjusted to pH 7.0 and held at 5°C. Unlike raw whole egg, albumen, and egg yolk, listeriae grew rapidly in corresponding cooked samples. Generation times for the pathogen in cooked whole egg, egg yolk, and albumen were 1.9, 2.3, and 2.4 days, respectively, at 5°C, and 2.6, 2.66, and 3.5 hours at 20°C. These authors speculated that loss of the aforementioned antilisterial properties of raw albumen resulted from inactivation of one or more binding proteins (i.e., ovotransferrin, ovoflavoprotein, avidin) during heating. Since *L. monocytogenes* can grow rapidly in cooked whole as well as separated eggs, investigators of foodborne outbreaks should not overlook these products as potential vehicles of infection.

In 1990 Sionkowski and Shelef (79) provided the first information concerning growth of *L. monocytogenes* in pasteurized egg products. To simulate postpasteurization contamination, pasteurized (64.4°C/2.5 minutes) samples of liquid egg and reconstituted dried egg were inoculated to contain ~10^4–10^5 *L. monocytogenes* CFU/ml and examined for numbers of listeriae during 7 days of storage at 4°C. As shown in Fig. 12.8, the pathogen grew similarly in both products, reaching populations > 10^7 CFU/ml after 7 days of refrigerated storage. While transmission of *L. monocytogenes* by pasteurized egg products has not yet been documented, these findings suggest that a possible public health problem could develop if *L. monocytogenes* enters pasteurized liquid egg, particularly since the shelf life of some of these refrigerated products has recently been extended to several months.

Growth of *L. monocytogenes* in commercially processed, liquid whole egg was most recently investigated by Foegeding and Leasor (31). In this study, commercially broken, liquid whole egg was ultrapasteurized (68°C/118 sec), homogenized, inoculated to contain one of five strains of *L. monocytogenes* [Scott A (clinical isolate), F5069 (milk isolate), ATCC 19111 (poultry isolate), NCF-U2K3, and NCF-F1KKr (raw liquid whole egg isolates)] at a level of 5×10^2 to 1×10^3 CFU/ml, overlaid with mineral oil to prevent oxygen transfer, and examined for numbers of listeriae during extended incubation at 4, 10, 20, and/or 30°C.

Generation times and maximum populations were generally similar to those previously observed in fluid milk products (see Chapter 9) with the exception that strain Scott A failed to grow in liquid whole egg during prolonged incubation at 4 and 10°C (Table 12.6). While growth of strain Scott A in fluid milk, cheese, and cabbage juice at refrigeration temperatures is well documented, Buchanan et al. (25) recently reported that this strain failed to grow in meat and poultry products incubated at 4°C. As shown in Table 12.6, generation times for the five *L. monocytogenes* strains ranged from 24 to 51, 8 to 31, 7.5 to 26, and 4.3 to 15 hours at 4, 10, 20, and 30°C, respectively. Maximum populations ranged from 5.00 to 7.00, 5.48 to 8.48, 6.85 to 8.00, and 7.00 to 8.00 *L. monocytogenes* $\log_{10}$ CFU/g in liquid whole eggs incubated at 4, 10, 20, and 30°C, respectively. Considering current distribution and marketing practices, it is likely that perishable products such as liquid whole egg occasionally will encounter periods of temperature abuse. Hence, from these data it follows that even brief exposure to temperatures $\geq$ 10°C can lead to a dramatic increase in both growth rate (i.e., decreased generation time) and maximum populations of *L. monocytogenes* attained in ultrapasteurized liquid whole egg. Since most *L. monocytogenes* strains can proliferate in ultrapasteurized liquid egg products at refrigeration temperatures, postpasteurization

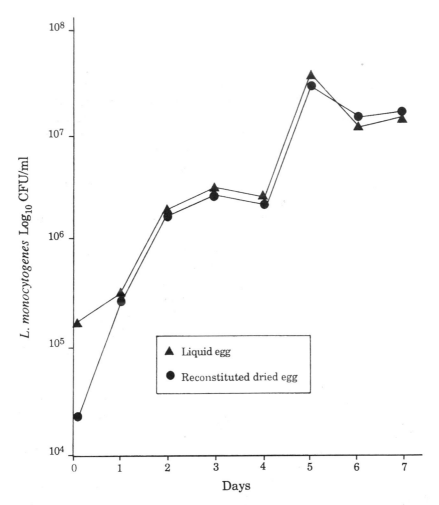

Figure 12.8 Growth of *L. monocytogenes* in liquid and reconstituted dried egg incubated at 4°C. (Adapted from Ref. 79.)

Table 12.6 Generation Times and Maximum Populations of *L. monocytogenes* in Ultrapasteurized Liquid Whole Egg Incubated at 4, 10, 20, and 30°C

Strain of *L. monocytogenes*	Incubation temperature (°C)			
	4	10	20	30
	Generation time (h)			
F5069	24	12	7.5	4.3
Scott A	NG[a]	NG	26	7.1
ATCC 19111	51	31	22	15
NCF-U2K3	26	7.8	ND[b]	ND
NCF-F1KK4	25	8.0	ND	ND
	Maximum population ($\log_{10}$ CFU/g)			
F5069	6.70	7.00	8.00	8.00
Scott A	NG	NG	7.00	7.85
ATCC 19111	5.00	5.48	6.85	7.00
NCF-U2K3	7.00	8.48	ND	ND
NCF-F1KK4	6.48	8.30	ND	ND

[a]No growth.
[b]Not determined.
Source: Adapted from Ref. 31.

contamination should be avoided and the product should be stored at temperatures close to, or preferably below, 0°C.

In the only other egg-related growth study thus far reported, Notermans et al. (65) examined the viability of several foodborne pathogens, including *L. monocytogenes*, in an eggnog-like product prepared from raw whole egg and sugar (25%, w/v) with/without ethanol (7%, v/v). When samples of ethanol-free product were inoculated to contain ~10^4–10^5 *L. monocytogenes* CFU/g, numbers of listeriae generally decreased 10-fold during the first 2 days of incubation at 4°C and then slowly increased to levels near or slightly above the original inoculum level after 5 additional days of refrigerated storage. Although *L. monocytogenes* generally exhibited similar behavioral patterns in nonalcoholic samples incubated at 22°C, initial population decreases were far more abrupt, with the pathogen then increasing to populations one to three orders of magnitude lower than the original inoculum after 7 days of incubation. Unlike alcohol-free samples, *L. monocytogenes* was slowly inactivated in product containing 7% ethanol with populations typically one to two and more than four orders of magnitude lower in 7-day-old samples held at 4 and 22°C, respectively, than were present initially. Hence, given the normal 2-week refrigerated shelf life of similar commercially available nonalcoholic eggnog-like products, recontamination of these beverages during packaging could lead to potential public health problems involving listeriae and other foodborne pathogens, with *Salmonella enteritidis* and *Salmonella typhimurium* reportedly also remaining viable in artificially contaminated samples during 63 days of refrigerated storage.

Thermal Inactivation

Interest in possible heat resistance of *L. monocytogenes* in eggs is of recent origin; however, concerns by European scientists regarding potential transmission of listeriae through eggs prompted a 1955 study by Urbach and Schabinski (86), which examined the ability of this pathogen to survive in artificially infected eggs that were fried. According to these authors, *L. monocytogenes* was isolated from fried eggs (congealed white, soft yolk) prepared from inoculated raw eggs in which the pathogen had previously grown to levels $> 5 \times 10^5$ CFU/g.

Whereas the aforementioned work appears to be fairly crude by current standards and is now primarily only of historical interest, Foegeding and Leasor (31) conducted a more sophisticated study in which D-values were determined for five strains of *L. monocytogenes* [Scott A (clinical isolate), F5069 (milk isolate), ATCC 19111 (poultry isolate), NCF-U2K3 and NCF-F1KK4 (raw liquid whole egg isolates)] in essentially sterile raw egg. Inoculated samples of raw liquid whole egg were added to glass capillary tubes which were heat-sealed and immersed in a water or oil bath at 51, 55.5, 60, and 66°C. After various times, tubes were removed and contents examined for survivors. Numbers of listeriae decreased linearly in raw egg during all four heat treatments, with D-values for the five *L. monocytogenes* strains ranging from 14.3 to 22.6, 5.3 to 8.2, 1.3 to 1.7, and 0.06 to 0.20 minute(s) at 51, 55.5, 60, and 66°C, respectively. Strain Scott A was generally less heat resistant than were the other four strains, particularly at the two lower temperatures; however, strain F5069 and the two isolates from raw egg exhibited moderate thermal tolerance at all four temperatures. Thus this pathogen appears to exhibit a similar degree of heat resistance in both raw whole milk (see Chapter 5) and raw liquid whole egg.

In more practical terms, USDA officials currently require that liquid whole egg be pasteurized at a minimum of 60°C for 3.5 minutes to effect a nine-order-of-magnitude (9-D) kill of *Salmonella* spp. (87). While results from the study just discussed indicate that minimum pasteurization of liquid whole egg would effect only a 2.1- to 2.7-D kill of *L. monocytogenes*, one must remember that current estimates place *L. monocytogenes* populations in liquid whole eggs at <100 CFU/g (31). Hence, as is true for milk pasteurization, current minimum pasteurization requirements for raw liquid whole egg appear adequate to inactivate normal levels of *Listeria* that might be present in the product. However, it is important to stress that current minimum pasteurization requirements for liquid whole egg, as specified in the USDA Egg Pasteurization Manual, indicate that the margin of safety is approximately six orders of magnitude lower for *L. monocytogenes* than for most *Salmonella* spp.

In 1987, Ball et al. (20) documented that ultrapasteurization (i.e., pasteurization at >60°C for <3.5 min) in combination with aseptic processing and packaging can be used to produce liquid whole egg with a refrigerated shelf life of 3–6 months. After results from this study were published, FDA officials issued a temporary permit allowing a North Carolina firm to market ultrapasteurized liquid whole eggs (12,74). Although two of the four objectives of the process were to "render the egg products free of *Salmonella* and *L. monocytogenes*," the exact time/temperature requirements to completely inactivate *L. monocytogenes* in liquid whole egg were not specified in the FDA temporary permit.

Based on extrapolations from the aforementioned survivor curves which showed no evidence of tailing, Foegeding and Leasor (31) predicted that the ultrapasteurization processes used by Ball et al. (20) would effect a 1- to 34-D (average of 14-D) kill of *L. monocytogenes* in liquid whole egg. Assuming that the ultrapasteurization times and temperatures used in conjunction with the temporary FDA permit are those values that were previously determined by Ball et al. (20), Foegeding and Leasor (31) went on to speculate that four of the 10 thermal treatments used by Ball and co-workers may not conform to the definition of ultrapasteurization in the temporary permit, depending on how one views the necessity for a 9-D reduction in numbers of listeriae. However, it appears that *Listeria*-free ultrapasteurized liquid whole egg having a refrigerated shelf life of one to several months can be produced, provided that the raw product is processed using one of the six more severe time/temperature treatments proposed by Ball et al. (20) and then is aseptically packaged to eliminate postpasteurization contamination.

Foegeding and Stanley (32) verified the previous predictions concerning heat resistance of listeriae by determining the thermal death time (F-value) for *L. monocytogenes* strain F5069 in liquid whole egg. Using their previously described submerged capillary tube method (31), they found *L. monocytogenes* was eliminated from inoculated samples (1.0×10^8 to 4.0×10^8 CFU/ml) of sterile liquid whole egg after processing at 62, 64, 66, 69, and 72°C for 16, 8, 4.5, 1.6, and 0.6 minute(s), respectively.

While results from this study confirm that minimum pasteurization (60°C/3.5 minutes) will not result in a *Listeria*-free product if initial populations are large, the need for a 9-D kill as currently required by the USDA may not be appropriate for *L. monocytogenes* since present estimates place the population of this pathogen at <100 CFU/g in raw liquid whole egg. Hence, based on maximum expected *L. monocytogenes* levels in raw liquid whole egg, pasteurization by current standards should render such products free of *Listeria*.

The situation regarding ultrapasteurization appears to be somewhat different since the thermal-death-time data obtained by Foegeding and Stanley (32) indicate that four of the 10 ultrapasteurization processes proposed by Ball et al. (20) (63.7°C/26.2 sec, 63.8°C/92.0 sec, 67.7°C/9.2 sec, and 71.5°C/2.7 sec) would likely fail to produce a 9-D decrease in numbers of listeriae in raw liquid whole egg. Nonetheless, the ≥9-D kill effected by the remaining six ultrapasteurization processes proposed by Ball et al. (20) indicates that ultrapasteurization processes can be designed to produce *Listeria*-free liquid whole egg with an anticipated refrigerated shelf life of 3–6 months.

REFERENCES

1. Al-Sheddy, I., and E. R. Richter. 1989. Microbiological quality/safety of zoo food. Ann. Mtg., Inst. Food Technol., Chicago, IL, June 26–29, Abstr. 476.
2. Anonymous. 1988. Code of Federal Regulations, Title 9, Section 381.150.
3. Anonymous. 1988. FSIS recommends 35°F for long-term storage of meat, poultry. *Food Chem. News 30*(12):25–28.
4. Anonymous. 1989. Chicken salad recalled in New England due to *Listeria*. *Food Chem. News 31(42):65–66.*
5. Anonymous. 1989. Current meat processing may not kill *Listeria*, study shows. *Food Chem. News 30*(52):57–58.

6. Anonymous. 1989. *Listeria*-contaminated chicken salad recalled from 3 states. *Food Chem. News 31*(35):51.

7. Anonymous. 1989. *Listeria* found by FSIS in small number but wide range of products. *Food Chem. News 31*(30):47–48.

8. Anonymous. 1989. *Listeria monocytogenes*: Paté. *Commun. Dis. Report 89*(27):1.

9. Anonymous. 1989. *Listeria* tolerances asked by meat, poultry group. *Food Chem. News 31*(14):46–48.

10. Anonymous. *Listeria* zero tolerance is warranted, USDA says. *Food Chem. News 31*(19):47–48.

11. Anonymous. 1989. Refrigerated fresh and frozen sandwiches recalled. FDA Enforcement Report, Dec. 20.

12. Anonymous. 1989. Temporary permit granted antimicrobial liquid eggs. *Food Chem. News 30*(47):49.

13. Anonymous. 1989. UK establishes committee to investigate food safety. *Food Chem. News 30*(51):39–40.

14. Anonymous. 1989. USDA to toughen regulatory policy on *Listeria* in meat, poultry. *Food Chem. News 31*(8):52–53.

15. Anonymous. 1990. Chicken, potato salad recalled by Campbell unit due to *Listeria*. *Food Chem. News 32*(9):61–63.

16. Anonymous. 1990. Irradiation in the production, processing and handling of food. *Fed. Reg. 55*:18538.

17. Anonymous. 1990. Prepared sandwiches recalled. FDA Enforcement Report, Jan. 31.

18. Anonymous. 1990. USDA monitoring finds *Listeria* in ready-to-eat products at 78 plants. *Food Chem. News 32*(7):71–73.

19. Bailey, J. S., D. L. Fletcher, and N. A. Cox. 1989. Recovery and serotype distribution of *Listeria monocytogenes* from broiler chickens in the southeastern United States. *J. Food Prot. 52*:148–150.

20. Ball, H. R., Jr., M. Hamid-Samimi, P. M. Foegeding, and K. R. Swartzel. 1987. Functionality and microbial stability of ultrapasteurized, aseptically packaged, refrigerated whole egg. *J. Food Sci. 52*:1212–1218.

21. Baranenkov, M. A. 1969. Survival rate of *Listeria* on the surface of eggs and the development of methods for disinfecting them. *Tr. Vses. Nauch.-Issled. Inst. Vet. Sanit. 32*:453–458.

22. Belding, R. C., and M. L. Mayer. 1957. Listeriosis in the turkey—two case reports. *J. Amer. Vet. Med. Assoc. 131*:296–297.

23. Bind, J.-L. 1988. Review of latest information concerning data about repartition of *Listeria* in France. WHO Working Group on Foodborne Listeriosis, Geneva, Switzerland, February 15–19.

24. Breer, C. 1988. Occurrence of *Listeria* spp. in different foods. WHO Working Group on Foodborne Listeriosis, Geneva, Switzerland, Feb. 15–19.

25. Buchanan, R. L., H. G. Stahl, and D. L. Archer. 1987. Improved plating media for simplified, quantitative detection of *Listeria monocytogenes* in foods. *Food Microbiol. 4*:269–275.

26. Carosella, J. 1989. Personal communication.

27. Carpenter, S. L., and M. A. Harrison. 1989. Survival of *Listeria monocytogenes* on processed poultry. *J. Food Sci. 54*:556–557.

28. Comi, G., and C. Cantoni. 1985. *Listeria* spp. in poultry from slaughterhouses of Lombardia. *Indust. Aliment. 24*:521–525.

29. Crawford, L. M. 1989. Food Safety and Inspection Service—Revised policy for controlling *Listeria monocytogenes*. *Fed. Reg. 54*:22345–22346.

30. Felsenfeld, O. 1951. Diseases of poultry transmissible to man. *Iowa State College Vet. 13*:89–92.

31. Foegeding, P. M., and S. B. Leasor. 1990. Heat resistance and growth of *Listeria monocytogenes* in liquid whole egg. *J. Food Prot. 53*:9–14.

32. Foegeding, P. M., and N. W. Stanley. 1990. *Listeria monocytogenes* F5069 thermal death times in liquid whole egg. *J. Food Prot. 53*:6–8, 25.

33. Genigeorgis, C. A., D. Dutulescu, and J. F. Garayzabal. 1989. Prevalence of *Listeria* spp. in poultry meat at the supermarket and slaughterhouse level. *J. Food Prot.* 52:618–624.
34. Genigeorgis, C. A., P. Oanca, and D. Dutulescu. 1990. Prevalence of *Listeria* spp. in turkey meat at the supermarket and slaughterhouse level. *J. Food Prot.* 53:282–288.
35. Gilbert, R. J. 1990. Personal communication.
36. Gilbert, R. J., S. M. Hall, and A. G. Taylor. 1989. Listeriosis update. *Public Health Lab Service Digest* 6:33–37.
37. Gilbert, R. J., K. L. Miller, and D. Roberts. 1989. *Listeria monocytogenes* and chilled foods. *Lancet i*:383–384.
38. Gitter, M. 1976. *Listeria monocytogenes* in "oven ready" poultry. *Vet. Rec.* 99:336.
39. Glass, K. A., and M. P. Doyle. 1989. Fate of *Listeria monocytogenes* in processed meat products during refrigerated storage. *Appl. Environ. Microbiol.* 55:1565–1569.
40. Gray, M. L. 1958. Listeriosis in fowls—A review. *Avian Dis.* 2:296–314.
41. Harrison, M. A., and S. L. Carpenter. 1989. Fate of small populations of *Listeria monocytogenes* on poultry processed using moist heat. *J. Food Prot.* 52:768–770.
42. Harrison, M. A., and S. L. Carpenter. 1989. Survival of large populations of *Listeria monocytogenes* on chicken breasts processed using moist heat. *J. Food Prot.* 52:376–378.
43. Harrison, M. A., and S. L. Carpenter. 1990. Survival of *Listeria monocytogenes* on microwave cooked poultry. *Food Microbiol.* (Accepted).
44. Hatkin, J. M., and W. E. Phillips, Jr. 1986. Isolation of *Listeria monocytogenes* from an eastern wild turkey. *J. Wildlife Dis.* 22:110–112.
45. Houston, D. L. 1987. Food Safety and Inspection Service—Testing for *Listeria monocytogenes*. *Fed. Reg.* 52:7464–7465.
46. Huang, D., A. E. Yousef, M. E. Matthews, and E. H. Marth. 1990. Growth of *Listeria monocytogenes* during cooling of chicken gravy. Unpublished data.
47. Hudson, W. R., and G. C. Mead. 1989. *Listeria* contamination at a poultry processing plant. *Lett. Appl. Microbiol.* 9:211–214.
48. Huhtanen, C. N., R. K. Jenkins, and D. W. Thayer. 1989. Gamma radiation sensitivity of *Listeria monocytogenes*. *J. Food Prot.* 52:610–613.
49. Ingham, S. C., J. M. Escude, and P. McCown. 1990. Comparative growth rates of *Listeria monocytogenes* and *Pseudomonas fragi* on cooked chicken loaf stored under air and two modified atmospheres. *J. Food Prot.* 53:289–291.
50. Kampelmacher, E. H. 1958. Berichten uit het Rijksinstitut voor de Volksgezondheit, Utrecht, The Netherlands. (In Seeliger, H. P. R. 1961. *Listeriosis*, Hafner Publ. Co., New York.)
51. Kampelmacher, E. H. 1962. Animal products as a source of listeric infection in man. In M. L. Gray (ed.), Second symposium on listeric infection, Montana State College, Bozeman, Montana, pp. 146–151.
52. Kampelmacher, E. H., and L. M. van Noorle Jansen. 1969. Isolation of *Listeria monocytogenes* from faeces of clinically healthy humans and animals. *Zbl. Bakteriol. I Abt. Orig.* 211:353–359.
53. Khan, M. A., I. A. Newton, A. Seaman, and M. Woodbine. 1975. Survival of *Listeria monocytogenes* inside and outside its host. In M. Woodbine (ed.), *Problems of Listeriosis*, Leicester University Press, Surrey, England, pp. 75–83.
54. Kwantes, W., and M. Isaac. 1971. Listeriosis. *Br. Med. J.* 4:296–297.
55. Kwantes, W., and M. Isaac. 1975. *Listeria* infection in West Glamorgan. In M. Woodbine (ed.), *Problems of Listeriosis*, Leicester University Press, Surrey, England, pp. 112–114.
56. Leasor, S. B., and P. M. Foegeding. 1989. *Listeria* species in commercially broken raw liquid whole egg. *J. Food Prot.* 52:777–780.
57. Lieval, F., J. Tache, and M. Poumeyrol. 1989. Qualité microbiologique et *Listeria* sp. dans les produits de la restauration rapide. *Sci. Aliment.* 9:111–115.
58. Lund, B. M., M. R. Knox, and M. B. Cole. 1989. Destruction of *Listeria monocytogenes* during microwave cooking. *Lancet i*:218.
59. McLauchlin, J., N. A. Saunders, A. M. Ridley, and A. G. Taylor. 1988. Listeriosis and food-borne transmission. *Lancet i*:177–178.

60. Mead, G. C., W. R. Hudson, and R. Ariffin. 1990. Survival and growth of *Listeria monocytogenes* on irradiated poultry carcasses. *Lancet i*:1036.
61. Morris, I. J., and C. D. Ribeiro. 1989. *Listeria monocytogenes* and paté. *Lancet ii*:1285–1286.
62. Mulder, R. W. A., S. Notermans, and E. H. Kampelmacher. 1977. Inactivation of salmonellae on chilled and deep frozen broiler carcasses by irradiation. *J. Appl. Bacteriol. 42*:179–185.
63. Nagi, M. S., and J. D. Verma. 1967. An outbreak of listeriosis in chickens. *Indian J. Vet. Med. 44*:539–543.
64. Nilsson, A., and K. A. Karlsson. 1959. *Listeria monocytogenes* isolations from animals in Sweden during 1948 to 1957. *Nord. Vet. Med. 11*:305–315.
65. Notermans, S., P. S. S. Soentoro, and E. H. M. Delfgou-van Asch. 1990. Survival of pathogenic microorganisms in an egg-nog-like product containing 7% ethanol. *Int. J. Food Microbiol. 10*:209–218.
66. Ozari, R. von, and F. A. Stolle. 1990. Zum Vorkommen von *Listeria monocytogenes* in Fleisch und Fleisch-Erzeugnissen einschliesslich Geflügelfleisch des Handels. *Arch. Lebensmittelhyg. 41*:47–50.
67. Palumbo, S., and A. C. Williams. 1989. Freezing and freeze-injury in *Listeria monocytogenes*. Ann. Mtg., Amer. Soc. Microbiol., New Orleans, LA, May 14–18, Abstr. P-1.
68. Paterson, J. St. 1937. *Listerella* infection in fowls—Preliminary note on its occurrence in East Anglia. *Vet. Rec. 49*:1533–1534.
69. Paterson, J. St. 1940. Experimental infection of the chick embryo with organisms of the genus *Listerella*. *J. Pathol. Bacteriol. 51*:437–440.
70. Patterson, M. 1989. Sensitivity of *Listeria monocytogenes* to irradiation on poultry meat and in phosphate-buffered saline. *Lett. Appl. Microbiol. 8*:181–184.
71. Pini, P. N., and R. J. Gilbert. 1988. A comparison of two procedures for the isolation of *Listeria monocytogenes* from raw chickens and soft cheeses. *Int. J. Food Microbiol. 7*:331–337.
72. Pini, P. N., and R. J. Gilbert. 1988. The occurrence in the U.K. of *Listeria* species in raw chickens and soft cheese. *Int. J. Food Microbiol. 6*:317–326.
73. Richmond, M. 1990. Report of the Committee on the Microbiological Safety of Food, HMSO, pp. 133–137.
74. Ronk, R. J. 1989. Liquid eggs deviating from the standard of identity; temporary permit for market testing. *Fed. Reg. 54*:1794–1795.
75. Schönberg, A., P. Teufel, and E. Weise. 1988. Isolates of *Listeria monocytogenes* and *Listeria innocua*. 10th International Symposium on Listeriosis, Pecs, Hungary, Aug. 22–26, Abstr. 45.
76. Seastone, C. V. 1935. Pathogenic organisms of the genus *Listerella*. *J. Exp. Med. 62*:203–212.
77. Seeliger, H. P. R. 1961. *Listeriosis*, Hafner Publishing Co., New York.
78. Seeliger, H. P. R., and D. Jones. 1987. *Listeria*. In *Bergy's Manual of Systematic Bacteriology*, 9th ed. Williams and Wilkins, Baltimore, pp. 1235–1245.
79. Sionkowski, P. J., and L. A. Shelef. 1990. Viability of *Listeria monocytogenes* strain Brie-1 in the avian egg. *J. Food Prot. 53*:15–17, 25.
80. Siragusa, G. R., and M. G. Johnson. 1988. Detection by conventional culture methods and a commercial ELISA test of *Listeria monocytogenes* added to cooked chicken. *Poultry Sci. 67* (Suppl. 1):157 (Abstr.)
81. Siragusa, G. R., K. J. Moore, and M. G. Johnson. 1988. Persistence on and recovery of *Listeria* from refrigerated processed poultry. *J. Food Prot. 51*:831–832.
82. Skovgaard, N., and C.-A. Morgen. 1988. Detection of *Listeria* spp. in faeces from animals, in feeds, and in raw foods of animal origin. *Int. J. Food Microbiol. 6*:229–242.
83. Steinmeyer, S. von, and G. Terplan. 1990. Listerien in Lebensmitteln—eine aktuelle Übersicht zu Vorkommen, Bedeutung als Krankheitserreger, Nachweis und Bewertung. *DMZ Lebensmittelindustrie und Milchwirtschaft 111*:150–155.
84. Steinmeyer, S. von, R. Schoen, and G. Terplan. 1987. Zum Nachweis der Pathogenität von aus Lebensmitteln isolierten Listerien am bebrüteten Hühnerei. *Arch. Lebensmittelhyg. 38*:95–99.
85. Ternström, A., and G. Molin. 1987. Incidence of potential pathogens on raw pork, beef and chicken in Sweden, with special reference to *Erysipelothrix rhusiopathiae*. *J. Food Prot. 50*:141–146, 149.

86. Urbach, H., and G. I. Schabinski. 1955. Zur Listeriose des Menschen. *Z. Hyg. 141*:239–248.
87. USDA. 1969. Egg Pasteurization Manual. ARS 74-48. Poultry Laboratory, Agriculture Research Service, USDA, Albany, CA.
88. Walker, S. J., P. Archer, and J. G. Banks. 1990. Growth of *Listeria monocytogenes* at refrigeration temperatures. *J. Appl. Bacteriol. 68*:157–162.
89. Wimpfheimer, L., N. S. Altman, and J. H. Hotchkiss. 1990. Predictive growth of *Listeria monocytogenes* and aerobic spoilage organisms in raw chicken packaged in modified atmospheres and air. *Int. J. Food Microbiol.* (Accepted).

13

Incidence and Behavior of *Listeria monocytogenes* in Fish and Seafood

INTRODUCTION

Since *L. monocytogenes* is ubiquitous in nature and many aquatic creatures including fin fish, oysters, shrimp, crabs, lobsters, squid, and scallops are harvested from natural environments, fish and seafoods also have been targeted as potential sources of listeriae in the human diet. Since the May 1987 discovery of *L. monocytogenes* in imported cooked crabmeat, at least 15 Class I recalls have been issued for nearly 45,000 pounds of domestic/imported fish and seafood, with this pathogen routinely found in 5–6% of all such products marketed in the United States. The first case of listeriosis positively linked to consumption of fish or seafood was not reported until 1989 when a 54-year-old Italian woman contracted listeric meningitis 4 days after consuming steamed fish from which *L. monocytogenes* was later isolated (43) (see Chapter 8). This case and the potential hazard associated with consumption of other *Listeria*-contaminated ready-to-eat food such as cooked crabmeat, cooked shrimp, and smoked salmon prompted studies on determining the incidence of listeriae in various seafoods and on means by which growth and survival of this pathogen can be sharply reduced in ready-to-eat as well as raw fish and seafood during refrigerated and frozen storage.

This chapter reviews data from a series of FDA surveys designed to determine the incidence of *L. monocytogenes* in domestic/imported shrimp, crab, and various other seafoods. As in previous chapters, Class I recalls that have been issued for *Listeria*-contaminated fish and seafoods also will be mentioned. While little information is currently available on behavior of *L. monocytogenes* in these foods, preliminary data concerning growth and thermal resistance of *L. monocytogenes* in seafood can be found in the remaining pages of this chapter along with several reports which address the use of lactic acid in controlling growth of listeriae in seafood. If current trends continue, additional information on incidence and behavior of *L. monocytogenes* in these foods will likely be generated by North American and European scientists in the future.

FDA SURVEYS FOR AND RECALLS BECAUSE OF *L. MONOCYTOGENES* IN DOMESTIC AND IMPORTED SEA FOOD

The notion that aquatic forms of life can harbor *L. monocytogenes* is not new. As early as 1957 Romanian workers (60) reported isolating *L. monocytogenes* from the viscera of pond-reared rainbow trout. Two years later, the pathogen also was detected in crustaceans gathered from a Russian stream (56). Until May of 1987, these were the only two accounts of *L. monocytogenes* in fish and seafood, probably a direct result of the poor isolation methods that were available at the time.

Immediately after the June 1985 outbreak of cheeseborne listeriosis in California, FDA officials rightly focused their attention on solving the many immediate problems that confronted the dairy industry. Despite a lack of evidence linking consumption of meat and poultry products to cases of human listeriosis before 1988, as early as December 1985 USDA-FSIS officials began taking an active interest in determining the incidence of *L. monocytogenes* in meat and poultry products. This information, along with the fact that the United States did not and presently (1990) still does not have a mandatory seafood inspection program, enables one to easily understand why *L. monocytogenes* was not detected in seafood products until nearly 2 years after the listeriosis outbreak in California became public knowledge.

Concern about the potential hazard of *Listeria*-contaminated seafood began in the spring of 1987 after a private testing laboratory in the United States isolated *L. monocytogenes* from frozen cooked crabmeat that was obtained from a Mexican supplier (3). Once proper authorities were informed of the positive finding, FDA officials in Baltimore, Maryland, confirmed the presence of *L. monocytogenes* in this product in May of 1987 (Fig. 13.1). In keeping with the FDA's "zero tolerance policy" for *L. monocytogenes* in cooked and ready-to-eat foods, the first in a series of Class I recalls involving *Listeria*-contaminated seafood was issued in May of 1987 to retrieve nearly 4 tons of tainted crabmeat that was marketed in four states (Table 13.1). These events also prompted an import alert on June 17, 1989 (6), which called for automatic detention and *Listeria/E. coli* testing of all frozen crabmeat shipped from Mexico.

Less than 1 month after this product was recalled without incident, FDA officials in Seattle, Washington, detected *L. monocytogenes* in samples of imported frozen raw shrimp (2) and lobster tails (37). While no recalls were issued for these products, which are almost invariably cooked before consumption, confirmation of listeriae in these seafoods together with the cooked crabmeat noted previously prompted the FDA to initiate two surveys in July of 1987 (Fig. 13.1).

In the first of these surveys, FDA officials at each district office collected and examined six imported samples of frozen raw shrimp per month for listeriae, with the samples representing as many different countries as possible (Table 13.2) (2). Additionally, each district also was requested to collect three domestic samples of frozen raw shrimp per month at the wholesale or retail level. The original FDA procedure (see Fig. 6.14) was used, and *Listeria* spp. were detected in 18 of 74 (24.3%) samples of frozen raw shrimp imported from 10 different countries between July and October of 1987 (Table 13.2). *Listeria monocytogenes* also was isolated from 4 of 74 imported samples of frozen raw shrimp, with all positive samples originating from Central or South American countries. Subsequently, three lots of raw shrimp imported from Ecuador and Honduras also were found to contain 10^3–10^5 *L. monocytogenes* or *L. innocua* CFU/g (53). However, since shrimp are normally not consumed in the raw state, FDA officials did not request the recall of any of these contaminated lots. Unfortunately, the results from the corresponding domestic survey have not yet (June 1990) been made public.

In the second of these FDA surveys, domestic and imported samples of cooked,

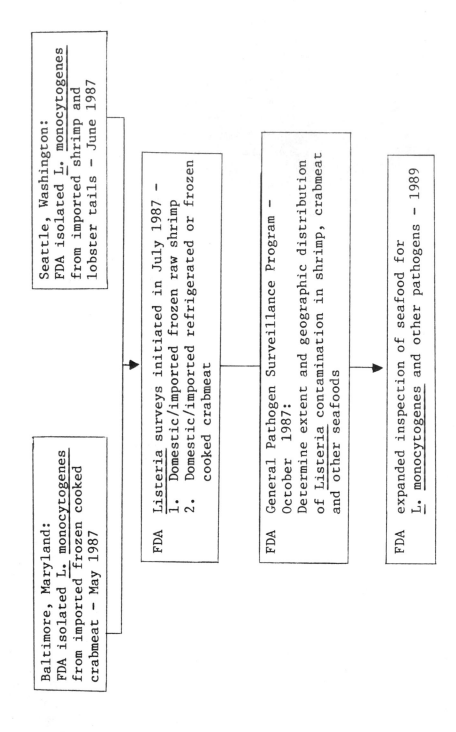

Figure 13.1 FDA surveys for *Listeria* spp. in domestic and imported seafood. (Adapted from Refs. 2, 20, 37.)

Table 13.1 Chronological List of Class I Recalls Issued in the United States for Domestic/Imported Fish and Seafood Contaminated with *L. monocytogenes*

Product	Date recall initiated	Origin of manufacture	Distribution	Quantity (lb.)	Ref.
Fresh frozen cooked crabmeat	5/28/87	Mexico	California, Pennsylvania, Texas, Virginia	7,500	3,5
Cooked, peeled shrimp	11/4/87	Florida	Florida, Illinois	79	1,7
Fresh crabmeat	12/2/87	Texas	Maryland, Pennsylvania, Washington, DC	700	4,9
Frozen crabmeat	6/10/88	Oregon	California, Washington	1,685	11,15
Frozen cooked shrimp	8/1/88	New York	New York	1,230	13,14
Frozen lobster meat	8/26/88	Canada	Maine, Massachusetts	264	16
Cooked, peeled shrimp	9/16/88	Washington	Washington	6,830	8,21
Smoked Nova Scotia salmon	12/1/88	Washington	Massachusetts, New York	12,000–15,000	10,22,33
Imitation crabmeat	12/9/88	Japan	Colorado, Michigan, Washington	Unknown	26
Fresh crabmeat	4/10/89	Mexico	Maryland, Washington, DC	Unknown	25
Nova lox	4/14/89	California	Massachusetts	11,640	29
Fresh crabmeat	8/8/89	Texas	Maryland, Texas	Unknown	23,24
Smoked salmon	8/14/89	Washington	California, Washington	132	32
Smoked salmon products	9/29/89	Illinois	Nationwide	6,975	31,34
Smoked cod and trout	11/10/89	Maryland	Ohio, Maryland, Virginia, Washington, DC	Unknown	35,36

Table 13.2 Results from an FDA Survey of Imported Frozen Raw Shrimp, July to October, 1987

Country of origin	Number of samples analyzed	Number of positive samples (%)	
		L. monocytogenes	Other *Listeria* spp.
Brazil	4	1 (25)	1 (25)
Ecuador	8	1 (12.5)	2 (25)
Guyana	1	1 (100)	0
Honduras	5	1[a] (20)	2 (40)
Hong Kong	1	0	0
India	4	0	1 (25)
Indonesia	1	0	0
Macau	1	0	0
Mexico	10	0	1 (10)
Nigeria	3	0	1 (33.3)
Norway	1	0	0
Pakistan	4	0	0
Panama	7	0	0
People's Republic of China	4	0	1 (25)
Peru	1	0	0
Philippines	3	0	0
Taiwan	9	0	4 (44.4)
Thailand	4	0	2 (50)
Venezuela	3	0	0
Total	74	4 (5.4)	15 (20.3)

[a]One sample contained *L. monocytogenes* and other *Listeria* spp.
Source: Adapted from Ref. 37.

frozen, and refrigerated crabmeat (i.e., picked or extracted) were examined for presence of *L. monocytogenes*, *Staphylococcus aureus*, *Vibrio cholerae*, *Vibrio parahaemolyticus*, *Vibrio vulnificus*, and *Yersinia enterocolitica* and numbers of *E. coli* (2). Again, samples of imported crabmeat from as many different countries as possible were collected. As of January 1988, 6 of 98 (6.1%) domestic samples of cooked crabmeat contained listeriae, with *L. monocytogenes* and *L. innocua* being recovered from 4 and 2 samples, respectively (Table 13.3). Similarly, *Listeria* spp. were detected in 3 of 24 (12.5%) imported samples of cooked crabmeat, with *L. monocytogenes* being discovered in 2 of 24 (8.3%) samples of product marketed in the United States. Hence, when these data are compared to those of other food surveys, the incidence of *L. monocytogenes* in raw and cooked seafood appears to be equal to or higher than that previously observed for raw milk, fermented dairy products (including certain varieties of cheese), and some types of ready-to-eat meat products. While further work is needed to confirm this observation, one must remember that as of June 1990 only one case of listeriosis has been positively linked to consumption of contaminated fish. Nonetheless, since presence of *L. monocytogenes* in any cooked or ready-to-eat product, including fish and seafood, is now recognized as

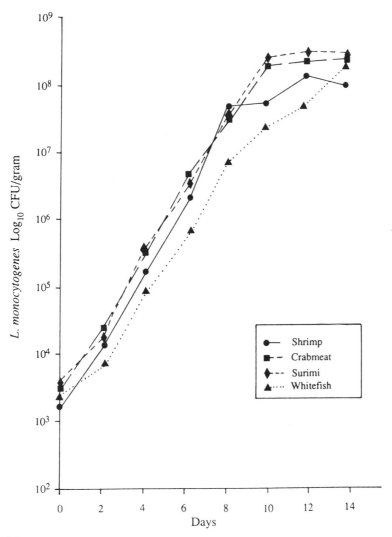

Figure 13.2 Growth of *L. monocytogenes* in raw shrimp, crabmeat, whitefish, and surimi during extended storage at 7°C. (Adapted from Ref. 52.)

Table 13.3 Results from an FDA Survey of Domestic/Imported
Refrigerated or Frozen Cooked Crabmeat, July 1987 to January 1988

Country of origin	Number of samples analyzed	Number of positive samples (%)	
		L. monocytogenes	Other *Listeria* spp.
United States	98	4 (4.1)	2 (2.0)
Canada	3	0	1 (33.3)
Chile	2	0	0
Korea	11	2 (18.2)	2[a] (18.2)
Japan	2	0	0
Mexico	3	0	0
Venezuela	3	0	0
Total (imported)	24	2 (8.3)	3 (12.5)

[a]One sample contained *L. monocytogenes* and *L. innocua.*
Source: Adapted from Ref. 37.

a potential health risk for certain groups of individuals, FDA officials have begun to detain, seize, and/or recall many contaminated lots of fish and seafood (Table 13.1) with 9 of the 15 Class I recalls issued thus far involving shrimp and crabmeat.

Discovery of listeriae in raw shrimp and crabmeat, coupled with an increased concern about the general safety of seafood, prompted FDA officials in October of 1987 to develop a compliance program for *L. monocytogenes* (and *Salmonella*) in domestic/imported shrimp (12) and to increase testing of many other domestically produced seafoods under the General Pathogen Surveillance Program (28,37) (Fig. 13.1). This program also seeks to determine the geographic distribution of listeriae in domestic/imported seafood and to identify the incidence of *L. monocytogenes, L. innocua, L. seeligeri, L. ivanovii,* and *L. welshimeri* in such products. In addition, the National Advisory Committee on Microbiological Criteria for Foods (NACMCF) met in April of 1988 to begin the laborious task of developing microbiological criteria for cooked shrimp and crabmeat (17). While a detailed discussion of proposed criteria for *L. monocytogenes* and other pathogens in seafoods has been reserved for Chapter 15, which deals in part with the incidence and control of listeriae in fish- and seafood-processing facilities, the reader should be aware that the NACMCF has recommended a "zero tolerance" for *L. monocytogenes* in cooked shrimp and crabmeat (27,30). Despite the recommended "zero tolerance" level, FDA district offices were instructed not to take immediate regulatory action if *L. monocytogenes* is discovered, but rather notify FDA's Center for Food Safety and Applied Nutrition for appropriate follow-up action in the form of a regulatory warning letter, seizure, or product recall (12). However, the "zero tolerance" and regulatory policies probably will be reviewed and revised periodically as new information concerning the incidence and behavior of *L. monocytogenes* in various seafoods becomes available.

While formal results from the aforementioned 1988/1989 FDA surveys have not yet been published, some preliminary data from these efforts have become available. According to Archer (37), *L. monocytogenes* was detected in 3 of 4, 2 of 6, and 2 of 5 samples of domestically produced crabmeat, shrimp. and fish, respectively, during the first 4 months of the Pathogen Surveillance Program, which began in October of 1987. Seafood products from which *L. monocytogenes* was isolated included frozen cooked snow crab, instant quick-frozen shrimp, frozen breaded pollock, and frozen mackerel (19,37). *Listeria innocua* also was discovered in 2 of 4, 1 of 6, 3 of 5, and 1 of 1 samples of crabmeat, shrimp, fish, and squid rings, respectively, with one sample each of crabmeat and shrimp contaminated with both *L. innocua* and *L. monocytogenes*. In addition to the recalled items listed in Table 13.1, FDA surveys associated with the various surveillance programs outlined in Fig. 13.1 have uncovered *L. monocytogenes* in shellfish (51), partially cooked scallop-flavored surimi fish cake (19,20,37), and a host of other cooked/ready-to-eat seafoods including blue crabmeat from the East and Gulf Coasts of the United States, Dungeness crab, cold smoked fish, analogue seafood products (11), and crawfish (54). [Independent investigators (11,20) have isolated *L. monocytogenes* from aquaculture products and catfish.]

Working at the FDA's District Laboratory in Seattle, Washington, Weagant et al. (62) can be credited with formally publishing the first results of a survey dealing with the incidence of *Listeria* spp. in imported/domestic frozen seafood products. While this survey presumably was made sometime during the second half of 1987, the exact relationship between this survey and the domestic/imported shrimp and crabmeat surveys as well as the General Pathogen Surveillance Program outlined in Fig. 13.1 remains unclear. Hence, the following results should be considered separately from those that were previously discussed. The FDA procedure outlined in Fig. 6.14 was used, and 31 of 50 (62%) imported and 4 of 7 (57%) domestic samples of frozen seafood tested positive for *Listeria* spp. with 15 of 57 (26.3%) and 26 of 57 (45.6%) samples containing *L. monocytogenes* and *L. innocua*, respectively (Table 13.4). Since no other *Listeria* spp. were found, it appears that 6 of the 35 (17%) *Listeria*-positive samples were contaminated with both *L. monocytogenes* and *L. innocua*. While 4 of 7 (57%) *Listeria*-positive domestic seafoods yielded only *L. monocytogenes*, the pathogen was detected in 3 of 18 (17%); 1 of 6 (17%), 2 of 8 (25%), 1 of 4 (25%), 3 of 7 (43%), and 1 of 2 (50%) samples of frozen seafood imported from Korea, the Philippines, Japan, Canada, Chile, and Taiwan, respectively, with single samples from The People's Republic of China, Ecuador, Mexico, Singapore, and Thailand testing negative for *L. monocytogenes*. With the exception of Ecuador, Mexico, and Thailand, one or more samples from the previously mentioned countries contained *L. innocua* alone or together with *L. monocytogenes* (six samples). While the number of samples examined from the various product categories was small, data in Table 13.4 do suggest that frozen seafood more frequently contains *L. innocua* than *L. monocytogenes*. Hence, as was true for raw milk, meat, and poultry products, it appears that both organisms also may occupy similar niches in seafood-processing environments. Therefore, presence of *L. innocua* in raw and particularly in cooked seafood should not be ignored but rather should be viewed as an indicator of possible contamination with *L. monocytogenes*.

In 1990 Motes (54) investigated the incidence of listeriae in raw oysters, shrimp, and crawfish as well as in estuarine and seawater samples collected along the Gulf Coast of the United States. Although preliminary findings indicate the *L. monocytogenes* was

Table 13.4 Incidence of *Listeria* spp. in Domestic and Imported Frozen Seafood

Product	Number of samples analyzed	Number of positive samples (%)	
		L. monocytogenes	Other *Listeria* spp.
Oysters	1	0	0
Shrimp (raw)	7	2 (29)	4 (57)
Shrimp (cooked, peeled)	8	2 (25)	3 (38)
Crabmeat (cooked)	24	7 (29)	12 (50)
Lobster tails (raw)	2	1 (50)	1 (50)
Squid	1	0	1 (100)
Langostinos	1	0	1 (100)
Scallops	2	0	1 (50)
Fin fish	4	1 (25)	2 (50)
Surimi-based seafood	7	2 (29)	1 (14)
Total	57	15 (26.3)	26 (45.6)

Source: Adapted from Ref. 62.

isolated from ~4% of 214 seafood samples, the pathogen was never detected in raw oysters. As part of the National Shellfish Sanitation Program, FDA personnel in Washington state (41) also failed to detect any listeriae in four oysters harvested from Puget Sound during August of 1987 even though one of these oysters contained 5400 coliforms/100 g. Additionally, no *Listeria* spp. were detected in water from tanks in which the four oysters were held. Unlike these findings, Motes (54) reported that some of the aforementioned estuarine and seawater samples contained low levels of listeriae with presence of these organisms unrelated to either water temperature or salinity. As in the previous study, further work failed to identify any correlation between presence of fecal coliforms and *Listeria* in shellfish. Hence, these results, like those from the raw milk surveys discussed in Chapter 9, suggest that coliform and *Listeria* counts in seafood are unlikely to be closely related.

OTHER SURVEYS FOR *LISTERIA* SPP. IN SEAFOOD

United States

In addition to the FDA surveys just discussed, Buchanan and co-workers (40) at the USDA made a limited survey of raw and cooked retail seafood products to (a) compare the ability of two selective plating media to recover *Listeria* spp. from different seafoods and (b) test a three-tube MPN (most probable number) enrichment procedure for quantitating listeriae in seafood. (Results concerning isolation, detection, and quantitation methods used in this study are discussed in Chapter 6.) Overall, *Listeria* spp. were detected in 5 of 18 (28%) seafood samples (Table 13.5) as compared to 8 and 52% of fresh and cured retail red meat products that were examined in the same study (see Table

Table 13.5 Limited Survey of Raw and Cooked Retail Seafood for *Listeria* spp.

Product	Number of samples analyzed	Number of positive samples	*Listeria* spp. identified[a]	Level of *Listeria* spp. (CFU/g)[b]
Shrimp (uncooked, frozen)	1	1	I	0.74
Shrimp (uncooked, refrig.)	3	0	—	ND[c]
Shrimp salad	1	0	—	ND
Seafood salad	1	0	—	ND
Crabmeat (cooked, nonpasteurized)	2	1	W	ND–>110
Crabmeat (surimi)	1	0	—	ND
Flounder (refrig.)	1	1	M	0.92
Haddock (refrig.)	1	0	—	ND
Scrod (refrig.)	1	0	—	ND
Monkfish (refrig.)	1	1	M	0.36
Catfish (refrig.)	1	1	W	23.98
Scallops (uncooked)	1	0	—	ND
Oysters (uncooked)	2	0	—	ND
Clams (uncooked)	1	0	—	ND
Total	18	5	I, M, W	ND–>110

[a]M = *L. monocytogenes*; I = *L. innocua*; W = *L. welshimeri*.
[b]Minimum detectable level = 0.03 *Listeria* spp. CFU/g using an MPN procedure.
[c]Not detected.
Source: Adapted from Ref. 40.

11.3). Low levels of *L. monocytogenes* were observed in 2 of 18 (11%) samples examined, namely flounder and monkfish, with a small number of *L. innocua* also detected in one sample of uncooked frozen shrimp. Unlike the aforementioned studies, *L. welshimeri* was identified in 2 of 18 (11%) samples (i.e., crabmeat, catfish) at levels many times higher than those previously observed for *L. monocytogenes* and *L. innocua*. Fortunately, since *L. innocua* and *L. welshimeri* are both widely regarded as nonpathogenic, their presence in raw and cooked seafood should not be considered as a direct threat to public health. Nonetheless, because of the potential indicator status of other *Listeria* spp. for *L. monocytogenes* in raw and particularly cooked seafood, discovery of any *Listeria* spp. in processed seafood should prompt manufacturers to review the adequacy of current cleaning and sanitation practices.

Other Countries

Thus far the United States appears to have taken the lead in determining the incidence of listeriae in fish and seafood; however, reports indicate that testing of these products for listeriae is underway in Canada and England (47). According to one such survey, *L. monocytogenes* was absent from 40 retail samples of cooked prawns, shrimp, and cockles that were sold in England and Wales between 1987 and 1989 (58). However, as of early

1990 officials at the Public Health Laboratory Service in London have recovered *L. monocytogenes* from retail raw, cooked, and smoked fish as well as fish fingers, shrimp, and shellfish (46), which suggests that England and the United States are experiencing somewhat similar problems regarding *Listeria*-contaminated fish and seafood. Although a report in February 1988 to the World Health Organization also indicated some activity in France (38) (i.e., 3 of 3 fish products were free of *Listeria* spp.), interest in the occurrence of listeriae in various raw and cooked seafoods marketed within Europe is likely to increase in the future, particularly if follow-up investigations of recent listeriosis cases are successful in linking this illness to consumption of contaminated seafood.

The aforementioned import alerts and accompanying recalls of *Listeria*-contaminated seafoods shipped to the United States have caused concern among seafood exporting nations. In 1989, Indian and British investigators (45) published results from a joint study in which fish and seafood products marketed in southern India were examined for listeriae. They used the original FDA procedure (see Figure 6.14) and detected only *L. innocua*, with this organism present in 3 of 10 (30%) fresh and 4 of 14 (28.6%) frozen fish/seafood samples, respectively, and 0 of 11 samples of dried and salted fish (Table 13.6). While listeriae would not be expected to grow in sun-dried and salted fish containing 20–25% moisture and 15–20% NaCl, exposure to the outdoor environment during drying provides ample opportunity for *Listeria* spp. to contaminate this product. Hence, sun-dried/salted fish should not automatically be considered as free of healthy and/or injured listeriae. While this study provides much needed information, progress

Table 13.6 Incidence of *L. innocua* in Fresh, Frozen, and Dried/Salted Fish and Seafood Products Marketed in Southern India

Product	Number of samples analyzed	Number of positive samples (%)
Fresh		
shrimp	5	2 (40)
cuttlefish	1	0
pearl spot	3	1 (33.3)
clam meat	1	0
Frozen		
seer	3	1 (33.3)
peeled prawn meat	4	2 (50)
black pomfret	2	2 (100)
pearl spot	3	0
vatta	1	0
mackerel	1	0
Dried/salted fish	11	0
Total	35	8 (22.9)

Source: Adapted from Ref. 45.

toward decreasing the incidence of listeriae in raw and cooked seafood will likely be very slow since, with a few exceptions (Iceland, Norway, Japan), most of the world's fish and seafood is harvested and processed by third world countries, which probably lack both the financial resources and technical personnel to implement and strictly enforce good manufacturing practices.

BEHAVIOR OF *LISTERIA* IN FISH AND SEAFOOD

Considering that nothing was known about the incidence of *Listeria* spp. in fish or seafood before 1987, it is not surprising that behavior of listeriae in these products also is only poorly understood with virtually all such information coming from studies initiated since 1987. Preliminary data from these studies, which have primarily focused on growth and thermal inactivation of *L. monocytogenes* in shrimp, will be briefly discussed on the following pages. However, first it is appropriate to examine the means by which this pathogen may be transmitted to various forms of aquatic life.

Modes of Transmission

Current data point to cross-contamination as the major source of listeriae in cooked or otherwise processed seafood, as evidenced by the recovery of healthy, noninjured cells of *L. monocytogenes* from the surface of many heat-processed/ready-to-eat seafood products. However, one also must consider the possibility that a small percentage of aquatic creatures may become contaminated through direct/indirect contact with listeriae in their natural environment. This appears even more plausible when one recalls the salt-tolerant nature of *L. monocytogenes* and that this pathogen has been isolated from sewage effluent entering the North Sea (42) and also from crustaceans that were harvested from stream water in which *L. monocytogenes* was previously identified (56).

In 1989, Fuad et al. (44) evaluated the ability of *L. monocytogenes* to survive in the estuarine environment. Since there appears to be a higher incidence of listeriae in chitinous seafood (i.e., shrimp, crab, lobster), samples of filtered and unfiltered seawater with and without chitin and chitin-free filtered and unfiltered stream water were inoculated with various strains of *L. monocytogenes*, many of which possessed chitinase activity. Although preliminary results indicate that *Listeria* populations decreased in chitin-free filtered and unfiltered seawater, addition of chitin to both types of seawater stimulated growth of listeriae. Moreover, the pathogen also grew in filtered stream water. These findings, along with those from a report in which *L. monocytogenes* was found on the exoskeleton but not in the digestive tract of shrimp that were exposed to high levels of *L. monocytogenes* in aquaculture tanks (61), suggest that this pathogen may be ecologically adapted to chitin. If this is true, then it is imperative that holding tanks for chitinous marine animals be properly set up and maintained to avoid potential microbiological problems involving *L. monocytogenes* and other foodborne pathogens including *Vibrio* spp. and *Aeromonas hydrophila*.

Growth and Survival

Raw and processed seafoods have long been regarded as excellent substrates for growth of most common agents of foodborne disease, particularly if seafoods are held at improper temperatures; however, interest in behavior of *L. monocytogenes* in these products is of recent origin with preliminary results from relatively few studies being thus far reported. According to data gathered by Lovett et al. (52) in 1988, *L. monocytogenes* grew readily (generation time $\cong$ 12 hours) in inoculated samples of raw shrimp, crab, surimi, and whitefish, with the pathogen attaining maximum populations of $>10^8$ CFU/g in all four products following 14 days of storage at 7°C (Fig. 13.2). Two years later, Brackett and Beuchat (39) also reported that *L. monocytogenes* grew and retained similar levels of pathogenicity on artificially contaminated crabmeat during 14 days of storage at 5 or 10°C. However, in contrast to what Lovett et al. (52) observed for shrimp and whitefish, Harrison et al. (48) found *L. monocytogenes* failed to grow in overwrapped/vacuum-packaged raw shrimp and fin fish, with numbers of listeriae generally decreasing <10-fold after 21 days of storage in an ice chest. During this same period, psychrotrophic populations increased from 10^3 to $>10^7$ CFU/g, thus reinforcing the notion that *L. monocytogenes* can readily survive in refrigerated raw foods, even when greatly outnumbered by natural contaminants. Since *L. monocytogenes* was recovered from laboratory-contaminated shrimp (initial inoculum $\cong 10^5$ CFU/g) after 90 days of storage at –20°C (53), it is evident that this pathogen also is fairly resistant to subfreezing temperatures.

Unlike the aforementioned products, preliminary results from Kaysner et al. (49) suggest that *L. monocytogenes* was unable to grow in artificially contaminated oysters, with *Listeria* populations remaining constant in shucked oysters and decreasing approximately 10-fold in shellstock oysters after 21 days at 4°C. Apparent inability of listeriae to grow in raw oysters may be related to difficulties in isolating listeriae from retail raw oysters. Nevertheless, considering the potential for rapid growth of *L. monocytogenes* in most raw seafood during extended storage at 7°C and the microbial populations on which current thermal processing requirements are based, it would be prudent to store such products at temperatures as close to or preferably below 0°C before commercial processing to prevent growth of listeriae to the point where the pathogen may survive cooking.

Recognizing that *L. monocytogenes* is more likely to contaminate the surface rather than interior of most seafoods, Noel et al. (55) investigated the possibility of using various lactic acid treatments to inactivate *L. monocytogenes* on the surface of processed seafoods and also to extend the shelf life of the products during refrigerated and frozen storage. In this study, samples of locally processed peeled and unpeeled shrimp were immersed in an *L. monocytogenes* broth culture, removed, thoroughly drained, and immersed in an aqueous solution of 1.5, 3.0, or 6.0% lactic acid for 1, 10, or 120 minutes. Lactic acid–treated and untreated shrimp were then frozen at –20°C and examined for numbers of listeriae during 28 days of storage.

While all lactic acid treatments decreased numbers of listeriae and natural contaminants on both peeled and unpeeled shrimp, exposure to 1.5% lactic acid for 10 minutes was deemed most appropriate since this treatment did not adversely affect the product's appearance or organoleptic quality. Overall, initial *L. monocytogenes* populations of 2.6×10^3 CFU/g in inoculated shrimp decreased to $<3.2 \times 10^2$ CFU/g following 10 minutes of exposure to 1.5% lactic acid. After 7 days of frozen storage, lactic acid–treated and untreated shrimp contained <100 *L. monocytogenes* CFU/g, which attests to the adverse effects of freezing on listeriae. Although *Listeria* populations continued to decrease in all samples, fewer listeriae were observed in lactic acid–treated (~10 CFU/g) rather than untreated shrimp (~40 CFU/g) after 28 days of frozen storage. Thus, despite the inability of this treatment to completely eliminate *L. monocytogenes* from shrimp, it appears that lactic acid dips can be used as an added safeguard during processing of frozen shrimp with recent field tests also showing that similar treatments will likely prove useful in decreasing levels of listeriae on lobster, crabs, and scallops before freezing.

Considering the innate ability of *L. monocytogenes* to survive in low moisture environments, Sikes (59) investigated the fate of this pathogen in surimi-based chowder bars, a United States Army ration product containing 10% freeze-dried surimi, 49% powdered cream, 15% maltodextrin, 21% corn oil, 4.7% other ingredients, and 2.3% moisture. After this product at pH 7.1 was inoculated to contain ~10^8 *L. monocytogenes* CFU/g, numbers of listeriae decreased >6 orders of magnitude during 80 days of storage at 25°C. As you will recall from Chapter 10, this organism was eliminated somewhat faster from similar yogurt-based bars having a pH value of 4.9. Hence, viability of *Listeria* in dried foods appears to be inversely related to pH of the product.

Thermal Resistance

As was true for dairy, meat, and poultry products, the recent rash of Class I recalls primarily involving cooked shrimp and crabmeat (Table 13.1) has prompted concerns about the adequacy of thermal processing treatments currently used for raw seafood. Hence, in early 1988 Pace et al. (57) reported results from a study in which freshly shucked oysters were exposed to 150 ppm chlorine for 30 minutes, pasteurized at an internal temperature of 72–74°C for 8 minutes, and then periodically examined for major bacterial groups during 5 months of refrigerated storage. According to these authors chlorination reduced initial aerobic plate counts of 4.5×10^5 CFU/g by 40–90%, with pasteurization reducing the population by an additional 99.9%. Despite these large reductions in microbial flora, survivors classified in eight different genera of aerobic or facultatively anaerobic bacteria were detected in the final product during extended incubation at refrigeration temperatures. While *Bacillus* spp. predominated in oysters throughout cold storage, organisms which were classified as nonpathogenic *Listeria* spp. emerged in 5-month old oysters and accounted for 8.8–37.6% of all facultatively anaerobic bacteria present in the product. However, at this point the oysters were unfit for consumption as evidenced by profuse gas production and swelling of plastic pouches in which the product was pasteurized.

In response to public and industry concerns, FDA officials at the Fishery Research Branch in Alabama (53) also examined the thermal resistance of *Listeria* in raw shrimp tails that were inoculated internally to contain ~10^4–10^5 *L. monocytogenes* CFU/g. Using a combination of cold (with/without broth) enrichment and warm (selective) enrichment, these investigators failed to recover the pathogen from shrimp tails that were boiled longer than 5 minutes. Although appreciable numbers of heat-stressed cells were detected in inoculated shrimp tails that were boiled for 3 minutes, frozen storage of the product at –20°C eventually led to complete inactivation of the pathogen. More important, when this study was repeated using naturally contaminated frozen shrimp from Ecuador and Honduras in which 10^3–10^5 *L. monocytogenes* or *L. innocua* CFU/g were presumably present only on the chitinous exoskeleton, all listeriae were eliminated after

1 minute of boiling. Hence, since shrimp are more likely to be contaminated externally than internally with relatively low levels of listeriae, these preliminary findings suggest that present cooking methods are adequate to eliminate these organisms from raw shrimp. If this is true, then the recent Class I recalls involving cooked shrimp (and probably cooked crabmeat as well) likely resulted from postprocessing contamination as has already been implied by Kvenberg (18,50) and other FDA officials (11,61). However, considering the possibility for an error during thermal processing, members of the Seafood Working Group of NACMCF agreed it would be prudent to consider certifying or licensing persons who are directly involved in thermally processing shrimp and crabmeat, as has been done for many years in the canned food industry (18).

REFERENCES

1. Anonymous. 1987. Cooked shrimp recalled. FDA Enforcement Report, Dec. 16.
2. Anonymous. 1987. FDA checking imported, domestic shrimp, crabmeat for *Listeria*. *Food Chem. News* 29(24):15–17.
3. Anonymous. 1987. First *Listeria* finding in crabmeat confirmed by FDA. *Food Chem. News* 29(14):38.
4. Anonymous. 1987. Fresh crabmeat recalled. FDA Enforcement Report, Dec. 23.
5. Anonymous. 1987. Fresh frozen crabmeat recalled. FDA Enforcement Report, June 10.
6. Anonymous. 1987. Mexican crabmeat, Greek pasta automatically detained. *Food Chem. News* 29(19):43.
7. Anonymous. 1987. Shrimp recalled because of *Listeria monocytogenes*. *Food Chem. News* 29(42):12.
8. Anonymous. 1988. Cooked and peeled shrimp recalled. FDA Enforcement Report, Oct. 19.
9. Anonymous. 1988. Crabmeat undergoes Class I recall because of *Listeria*. *Food Chem. News* 29(44):51.
10. Anonymous. 1988. FDA investigates *Listeria* problem in Nova Scotia salmon. *Food Chem. News* 30(40):38–39.
11. Anonymous. 1988. FDA regional workshops to discuss microbial concerns in seafoods. *Food Chem. News* 30(43):27–31.
12. Anonymous. 1988. FDA to sample shrimp for *Salmonella*, *Listeria*. *Food Chem. News* 30(36):9–10.
13. Anonymous. 1988. Frozen cooked shrimp recalled. FDA Enforcement Report, Aug. 10.
14. Anonymous. 1988. Frozen cooked shrimp recalled due to *Listeria* contamination. *Food Chem. News* 30(24):37.
15. Anonymous. 1988. Frozen crabmeat recalled. FDA Enforcement Report, July 20.
16. Anonymous. 1988. Frozen lobster meat recalled. FDA Enforcement Report, Oct. 5.
17. Anonymous. 1988. Hot dogs, shrimp, crab targeted for microbiological criteria. *Food Chem. News* 30(6):43–45.
18. Anonymous. 1988. Micro criteria for crabmeat, shrimp would have 3-class attributes. *Food Chem. News* 30(24):25–27.
19. Anonymous. 1988. Ongoing CDC/FDA study shows listeriosis rate at 0.7 per million. *Food Chem. News* 30(14):5–8.
20. Anonymous. 1988. Seafood industry faces major challenge in *Listeria*, Kvenberg says. *Food Chem. News* 30(25):6–9.
21. Anonymous. 1988. Shrimp undergo Class I recall because of *Listeria*. *Food Chem. News* 30(34):20–21.
22. Anonymous. 1988. Smoked Nova Scotia salmon recalled. FDA Enforcement Report, Dec. 28.
23. Anonymous. 1989. Class I recall made of crabmeat because of *Listeria*, *Vibrio*. *Food Chem. News* 31(32):39.
24. Anonymous. 1989. Crabmeat recalled. FDA Enforcement Report, Oct. 4.

25. Anonymous. 1989. Fresh crabmeat recalled. FDA Enforcement Report, May 24.

26. Anonymous. 1989. Imitation crabmeat recalled. FDA Enforcement Report, Jan. 18.

27. Anonymous. 1989. *Listeria, Salmonella* zero tolerance in cooked crab, shrimp proposed. *Food Chem. News 31*(1):11–14.

28. Anonymous. 1989. Monitoring of changes to listeriosis problem urged. *Food Chem. News 31*(20):13–17.

29. Anonymous. 1989. Nova lox bits recalled. FDA Enforcement Report, May 24.

30. Anonymous 1989. Seafood micro group publishes pathogen criteria. *Food Chem. News 31*(19):31–34.

31. Anonymous. 1989. Smoked salmon products recalled. FDA Enforcement Report, Nov. 8.

32. Anonymous. 1989. Smoked salmon recalled. FDA Enforcement Report, Nov. 1.

33. Anonymous. 1989. Smoked salmon recalled because of *Listeria. Food Chem. News 30*(45):27.

34. Anonymous. 1989. Smoked salmon recalled because of *Listeria. Food Chem. News 31*(34):26.

35. Anonymous. 1990. Smoked fish recalled. FDA Enforcement Report, Jan. 24.

36. Anonymous. 1990. Smoked fish recalled due to *Listeria* contamination. *Food Chem. News 31*(48):34.

37. Archer, D. L. 1988. Review of the latest FDA information on the presence of *Listeria* in foods. WHO Working Group on Foodborne Listeriosis, Geneva, Switzerland, Feb. 15–19.

38. Bind, J.-L. 1988. Review of latest information concerning data about repartition of *Listeria* in France. WHO Working Group on Foodborne Listeriosis, Geneva, Switzerland, February 15–19.

39. Brackett, R. E., and L. R. Beuchat. 1990. Changes in the pathogenicity of *Listeria monocytogenes* grown in crabmeat. Ann. Mtg. Amer. Soc. Microbiol., Anaheim, CA, May 13–17, Abstr. P-60.

40. Buchanan, R. L., H. G. Stahl, M. M. Bencivengo, and F. del Corral. 1989. Comparison of lithium chloride-phenylethanol-moxalactam and modified Vogel Johnson agars for detection of *Listeria* spp. in retail-level meats, poultry and seafood. *Appl. Environ. Microbiol. 55*:599–603.

41. Colburn, K. G., C. A. Kaysner, M. M. Wekell, J. R. Matches, C. Abeyta, Jr., and R. F. Stott. 1989. Microbiological quality of oysters (*Crassostrea gigas*) and water of live holding tanks in Seattle, WA markets. *J. Food Prot. 52*:100–104.

42. Dijkstra, R. G. 1982. The occurrence of *Listeria monocytogenes* in surface water of canals and lakes, in ditches of one big polder and in the effluents and canals of a sewage treatment plant. *Zbl. Bakteriol. Hyg., I Abt. Orig. B 176*:202–205.

43. Facinelli, B., P. E. Varaldo, M. Toni, C. Casolari, and U. Fabio. 1989. Ignorance about *Listeria. Brit. Med. J. 299*:738.

44. Fuad, A., S. Weagant, M. Wekell, and J. Liston. 1989. Survival of *Listeria monocytogenes* in the estuarine environment. Ann. Mtg., Amer. Soc. Microbiol., New Orleans, LA, May 14–18, Abstr. Q-243.

45. Fuchs, R. S., and P. K. Surendran. 1989. Incidence of *Listeria* in tropical fish and fishing products. *Lett. Appl. Microbiol. 9*:49–51.

46. Gilbert, R. J. 1990. Personal communication.

47. Gilbert, R. J., and P. N. Pini. 1988. Listeriosis and food-borne transmission. *Lancet i*:472–473.

48. Harrison, M., Y. Huang, C. Chao, and T. Shineman. 1990. Fate of *Listeria monocytogenes* on packaged, refrigerated seafood products. Ann. Mtg., Amer. Soc. Microbiol., Anaheim, CA, May 13–17, Abstr. P-56.

49. Kaysner, C., K. Colburn, C. Abeyta, and M. Wekell. 1990. Survival of *Listeria monocytogenes* in shellstock and shucked oysters, *Crassostrea gigas*, stored at 4°C. Ann. Mtg., Amer. Soc. Microbiol., Anaheim, CA, May 13–17, Abstr. P-52.

50. Kvenberg, J. E. 1988. Ocurrence of *Listeria monocytogenes* in seafood. Society for Industrial Microbiology–Comprehensive Conference on *Listeria monocytogenes*, Rohnert Park, CA, Oct. 2–5.

51. Kvenberg, J. E. 1988. Outbreaks of listeriosis/*Listeria*-contaminated foods. *Microbiol. Sci. 5*:355–358.

52. Lovett, J., D. W. Francis, and J. G. Bradshaw. 1988. Outgrowth of *Listeria monocytogenes* in foods. Society for Industrial Microbiology–Comprehensive Conference on *Listeria monocytogenes*, Rohnert Park, CA, Oct. 2–5.
53. McCarthy, S. A., M. L. Motes, and M. McPhearson. 1990. Recovery of heat-stressed *Listeria monocytogenes* from experimentally and naturally contaminated shrimp. *J. Food Prot. 53*:22–25.
54. Motes, M. 1990. Recovery of *Listeria* spp. from seafoods and their ambient environments. Ann. Mtg., Amer. Soc. Microbiol., Anaheim, CA, May 13–17, Abstr. Q-76.
55. Noel, D., G. E. Rodrick, W. S. Otwell, and J. Bacus. 1989. Lactic acid use in seafood microbial control. Ann. Mtg., Inst. Food Technol., Chicago, IL, June 25–29, Abstr. 355.
56. Olsufjew, N. G., and V. G. Petrow. 1959. Detection of *Erysipelothrix* and *Listeria* in stream water. *Zh. Mikrobiol. Epidemiol. Immunobiol. 30*:89–94.
57. Pace, J., C. Y. Wu, and T. Chai. 1988. Bacterial flora in pasteurized oysters after refrigerated storage. *J. Food Sci. 53*:325–327, 348.
58. Richmond, M. 1990. Report of the Committee on the Microbiological Safety of Food, HMSO, pp. 133–137.
59. Sikes, A. 1989. Fate of *Staphylococcus aureus* and *Listeria monocytogenes* in certain low moisture military rations during processing and storage. Ann. Mtg., Inst. Food Technol., Chicago, IL, June 25–29, Abstr. 466.
60. Stamatin, N., C. Ungureanu, E. Constantinescu, A. Solnitzky, and E. Vasilescu. 1957. Infectia naturala cu *Listeria monocytogenes* la pastravul curcubeu *Salmo irideus. Anuar. Inst. Animal Pathol. Hyg. Bucuresti 7*:163–180. (Cited from Gray, M. L., and A. H. Killinger. 1966. *Listeria monocytogenes* and listeric infections. *Bacteriol. Rev. 30*:309–382.)
62. Van Wagner, L. R. 1989. FDA takes action to combat seafood contamination. *Food Proc. 50*:8–12.
62. Weagant, S. D., P. A. Sade, K. G. Colburn, J. D. Torkelson, F. A. Stanley, M. H. Krane, S. C. Shields, and C. F. Thayer. 1988. The incidence of *Listeria* species in frozen seafood products. *J. Food Prot. 51*:655–657.

14

Incidence and Behavior of *Listeria monocytogenes* in Products of Plant Origin

INTRODUCTION

It should now be evident that use of adequate isolation procedures, enough time, and a little perseverance by investigators make it possible to isolate *Listeria* spp., including *L. monocytogenes*, from most forms of animal life. A similar situation also exists with products of plant origin. Chapter 3 describes the apparent association between consumption of silage and occurrence of an illness resembling listeriosis in ruminants, which was observed as early as 1922; however, this link between silage consumption and listeriosis in domestic livestock was not confirmed until 1960 (23). While three papers published during the next 15-year period documented the presence of *L. monocytogenes* in vegetation grown primarily for consumption by animals (39–41) (see Chapter 2), scientists at the time were generally unconcerned about the incidence of listeriae in produce destined for human consumption, primarily since such products had not been positively linked to human listeriosis. In fact, the only instance in which listeriae were recovered from raw retail produce before the 1981 listeriosis outbreak in Canada involving contaminated coleslaw occurred in 1975 when the successful isolation of three untypable *Listeria* strains from lettuce marketed in Brazil was reported (27).

Although 18 of 41 Canadians contracted a fatal listeric infection in 1981 after consuming coleslaw from which *L. monocytogenes* was isolated and positively identified (35), it was not until the 1985 cheese-related listeriosis outbreak in California that researchers began to develop more than a passive interest in the public health significance of *L. monocytogenes* in vegetables, fruits, and other products of plant origin. Nevertheless, with the exception of one isolated listeriosis case in Finland involving homemade salted mushrooms (30), no additional cases of listeriosis have been positively linked to consumption of products of plant origin produced in North America or elsewhere.

This final chapter devoted to food products will specifically address the incidence of *Listeria* spp. in raw retail vegetables and fruits. As in earlier chapters, information concerning behavior of *L. monocytogenes* in fresh produce and related products (orange juice/serum, soymilk, pasta, beet pigment) will also be presented along with some possible means by which listeriae can be inactivated in some of these products.

INCIDENCE OF *LISTERIA* ON RAW VEGETABLES

Unless fertilized with human and/or animal waste or irrigated with water containing such waste, raw vegetables (and fruits) normally should be free of most human and animal enteric pathogens. While presence of soilborne spore-forming organisms such as *Clostridium perfringens* and *Bacillus cereus* are of little consequence on raw vegetables, these organisms can pose potential health problems in cooked vegetables that have been held at inappropriate temperatures. However, relatively few outbreaks of foodborne illness have been associated with consumption of vegetables.

When one considers the enormous variety and quantity of produce being marketed annually, routine microbiological examination of raw vegetables (and fruits) seems highly impractical and probably unnecessary if good agricultural practices are used in growing crops along with acceptable hygienic practices while harvesting, packaging, and transporting raw produce to market. Although consumption of coleslaw prepared from contaminated cabbage was linked to a large Canadian outbreak of listeriosis in 1981 (36), in retrospect it appears that this outbreak could have been easily avoided if the coleslaw manufacturer had realized that the cabbage farmer had fertilized the cabbage with sheep manure from a flock that was previously diagnosed as having listeriosis. (The role of manure and sewage as vehicles for listeriae is discussed in Chapter 2.) Hence, in spite of this outbreak, which resulted in 18 fatalities, it is not surprising that, unlike dairy, meat, poultry, and seafood, no surveillance and/or regulatory programs have been initiated to assess the incidence of listeriae in raw vegetables (or fruits) marketed in the United States, Canada, or elsewhere. Nevertheless, inadvertent isolation of *L. monocytogenes* from potato salad in April 1990 prompted a Virginia-based manufacturer to recall 5700 pounds of product that had been distributed in the southeastern United States (2). While the risk of contracting listeriosis from such products is generally thought to be quite low, lack of routine microbiological analysis of raw produce should not be interpreted to mean that fresh vegetables and fruits will always be free of listeriae, including *L. monocytogenes*.

United States

In response to heightened concern about foodborne listeriosis, several small surveys were conducted after the 1985 outbreak in California to determine the extent of *Listeria* contamination in raw fresh and frozen vegetables destined for human consumption. During 1986 and 1987, Petran et al. (35) used the FDA procedure in an attempt to isolate *Listeria* spp., including *L. monocytogenes*, from 23 retail samples of vegetables, including fresh beet peels, broccoli, cabbage (outer leaves), carrot peels, cauliflower stems, corn husks, head lettuce, leaf lettuce, mushroom stems, potato peels, and spinach as well as frozen green beans, pea pods, green peas, and spinach. Using FDA and CDC procedures along with direct plating, officials at the CDC (3) tried to isolate listeriae from 22 samples of broccoli, carrots, celery, lettuce, green peppers, and potatoes in conjunction with several clusters of listeriosis cases in Los Angeles County and Philadelphia, Pennsylvania. Finally, as part of a much larger survey dealing with the incidence of *Listeria* spp. in retail meat, poultry, and seafood products, Buchanan et al. (13) used an MPN method to examine two samples of potato salad for listeriae. As implied previously, no *Listeria* spp. were isolated from any samples examined in the three surveys just described. However, when one considers the small number of samples examined, these findings cannot assure consumers that these products will always be free of listeriae.

In the only truly definitive survey thus far reported, Heisick et al. (25) used the FDA procedure to determine the incidence of various *Listeria* spp., including *L. monocytogenes*, in 10 different varieties of raw unwashed vegetables (total of 1000 samples) obtained from two Minneapolis-area supermarkets between October 1987 and August 1988. As shown in Table 14.1, *Listeria* spp. were detected in one or more samples of cabbage, cucumbers, lettuce, mushrooms, potatoes, and radishes, but were never found in broccoli, carrots, cauliflower, or tomatoes. While *L. monocytogenes*, *L. innocua*, *L. welshimeri*, and *L. seeligeri* were recovered from 5.0, 2.6, 0.8, and 1.3% of all raw produce examined, respectively, with 41 of 50 (82%) and 9 of 50 (18%) *L. monocytogenes* strains classified as serotypes 1a and 4a/4ab, respectively, the overall incidence of *Listeria* spp. as well as *L. monocytogenes* was markedly higher in radishes and potatoes than in other types of vegetables. Thus, keeping in mind that carrots recently were shown to possess some kind of inherent antilisterial activity (9,19), it appears that root crops such as potatoes and radishes more frequently carry viable listeriae than other vegetables because of their close association with soil. Interestingly, the fact that contamination rates for most raw vegetables were fairly consistent throughout the year reinforces the belief that listeriae populations remain relatively constant in soil. These findings also are supported by those from a similar study in which Heisick et al. (26) used four procedures to ultimately identify *Listeria* spp. in 19 of 70 (27.1%) and 25 of 68 (36.8%) potato and radish samples, respectively, with no listeriae being detected in mushrooms, carrots, cabbage, broccoli, cauliflower, lettuce, tomatoes, or cucumbers obtained from the same two Minneapolis supermarkets.

Given an adequate isolation procedure and sufficient time to examine large numbers of samples, it is now clear that a small percentage of raw vegetables marketed in the United States is likely to harbor *Listeria* spp., including *L. monocytogenes*, with the incidence of this pathogen highest in root crops. Hence, it appears that the inability to detect listeriae in raw vegetables examined in the three aforementioned surveys probably resulted because only small numbers of samples were examined. In support of this observation, Steinbruegge et al. (38) isolated *L. monocytogenes* from only 2 of 43 retail samples of head lettuce purchased in Nebraska. While the occasional presence of listeriae in retail raw vegetables should not be viewed with alarm, careful handling and washing of all produce to be consumed raw is recommended, particularly for pregnant women, the elderly, and other individuals at greater than normal risk of developing listeriosis.

Canada

Despite the Canadian coleslaw outbreak of 1981, the incidence of listeriae in fresh produce has received relatively little attention in Canada, with only one formal Canadian publication on the subject presently recorded in the scientific literature. Using the original FDA procedure (see Fig. 6.14), Farber et al. (20) failed to recover any *Listeria* spp. from lettuce (50 samples), celery (30 samples), or tomatoes (20 samples) purchased in Ottawa during 1988. However, *L. innocua* was detected in 1 of 10 radish samples,

Table 14.1 Incidence of Various *Listeria* spp. in Unwashed Raw Retail Vegetables Marketed in the Minneapolis, Minnesota, Area Between October 1987 and August 1988

Type of vegetable	Number of samples analyzed	Number of positive samples (%)				
		L. monocytogenes	*L. innocua*	*L. welshimeri*	*L. seeligeri*	Total
Broccoli	92	0	0	0	0	0
Cabbage	92	1 (1.1)	0	0	1 (1.1)	2 (2.2)
Carrots	92	0	0	0	0	0
Cauliflower	92	0	0	0	0	0
Cucumbers	92	2 (2.2)	5 (5.4)	2 (2.2)	0	9 (9.8)
Lettuce	92	0	1 (1.1)	0	0	1 (1.1)
Mushrooms	92	0	11 (12.0)	0	0	11 (12.0)
Potatoes	132	28 (21.2)	5 (3.8)	1 (0.8)	0	34 (25.8)
Radishes	132	19 (14.4)	4 (3.0)	5 (3.8)	12 (9.1)	40 (30.3)
Tomatoes	92	0	0	0	0	0
Total	1,000	50 (5.0)	26 (2.6)	8 (0.8)	13 (1.3)	97 (9.7)

Source: Adapted from Ref. 25.

which again suggests that the incidence of listeriae may be somewhat higher in root crops than in other vegetables.

Western Europe

Information concerning the incidence of listeriae in raw vegetables marketed in Western Europe also is of relatively recent origin, and to our knowledge is confined to a few scattered reports from England, Switzerland, Finland, and The Netherlands.

A recent increase in the number of listeriosis cases in England, along with the possibility that some of these cases may have been food-related, prompted several surveys to determine the incidence of listeriae in various foods including dairy, meat, poultry and seafood products, raw vegetables, and prepacked salads. Working at Cambridge, Sizmur and Walker (37) examined 10 different varieties of prepacked salads obtained at two leading area supermarkets. Overall, *L. monocytogenes* serotype 1/2 was isolated from 4 of 60 (6.7%) samples with *L. monocytogenes* serotype 4b also present in one of these positive samples. Prepacked salads from which the pathogen was recovered consisted of two varieties that contained either (a) cabbage, celery, sultanas, onions, and carrots or (b) lettuce, cucumbers, radishes, fennel, watercress, and leeks. Both of these salad varieties contained cabbage, cucumbers, and/or radishes—three of four raw vegetables from which *L. monocytogenes* (predominantly serotype 1a) was isolated in the United States (Table 14.1). Although no *Listeria* spp. were recovered from plain beansprout salads or those that contained nuts, possibly because of a low pH, *L. innocua* was discovered in 13 of 60 (21.7%) samples representing five different varieties of mixed vegetables and/or fruit salad. In addition to these findings, English investigators (22) also have isolated *L. monocytogenes* from coleslaw. Thus raw salad vegetables can serve as a potential source of *L. monocytogenes* in the human diet.

Bendig and Strangeways (4) recently proposed that a 74-year-old postoperative patient in a London hospital may have acquired listeric septicemia and meningitis from consuming contaminated lettuce. While different serotypes of *L. monocytogenes* (1/2a and 1/2c) were isolated from the patient and 1 of 11 (9.1%) samples of washed English round lettuce, recovery of the pathogen from washed lettuce prepared in the hospital's kitchen, but not from 44 other food samples examined, suggests that consumption of washed raw vegetables may pose a potential health threat to hospital patients, many of whom are debilitated and/or immunocompromised.

Consumption of homemade uncooked salted mushrooms containing 10^6 *L. monocytogenes* serotype 4b CFU/g has been positively linked to a nonfatal case of listeric septicemia in an 80-year-old apparently healthy Finnish man (30) (see Chapter 8). [Working in The Netherlands, van Netten et al. (32) also isolated *L. monocytogenes* from 2 of 20 raw mushroom samples obtained from area markets.] During this investigation, low levels ($<10^2$ CFU/g) of an unrelated *L. monocytogenes* strain belonging to serotype 1/2a also were detected in carrots that were stored in the same cow barn with the tainted mushrooms, thus making this the first account in which this pathogen has been recovered from raw carrots, a vegetable that reportedly possesses listericidal properties (7,29).

In the only other European survey reported thus far (12), 27 raw vegetable samples obtained from a group of retail markets in Switzerland were free of listeriae. However, *L. monocytogenes* was detected in 3 of 64 (4.7%) raw salads (two mixed salads and one parsley salad) obtained from the same group of markets. Similarly, *L. innocua* was recovered from 4 of 64 (6.3%) raw salads. Thus, as was true for England, preliminary data from Switzerland indicate the presence of *Listeria* spp. in a small percentage of raw vegetable salads. From these findings and the fact that *L. monocytogenes* is ubiquitous in the environment, it appears likely that forthcoming surveys conducted in other industrialized Western European nations will yield generally similar results.

BEHAVIOR OF *L. MONOCYTOGENES* ON VEGETABLES

Despite the 1981 listeriosis outbreak in Canada directly linked to consumption of contaminated coleslaw (35) and an earlier cluster of listeriosis cases in Massachusetts that appears to have been epidemiologically linked to raw celery, lettuce, and tomatoes, until recently scientists were generally unconcerned about behavior of *L. monocytogenes* in raw produce. This lack of concern probably existed because vegetables grown in modern industrialized nations only rarely have been associated with any type of bacterial foodborne illness. Furthermore, the source of contamination in the Canadian coleslaw outbreak was readily traced to a farmer who fertilized cabbage with untreated manure obtained from a flock of sheep that was previously diagnosed as having listeriosis. Consequently, most individuals in the scientific community probably viewed this outbreak as an isolated incident which could have been easily prevented if better agricultural practices had been followed in growing cabbage.

Interest in *L. monocytogenes* as a serious foodborne pathogen increased in 1985 following reports from California that at least 40 individuals died after consuming contaminated Mexican-style cheese. This outbreak sparked a renewed interest in the Canadian coleslaw outbreak and also prompted a series of investigations to determine both the incidence and behavior of *L. monocytogenes* in raw vegetables including cabbage. Results from these studies will now be reviewed along with some data concerning thermal inactivation of *L. monocytogenes* in cabbage and the effect of modified atmospheric storage, chlorine, and lysozyme on growth and survival of this pathogen in various raw vegetables. As was true for meat, poultry, and seafood, behavior of listeriae in raw produce is becoming an active area of research. Hence, additional information regarding various means to inactivate *Listeria* in raw vegetables and particularly prepacked refrigerated salads will probably be available in the near future.

Growth and Survival

Since coleslaw was and presently still is the only vegetable that has been directly linked to an actual outbreak of listeriosis in humans, it is not surprising that growth and survival of *L. monocytogenes* in cabbage was initially investigated. In the first such study published in 1986, Beuchat et al. (10) determined behavior of *L. monocytogenes* strains Scott A (clinical isolate) and LCDC 81-861 (Canadian cabbage isolate) on inoculated samples of shredded and raw and autoclaved (121°C/20 min) cabbage as well as in autoclaved (121°C/15 min) salted and unsalted cabbage juice during extended storage at 5 and 30°C. According to the authors, both test strains of the pathogen exhibited relatively similar patterns of behavior on sterile cabbage with populations decreasing from approximately 10^7 to 10^4 or 10^5 CFU/g during 42 days of refrigerated storage.

This apparent inability of *L. monocytogenes* to grow on heat-sterilized cabbage at 5°C suggests that heating either decreases the availability of essential nutrients or leads to development of toxic and/or inhibitory constituents in cabbage. In sharp contrast, *L. monocytogenes* competed well with the normal aerobic flora and lactic acid bacteria of raw cabbage with *Listeria* populations increasing approximately four orders of magnitude on raw cabbage during the first 25 days of refrigerated storage (Fig. 14.1). Thereafter, numbers of listeriae failed to decrease appreciably on raw cabbage stored up to 64 days. Similar results also were observed in subsequent studies by Hao et al. (24) and Lovett et al. (31). Thus these findings demonstrate that *L. monocytogenes* can grow under conditions normally encountered during shipping and distribution of cabbage. While both *Listeria* strains failed to grow in autoclaved cabbage juice containing >5% NaCl during 2 weeks of storage at 30°C, *L. monocytogenes* grew to levels of 10^6 CFU/g in the aforementioned homemade salted mushrooms (~7.5% NaCl) during 5 months of cold storage (30). Hence, behavior of listeriae in raw vegetables appears to be greatly affected by incubation temperature as well as the concentration of salt and various growth constituents.

Subsequently, Conner et al. (15) more closely examined the influence of temperature, NaCl, and pH on growth of *L. monocytogenes* in cabbage juice. In this study, samples of cabbage juice, obtained by grinding and pressing retail heads of fresh

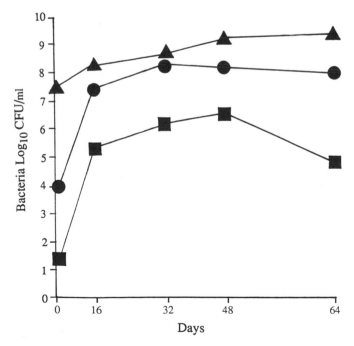

Figure 14.1 Behavior of *L. monocytogenes* (●), lactic acid bacteria (■), and total aerobic microorganisms (▲) on raw cabbage incubated at 5°C. (Adapted from Ref. 10.)

cabbage, were prepared to contain 0–5.0% NaCl (12 different concentrations), auto-claved at 121°C for 15 minutes, cooled, inoculated to contain ~10^4 *L. monocytogenes* strain Scott A or LCDC 81-861 CFU/ml and incubated at 5 and 30°C. This experiment also was repeated using sterile clarified (centrifuged) cabbage juice supplemented with 0, 0.5, 1.0, 1.5, or 2.0% NaCl. Finally, the effect of pH on growth of *L. monocytogenes* was studied using sterile unclarified cabbage juice adjusted to pH 3.8–5.6 (0.2-unit increments) with lactic acid.

As in the previous study, salt-free unclarified cabbage juice again was an excellent growth medium for *L. monocytogenes*, with populations increasing to ~10^9 CFU/ml after 8 days of incubation at 30°C. Beyond 8 days, populations in cabbage juice containing low levels of salt decreased rapidly and viable cells were no longer detected after 20 days of incubation at 30°C. Growth rates of both *Listeria* strains at 30°C decreased markedly in cabbage juice containing low levels of salt, with inactivation of strains Scott A and LCDC 81-861 occurring in the presence of ≥1.5 and ≥2.5% NaCl, respec-tively. As expected, behavior of both strains was strongly influenced by development of acid with the pH of samples in which growth had occurred decreasing from 5.6 to ≤4.3 after 8 days of incubation at 30°C. While numbers of both *Listeria* strains failed to increase in salted and unsalted cabbage juice when the experiment was repeated at 5°C, populations remained relatively stable, generally decreasing only 10- to 100-fold in cabbage juice containing 3.5–5.0% NaCl during 70 days of refrigerated storage. A relatively constant pH of ~5.6 in these samples undoubtedly contributed to enhanced survival of listeriae in refrigerated unclarified cabbage juice. However, preliminary results from another study (14) suggest that viability of *Listeria* in similar samples of salted and unsalted cabbage juice was reduced by adding extracts from several Chinese medicinal plants.

Interestingly, growth patterns for *L. monocytogenes* differed dramatically in clari-fied cabbage juice with both strains growing well at 30°C in the presence of up to 2.0% NaCl. Since similar changes were observed between pH and growth of listeriae in clarified and unclarified cabbage juice, these findings suggest that solid material in unclarified cabbage juice may be partly inhibitory to *L. monocytogenes* in the presence of salt.

Using pH-adjusted unclarified cabbage juice, these researchers further demon-strated that *L. monocytogenes* failed to initiate growth at pH values <5.0 when inoculated samples were incubated at 30°C. Although more acidic environments (pH ≤ 4.8) proved to be lethal, complete inactivation of both *Listeria* strains did not occur until the pH was reduced to ~4.1. When the incubation temperature was lowered to 5°C, *L. monocytogenes* populations gradually decreased in cabbage juice adjusted to pH ≤ 5.2, with the pathogen surviving >63, 49, <21, and <21 days in samples adjusted to pH values of 5.2, 5.0, 4.8, and 4.6, respectively. In contrast, *Listeria* populations remained relatively constant during extended cold storage of cabbage juice adjusted to pH values > 5.2. Since inactivation rates were markedly slower at 5 than at 30°C, it appears that lower temperatures help protect *L. monocytogenes* from the harmful effects of low pH, as noted in Chapter 5.

Concern about behavior of *L. monocytogenes* in fresh produce has extended beyond cabbage and now includes an ever increasing variety of fresh salad vegetables. In 1988, Steinbruegge et al. (38) reported results of a study which examined the ability of *L.*

monocytogenes to survive and grow on inoculated (10^3–10^5 CFU/g) samples of washed retail head lettuce during storage in sealed and open plastic bags at 5, 12, and 25°C.

While behavior of *L. monocytogenes* on lettuce was somewhat variable, the pathogen generally grew under conditions simulating proper refrigeration, normal mishandling, and ambient serving temperatures with the pathogen increasing one to four orders of magnitude following 2 weeks of storage. Similar results also were observed when inoculated samples of fresh lettuce juice were held at 5°C for 2 weeks.

Information regarding fate of *L. monocytogenes* in or on other types of salad vegetables also is limited; however, results from several studies indicate that with the exception of raw carrots, this pathogen will grow and/or survive on most other types of fresh produce including asparagus (5), broccoli (5,31), cauliflower (5), corn (29), green beans (29), lettuce (8,29), and radishes (31) during the normal refrigerated shelf life of the product. In addition, Sizmur and Walker (37) reported that *L. monocytogenes* populations in several naturally contaminated vegetable salads purchased from two supermarkets in England increased approximately twofold after 4 days of refrigerated storage. Given the apparent ability of *L. monocytogenes* to survive and/or grow on most raw salad vegetables and the possible presence of this pathogen on many types of raw produce, health officials need to consider raw vegetables as another possible source of listeric infections.

Modified Atmosphere Storage

The widespread practice of packaging and/or storing fresh produce with a modified atmosphere has led to dramatic increases in the types of produce available to consumers and in the shelf life of these products so that most fresh vegetables (and fruits) are now available throughout the year. However, with the occasional presence of *L. monocytogenes* on raw produce, the ability of this pathogen to multiply relatively rapidly under microaerobic conditions at refrigeration temperatures and the present popularity of modified atmosphere packaging, legitimate questions have been raised about the safety of refrigerated produce during long-term storage with modified atmospheres.

In response to these concerns, Berrange et al. (5,6) recently investigated behavior of *L. monocytogenes* on inoculated (10^3–10^5 CFU/g) samples of fresh asparagus, broccoli, and cauliflower during extended refrigerated storage in glass jars containing (a) 15% O_2:6% CO_2:79% N_2, (b) 11% O_2:10% CO_2:79% N_2, (c) 18% O_2:3% CO_2:79% N_2, or (d) air. *Listeria monocytogenes* behaved similarly on each vegetable when the product was stored in a modified atmosphere or air. All three vegetables supported growth of *L. monocytogenes* at 15°C, with the pathogen attaining populations of ~10^6 to nearly 10^9/g when these products were first deemed to be unfit for human consumption 6–10 days after the start of incubation. While storage in a modified atmosphere at 15°C did not appreciably affect growth of listeriae on any of the three vegetables examined, the ability of such storage conditions to increase the shelf life of these products by 2–4 days beyond that of the products packaged in air led to higher *Listeria* populations when these vegetables were first declared inedible by subjective evaluations. In contrast, only asparagus supported growth of *L. monocytogenes* at 4°C, with initial numbers approximately 10- to 100-fold higher at the end of the product's 21-day shelf life. However, numbers of listeriae remained relatively constant on broccoli and cauliflower during 21 days at 4°C, regardless of the storage atmosphere. Since these findings and those of the previous study indicate that *L. monocytogenes* is basically unaffected by controlled atmosphere storage, the extended shelf life gained with such storage conditions provides additional time for growth of this pathogen which, in turn, increases the public health hazard associated with consumption of raw vegetables.

Subsequently, Beuchat and Brackett (8) observed that *L. monocytogenes* behaved similarly when inoculated samples of iceberg lettuce were stored at 5 or 10°C in 3% O_2:97% N_2 or air. As with cabbage and asparagus, the pathogen grew on lettuce reaching populations of 10^8–10^9 CFU/g after 10 days of storage at 10°C, with only slight growth observed in identical samples held at 5°C. Therefore it appears prudent for handlers of raw produce to be stored in a modified atmosphere to institute sanitation and quality control programs that will decrease the incidence of listeriae in incoming raw vegetables. It also may be necessary to shorten the marketable period for such products, even though the food may appear to be acceptable.

Inactivation

As a follow-up to the aforementioned studies dealing with growth and survival of *L. monocytogenes* in raw vegetables, scientists also examined different methods by which *L. monocytogenes* can be eliminated from raw vegetables. While these methods, which will now be discussed, involve use of heat, chlorine, and lysozyme, information concerning the effect of other methods such as irradiation should be available in the future.

In response to the 1981 listeriosis outbreak in Canada involving consumption of contaminated coleslaw, Beuchat et al. (10) investigated thermal inactivation of *L. monocytogenes* in cabbage juice. Flasks of sterile, clarified cabbage juice adjusted to pH 4.0, 4.6, and 5.6 were inoculated to contain approximately 4×10^6 *L. monocytogenes* CFU/ml, placed in a shaking water bath at 50, 52, 54, 56, or 58°C, and sampled for listeriae at 10-minute intervals for up to 60 minutes. As expected, thermal inactivation rates for *Listeria* in cabbage juice at 50, 52, 54, and 56°C were faster at lower pH values, with D-values of 25, 14, 6.7, and 3.6 minutes at pH 4.6 as compared to D-values of 60, 34, 8.4, and 6.8 minutes at pH 5.6, respectively. No viable cells were detected in any cabbage juice held at 58°C for 10 minutes. Although inactivation rates were unaffected by addition of 1 or 2% NaCl to cabbage juice, sublethally injured cells were more sensitive to NaCl on a nonselective plating medium (Tryptic Soy Agar) than were uninjured cells. As shown by data in Fig. 14.1, *L. monocytogenes* can multiply on raw cabbage during extended refrigerated storage; however, results from the study just discussed suggest that normal pasteurization treatments given to cabbage juice and sauerkraut are probably sufficient to eliminate any viable listeriae that may be present. Hence, unlike unfermented raw vegetables, the risk of contracting listeriosis from sauerkraut and other pasteurized fermented vegetable products appears to be minimal.

Brackett (11) investigated the possibility of using hypochlorite solutions to inactivate *L. monocytogenes* on the surface of Brussels sprouts. In this study, fresh retail Brussels sprouts were inoculated to contain ~10^6 *L. monocytogenes* CFU/g, immersed in a hypochlorite solution containing 200 mg of chlorine/L, removed, air-dried for 30 minutes, and examined for numbers of surviving listeriae. The procedure just described decreased populations of *L. monocytogenes* on Brussels sprouts approximately 100-fold.

However, since dipping inoculated Brussels sprouts in sterile chlorine demand-free water reduced the number of viable listeriae by approximately 10-fold, the authors concluded that many cells were simply washed off the surface rather than inactivated by chlorine. In a follow-up study with fresh retail lettuce, Beuchat and Brackett (8) also found that *L. monocytogenes* was still present at levels of 10^5–10^6 and 10^7–10^8 CFU/g after extended storage at 5 and 10°C, respectively, regardless of whether or not the lettuce was pretreated with a sodium hypochlorite solution to reduce the population of naturally occurring microflora. As indicated in Chapter 5, hypochlorite can be used very effectively to inactivate *L. monocytogenes* in water supplies and on the surface of previously cleaned equipment. However, current evidence indicates that chlorine dips are relatively ineffective for eliminating *L. monocytogenes* from contaminated raw vegetables.

After demonstrating that egg white lysozyme—a GRAS (generally recognized as safe) food additive—inhibited growth of several foodborne pathogens, including *L. monocytogenes*, in laboratory media and phosphate buffer (28), Hughey et al. (29) investigated the possibility of using this enzyme during refrigerated storage to inactivate *L. monocytogenes* on various retail vegetables including fresh lettuce, cabbage, sweet corn, green beans, and carrots as well as previously frozen corn and green beans. In this study, 1.8-kg portions of coarsely shredded or cut fresh and thawed frozen vegetables were treated to contain 100 mg of lysozyme/kg of vegetables and/or 5 mM of EDTA, inoculated to contain ~10^3–10^4 *L. monocytogenes* CFU/g, mixed by hand, and examined for numbers of listeriae during extended storage at 5°C.

Overall, lysozyme was fairly effective in decreasing populations of *L. monocytogenes* on the surface of fresh vegetables, particularly when used in conjunction with EDTA, which presumably facilitated cell lysis by increasing contact between lysozyme and peptidoglycan in the cell wall. Listericidal effects from the combined use of lysozyme and EDTA were most pronounced on lettuce, with the pathogen no longer being detected after 12 days of refrigerated storage (Fig. 14.2). While lysozyme alone was listeriostatic, use of EDTA alone failed to prevent growth of *L. monocytogenes*, with the pathogen eventually attaining levels only slightly lower than those observed in untreated lettuce. *Listeria* behaved similarly on fresh green beans and sweet corn with two exceptions: (a) growth occurred on lysozyme-treated sweet corn, and (b) combined use of lysozyme and EDTA never completely eliminated the pathogen from either product. In contrast to fresh lettuce, green beans, and sweet corn, numbers of listeriae on EDTA- and lysozyme-treated raw cabbage increased during the first 20 days of refrigerated storage and then decreased four to five orders of magnitude during 28 days of incubation at 5°C. Although combined use of lysozyme and EDTA again was most listericidal, 41 days of refrigerated storage were required to rid this lettuce of listeriae. Unlike other fresh vegetables, the pathogen was eliminated within 9 days from untreated raw carrots as well as from those that were treated with lysozyme alone or in combination with EDTA (Fig. 14.3). Hence, these findings support the notion that carrots probably contain one or more naturally occurring listericidal substances (9).

In contrast to fresh vegetables, numbers of listeriae remained relatively constant on previously frozen green beans and corn that were treated with lysozyme alone or in combination with EDTA. This apparent failure of lysozyme to inactivate listeriae on frozen vegetables may be related to loss of certain lysis-enhancing substances during processing of vegetables. These findings, together with the current use of lysozyme to

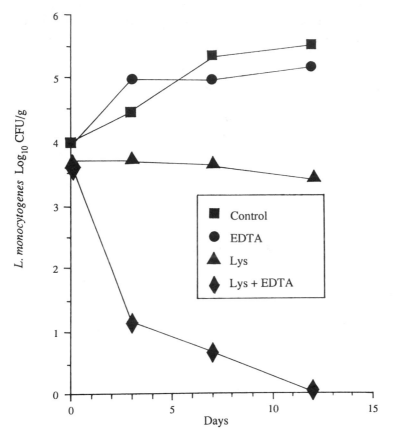

Figure 14.2 Behavior of *L. monocytogenes* on fresh lettuce treated with lysozyme (Lys) and EDTA. (Adapted from Ref. 29.)

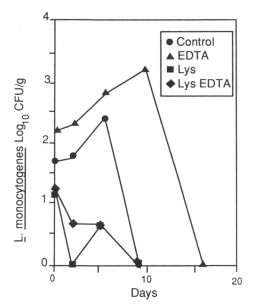

Figure 14.3 Behavior of *L. monocytogenes* on fresh carrots treated with lysozyme (Lys) and EDTA. (Adapted from Ref. 29.)

prevent growth of gas-producing spore-forming bacteria in certain European cheeses, suggest that commercial use of lysozyme in combination with other previously discussed measures should help to inhibit *Listeria* and other foodborne pathogens on fresh vegetables.

INCIDENCE OF *LISTERIA* ON RAW FRUITS

Unlike raw vegetables, information concerning the incidence of *Listeria* spp. on raw fruit is virtually nonexistent and is presently limited to one preliminary report (3) in which CDC officials failed to recover listeriae from seven fruit samples (e.g., cherries, pears, peach, avocado, and tomato) during an investigation of two clusters of foodborne listeriosis cases in Los Angeles County, California, and Philadelphia, Pennsylvania. While scientific evidence is lacking, two observations, namely, (a) absence of an association between consumption of raw fruit and listeriosis in any case presently recorded in the literature and (b) the fact that most fruits grow well above ground and are therefore not subject to frequent contact with *Listeria*-contaminated soil or feces, lead one to speculate that the incidence of listeriae on raw fruit may well be as low or lower than that observed for raw vegetables.

Given the probable low incidence of listeriae on raw fruits, it may seem somewhat surprising to learn that FDA officials prompted an Oregon firm to issue a Class I recall for over 500,000 flavored frozen ice and juice bars that were contaminated with *L. monocytogenes* during the latter stages of manufacture (1), which suggests postpasteurization contamination. Since raw milk also was routinely processed into frozen dairy products at this same facility, *L. monocytogenes* was most likely introduced into the factory environment through the raw milk supply rather than fruit juice. If this is true, then it follows that the incidence of listeriae in highly acidic fruit juice is likely to be extremely low. This view is further supported by results from a recent survey in which Parish and Higgins (33) failed to detect any *Listeria* spp. in 100 retail samples of reconstituted single-strength orange juice (pH 3.63–3.84) that were pasteurized at 30 geographically distinct dairy and nondairy facilities located across the United States and Canada.

BEHAVIOR OF *L. MONOCYTOGENES* IN FRUIT JUICES

Since presently we lack information on the incidence of listeriae in raw fruits, it is not surprising that our knowledge of *Listeria* behavior in these products also is extremely limited. Thus far (June 1990) results from only two studies dealing with viability of listeriae in orange serum and juice have appeared in the scientific literature.

In 1989, Parish and Higgins (34) published data from the first of two studies in which orange serum was adjusted to pH values of 3.6–5.0 with hydrochloric acid, inoculated to contain ~10^6 *L. monocytogenes* CFU/ml and examined for numbers of listeriae during prolonged incubation at 4 and 30°C. As was true for cabbage juice (15), behavior of listeriae in orange serum also was markedly influenced by incubation temperature and pH. Overall, *L. monocytogenes* failed to grow in refrigerated orange serum adjusted to pH ≤ 4.6 and was completely eliminated from these samples after 18 to 70 days of storage, with lowest pH values proving most detrimental to survival of *Listeria* (Fig. 14.4). However, modest growth of listeriae was observed in orange serum samples at pH 5.0, with the pathogen still present at levels of 10^2–10^3 CFU/ml in the

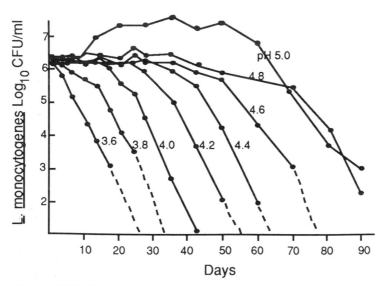

Figure 14.4 Behavior of *L. monocytogenes* in pH-adjusted orange serum during extended incubation at 4°C. (Adapted from Ref. 34.)

two least acidic samples after 90 days of refrigerated storage. Incubation at 30°C led to *Listeria* increases of approximately 10- and 100-fold in orange serum samples adjusted to pH values of 4.8 and 5.0, respectively. As was true for unclarified cabbage juice (15), overall viability of listeriae again was greatly reduced by raising the incubation temperature, with the pathogen generally eliminated from orange serum samples at pH 3.6–4.0 and 4.2–5.0 after 5 and 8 days of incubation at 30°C, respectively.

These same authors (33) subsequently used several enrichment procedures to determine the viability of listeriae in single-strength reconstituted samples of commercial frozen concentrated orange juice that were inoculated to contain ~1–10 *L. monocytogenes* CFU/ml. While numbers of inherent microorganisms (primarily lactic acid bacteria and yeast) increased from ~10^2–10^8 CFU/ml after 4 weeks of incubation at 4°C, *L. monocytogenes* was eliminated from reconstituted frozen orange juice having an average pH of 4.06 after 42 days of refrigerated storage. Thus these findings appear to be consistent with those from the previous study involving orange serum.

BEHAVIOR OF *L. MONOCYTOGENES* IN OTHER PRODUCTS OF PLANT ORIGIN

Increased consumer demand for precooked, long shelf life, ready-to-eat foods containing a minimum of preservatives is making the development of microbiologically safe products increasingly difficult. Not too many years ago it was thought that no foodborne pathogen could multiply in properly refrigerated food. However, this belief has been proven as invalid by emergence of *L. monocytogenes* and *Yersinia enterocolitica*, in particular, as causes of foodborne illness. Thus public health officials have become concerned about the safety of many cook-chilled and ready-to-eat foods of animal origin, including fermented and unfermented dairy products, luncheon meats, sausage, and precooked chicken as well as peel-and-eat shrimp. These concerns have since spread to products of plant origin including soymilk, precooked delicatessen products such as ravioli (prepared in part from flour), and food colorants derived from red beets.

Since there is an increased use of soymilk by individuals who cannot tolerate cow's milk, the ability of *Listeria* to proliferate in this product should be known. Hence, Ferguson and Shelef (21) inoculated commercially available pasteurized and sterile soymilk to contain 10^2 or 10^4 *L. monocytogenes* CFU/ml and incubated them at 5 and 22°C. The pathogen attained maximum populations similar to those previously observed in cow's milk, reaching levels of 7×10^8 to 3×10^9 and 8×10^8 CFU/ml in both soymilks following 3 and 30 days of incubation at 5 and 22°C, respectively. Not surprising, generation times for *L. monocytogenes* in soymilk—1 hour and 33 minutes at 22°C and 37 hours and 41 minutes at 4°C—are similar to those previously reported for the same strain of *L. monocytogenes* in cow's milk (see Chapter 9). No one has yet investigated the incidence of *Listeria* spp. on soybeans; however, since listeriae are relatively common in soil, the potential exists that these organisms can find their way into soymilk-processing factories and also into the finished product as a postpasteurization contaminant. If this is true, then rapid growth of *L. monocytogenes* in soymilk at refrigeration temperatures suggests that this product should not be overlooked as a possible vehicle of human listeric infections.

Recent concern about behavior of *Listeria* in delicatessen products marketed in England and the United States prompted Beuchat and Brackett (7) to investigate viability and thermal inactivation of *L. monocytogenes* in commercially prepared meat, cheese, and egg ravioli purchased from Atlanta-area delicatessens. The growth portion of this study involved quantitation of *L. monocytogenes* in inoculated (approx. 10^4 and 10^6 CFU/g) samples of ravioli during 14 days of incubation at 5°C. For thermal inactivation studies, the three types of ravioli were inoculated to contain 3×10^5 *L. monocytogenes* CFU/g, stored 0 or 9 days at 5°C, and then boiled up to 7 minutes using cooking procedures that might be practical in the home. Overall, numbers of viable listeriae remained relatively constant during the 9-day refrigerated shelf life of ravioli, with populations decreasing <10-fold in all three types of ravioli. Results of thermal inactivation studies indicated that normal cooking procedures (7 minutes of boiling) were sufficient to destroy *L. monocytogenes* populations of ~10^5 CFU/g in all three types of ravioli, regardless of whether or not ravioli was refrigerated 0 or 9 days before cooking. While this study provides valuable information concerning behavior of *Listeria* in ravioli, there appears to be an urgent need for more work of this type to address the microbiological safety of precooked and/or ready-to-eat delicatessen products such as sandwiches, filled rolls, pizza, garlic bread, desserts, confectionery products, and chocolate since work in England (22) and elsewhere has shown that all of these products can harbor *L. monocytogenes*.

Finally, increased use of plant-based food colorants prompted El-Gazzar and Marth (19) to investigate behavior of *Listeria* in a commercial aqueous extract from the red beet root (*Beta vulgaris*) to which vitamin C, citric acid, and sodium propionate (≤1.5%) were added as preservatives. As in their previous work with milk coagulants (17,18) and annatto colorants (16), samples of beet extract were inoculated to contain 10^3–10^7 *L. monocytogenes* strain CA, V7, or Scott A CFU/ml and examined for numbers of survivors during prolonged storage at 7°C. Not surprisingly, the combined effect of a relatively low pH of 4.3–4.8 and sodium propionate prevented growth of listeriae in all samples. However, while 42–56 days of incubation at 7°C was sufficient to rid these extracts of 10^3–10^4 strain CA CFU/ml, this strain was still detected in 56-day-old samples that contained larger initial populations. In contrast, strains V7 and Scott A were far more resistant to the listericidal action of beet extract, with both strains recovered at levels of 10^1–10^4 CFU/ml, depending on initial inoculum, following 56 days of storage. Hence, unlike highly alkaline annatto extracts in which *L. monocytogenes* was inactivated almost instantaneously (see Chapter 10), prolonged survival of listeriae in beet colorants makes it imperative that these extracts be processed and handled carefully to prevent their contamination with this pathogen.

REFERENCES

1. Anonymous. 1987. Frozen ice, juice and fudge bars recalled. FDA Enforcement Report, June 3.
2. Anonymous. 1990. Chicken, potato salads recalled by Campbell unit due to *Listeria*. *Food Chem. News 32*(9):61.
3. Archer, D. L. 1988. Review of the latest FDA information on the presence of *Listeria* in foods. WHO Working Group on Foodborne Listeriosis. Geneva, Switzerland, Feb. 15–19.
4. Bendig, J. W. A., and J. E. M. Strangeways. 1989. *Listeria* in hospital lettuce. *Lancet i*:616–617.

5. Berrange, M. E., R. E. Brackett, and L. R. Beuchat. 1989. Growth of *Aeromonas hydrophila* and *Listeria monocytogenes* on controlled atmosphere stored refrigerated fresh vegetables. Ann. Mtg., Inst. Food Technol., Chicago, IL, June 25–29, Abstr. 470.

6. Berrange, M. E., R. E. Brackett, and L. R. Beuchat. 1989. Growth of *Listeria monocytogenes* on fresh vegetables stored under controlled atmosphere. *J. Food Prot.* 52:702–705.

7. Beuchat, L. R., and R. E. Brackett. 1989. Observations on survival and thermal inactivation of *Listeria monocytogenes* in ravioli. *Lett. Appl. Microbiol.* 8:173–175.

8. Beuchat, L. R., and R. E. Brackett. 1990. Survival and growth of *Listeria monocytogenes* on lettuce as influenced by shredding, chlorine treatment, modified atmosphere packaging and temperature. *J. Food Sci.* 55:755–758, 870.

9. Beuchat, L. R., and R. E. Brackett. 1990. Inhibitory effects of carrots on *Listeria monocytogenes*. Ann. Mtg., Inst. Food Technol., Anaheim, CA, June 16–20, Abstr. 391.

10. Beuchat, L. R., R. E. Brackett, D.Y.-Y. Hao, and D. E. Conner. 1986. Growth and thermal inactivation of *Listeria monocytogenes* in cabbage and cabbage juice. *Can. J. Microbiol.* 32:791–795.

11. Brackett, R. E. 1987. Antimicrobial effect of chlorine on *Listeria monocytogenes. J. Food Prot.* 50:999–1003.

12. Breer, C. 1988. Occurrence of *Listeria* spp. in different foods. WHO Working Group on Foodborne Listeriosis, Geneva, Switzerland, Feb. 15–19.

13. Buchanan, R. L., H. G. Stahl, M. M. Bencivengo, and F. del Corral. 1989. Comparison of lithium chloride-phenylethanol-moxalactam and modified Vogel Johnson agars for detection of *Listeria* spp. in retail-level meats, poultry and seafood. *Appl. Environ. Microbiol.* 55:599–603.

14. Chung, K.-T., W. R. Thomasson, and C. D. Wu-Yuan. 1990. Growth inhibition of selected food-borne bacteria by plant extracts. Ann. Mtg., Amer. Soc. Microbiol., Anaheim, CA, May 13–17, Abstr. p. 24.

15. Conner, D. E., R. E. Brackett, and L. R. Beuchat. 1986. Effect of temperature, sodium chloride, and pH on growth of *Listeria monocytogenes* in cabbage juice. *Appl. Environ. Microbiol.* 52:59–63.

16. El-Gazzar, F. E., and E. H. Marth. 1989. Fate of *Listeria monocytogenes* in some food colorants and starter distillate. *Lebensm. Wiss. Technol.* 22:406–410.

17. El-Gazzar, F. E., and E. H. Marth. 1989. Loss of viability by *Listeria monocytogenes* in commercial bovine-pepsin rennet extract. *J. Dairy Sci.* 72:1098–1102.

18. El-Gazzar, F. E., and E. H. Marth. 1989. Loss of viability by *Listeria monocytogenes* in commercial microbial rennet. *Milchwissenschaft* 44:83–86.

19. El-Gazzar, F. E., and E. H. Marth. 1991. Survival of *Listeria monocytogenes* in food colorant derived from red beets. *J. Dairy Sci.* 74:81–85.

20. Farber, J. M., G. W. Sanders, and M. A. Johnston. 1989. A survey of various foods for the presence of *Listeria* species. *J. Food Prot.* 52:456–458.

21. Ferguson, R. D., and L. A. Shelef. 1990. Growth of *Listeria monocytogenes* in soymilk. *J. Food Prot.* (submitted).

22. Gilbert, R. J. 1990. Personal communication.

23. Gray, M. L. 1960. A possible link in the relationship between silage feeding and listeriosis. *J. Am. Vet. Med. Assoc.* 136:205–208.

24. Hao, D.Y.-Y., L. R. Beuchat, and R. E. Brackett. 1989. Comparison of media and methods for detecting and enumerating *Listeria monocytogenes* in refrigerated cabbage. *Appl. Environ. Microbiol.* 53:955–957.

25. Heisick, J. E., D. E. Wagner, M. L. Nierman, and J. T. Peeler. 1989. *Listeria* spp. found on fresh market produce. *Appl. Environ. Microbiol.* 55:1925–1927.

26. Heisick, J. E., F. M. Harrell, E. H. Peterson, S. McLaughlin, D. E. Wagner, I. V. Wesley, and J. Bryner. 1989. Comparison of four procedures to detect *Listeria* spp. in foods. *J. Food Prot.* 52:154–157.

27. Hofer, E. 1975. Study of *Listeria* spp. on vegetables suitable for human consumption. VI Congresso Brazil de Microbiologia, Salvador, July 27–31, Abstr. K-11. Cited in Ralovich, B. 1984. Listeriosis Research—Present Situation and Perspective, Akadémiai Kiado, Budapest, p. 73.
28. Hughey, V. L., and E. A. Johnson. 1987. Antimicrobial activity of lysozyme against bacteria involved in food spoilage and food-borne disease. *Appl. Environ. Microbiol. 53*:2165–2170.
29. Hughey, V. L., P. A. Wilger, and E. A. Johnson. 1989. Antibacterial activity of hen egg white lysozyme against *Listeria monocytogenes* Scott A in foods. *Appl. Environ. Microbiol. 55*:631–638.
30. Junttila, J., and M. Brander. 1989. *Listeria monocytogenes* septicemia associated with consumption of salted mushrooms. *Scand. J. Infect. Dis. 21*:339–342.
31. Lovett, J., D. W. Francis, and J. G. Bradshaw. 1988. Outgrowth of *Listeria monocytogenes* in foods. Society for Industrial Microbiology—Comprehensive Conference on *Listeria monocytogenes*, Rohnert Park, CA, Oct. 2–5, Abstr. I-26.
32. Netten, P. van, I. Perales, A. van de Moosdijk, G. D. W. Curtis, and D. A. A. Mossel. 1989. Liquid and solid selective differential media for the detection and enumeration of *L. monocytogenes* and other *Listeria* spp. *Int. J. Food Microbiol. 8*:299–316.
33. Parish, M. E., and D. P. Higgins. 1989. Extinction of *Listeria monocytogenes* in single-strength orange juice: Comparison of methods for detection in mixed populations. *J. Food Safety 9*:267–277.
34. Parish, M. E., and D. P. Higgins. 1989. Survival of *Listeria monocytogenes* in low pH model broth systems. *J. Food Prot. 52*:144–147.
35. Petran, R. L., E. A. Zottola, and R. B. Gravani. 1988. Incidence of *Listeria monocytogenes* in market samples of fresh and frozen vegetables. *J. Food Sci. 53*:1238–1240.
36. Schlech, W. F., P. M. Lavigne, R. A. Bortolussi, A. C. Allen, E. V. Haldane, A. J. Wort, A. W. Hightower, S. E. Johnson, S. H. King, E. S. Nichols, and C. V. Broome. 1983. Epidemic listeriosis—evidence for transmission by food. *N. Engl. J. Med. 308*:203–206.
37. Sizmur, KI., and C. W. Walker. 1988. *Listeria* in prepackaged salads. *Lancet i*:1167.
38. Steinbruegge, E. G., R. B. Maxcy, and M. B. Liewen. 1988. Fate of *Listeria monocytogenes* on ready to serve lettuce. *J. Food Prot. 51*:596–599.
39. Weis, J. 1975. The incidence of *Listeria monocytogenes* on plants and in soil. In M. Woodbine (ed.), *Problems of Listeriosis*, Leicester University Press, Surrey, England, pp. 61–65.
40. Weis, J., and H. P. R. Seeliger. 1975. Incidence of *Listeria monocytogenes* in nature. *Appl. Microbiol. 30*:29–32.
41. Welshimer, W. J. 1968. Isolation of *Listeria monocytogenes* from vegetation. *J. Appl. Bacteriol. 95*:300–303.

15

Incidence and Control of *Listeria* in Food-Processing Facilities

INTRODUCTION

Overwhelming evidence indicates that when *L. monocytogenes* and other *Listeria* spp. occur in commercially processed foods, this happens primarily because the product was contaminated after processing rather than because these organisms survived heat treatments that normally render the product safe. This view is strongly supported by the lack of scientific evidence indicating that minimum required heat treatments given to dairy, meat, poultry, seafood, and other products are inadequate to inactivate levels of listeriae that might be reasonably expected to occur in such products before heat processing. Furthermore, while *L. monocytogenes* is clearly more heat-tolerant than most other non–spore-forming foodborne pathogens, to our knowledge no recalls of commercially prepared, *Listeria*-contaminated products have been unequivocally linked to inadequacy of minimum required heat treatments. However, the clearest indication that *L. monocytogenes* and other *Listeria* spp. enter commercially produced foods as postprocessing contaminants comes from the fact that apparently healthy, non–thermally injured cells have been routinely recovered from many thermally processed dairy, meat, poultry, and seafood products and that these organisms have been found in working environments of virtually all processing facilities that have yielded foods involved in *Listeria*-related recalls.

This final chapter has been specifically designed for plant managers, sanitation workers, and quality control/quality assurance personnel employed in the food industry. In keeping with the format of Chapters 9 through 14, results from recent American and European surveys concerning the incidence of listeriae in environments of dairy-, meat-, poultry-, seafood-, and vegetable-processing facilities as well as household kitchens will be described first. This will be followed by some general guidelines for reducing levels of listeriae and other microbial contaminants in working areas that are common to virtually all food-processing facilities.

The wide variations in microbial load and types of microorganisms present in similar raw and finished products manufactured at different facilities along with the fact that no two factories are exactly alike in terms of design, equipment, product flow, sanitation standards, distribution patterns, and managerial policies suggest that a discussion of current cleaning/sanitation programs used at particular food-processing facilities would be of little benefit. Instead, we will try to identify specific problem areas (e.g., pasteurization, sausage peelers) associated with manufacture of particular products and then briefly discuss how the Hazard Analysis Critical Control Point (HACCP) approach can be used to sharply decrease the microbial load in any given food, thereby reducing the possibility of producing a product contaminated with *L. monocytogenes* or any other foodborne pathogen.

INCIDENCE OF *LISTERIA* SPP. IN VARIOUS TYPES OF FOOD-PROCESSING FACILITIES IN THE UNITED STATES

Interest in the extent of *Listeria* contamination in various food-processing facilities is of recent origin since *L. monocytogenes* was not identified as a serious foodborne pathogen until 41 cases of listeriosis in Canada, including 17 deaths, were linked to consumption of contaminated coleslaw in 1981. Despite further evidence 2 years later suggesting possible involvement of pasteurized milk in an outbreak of listeriosis in Massachusetts, public health officials in the United States and elsewhere did not yet regard the presence of *L. monocytogenes* in food as a major threat to public health. However, this situation changed dramatically in June of 1985 when up to 300 cases of listeriosis, including 40 deaths, were eventually linked to consumption of contaminated Mexican-style cheese in southern California. This listeriosis outbreak, along with America's worst outbreak of salmonellosis in which over 16,000 individuals in the Chicago area became ill during March and April of 1985 after consuming a particular brand of pasteurized milk contaminated with *Salmonella typhimurium* (59), prompted FDA officials to begin testing various types of domestic and imported cheese for *Listeria*. FDA officials also developed the Dairy Safety Initiative Program, which included microbiological surveillance of finished dairy products and the factory environment in which they were produced along with in-depth inspection of fluid milk factories and eventually all types of dairy-processing facilities located throughout the United States. With the subsequent discovery of *L. monocytogenes* in cooked, ready-to-eat meat, poultry, and seafood products by FDA and USDA officials, manufacturers of foods other than dairy products also became concerned about the incidence of listeriae in their products and processing facilities.

Once FDA and USDA officials announced their plans to review Good Manufacturing Practices that were presumably being used by most American firms, the food industry launched a Herculean effort to identify *Listeria* spp. and eliminate such problems within the factory environment before governmental inspectors arrived. Considering the adverse publicity and potential monetary losses that could result from discovery of *L. monocytogenes* in finished product and the factory environment, it is not surprising that very little information concerning the incidence of listeriae and other microbial contaminants in food (except Class I recalls) and food-processing facilities has been released to the scientific community. Hence, while vast amounts of data have been generated since 1985 by local, state, and federal government inspectors as well as private microbiological testing/consulting laboratories and the food manufacturers themselves, much of the information which now follows is either of a general nature describing particular niches within food-processing facilities from which listeriae have been isolated or consists of limited results from academic surveys which describe the actual incidence of *Listeria* contamination in a relatively small number of food-processing facilities.

Dairy-Processing Facilities

Following the aforementioned dairy-related outbreaks of salmonellosis and listeriosis, FDA officials in cooperation with state governments and the dairy industry intensified surveillance of various types of dairy-processing facilities under the Dairy Safety Initiative Program which began April 1, 1986 (57). Under this program, state officials were requested to sponsor a series of statewide meetings to discuss foodborne illness associated with Grade A and non–Grade A dairy products and to intensify their present surveillance/inspection efforts in dairy-processing facilities. Nationally, FDA officials vowed to (a) conduct intensified check ratings in every interstate milk shipment (IMS) milk pasteurization factory, (b) conduct similar inspections at non–Grade A (non-IMS) milk pasteurization factories, (c) initiate a microbiological surveillance program designed to detect pathogenic microorganisms in finished product (see Chapters 9 and 10), (d) intensify and upgrade training and standardization practices for federal and state milk specialists, rating officers, and sanitarians, and (e) regularly prepare national reports which summarize the status of the United States dairy industry.

In the first of these reports (4) covering the 6-month period from April to September 1986, 9 of 357 (2.5%) milk pasteurization factories examined produced various dairy products contaminated with *L. monocytogenes*. A subsequent report in February 1987 indicated generally similar contamination rates with 16 of 620 (2.6%) and 3 of 620 (0.48%) dairy-processing facilities manufacturing finished products containing *L. monocytogenes* and *L. innocua*, respectively (5). Eight months later, FDA officials reported that 11 of 604 (1.8%) IMS and 18 of 412 (4.4%) non-IMS milk pasteurization factories had produced products contaminated with *Listeria* spp., principally *L. monocytogenes* (6).

Extensive follow-up efforts in milk pasteurization factories producing *Listeria*-contaminated products uncovered various defects in pasteurization equipment and factory design. Nevertheless, FDA officials have maintained that listeriae entered these products as postpasteurization contaminants. This view is strongly supported by FDA's success in isolating *Listeria* from numerous floor drains in processing and other areas, wooden (porous) walls, floors and ceilings, wooden pallets, external surfaces of milk cartons, and sweetwater (refrigerated water) from leaking pasteurizer plates. While not clearly identified in FDA's "list" of environmental samples that harbored *Listeria*, FDA officials (75) noted the following problem areas related to environmental, postpasteurization contamination of dairy products with listeriae: (a) improperly operating HTST and/or vat pasteurizers, (b) leaking and/or cracked storage tanks, jacketed vessels, and valves, (c) inadequate sanitizing regimens, (d) cross-connecting pipes which allow commingling of raw and pasteurized product, (e) use of contaminated rags and sponges, (f) exposure to contaminants in unfiltered air and condensate, (g) filling/packaging operations, (h) conveyor belts, (i) use of returned product and reclaiming operations, (j) walls, floors, and ceilings particularly in walk-in refrigerators, (k) formation of aerosols, (l) traffic patterns within the factory, (m) entrances and floor mats, and (n) personal cleanliness of employees and others in the factory. In reality, *L. monocytogenes* and other foodborne pathogens have been detected in environmental samples from many of these problem areas as indicated in the following surveys of dairy factories in California and Vermont.

In response to the aforementioned federal programs, officials of the Milk and Dairy Foods Control Branch of the California Department of Food and Agriculture published (38) results from a statewide survey in which 597 environmental samples were collected from 156 milk-processing facilities during the first half of 1987 and analyzed for listeriae. Overall, *Listeria* spp. were identified in the working environment of 46 (29.5%) milk-processing facilities with 31 of these 46 (67.4%) *Listeria*-positive factories contaminated with *L. monocytogenes* (Table 15.1). Furthermore, *L. monocytogenes* and other *Listeria* spp. were most frequently observed in factories producing fluid milk products followed by those that manufactured frozen dairy products (i.e., ice cream and novelty desserts) and cultured milk products (i.e., yogurt and cottage cheese), with lowest contamination rates associated with production of miscellaneous products and cheese. In all likelihood, this unusually low incidence of listeriae in California cheese factories was a direct result of massive clean-up efforts that were instituted following the 1985 listeriosis outbreak in the Los Angeles area involving Mexican-style cheese.

A comparison of the incidence of listeriae in different milk-processing areas and sample sites (Table 15.2) supports the widespread belief that listeriae most frequently enter products after rather than before pasteurization, with the prevalence of these organisms in the factory environment increasing as the product passes through processing, packaging/filling, and storage areas. This apparent movement of listeriae through milk-processing facilities is most readily seen in results obtained from conveyor belts and floor drains. However, sporadic isolation of listeriae from condensate as well as wooden blocks, pallets, case dollies, and utility tables points to additional routes by which these organisms can be disseminated in dairy factories. While the low incidence of listeriae in raw milk receiving rooms as compared to other areas of the factory may at first seem surprising, these findings most likely reflect difficulties encountered in adequately cleaning and sanitizing equipment in processing and packaging/filling areas of factories rather than what could be interpreted as a near absence of listeriae in California raw milk.

Table 15.1   Incidence of *Listeria* in Various Types of Milk-Processing Facilities in California, January to July 1987

Type of facility	Number of facilities examined	Number (%) of positive facilities	
		L. monocytogenes	All *Listeria* spp.
Fluid milk	63	19 (30.2)	27 (42.9)
Frozen milk products	30	7 (23.3)	11 (36.7)
Cheese	41	2 (4.9)	4 (9.8)
Cultured milk products	9	2 (22.2)	3 (33.3)
Miscellaneous products[a]	13	1[b] (7.7)	1[b](7.7)
Total	156	31 (19.9)	46 (29.5)

[a]Includes butter, nonfat dry milk, whey products, and condensed milk.
[b]Positive sample from a butter factory.
Source: Adapted from Ref. 38.

Table 15.2 Incidence of Listeriae in Different Milk-Processing Areas
and Sample Sites

Facility working area and sample site	Number of samples examined	Number (%) of positive samples	
		L. monocytogenes	All *Listeria* spp.
Raw milk receiving room			
Drain	30	1 (3.3)	1 (3.3)
Condensate	32	0	1 (4.5)
Other[a]	1	0	0
Processing room			
Drain	150	4 (2.7)	14 (9.3)
Condensate	76	1 (1.3)	3 (3.9)
Other[a]	21	3 (14.3)	6 (28.6)
Packaging/Filling room			
Drain	60	7 (11.7)	12 (20.0)
Condensate	36	1 (2.8)	1 (2.8)
Conveyor	15	5 (33.3)	7 (20.0)
Other[a]	10	0	2 (20.0)
Cold storage room			
Drain	105	12 (11.4)	17 (16.2)
Condensate	44	0	1 (2.3)
Conveyor	14	4 (28.6)	9 (64.3)

[a]Includes wooden blocks, pallets, case dollies, and utility tables.
Source: Adapted from Ref. 38.

Working at the University of Vermont, Klausner and Donnelly (56) made a large-scale survey to identify sources of *Listeria* (and *Yersinia*) contamination in fluid milk–, cheese-, and non–cheese-producing facilities. Overall, 66.7, 9.5, and 23.8% of samples collected from floors and other non–food contact surfaces at 34 fluid milk, cheese, and non–cheese factories were positive for *Listeria* spp., with *L. monocytogenes* and *L. innocua* being identified in 1.4 and 16.1%, respectively, of 361 samples examined. As expected, the percentage of *Listeria*-positive samples was higher among those from floors (12.0–27.9%) than from other non–food contact surfaces (8.1%) (Table 15.3) and wet (85.7%) rather than dry (14.3%) areas. According to these investigators, paper filler beds, whey drainage pans on cheese presses, and case-washing areas were particularly prone to contamination with *Listeria* and *Yersinia*. The fact that 20.9% of all positive samples contained both *Listeria* and *Yersinia* suggests that yersiniae might be somewhat useful as a potential indicator of *Listeria* contamination within the dairy-processing environment.

As just noted, *L. monocytogenes*, *Yersinia* spp., and most other foodborne pathogens are more commonly found in wet than dry processing areas. However, the fact that listeriae (a) were recovered from whey drainage pans, (b) were routinely shed in whey during cheesemaking experiments, (c) grew in samples of refrigerated milk/whey, and

Table 15.3 Incidence of *Listeria* and *Yersinia* on Floors and Non–Food Contact Surfaces of 34 Fluid Milk, Cheese, and Non–Cheese Factories in Vermont

Type of sample	Number of samples analyzed	Number (%) of positive samples	
		Listeria	*Yersinia*
Floor areas			
Coolers	43	12 (27.9)	9 (20.9)
Processing	117	21 (17.9)	14 (12.0)
Entrances	64	11 (17.2)	18 (27.7)
Mats/Footbaths	25	3 (12.0)	1 (4.0)
Other areas	38	10 (26.3)	6 (15.8)
Non–food contact surfaces	74	6 (8.1)	4 (5.4)
Total	361	63 (17.5)	52 (14.4)

Source: Adapted from Ref. 56.

Table 15.4 Incidence of *Listeria* in the Working Environment of 18 Nonfat Dry Milk/Whey-Processing Facilities Located Throughout the United States

Work area	Number of samples analyzed	Number (%) of positive samples	
		L. monocytogenes	Other *Listeria* spp.
Raw milk receiving	62	1 (1.6)	0
Wet processing	151	0	0
Cheese factory	22	0	0
Whey factory	23	0	1 (4.3)
Dryer room	38	0	0
Bagging room	27	0	0
Heating, ventilating and air conditioning system	53	0	0
Miscellaneous	34	0	0
Total	410	1 (0.24)	1 (0.24)

Source: Adapted from Ref. 44.

(d) survived the typical spray-drying process used to manufacture nonfat dry milk suggests that these organisms should be of concern to manufacturers of dry dairy products.

In the light of these concerns, Gabis et al. (44) determined the incidence of *Listeria* in the working environment of 18 dry milk/whey-processing facilities throughout the United States. The authors supplied environmental sampling kits containing sterile cellulose sponges, fabric-tipped swabs, and other necessities to all firms participating in the survey along with instructions as to how and where to collect samples. All samples were then sent to a central laboratory and within 48 hours of collection were analyzed for listeriae according to the FDA procedure. Overall, only 2 of 410 (0.24%) samples examined were positive for *Listeria* spp. with *L. monocytogenes* and a species other than *L. monocytogenes* isolated from floor drains in a raw milk receiving area and from a composite sample from several floor drains and trenches in a powder production area, respectively (Table 15.4). Allowing factory employees to choose specific sampling sites as well as the number of samples to be analyzed may have somewhat biased these results; however, the incidence of listeriae and hence the risk of postprocessing contamination appears to be many times lower in dry rather than wet dairy-processing facilities. Nevertheless, since manufacturers of nonfat dry milk and dry whey are not immune to the *Listeria* problem, they should take appropriate action to eliminate this organism from the processing environment, thereby greatly reducing the chance of producing a contaminated product.

Meat-Processing Facilities

Unlike dairy-processing facilities in which raw milk is pumped into the factory, pasteurized, and then either packaged immediately or pumped to closed vats for processing into cream, butter, ice cream, cheese, or other dairy products, meat-processing factories are in actuality "open-air disassembly line operations" in which animals are slaughtered, eviscerated, and taken apart to obtain various cuts of meat, hides for leather, and other items of commercial value. Thus, considering that domestic cattle, sheep, and pigs frequently shed *L. monocytogenes* asymptomatically in fecal material, it is not surprising that recent surveys have shown this pathogen to be not only ubiquitous but also endemic to slaughterhouses and meat-packing facilities.

Initiation of the USDA-FSIS testing program for listeriae in cooked and ready-to-eat meat products in September of 1987 (see Fig. 11.1) prompted immediate action by the meat industry. However, even before government testing began, meat processors became concerned about the incidence of listeriae in the working environment. In June of 1987, Flowers (9) reported results of a large-scale survey in which nearly 2300 environmental samples were collected from over 40 meat-processing facilities nationwide and analyzed for listeriae. Fourteen processing areas within these factories yielded evidence of being contaminated with *L. monocytogenes* or other *Listeria* spp. Overall, listeriae were recovered from ~21% of all environmental samples examined. [These results also compare favorably to those of a much smaller survey (15) in which *Listeria* spp. were detected in 9 of 27 (33%) meat-processing environmental samples.] Problem areas in which ≥20% of the samples were positive included drains, trenches, floors, exhaust hoods, cleaning aids (sponges, brooms, hoses, mops), product contact surfaces (peelers, conveyors, slicers), and wash areas. Sampling of surfaces in contact with sliced luncheon meat revealed *Listeria* contamination rates of 9.3, 32.3, and 23.6% before, during, and after production, respectively. Similarly, listeriae were recovered from 2.8, 14.5, and 25.5% of food contact surfaces examined before, during, and after production of frankfurters.

As of April 1990, USDA-FSIS inspectors have documented the presence of *L. monocytogenes* in at least 78 meat-processing facilities of which 34, 16, 12, and 12 of the factories were cited for production of *Listeria*-contaminated cooked beef, cooked sausage, cooked poultry, and ready-to-eat salads/spreads, respectively (30). Although government officials have not yet released any additional information concerning specific work areas from which listeriae were isolated, results from a large-scale 1987 survey sponsored by the American Meat Institute (2,15) support the notion that *Listeria* spp. are widely distributed within the environment of many meat-processing facilities, and as in the earlier study by Flowers (9), also point to floors, drains, cleaning aids, wash areas, sausage peelers, and food contact surfaces as significant problem areas, with between 20 and 37% of such samples harboring listeriae (Table 15.5). With the identification of listeriae as present in condensate, compressed air, and on walls and ceilings, there can be no doubt that these organisms are ubiquitous in at least some meat-processing facilities.

Recognizing the potential opportunity for *Listeria* to contaminate meat during packaging, one major manufacturer of processed meat products attempted to obtain "near-operating room conditions" in its packaging room by cleaning the area for 3 days and then fogging the entire packaging room with 200 ppm quaternary ammonium compound (8,9). In spite of this, listeriae were still detected in 1 of 19 environmental samples obtained from the packaging room. After this exercise, the firm packaged processed meat products in this room over a 2-week period. Despite adherence to normal cleaning/sanitizing procedures at the end of each working day, the overall incidence of listeriae in the packaging room increased, with 3 of 20 (15%), 6 of 20(30%), and 8 of 20 (40%) samples positive for *Listeria* spp. 3, 6, and 8 days after the room was initially cleaned and fogged, respectively.

Table 15.5 Incidence of *Listeria* spp. in Post–Heat-Processing Areas of 41 Meat Factories Examined in the United States During 1987

Area	Positive samples (%)
Floors	37
Drains	37
Cleaning aids	24
Wash areas	24
Sausage peelers	22
Food contact surfaces	20
Condensate	7
Walls and ceilings	5
Compressed air	4

Source: Adapted from Ref. 2.

Since *Listeria* spp., including *L. monocytogenes*, have been found in up to 50% of raw beef, pork, and lamb marketed in the United States, complete elimination of listeriae from meat-processing environments appears highly improbable. However, the American Meat Institute has developed a series of interim guidelines (2), which, if followed, will reduce the incidence of listeriae and decrease the overall microbial load in the working environment. A detailed description of these guidelines appears later in this chapter.

Poultry-Processing Facilities

Current reports show that up to 50% of all raw poultry sold in the United States contains various *Listeria* spp., including *L. monocytogenes*, with fecal material from infected flocks cited most frequently as the source of contamination. Unfortunately, information concerning the incidence of listeriae in American poultry-processing facilities is presently limited to results from two recent California surveys. In these studies, researchers at the University of California-Davis investigated the prevalence of listeriae in processing samples from one chicken (46) and one turkey slaughterhouse (47) during three or four separate visits. According to these investigators, no *Listeria* spp. were isolated from feathers, incoming chiller water, or scalding water, the latter of which aids in feather removal (Table 15.6). Nonetheless, *L. monocytogenes* and *L. innocua* were identified in samples of overflow chiller water and feather picker drip water obtained from the chicken slaughterhouse, with both organisms detected in recycled water used to clean gutting equipment. Incidence rates for *L. monocytogenes* in chicken- and turkey-processing facilities were generally similar, with the percentage of *Listeria*-positive samples increasing approximately 2- to 2.5-fold during the latter stages of processing. However, *L. welshimeri* and *L. innocua* were absent from all chicken- and turkey-processing samples, respectively. While only two poultry slaughterhouses were examined in this survey, inability of these researchers to routinely detect *L. welshimeri* in fresh chicken meat and *L. innocua* in fresh turkey meat processed at these facilities suggests that *L. welshimeri* and *L. innocua* might be able to preferentially colonize the gastrointestinal tract of turkeys and chickens, respectively. These findings, along with the ability of these investigators to further demonstrate an increasing incidence of *Listeria* spp. on gloves/hands of poultry workers from the beginning to the end of processing (Table 15.7) confirms that these contaminants move along the processing line with the raw product.

Unfortunately, neither the USDA nor the poultry industry have released any data regarding the incidence of listeriae within the general working environment of poultry-processing facilities. However, considering the fecal carriage rate for listeriae in domestic birds, the current assembly line methods for processing poultry, and the fact that *Listeria* spp. (including *L. monocytogenes*) and salmonellae have been isolated from up to about half of all raw chickens marketed in the United States, one can speculate that the poultry and meat industries face similar problems in controlling the spread of listeriae and other organisms in the work environment. If one draws a parallel between methods used to process meat and poultry, then floors, drains, cleaning aids, wash areas, and food contact surfaces emerge as likely niches for *Listeria* spp., including *L. monocytogenes*, in poultry-processing facilities. These predictions may be supported by published scientific data in the future.

Table 15.6 Incidence of *Listeria* spp. in One Chicken and One Turkey Slaughterhouse in California

Sample	Number of chicken/turkey slaughterhouse samples analyzed	Number (%) of positive samples			
		L. monocytogenes	*L. innocua*	*L. welshimeri*	Total
Scalding water overflow	16/15	0/0	0/0	0/0	0/0
Feather picker drip water	16/15	0/1 (6.7)	3 (18.8)/0	0/1 (6.7)	3 (18.8)/2 (13.3)
Incoming chiller water	16/0	0/0	0/0	0/0	0/0
Overflow chiller water	16/15	2 (12.5)/0	0/0	0/1 (6.7)	2 (12.5)/1 (6.7)
Recycled water for cleaning gutters	16/15	1 (6.3)/2 (13.3)	5 (31.3)/0	0/3 (20.0)	6 (37.5)/5 (33.3)

Source: Adapted from Refs. 46, 47.

Table 15.7 Incidence of *L. monocytogenes* and *L. innocua* on the Hands and Gloves of Poultry Meat Processors Assigned to Three Different Stations in a Slaughterhouse

Sample	Number of chicken/turkey slaughterhouse samples analyzed	Number (%) of positive samples			
		L. monocytogenes	*L. innocua*	*L. welshimeri*	Total
Postchilling handlers	20/30	2 (10.0)/3 (10.0)	2 (10.0)/0	0/2 (6.7)	4 (20.0)/5 (16.7)
Leg/Wing cutters	11/30	4 (36.4)/3 (10.0)	1 (9.1)/0	0/7 (23.3)	5 (45.5)/10 (33.3)
Leg/Wing packers	44/30	20 (45.5)/5 (16.7)	11 (25.0)/0	0/7 (23.3)	31 (70.5)/12 (40.0)

Source: Adapted from Refs. 46, 47.

Egg-Processing Facilities

Isolation of listeriae from the surface of intact whole eggs remains to be documented (see Chapter 12). However, recent discovery of *L. innocua* and, to a lesser extent, *L. monocytogenes* in 15 of 42 (36%) samples of frozen, raw, commercial liquid whole egg obtained from 6 of 11 manufacturers located throughout the United States suggests that listeriae- as well as salmonellae-contaminated poultry feces may contaminate the surface of eggs before breaking, and that these organisms, in turn, may be spread to various areas within the egg-processing environment. Fortunately, the Egg Products Inspection Act of 1970 led to regulations which now require that all egg products be pasteurized to eliminate salmonellae (and *L. monocytogenes*). However, as is true for fluid milk, ample opportunity exists after pasteurization for recontamination of liquid egg products with listeriae, salmonellae, and nonpathogenic organisms which can greatly decrease the shelf life and/or microbial quality of the finished product. Although *Listeria* spp. have not yet been recovered from commercially prepared pasteurized egg products or the associated manufacturing environment, prudent producers of such products should be certain that floors, drains, cleaning aids, wash areas, and food contact surfaces as well as egg-breaking/egg-separating, pasteurization, and packaging equipment are thoroughly cleaned and sanitized on a regular basis to eliminate potential problems involving listeriae, salmonellae, and high levels of spoilage organisms.

Seafood-Processing Facilities

After *L. monocytogenes* was recovered from fresh frozen crabmeat in May of 1987, FDA officials began testing a wide range of domestic/imported fish and seafood products for listeriae and other organisms of public health significance. Whereas results from these efforts, which led to numerous Class I recalls of *Listeria*-contaminated products, are described in the first half of Chapter 13, government officials also released additional findings that were obtained during visits to various seafood-processing facilities.

Between January and April of 1988, inspectors from the Oregon Department of Agriculture analyzed 480 environmental swab samples from 17 seafood-processing facilities located throughout Oregon (10,43,77). While only 4% of all samples were positive for *Listeria* spp., 10 of 17 (60%) of the factories yielded evidence of *Listeria* contamination in the work environment. Specific locations from which listeriae were isolated included (a) a fiberglass tote in a walk-in cooler, (b) a drain in a walk-in cooler, (c) a phosphate recirculation system on a shrimp-processing line, (d) an ice tote in a cold room, (e) a floor gutter near a shrimp peeler, (f) a wooden door frame in a crab-freezing room, (g) tires on heavy machinery, (h) a cold saturated (~23%) brine solution, (i) the framework of a fish dumpster, (j) floor/wall junctions in a cooler, and (k) seagull droppings on an office manager's window. While not yet confirmed in the literature, additional niches within the working environment that are strongly suspected of harboring listeriae include walls, floors, ceilings, condensate, pooled water, and processing wastes. Hence, this information along with recent observations that virtually all *Listeria* cells recovered from processed seafoods have been healthy rather than thermally or otherwise injured suggest that presence of listeriae in processed seafood is almost exclusively the result of recontamination after processing. Information on preventing postprocessing contamination of fish, seafood, and other products discussed thus far appears in the second half of this chapter.

Vegetable/Fruit-Processing Facilities

Although consumption of coleslaw prepared from contaminated cabbage was directly linked to the first documented outbreak of foodborne listeriosis in 1981, the incidence of listeriae in raw vegetables/fruits and particularly the prevalence of these organisms in work environments of vegetable/fruit-processing facilities have received little attention. Nevertheless, the long-recognized association of listeriae with soil and the discovery of *Listeria* spp., including *L. monocytogenes*, on raw vegetables suggest that these organisms are almost certainly in vegetable/fruit-processing facilities. Unfortunately, the extent of *Listeria* contamination in such facilities in the United States is currently unknown. However, soil and production-area samples from one potato-processing factory in The Netherlands have yielded *L. monocytogenes*, *L. innocua*, and *L. seeligeri* (see Tables 15.11 and 15.12).

INCIDENCE OF *LISTERIA* SPP. IN WESTERN EUROPEAN AND AUSTRALIAN FOOD-PROCESSING FACILITIES

As is true for the United States, information concerning the extent of *Listeria* contamination in European food-processing facilities also is relatively scarce. However, data generated thus far indicate that European and American food companies are experiencing similar problems regarding listeriae in the manufacturing environment. Furthermore, since similar food production/processing/packaging methods and cleaning/sanitation practices are employed in both Western Europe and North America, much of the following information regarding the incidence of *Listeria* contamination within Western European food-processing facilities will probably be applicable to manufacturers of similar products in the United States and Canada.

Western Europe

Interest in the incidence of listeriae within European food-processing facilities has developed in parallel with discovery of these organisms in foods destined for human consumption. As you will recall from Chapter 10, large quantities of French Brie cheese were contaminated with *L. monocytogenes* in 1986. Therefore, emphasis was first placed on determining the prevalence of listeriae in cheese factories. While much work has been done in France during the past 4 years, as of June 1990 results from only one small-scale environmental survey of French cheese factories has formally appeared in the scientific literature (32), with *L. monocytogenes* identified in one floor sample and *L. innocua* recovered from boards/wheels on equipment (7 of 22 samples), brushes (1 of 6 samples), and filtered air (1 of 19 samples). During a survey of West German factories producing soft smear-ripened cheese, Terplan (74) also isolated nonpathogenic *Listeria* spp. from smear liquid, various pieces of machinery (especially smearing machines), and floor drains, with *L. monocytogenes* detected far less frequently than other listeriae (Table

Table 15.8 Prevalence of *L. monocytogenes* and Nonpathogenic *Listeria* spp. Within the Working Environment of West German Factories Producing Soft Smear-Ripened Cheese

Environmental sample	Number of samples analyzed	Number (%) of positive samples		
		L. monocytogenes	Nonpathogenic *Listeria* spp.	Total
Smear liquid and smearing machines	210	2 (0.9)	33 (15.7)	35 (16.7)
Other machinery	251	12 (4.8)	31 (12.3)	43 (17.1)
Ripening boards	69	0	2 (2.9)	2 (2.9)
Condensate and cooling water	36	1 (2.8)	2 (5.6)	3 (8.3)
Floor drains	74	3 (4.1)	29 (39.2)	32 (43.2)

Source: Adapted from Ref. 74.

15.8). Hence, opportunity exists for contamination of both mold and bacterial surface-ripened cheese during latter stages of manufacture and storage.

While such published information is scarce, some unpublished data are available on prevalence of listeriae in other Western European cheese factories. As mentioned in Chapter 8, Swiss officials who were tracing the source of contamination in the 1987 listeriosis outbreak involving consumption of Vacherin Mont d'Or soft-ripened cheese recovered the epidemic strain of *L. monocytogenes* from smear brine, curing brine, waste water sinks, wooden cheese hoops, and wooden boards used in 10 different cheese factories that manufactured *Listeria*-contaminated cheese (37). Additionally, nearly half of the 12 cellars used to ripen cheese contained listeriae, with the pathogen detected on 6.8% of the wooden shelves and 19.8% of the brushes used in the ripening cellars. Although not noted in the report, one would suspect that *L. monocytogenes* also was present in commonly recognized environmental niches such as drains, floors, stagnant water, and various food contact surfaces within cheese factories and ripening cellars. Thus brushing cheese with salt water and ripening hooped cheese on wooden shelves appear to be two important means for dissemination of listeriae within the cheese factories.

In 1988, Cox (39,40) presented some preliminary data concerning the prevalence of *Listeria* spp. within one blue and six soft cheese factories in Western Europe as well as in one ice cream factory and eight chocolate factories. As expected, listeriae generally occupied similar environmental niches in both soft and blue cheese factories; however, *Listeria*-contamination was far more common in ripening than production areas of the one blue cheese factory examined (Table 15.9). Ripening practices for blue cheese, including maintenance of a relatively moist environment, appear to be the likely reason for higher rates of *Listeria* contamination in ripening than production areas. Although

Table 15.9 Incidence of *Listeria* spp. in Several Western European Blue and Soft Cheese Factories

Environmental sample	Percent of samples yielding *Listeria* spp.	
	Soft cheese factory	Blue cheese factory
Drains	22	71[a]/80[b]
Floors	20	5/83
Residues	NA[c]	23/46
Equipment	0	0/NA
Walls	33	NA/NA
Air coolers	22	NA/NA
Stagnant water	14	NA/NA
Condensate	5	NA/NA
Brine	NA	0/NA
Miscellaneous	19	NA/NA

[a]Production areas.
[b]Ripening areas.
[c]Not analyzed.
Source: Adapted from Refs. 39, 40.

Table 15.10 Incidence of *Listeria* spp. in the Production Environment
of One Western European Ice Cream Factory

Environmental sample	Percent of samples yielding *Listeria* spp.	*Listeria* populations (CFU/g or ml)
Drains	100	$\geq 10^6$
Conveyors	75	10^2
Stagnant water	66	NR[a]
Floors	63	$10–10^6$
Residues/waste products	50	$10–10^4$

[a]Not reported.
Source: Adapted from Refs. 39, 40.

some environmental niches in this blue cheese factory were not sampled, results for soft cheese factories point to walls, air coolers, stagnant water, and condensate as possible problem areas in blue cheese factories as well.

During a similar investigation, samples of at least half of the drains, conveyors, stagnant water, floors, and residue/waste products from one Western European ice cream factory contained populations of *Listeria* spp. ranging from 10 to $\geq 10^6$ CFU/g or ml (Table 15.10). This factory manufactured all of its ice cream from commercially produced reconstituted powdered milk (a product from which *Listeria* has not yet been isolated) rather than fresh milk. Hence, these findings strongly suggest that *Listeria* contamination in dairy-processing facilities is not always linked to incoming raw milk or milk haulers.

Listeria spp., including *L. monocytogenes*, also have been detected in commercially produced chocolate that was marketed in England (48). Furthermore, a 1988 report by Cox (39) indicated that 8 of 32 (25%) and 10 of 59 (17%) samples obtained from damp, wet, and dry areas of eight Western European chocolate factories were positive for *Listeria* spp. While growth of listeriae in chocolate is very unlikely, contamination of the finished product during packaging is clearly possible. The relatively low risk of producing *Listeria*-contaminated chocolate can be further reduced by development of adequate cleaning/sanitation programs and by maintaining production and packaging areas as dry as possible.

In the largest European survey reported thus far, Cox et al. (41), during the latter half of 1986, investigated the incidence of *Listeria* spp. in the processing environment of 17 establishments in The Netherlands that produced fluid dairy products, ice cream, Italian-style cheese, frozen food, potato products, and dry culinary foods. A total of 608 samples were collected from drains, floors, condensed/stagnant water, residues, processing equipment, and/or other areas and were analyzed for listeriae using the original USDA or FDA method with or without modification. All presumptive *Listeria* isolates were then speciated according to results from conventional biochemical tests.

Despite use of Good Manufacturing Practices in these factories, *Listeria* spp. were recovered from all types of food-processing facilities examined with the exception of two that produced dry culinary products. Overall, 181 of 608 (29.8%) samples yielded

Listeria spp. with *L. innocua*, *L. monocytogenes*, and *L. seeligeri* identified in 87.3, 14.9, and 0.5% of all positive samples, respectively. Although only five samples contained both *L. monocytogenes* and *L. innocua*, the actual number of such samples is probably somewhat greater since a limited number of presumptive *Listeria* isolates from each sample were chosen for confirmation. As shown in Table 15.11, *L. innocua* was most prevalent in establishments that produced processed potato products followed by those that produced ice cream, frozen food, Italian-style cheese, and fluid dairy products, with the organism generally isolated most frequently from drains, floors, and condensed/stagnant water.

In contrast, *L. monocytogenes* was detected in 11.8% of all environmental samples obtained from one ice cream factory but was found in 2.9, 3.0, 3.3, and 3.7% of similar samples from establishments that manufactured fluid dairy products, potato products, frozen food, and Italian-style cheese, respectively (Table 15.12). Although only one ice cream factory was examined in this survey, the results are as expected when one recalls that Cox (39,40) previously found listeriae were widespread in another Western European ice cream factory and also were present in very large numbers particularly in floor drains (Table 15.10). Given such populations of listeriae in ice cream factories and the current extruding, molding, and freezing methods used to produce ice cream and particularly ice cream novelties, one can easily postulate many routes whereby listeriae may recontaminate the finished product, as has been reported in the United States.

Results concerning the incidence of *Listeria* spp. as well as *L. innocua* and *L. monocytogenes* in various work environments of all 15 food-processing facilities are summarized in Table 15.13. Overall, these findings are comparable to what has been previously noted for similar food-processing facilities in the United States, e.g., *Listeria* spp. and *L. innocua* were most frequently recovered from drains followed by condensed/stagnant water, floors, residues, and processing equipment. With a few minor exceptions, which probably resulted from the number of samples analyzed, this same trend is readily apparent for all five types of food-processing facilities listed in Table 15.11. Thus a logical pattern emerges in which *L. innocua* moves from floor drains to pools of condensed/stagnant water, which then come into direct contact with floors and residues. Once present in open areas of the work environment, *L. innocua* is spread by employees to processing equipment that comes into direct contact with the product. Unlike *L. innocua*, *L. monocytogenes* was far less prevalent in all types of food-processing facilities and was distributed fairly evenly within the factory environment with incidence rates ranging between 2.3 and 7.7%. Although *L. innocua* is by definition nonpathogenic, the fact that *L. innocua* and *L. monocytogenes* (and possibly other *Listeria* spp.) occupy similar environmental niches indicates that detection of listeriae anywhere within the manufacturing environment should prompt immediate corrective action, the details of which will be discussed shortly.

In the only other Western European survey thus far reported, Hudson and Mead (51) determined the incidence of *Listeria* spp. at 10 different sites within one large English poultry-processing facility. According to these authors, scald water, feathers, and chill water as well as swab samples from defeathering machines and conveyors leading to the chiller were free of listeriae; however, *L. monocytogenes* was routinely isolated from automatic carcass openers and also was present in samples from evisceration-line drains, neck-skin trimmers, and conveyors on which carcasses travel to the packing

Table 15.11 Incidence of *L. innocua* in Working Environments of 15 Food-Processing Facilities in The Netherlands

Environmental sample	Number of positive samples/Number of samples analyzed (%)				
	Fluid dairy factory $n^a = 5$	Ice cream factory $n = 1$	Italian-style cheese factory $n = 5$	Frozen food factory $n = 3$	Potato-processing factory $n = 1$
Drains	2/4 (50.0)	4/4 (100.0)	19/42 (45.2)	2/3 (66.7)	7/13 (53.8)
Condensed/Stagnant water	2/5 (40.0)	4/8 (50.0)	7/20 (35.0)	NA	7/10 (70.0)
Floors	0/2	8/16 (50.0)	14/44 (31.8)	2/4 (50.0)	9/13 (69.2)
Residues	NA[b]	4/12 (33.3)	16/71 (22.5)	NA	5/15[c] (33.3)
Processing equipment	0/10	7/20 (35.0)	6/68 (8.8)	1/6 (16.7)	NA
Miscellaneous	0/13	2/8[d] (25.0)	12/103[e] (11.7)	15/78 (19.2)	4/17[f] (23.5)
Total	4/34 (11.8)	29/68 (42.6)	74/348 (21.3)	20/91 (22.0)	32/68 (47.1)

[a]Number of factories analyzed.
[b]Not analyzed.
[c]Includes one sample positive for *L. seeligeri*.
[d]Conveyor belt (2 of 2 positive).
[e]Raw milk (2 of 2 positive), untreated effluent.
[f]Potato delivery soil (2 of 3 positive), sand from effluent treatment (2 of 2 positive).
Source: Adapted from Ref. 41.

Table 15.12 Incidence of *L. monocytogenes* in Working Environments of 15 Food-Processing Facilities in The Netherlands

Environmental sample	Number of positive samples/Number of samples analyzed (%)				
	Fluid dairy factory $n^a = 5$	Ice cream factory $n = 1$	Italian-style cheese factory $n = 5$	Frozen food factory $n = 3$	Potato-processing factory $n = 1$
Drains	0/4	0/4	2/42 (4.8)	1/3 (33.3)	0/13
Condensed/Stagnant water	0/5	0/8	0/20	NA	0/10
Floors	0/2	1/16 (6.3)	2/44 (4.5)	0/4	1/13 (7.7)
Residues	NA[b]	0/12	7/71 (9.9)	NA	0/15
Processing equipment	0/10	6/20 (30.0)	2/68 (2.9)	0/6	NA
Miscellaneous	1/13 (7.7)	1/8[c] (12.5)	0/103	2/78 (2.6)	1/17[d] (5.9)
Total	1/34 (2.9)	8/68 (11.8)	13/348 (3.7)	3/91 (3.3)	2/67 (3.0)

[a]Number of factories analyzed.
[b]Not analyzed.
[c]Sponge (1 of 1 positive).
[d]Potato delivery soil (1 of 3 positive).
Source: Adapted from Ref. 41.

Table 15.13 Overall Incidence of *Listeria* spp. in Working Environments of 15 Food-Processing Facilities in The Netherlands

Environmental sample	Number of samples analyzed	Number (%) of positive samples[a]		
		Listeria spp.	*L. innocua*	*L. monocytogenes*
Drains	66	36 (54.5)	34 (51.5)	3 (4.5)
Condensed/Stagnant water	43	20 (46.6)	20 (46.5)	0
Floors	79	36 (45.6)	33 (41.8)	4 (5.1)
Residues	97	32[a] (33.0)	24 (24.7)	7 (7.2)
Processing equipment	104	20 (19.2)	14 (13.5)	8 (7.7)
Miscellaneous	219	37 (16.9)	33 (15.1)	5 (2.3)
Total	608	181[b](29.8)	158 (26.0)	27 (4.4)

[a]One sample yielded *L. seeligeri*.
[b]Five samples yielded both *L. monocytogenes* and *L. innocua*.
Source: Adapted from Ref. 41.

Table 15.14 Incidence of *Listeria* spp. in the Working Environment of One Poultry-Processing Facility in England

Type of sample	Number of samples analyzed	Number (%) of positive samples	
		L. monocytogenes	*L. innocua*
Transport crates	9	0	1 (11.1)
Automatic carcass opener	3	3 (100)	0
Evisceration-line drain	3	2 (66.7)	0
Neck-skin trimmer	3	2 (66.7)	0
Conveyor to packing area	3	1 (33.3)	0

Source: Adapted from Ref. 51.

area (Table 15.14). While only one to three samples from each site were analyzed in three successive visits, the areas from which *L. monocytogenes* was recovered in this poultry-processing facility are generally similar to those observed by Genigeorgis et al. (46,47) for chicken and turkey slaughterhouses in California (Table 15.6).

Australia

Information concerning the prevalence of listeriae in food-processing facilities located in other parts of the world is currently limited to one Australian study. Following the isolation of *L. monocytogenes* from ricotta cheese in 1987, the Victorian Dairy Industry Authority and the Department of Agriculture and Rural Affairs conducted a joint survey to determine the extent of *Listeria* contamination in the working environments of 52 Melbourne-area factories producing pasteurized milk and various types of cheese (76). Overall, various *Listeria* spp. were detected in 141 of 763 (18.5%) environmental samples from 21 of 52 (40.4%) factory environments, with *L. monocytogenes*, *L. seeligeri*, and *L. ivanovii* identified in 132 (93.6%), 8 (5.7%), and 1 (0.7%) of these *Listeria*-positive samples, respectively. More important, *L. monocytogenes* was present in all but one of the *Listeria*-positive factories. As expected from other surveys conducted in the United States and Western Europe, factory sites most frequently contaminated with listeriae once again included drains/floors in coolers, surfaces of manufacturing/packaging equipment, and conveyors. Even though strict cleaning and sanitizing programs were implemented at many of these facilities, *Listeria* spp. were very difficult to eliminate from the working environment, with these organisms continuously isolated from one factory over a period of 5 months. Complete elimination of listeriae from dairy-processing facilities may, in some instances, be nearly impossible; however, the likelihood of producing *Listeria*-contaminated products can be greatly reduced by following Good Manufacturing Practices, which include implementation of rigorous cleaning and sanitizing programs for equipment used at critical points during manufacture and packaging of the foods in question.

INCIDENCE OF *LISTERIA* IN HOUSEHOLD KITCHENS

Thus far this chapter has dealt exclusively with *Listeria* contamination in commercial food-processing facilities; however, because of the relatively high incidence of *Listeria* spp. (including *L. monocytogenes*), salmonellae, and other foodborne pathogens in fresh beef, pork, lamb, and poultry available to the general public at butcher shops and supermarkets, safe home preparation of these foods must be reemphasized. In 1989, Cox et al. (41) isolated nine strains of listeriae from 7 of 35 (20%) household kitchens surveyed in The Netherlands. Overall, *L. monocytogenes* was recovered from four dishcloths and one refrigerator, with two dishcloths and two dustbins from two other households yielding *L. innocua* and *L. welshimeri*, respectively. Considering results from commercial food-processing facilities, one might expect to recover *Listeria* spp. from such household kitchen areas as drains, U-tubes, and drain boards. If this is true, then garbage disposal systems could conceivably lead to problems from production of aerosols. Although further work is needed to clarify the public health significance of listeriae in the kitchen environment, you may recall from Chapter 8 that *L. monocytogenes* was found in many refrigerated foods belonging to an Oklahoma woman who contracted listeriosis after consuming contaminated turkey frankfurters that were eventually recalled nationwide.

In 1989, CDC officials also isolated *L. monocytogenes* from 15 of 25 (60%) refrigerators that were used by apparent victims of foodborne listeriosis (25). Hence, consumers should regularly clean and sanitize kitchen areas, sinks, and refrigerators. Such efforts should help prevent potential problems involving listeriosis and other forms of foodborne illness in the home.

CONTROL OF *LISTERIA* IN FOOD-PROCESSING FACILITIES

The discovery of *Listeria* spp., including *L. monocytogenes*, in various fermented and unfermented dairy products, raw and ready-to-eat meats, poultry products, seafoods, and vegetable products has prompted food manufacturers to renew their concern about factory hygiene and product safety. Although failsafe procedures for production of *Listeria*-free foods largely do not yet exist, specific guidelines have been developed for controlling listeriae and other microbial contaminants within American dairy- (4,18,36,49,57,68,73,75), meat- (1,2), poultry- (19) and seafood- (43,45,77) processing facilities with Denmark (21), England (53,58,67), and France (17) also addressing the elimination of listeriae from fluid milk and cheese operations during all facets of production, distribution, and retail sale of the foods.

In response to the discovery of *L. monocytogenes* in ready-to-eat foods and delicatessen products, European public health officials have expressed particular concern about contamination of these products during retail slicing and storage. They also have warned grocery store managers to give particular attention to storage temperatures for refrigerated foods in display cases and the potential sale of products beyond their normal code dates. Most of these guidelines stress the need to (a) decrease the possibility that raw products will contain listeriae, (b) minimize environmental contamination in food-processing facilities, and (c) use processing methods that will eliminate listeriae from food. Benefits from following these proposed guidelines, which will be discussed in detail shortly, will decrease the possibility of producing foods contaminated with *L. monocytogenes* and other foodborne pathogens. In addition, diligent attention to cleaning and sanitation and overall Good Manufacturing Practices will lead to lower microbial populations in processed foods which will, in turn, increase the shelf life of the finished products.

Any approach to controlling the spread of listeriae and other microorganisms in food-processing facilities is complicated by the enormous variety of foods being processed today along with variability in quality of incoming raw products, design of the factory, and processing methods. However, this subject can be simplified by first focusing on problem areas such as factory design, general factory environment, heating/air-conditioning systems, traffic patterns, and personnel cleanliness that are common to all food-processing facilities. Once *Listeria*-control measures for these problem areas are understood, attention can be given to specific processing steps which are unique to the dairy, meat, poultry, seafood, and vegetable industries.

General Guidelines

Factory Design

Every food processor should be firmly committed to the long-term production of safe, wholesome food. The first step toward such a goal is an adequately designed factory to produce the particular product. While newly constructed buildings offer countless advantages in that they can be designed for production of specific products, existing buildings also can be used for safe production of food provided that such facilities have been properly modified to meet certain basic requirements.

Design features that are widely considered to be essential for all types of food-processing facilities include (a) a raw product receiving area that is completely isolated from processing and packaging areas of the factory, (b) tight-fitting exterior windows and doors that will prevent animals and insects from entering processing and packaging areas, (c) readily cleaned and sanitized walls, floors, and ceilings that are constructed of tile, metal, or concrete, not porous materials such as wood, (d) floors designed to drain rapidly, thus preventing pooling of water, (e) floor drains located away from packaging equipment, especially if processed foods are exposed to factory air, (f) proper screens, debris baskets, and traps on floor drains, (g) a quality control/quality assurance laboratory that is well isolated from other areas of the factory, and (h) proper means of waste disposal outside the factory to discourage congregation of insects, rodents, birds, and other animals that may harbor *Listeria* and other pathogenic microorganisms.

In addition to these concerns, the heating/ventilating/air-conditioning (HVAC) system also must be properly designed to minimize airborne contamination (68). Features considered to be essential for such a system include (a) intake air vents on the roof of the building that are located upwind from prevailing air currents but away from dumpsters, raw product receiving areas, and vents that are discharging factory air, (b) installation of screens and filters inside incoming air vents to remove particulate matter and condensate, (c) easily cleaned HVAC systems, and (d) proper location of dehumidifiers and air conditioning systems so that these units drain away from processing/packaging areas. Most important, all HVAC systems must be designed to produce a higher positive air pressure in processing/packaging rather than receiving areas. This design readily prevents movement of airborne contaminants from raw product areas to the cleanest areas of the factory where foods are processed and packaged.

Factory Environment

Various bacteria, yeasts, and molds can be found in most food-processing areas other than those associated with aseptic packaging, with populations normally many times higher in receiving than in processing/packaging areas. Furthermore, most of these microorganisms will grow in the factory environment if given a suitable temperature and enough time along with an adequate supply of nutrients and water. While microbial contamination will always occur in food-processing facilities, eliminating microbial growth by altering (a) temperature, (b) time that the organism is present in the environment, (c) availability of nutrients, and/or (d) availability of water will sharply decrease the incidence of *L. monocytogenes* and other foodborne pathogens as well as spoilage organisms in the factory environment. Hence, production of a safe food product with a long shelf life depends largely on control of time/temperature constraints and elimination of available nutrients and/or water through the concerted effort of everyone involved.

Since air, water, waste products, and anything else that comes in contact with the finished product must be considered as a potential source of contamination, food processors must strive to prevent spread of microbial contaminants from heavily contaminated raw product receiving areas to processing/packaging areas. In addition to construction of physical barriers between such areas in the factory, all incoming cases, pallets, containers, forklifts, and cleaning materials such as brushes and other equipment must be assumed to harbor listeriae along with other microbial contaminants and therefore should never be allowed to enter processing/packaging areas. Ideally, separate equipment, including tools employed by maintenance persons, should be available for use in raw and finished product areas. If this is not possible, then all equipment should be cleaned and sanitized before entering processing/packaging areas.

As previously stressed, all areas within food-processing facilities should be kept dry and as free as possible from processing waste to minimize microbial growth. Also, floor drainage problems that lead to pooling of water must be eliminated as well as cracks and holes in floor tiles and grouting in which water and food particles can accumulate. Since *L. monocytogenes* has been recovered from condensate in dairy factories, it is imperative to keep all processing/packaging equipment and walls, floors, and ceilings as condensate-free as possible. In the event that dripping condensate cannot be prevented by manipulation of temperature and humidity in processing/packaging areas, deflector shields should be installed to prevent direct contact between exposed product and dripping condensate. Aerosols provide another ready means for disseminating listeriae and other microbial contaminants throughout critical areas of food-processing facilities (55), with *L. monocytogenes* surviving 3.42 hours in experimentally produced aerosols of reconstituted skim milk (71). Therefore, high pressure sprays should never be used in processing/packaging areas for cleaning floors or drains since both are major sources of listeriae and other microbial contaminants and resulting aerosols can contaminate food contact surfaces of equipment. Operation of unshielded centrifugal pumps in such areas also is discouraged.

In addition to the building itself, all equipment within the factory should be designed to minimize cross-contamination between the factory environment and product and also should be constructed of stainless steel or other readily cleaned/sanitized nonabsorbent, nontoxic materials such as certain types of bonded rubber and plastic. All piping in food-processing facilities should be free-draining and designed to eliminate trapping of food and cleaning and sanitizing solutions used in clean-in-place (CIP) systems. It also is important that equipment such as product conveyors is positioned high enough above the floor to minimize cross-contamination from floors and drains.

The air supply within the factory must be considered as a potential source of *Listeria* and other microbial contaminants. Hence, all HVAC ducts and accompanying air filters should be kept in good repair and cleaned regularly to eliminate excessive dust and dirt. Compressed air lines and filters should also be inspected regularly and be free of moisture, oil, and debris.

Cleaning and Sanitizing

Cleaning can be defined as the physical removal of visible dirt, impurities, and other extraneous matter (i.e., nutrients for growth of microorganisms including *Listeria*) through proper use of solutions of soaps, detergents, surfactants, and abrasive agents. In contrast, sanitizing causes inactivation of most microorganisms left on cleaned surfaces through exposing them to heat or chemical agents such as chlorine, iodine (iodophor), acid anionic, or quaternary ammonium compounds. Hence, routine use of good cleaning and sanitizing practices is of utmost importance in controlling microbiological safety and quality of finished products. In establishments such as those that produce fluid milk and ice cream, adherence to good cleaning and sanitation practices that involve both equipment and the factory environment is the only means of preserving product quality beyond initial pasteurization of ingredients.

Each food-processing facility needs to institute and enforce a cleaning/sanitizing program that will ensure production of safe products. As part of this program, management personnel need to develop standard operating procedures for every job in the factory so that the workers will recognize their individual responsibilities and will maintain accurate records regarding routine sanitation practices. Management personnel also need to instill in their employees the great importance of good cleaning and sanitizing practices through use of continuing education programs that deal with current issues such as *Listeria*. Such cleaning and sanitizing responsibilities should never be assigned to new untrained employees.

Floors, drains, walls, ceilings, and each piece of equipment in the factory should be cleaned and/or sanitized on a regular basis with the frequency of cleaning and sanitizing dependent on the extent to which the particular item becomes contaminated during normal operation and whether or not a product is likely to come in contact with the item during processing and/or packaging. All food contact surfaces such as tables, peelers, slicers, collators, overhead shielding, conveyors, conveyor belts, chain rollers, supports, and other intricate equipment directly associated with processing, filling, and packaging operations need to be cleaned and sanitized daily and in some instances more often, particularly around filling and packaging operations. A regular cleaning and sanitizing schedule also must be adopted for non–food contact surfaces such as floors, walls, ceilings, floor drains, pipes, blowers, HVAC ducts, coils and pans from dehumidifying and air-conditioning units, light fixtures, material handling equipment, and wet/dry vacuum canisters. As indicated in the first half of this chapter, *Listeria* spp., including *L. monocytogenes*, have been most frequently isolated from floor drains and floors, thus suggesting that these areas may function as reservoirs for listeriae in food-processing facilities. Although all floors and drains in production and refrigerated storage areas should be thoroughly cleaned, including drain covers and baskets, and sanitized daily, high pressure hoses should never be used in these areas since such practices readily promote the spread of listeriae to nearby equipment and other areas of the factory by way of splashing and aerosols.

Managers of food-processing facilities must be sure that proper equipment is available for daily cleaning and sanitizing operations. Absorbent articles such as sponges and rags should never be used in the factory environment since these items function as virtual "microbial zoos." Various types of metal scrappers can be used for removing hard mineral deposits, with disposable paper towels best suited for eliminating excess moisture and accidental spills. Unlike sponges and rags, brushes are readily cleaned and sanitized and are therefore suitable for widespread use in the factory. However, to avoid cross-contamination, separate color-coded brushes with nonporous plastic or metal handles should be used for scrubbing (a) exterior and interior surfaces of equipment, (b) raw and finished product areas, (c) food contact and non–food contact equipment surfaces, and (d) floor drains. Brushes, particularly those used to scrub floor drains, are best cleaned and stored in sanitizing solution after use.

Sanitizing is the final step in eliminating *L. monocytogenes*, other foodborne pathogens, and the myriad of spoilage organisms present in the production environment. Since presence of organic debris, particularly if proteinaceous, readily decreases the effectiveness of sanitizing agents against most microorganisms including listeriae (33), it is important to remember that every item to be sanitized must first be thoroughly cleaned.

As discussed in Chapter 5, research has demonstrated that *L. monocytogenes* is sensitive to sanitizing agents commonly employed in the food industry. According to several authors (61,65), chlorine-based, iodine-based, acid anionic, and/or quaternary ammonium-type sanitizers were effective against *L. monocytogenes* when used at concentrations of 100 ppm, 25–45 ppm, 200 ppm, and 100–200 ppm, respectively. Although these concentrations may have to be adjusted to compensate for in-plant use as well as oxidation/reduction factors relating to water quality and hardness, recommended concentrations should not be markedly exceeded since use of extremely concentrated sanitizing solutions heightens the danger to employees, increases the risk of chemical contamination of food and, in some instances, causes corrosion of equipment. Since foaming chlorine-based sanitizers are corrosive, their use should be primarily confined to floors, floor drains, walls and ceilings. Alternatively, these areas can be flooded or foamed with quaternary ammonium-type sanitizers (~300 ppm); however, fogging exterior surfaces with quaternary ammonium-type sanitizers is frequently regarded as ineffective and dangerous for employees. Quaternary ammonium-based sanitizers also are not recommended for use on food-contact surfaces and should never be used in cheese or sausage factories since lactic acid starter culture bacteria are rapidly inactivated by small residues of these sanitizers. In contrast, acid anionic and iodine-type sanitizers are best suited for equipment surfaces, with the former readily neutralizing excess alkalinity from cleaning compounds and preventing formation of alkaline mineral deposits. While also effective, use of steam should be confined to closed systems because of potential hazards associated with aerosol formation. Sanitizing with hot water is not advised since sufficiently high water temperatures cannot be easily maintained.

Custom-designed clean-in-place (CIP) systems have been installed in many food-processing facilities, particularly dairies, for automated cleaning and sanitizing of pipelines, tanks, vats, heat exchangers, homogenizers, and other equipment in processing lines. Although presumably adequate by design, CIP systems also should be reviewed for proper timing, flow rate, temperature, pressure, and sanitizer strength as recommended by chemical suppliers. Furthermore, proper operation of the entire system should be verified from data collected on recording charts, which can be stored for future reference.

Regardless of how well the aforementioned recommendations regarding cleaning and sanitizing are followed, every food-processing facility should verify the effectiveness of its cleaning and sanitation program through daily microbiological analysis of both product and environmental samples gathered from all areas of the factory. Particular attention should be given to floor drains, floors, filling/packaging areas, and any processing equipment that is difficult to clean. While environmental samples are most easily collected using swabs or sponges, only polyurethane or expanding cellulose sponges should be used for such purpose since other types, including retail cellulose sponges, contain inhibitory agents that not only prevent recovery of *L. monocytogenes* and *Staphylococcus aureus*, but also interfere with recovery of *Bronchothrix thermosphacta*, *Aeromonas hydrophila*, *Pseudomonas putrefaciens* and *Pseudomonas fluorescens* as well as *Escherichia coli*, *Serratia marcescens*, and *Enterobacter cloacae* (60). However, it must again be stressed that laboratory personnel should never attempt to isolate pathogenic microorganisms from such samples unless the laboratory is in a separate building, completely removed from the factory. Although analysis of environmental and, if necessary, food samples for microbial pathogens is best left to outside commercial testing laboratories that are FDA-approved or otherwise certified, coliform and standard aerobic plate counts should be obtained for samples from the factory environment and the food during all stages of production to monitor the extent of postprocessing contamination and thus to quickly identify any problems associated with inadequate cleaning and sanitizing. Coliform organisms are commonly regarded as indicators of postprocessing contamination and possible presence of pathogens; however, presence or absence of coliforms in food or environmental samples does not guarantee the presence or absence of foodborne pathogens. In fact, often little if any correlation has been observed between presence of coliforms and *Listeria* in finished product. Therefore, routine testing of environmental samples for *Listeria* spp. and other foodborne pathogens by outside laboratories remains a critical component of any sanitation verification program.

Traffic Patterns

Employee movement within food-processing facilities also can have a major impact on the microbiological quality of finished products. Therefore, traffic patterns need to be developed that restrict or preferably eliminate movement of workers, between raw, processing, filling, packaging, and shipping areas. Managers need to educate employees about the spread of *Listeria* and other microbial contaminants from clothing, boots, and tools to all areas of the factory, and need to situate locker rooms, changing areas, and lunch/break rooms to minimize traffic through production areas. Issuing different-colored outer garments to workers in various areas of the factory has proven helpful in monitoring employee movement. Since *L. monocytogenes* and other microbial pathogens are commonly associated with raw products of both plant and animal origin, employees working in raw product receiving areas (including maintenance personnel) and individuals who deliver raw products, particularly milk haulers, should be denied access to all processing areas. When necessary, employee movement between raw product and processing areas of the factory should only be allowed after completely changing outer garments as well as scrubbing and disinfecting boots. All workers should be encouraged to use disinfectant-containing footbaths that should be placed in all doorways leading into the factory as well as between raw product and production areas.

These footbaths need to be monitored daily for sanitizer strength and cleanliness. Since a great variety of microorganisms are carried on street clothing, it also may be prudent for managers to consider limiting the number of visitors and tour groups going through the factory. Large glass observation windows provide ample opportunity for visitors to view processing areas, while at the same time prevent introduction of additional microbial contaminants.

Personnel Cleanliness

Factory managers and supervisors must stress good employee hygiene and also set a good example for other workers. All individuals with obvious illnesses, infected cuts, or abrasions need to be excluded from working in processing areas or from doing other tasks that may lead to contamination of food, food-contact surfaces, or packaging materials. Furthermore, use of tobacco and chewing gum as well as consumption of food should be banned in processing areas along with the wearing of hairpins, rings, earrings, and watches. Above all, employees should always wash their hands thoroughly before starting work, upon returning to work, and after touching floors, walls, light switches, or any other unclean surface. To further promote their use, handwashing facilities should be properly designed and conveniently located near work stations. All factory workers need to be provided with hair and/or beard nets as well as clean clothes, suitable footwear, and disposable gloves. Special attention also is needed to assure that street clothes do not enter processing areas and that factory clothing, including footwear, remain inside the factory. All factory clothing should be changed daily or more often if soiled, with the responsibility of laundering left to the employer. While the aforementioned recommendations may, in some instances, be difficult for food processors to follow and enforce, this task will be made much easier if management can instill in workers the conviction that each employee is personally responsible for both the quality and safety of the foods that are produced and ultimately consumed by the general public.

INDUSTRY-SPECIFIC EQUIPMENT, PROCESSING METHODS, AND PRODUCTS

It now is appropriate to briefly examine some of the industry-specific equipment and processing methods, many of which have been cited as critical control points for production of *Listeria*-free dairy, meat, poultry, seafood, and vegetable products. While this information will be useful to enhance the effectiveness of preexisting cleaning and sanitation programs, the reader is reminded that food-processing facilities, even though they manufacture similar products, are all unique in terms of factory design, raw product quality, and product-handling/processing methods. Therefore, no universally acceptable cleaning/sanitation program can be developed for the safe production of a given product.

Dairy Industry

Farm Environment

Since listeriae are widespread in the environment, any quality control program should first contain a plan to minimize contamination of raw milk with *Listeria* and other microorganisms on the dairy farm. Along with good animal husbandry practices, including use of only high quality feed and silage, farm workers also should give attention to cleanliness of the milkhouse and milking equipment. Most important, teats and udders of all cows should be properly sanitized and dried before milking equipment is attached. Bulk tanks in which raw milk is stored also need to be properly maintained and inspected regularly.

Clarifiers/Separators

All raw milk should be filtered and subsequently clarified/separated by centrifugation to remove extraneous matter and somatic cells (i.e., leukocytes) before pasteurization. Since *L. monocytogenes* is sometimes found in leukocytes, clarifiers and separators should be well isolated from the pasteurizer and all finished product areas of the factory. Sealed containers should be used to dispose of all clarifier and separator waste, both of which may contain high levels of listeriae. Special care also should be used in cleaning and sanitizing separators, clarifiers, and surrounding areas.

Pasteurization

Proper pasteurization using a vat or high-temperature short-time (HTST) pasteurizer is the only commercially practical means by which all non–spore-forming pathogens, including *L. monocytogenes*, in raw milk can be inactivated. Thus it is imperative that all pasteurization equipment be designed, installed, maintained, and operated properly.

Although continuous-flow HTST pasteurization is used to process virtually all fluid milk and ice cream mix, vat (or batch) pasteurization is employed by many smaller firms, particularly those involved in cheesemaking, when the volume of incoming raw milk is too small to justify use of a continuous flow HTST system. If vat pasteurization is used, raw milk must be heated to a minimum of 62.8°C (145°F) and then held at that temperature for at least 30 minutes. In theory, vat pasteurization is a relatively simple process with raw milk pumped into a steam- or hot water–jacketed vat and held for the prescribed time. However, FDA inspections conducted as part of the Dairy Initiative Program mentioned earlier have uncovered numerous problems with vat pasteurizers, including improper equipment design, absence of proper outlet valves and airspace thermometers, and improperly operated airspace heaters. The latter problem is particularly critical since the airspace temperature above the product in the vat must be at least 2.8°C (5°F) higher than that of the product at all times to assure proper pasteurization. Operators of such pasteurizers should be made accountable for proper performance as well as proper cleaning and sanitizing of the equipment. In addition, recording charts showing time/temperature relationships along with other data for each vat of product pasteurized should be preserved for at least 3 months.

As mentioned earlier, continuous-flow HTST pasteurization at 71.7°C (161°F) for a minimum of 15 seconds is the principal method for processing raw milk. Although an in-depth discussion of the many intricate problems associated with HTST pasteurization equipment is beyond the scope of this book, a basic knowledge of HTST pasteurization is essential to appreciate the seriousness of some of the recently identified problems that have been linked to faulty maintenance and/or operation of the equipment. Interested readers may consult the *HTST Pasteurizer Operation Manual* (50) for more detailed information on HTST pasteurization.

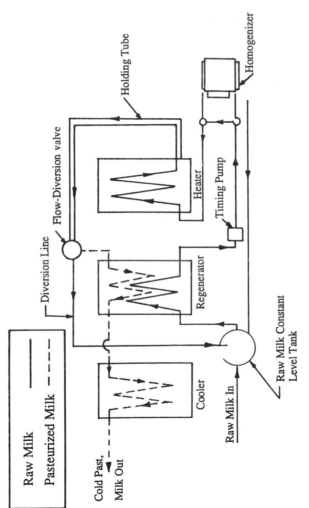

Figure 15.1 Schematic diagram of milk flow through an HTST pasteurizer. (Adapted from Ref. 50.)

All HTST pasteurizers consist of five basic components as shown in Fig. 15.1: (a) plate heat exchanger—a series of thin, gasketed stainless steel plates divided into three sections (heater, regenerator, and cooler) for heating incoming raw milk and cooling outgoing pasteurized milk, (b) constant level tank—provides a constant level of raw milk to the HTST system, (c) timing pump—a positive displacement pump that establishes the holding time of the time/temperature relationship for pasteurization, (d) holding tube—a length of pipe in which fully heated milk is held for the required holding time, and (e) flow diversion valve—a three-way valve that will allow properly pasteurized milk to enter the regenerator section of the plate heat exchanger or divert improperly pasteurized milk to the constant level tank for repasteurization. In addition to these five components, a source of steam and/or hot water is required to heat incoming raw milk, a safety thermal limit recorder is needed to activate the flow diversion value in the event of improper pasteurization and a cold milk recorder is required to record the temperature of outgoing pasteurized milk. Finally, auxiliary components that may be added to HTST units for additional processing of milk or milk products include a booster pump, homogenizer as a timing pump, stuffing pump, and flavor treatment or vacuum units.

Inspections of HTST pasteurizers conducted in conjunction with the FDA Dairy Initiative Program uncovered numerous problems relating to proper installation and maintenance of these units. Problems most commonly associated with HTST pasteurization equipment have included stress cracks and/or pinholes in the heat exchanger plates, leaking gaskets, improper flow diversion valves, and inadequate cleaning/sanitizing of the pasteurization unit. While not a strict regulatory requirement, positive pressure should be maintained between the product and heating medium as well as the product and cooling medium (sweetwater) to prevent *Listeria*-contaminated raw milk or sweetwater from mixing with pasteurized product in the event that some of the heat exchanger plates contain stress cracks or pinholes. Operators should examine all pasteurization plates for defects every 6 months using the standard dye test. Sweetwater and glycol solutions also should be routinely examined for microbial contaminants since these coolants may harbor *L. monocytogenes*, *Yersinia enterocolitica*, and *Salmonella typhimurium* for extended periods along with large populations of psychrotrophs (18,66); the latter are particularly detrimental to product shelf life. As was true for vat pasteurization, operators of HTST pasteurizers must be responsible for proper operation of these units and retain accurate records/chart recordings for each lot of pasteurized product for at least 3 months. Although the inability of *L. monocytogenes* to survive the minimum allowable HTST heat treatment given to commercially available raw milk (71.7°C/15 sec) is now generally accepted, most fluid milk processors in the United States are pasteurizing milk at ~76.7°C for 20 seconds, well above the minimum requirements established in the Pasteurized Milk Ordinance. While this more severe heat treatment markedly extends the shelf life of the finished product by inactivating larger numbers of spoilage organisms than does minimal HTST pasteurization, the psychrotrophic nature of *L. monocytogenes* increases the need to prevent introduction of listeriae into the product after pasteurization.

Pipeline and Cross-Connections

Many large dairy processors have installed up to several miles of pipeline in the factory to handle movement of raw milk from storage tanks to the pasteurizer and pasteurized milk from the pasteurizer to various holding tanks, mixing tanks, and product areas located throughout the factory. Considering the enormous quantities of product that can be manufactured at such facilities during one production period, careful attention must be given to each stage of manufacture since an error made during operations could adversely affect thousands of people, as was true for the 1985 outbreak of milkborne salmonellosis in Chicago.

FDA inspections have uncovered numerous violations related to pipelines, including cross-connections between raw and pasteurized milk lines and/or storage/holding tanks as well as cross-connections between CIP and product lines and other potentially hazardous circuits. Since many of these lines allow easy bypass of raw product around the pasteurizer thus permitting postpasteurization contamination in the event of equipment failure or operator error, factory managers, engineers, or other qualified people need to walk through the factory and construct an up-to-date detailed blueprint of raw and pasteurized product flow throughout the entire factory. Once the blueprint is constructed, any unwanted piping, dead ends, illegal cross-connections, or unauthorized changes made to initial installations should be promptly identified and eliminated. Most important, all pasteurized product lines need to be separated from raw and CIP lines by a physical break. To be of continued use, blueprints must be routinely updated and reviewed for accuracy by "walking" the blueprints through the factory. Finally, no piping changes should ever be made without prior review by qualified authorities.

Filling and Packaging

Postpasteurization contamination frequently occurs during filling and packaging operations when products are exposed to difficult-to-clean surfaces on equipment, the manufacturing environment, and airborne contaminants (54). Areas associated with product contamination have included mandrels, drip shields, bottom and top breakers, prefilling coding equipment, deflecter bars, and cutting blades as well as overhead shielding, conveyors, conveyor belts, chain rollers, supports, and lubricants. Product extruder heads are particular prone to contamination and therefore should be sanitized frequently during filling operations. Such practices will lead to production of safe products with markedly increased shelf lifes.

Reclaimed and Reworked Product

Salvage programs, by their nature, are high risk operations that can put an entire company in jeopardy if not done in a sanitary manner. Potential hazards associated with such salvage operations include (a) failure to repasteurize returned product before reuse, (b) inadvertently pumping returned but not repasteurized product through pasteurized product lines without proper cleaning and sanitizing between use, (c) accidental reuse of outdated product, (d) reuse of product returned from retail stores that may have been temperature-abused, tampered with, or exposed to chemical or biological contamination, and (e) use of product from contaminated, leaking, or otherwise damaged containers. Therefore, any product that left the possession and control of the processor or has been mishandled, inadequately protected from contamination, or exposed to temperatures $\geq 7.2°C$ (45°F) should be discarded. Dairy processors also should seriously consider confining use of reclaimed/repasteurized milk to dairy products prepared from non–Grade A milk.

According to the Pasteurized Milk Ordinance, American dairies involved in reclaiming programs now must have separate areas or rooms isolated from Grade A milk operations for receiving, handling, and storing all returned products. Outdated products and those which have left control of the processor and later are returned to the dairy for disposal should never reenter the factory. Given the recent isolation of *L. monocytogenes* and other microbial contaminants from the external surface of cartons containing returned product, along with the proven ability of *L. monocytogenes* and *Salmonella* spp. to survive up to 14 days on the external surface of both waxed cardboard and plastic-type milk containers (72), the process of opening containers and emptying reclaimed product into vats for reprocessing will likely introduce many new unwanted microbial contaminants into the factory environment. Therefore, it is imperative that all returned products be handled similar to raw milk and be repasteurized, preferably using times and temperatures well above the required minima. After reprocessing, all equipment including tanks, pumps, and pipelines used in the reclaiming operation should be thoroughly cleaned and sanitized. In view of the aforementioned problems associated with salvage operations, each dairy processor needs to reevaluate the advantages and disadvantages involved in reclaiming products and then decide whether or not the monetary benefits gained by such practices will outweigh the potential public health and other risks.

Frozen Dairy Products

Although few bacterial species can grow at temperatures below 0°C, most microorganisms including listeriae can survive for long times in frozen dairy products such as ice cream, ice cream novelties, and sherbet. Unlike fluid milk, frozen dairy products are particularly susceptible to microbial contamination during freezing and filling operations. All barrel freezers used to make frozen dairy products should be thoroughly sanitized before use since hand assembly of the many intricate freezer parts is likely to introduce numerous contaminants. The source of air for the barrel freezer is another likely source of contamination. Hence, in addition to maintaining positive air pressure in this area and keeping the surrounding area as clean and sanitary as possible, all air lines connected to the barrel freezer should be equipped with dryers and bacterial filters to prevent airborne contaminants from entering the product.

Ingredient feeders are perhaps the greatest source of contaminants in frozen dairy products. Therefore, fruits, nuts, candy, and other ingredients that are added directly to frozen ice cream mix need to be closely monitored for coliforms, pathogens, and other microbial contaminants. Exposure of ingredients to the factory environment also should be minimized. Strict adherence to Good Manufacturing Practices is necessary during production of molded, extruded, and/or dipped ice cream novelties since many such products have been recently recalled because of contamination with *L. monocytogenes* (see Table 9.3). Condensate in and around hardening rooms as well as conveyor belts appear to be likely sources of such contamination.

Finally, handling of product rerun exiting the freezer needs to be assessed at each factory. Although rerun product should never be added directly back to tanks containing unfrozen mix, frozen rerun product can be reclaimed by blending it with fresh mix, which is then repasteurized. Any rerun that is not reclaimed should be clearly separated from reclaimable material and properly disposed.

Fermented Dairy Products

Fortunately, the incidence of *Listeria* contamination in yogurt, cultured cream, cultured buttermilk, and other fermented fluid milk products appears to be quite low with very few recalls thus far issued for these products. The species of lactic acid bacteria used in manufacturing these products as well as the bacteriostatic/bactericidal effect of various organic acids produced during fermentation and the resultant lowering of pH are undoubtedly responsible for the near-absence of such recalls. However, since bacterial pathogens (including *L. monocytogenes*) and various spoilage organisms may inadvertently contaminate fermented milk products during any stage of manufacture, producers of such products need to follow Good Manufacturing Practices and be readily aware of potential problems regarding improper cleaning/sanitizing of equipment and the factory environment as well as potential sources of postpasteurization contamination (e.g., filling/packaging areas) discussed earlier in this chapter.

Production of *Listeria*-free cheese, particularly soft/semi-soft varieties surface-ripened with mold (e.g., Brie, Camembert) or bacteria (e.g., brick, Limburger), is difficult since environmental conditions required for proper cheese ripening also promote growth of *L. monocytogenes* and other unwanted organisms. Swiss officials who investigated the 1987 listeriosis outbreak involving consumption of Vacherin Mont d'Or soft-ripened cheese (see Chapter 8) eventually isolated the epidemic strain of *L. monocytogenes* from wooden shelves and cheese hoops found in over half of the caves used to ripen the tainted cheese. Thus the basic problem associated with soft cheese manufacture is to prevent postprocessing contamination by eliminating *L. monocytogenes* from the ripening room and particularly the shelves on which such cheese must be ripened. Considering the ability of *L. monocytogenes* to grow very rapidly both inside and on the surface of Brie, Camembert, brick, Limburger, and other similar cheeses during ripening, manufacturers of such products should test a portion of each lot for listeriae before releasing the product for sale.

In addition to these concerns, several studies have demonstrated that *L. monocytogenes* can survive well beyond 60 days in brick, Cheddar, and other varieties of cheese that were prepared from pasteurized milk inoculated with the pathogen. Certain cheeses, primarily hard and semi-hard varieties, can be manufactured from raw milk in the United States and elsewhere if the finished product is aged a minimum of 60 days at or above 1.7°C (35°C) to eliminate pathogenic microorganisms. However, since experimental evidence has indicating that this process in inadequate to free contaminated cheese from viable cells of *L. monocytogenes*, cheesemakers should prepare cheese from pasteurized milk whenever possible.

Meat Industry

Since *Listeria* spp., including *L. monocytogenes*, are virtually endemic to slaughterhouse environments, meat processors are faced with an almost impossible challenge of producing *Listeria*-free raw meats. Direct application of lactic and/or acetic acid to animal carcasses is one of the few economically feasible means by which meat processors can effectively reduce populations of listeriae and other surface contaminants, including common spoilage organisms (16,28,62). Nevertheless, while adoption of this procedure and the aforementioned general guidelines for controlling listeriae in food-processing establishments will benefit slaughterhouse operators, it appears unlikely that rigid enforcement of even the most stringent slaughter, dressing, cleaning, and sanitizing procedures will completely eliminate *L. monocytogenes* from wholesale and retail cuts of raw beef, pork, and lamb. Therefore, consumers of such products need to understand the potential health hazards associated with consumption of less than thoroughly cooked meats and also must follow appropriate hygienic practices in the kitchen to prevent the spread of listeriae from raw meats to ready-to-eat foods.

Firms producing processed meat products must assume that all incoming raw meat is potentially contaminated with listeriae, including *L. monocytogenes*. Since most *Listeria* contamination of finished product appears to result from postprocessing contamination rather than from the organism surviving various processing treatments, it is essential to segregate raw and finished products as well as employees working in raw and finished product areas of the factory. Although there is no "magic bullet" for *Listeria*, the incidence of listeriae in all areas of the factory can be greatly reduced through conscientious enforcement of a stringent cleaning and sanitation program. One six-step program that has been recommended for cleaning food contact surfaces (7) includes an initial dry clean-up step to remove as much product residue as possible, followed by (a) a warm water rinse (with minimum splashing) to mobilize fat and remove product, (b) cleaning with an appropriate foaming detergent, (c) warm or hot water rinse with minimum splashing, (d) disinfecting with an appropriate sanitizing agent (i.e., chlorine or quaternary ammonium compound), and finally (e) thorough drying of the cleaned and sanitized area. According to Boyle et al. (34,35), *L. monocytogenes* populations in inoculated samples of carcass rinse fluid, Hobart meat grinder rinse fluid, and floor drain waste water obtained from a beef and lamb processing facility increased one to four orders of magnitude during 24 hours of incubation at 8 and 35°C with the pathogen exhibiting shorter generation times in waste fluids containing 3.1 rather than ≤1.4% protein. Hence, while the procedure just described may seem adequate, routine random testing for *Listeria* and coliforms as well as an estimation of the general microbial load on cleaned and sanitized food contact surfaces should be done as an integral part of any sanitation program.

In 1987, the American Meat Institute published some interim guidelines for controlling the incidence of listeriae and other pathogenic/nonpathogenic microbial contaminants during production of ready-to-eat meat products (2). While the recommendations in this report regarding facility requirements, factory environment, food contact/non-food contact surfaces, cross-contamination, airborne contamination, condensation control, cleaning/sanitizing, traffic patterns, and personnel cleanliness are generally similar to those already presented in this chapter as General Guidelines, this report also outlined some of the critical operations associated with production of specific categories of ready-to-eat meat products

Roast Beef, Corned Beef, and Other Rebagged Products

Products such as roast beef and corned beef that are repackaged after cooking are particularly prone to contamination with listeriae and other microorganisms. Therefore, attention must be given to proper sanitation and prevention of cross-contamination when these products are removed from bags in which they were cooked. The outside surface of all bags should be thoroughly washed and sanitized before the bags are opened. In addition to a sanitary working environment, repackaging of cooked product requires use of clean clothing as well as frequently sanitized utensils and gloves. Trimming and cutting of cooked product just before rebagging are two more critical steps where listeriae and other contaminants can enter and compromise the integrity of the final product. Therefore, contact between cooked product and unsanitized surfaces must be avoided during rebagging operations. Since repackaging is by nature a wet process, this operation also needs to be well isolated from other processing areas to reduce cross-contamination.

Frankfurters and Other Link Products

Sausages such as frankfurters and other link varieties are typically prepared from a finely ground mixture (or emulsion) of beef and/or pork, which is stuffed into artificial or natural casings. After twisting the casing at approximately 6-inch intervals, the links are cooked using steam or hot water and then hung for smoking. To obtain skinless frankfurters, the artificial casing must be mechanically peeled from the congealed meat mixture. While prompt attention to cleaning, sanitizing, and cross-contamination problems is required during all stages of frankfurter production, the product is particularly vulnerable to contamination with listeriae and other microorganisms during the peeling process. It is imperative to keep the area around peeling machines as dry and as free from meat scraps and juices as possible. Peeling machine operators also need to change protective garments and gloves frequently. Hoods on peeler machines have been cited as a source of listeriae and should therefore be eliminated if at all possible.

Manufacturing practices also should be reviewed to ensure that losses from floor contamination and reworked product are minimized. While unpeeled frankfurters that touch the floor or other unclean surfaces can be reworked (i.e., washed and peeled after all other frankfurters have been peeled), any peeled frankfurters that come in contact with the floor or other unclean surfaces should be destroyed. This latter recommendation is supported by data indicating that *L. monocytogenes* is difficult to destroy on the surface of frankfurters during cooking without making the product organoleptically unacceptable (13). In addition to these concerns, brine chillers also have been cited as a potential source of listeriae, thus leading to contamination of casings and product surfaces. Finally, all packaging/heat shrinking equipment should be cleaned and sanitized daily to avoid spreading contaminants from steam and water to packaging lines.

Luncheon Meats

Concerns regarding control of listeriae and other contaminants in luncheon meats are generally similar to those just discussed for frankfurters and other link products. However, in addition slicing equipment should be kept dry and free of scraps and juices that may serve as potential nutrients for microbial contaminants, including listeriae.

Poultry Industry

Potential sources of listeriae contamination during processing of raw poultry are in many ways similar to those just discussed for the meat industry. Since a substantial percentage of birds harbor *Listeria* spp. (including *L. monocytogenes*) and *Salmonella* in their intestinal tract, enforcement of proper clean-up (i.e., elimination of water, condensate, and waste) and cleaning/sanitizing programs will likely decrease the incidence of contamination but never completely eliminate these pathogens from raw poultry-processing facilities or the raw product.

Most modern poultry-processing facilities are continuous line operations in which incoming birds are shackled, electrically stunned, bled, scalded to facilitate feather removal, plucked of feathers, eviscerated, inspected, washed, chilled, dried, and packaged for sale. Processing steps during which *L. monocytogenes*, *Salmonella* spp., and other pathogens are most likely to contaminate the product include scalding, defeathering, evisceration, and chilling (63,64). In 1988, USDA officials proposed processing changes that may be helpful in decreasing the incidence of *Salmonella* (and presumably *Listeria*) in raw poultry (19). These changes included (a) segregating and processing pathogen-infected flocks at different times from noninfected flocks, (b) examining potential benefits of adding bactericidal concentrations of organic acids to chill water tanks, (c) experimentation with different scalding methods, e.g., hot water sprays, steam scalders, or scald additives, (d) routine sanitizing of all equipment and utensils with hot water or bactericidal agents, (e) reemphasis of employee hygiene programs with routine handwashing/sanitizing required by all evisceration line workers, (f) elimination of off-line processing, and (g) installation of equipment designed to automatically transfer carcasses from the picking line to the evisceration line. Additional work is needed to further streamline processing of poultry carcasses and minimize cross-contamination during their processing.

With increasing consumption of poultry both in and outside the home, food handlers must take special precautions to prevent the spread of *L. monocytogenes*, *Salmonella* spp., and other foodborne pathogens from raw poultry to other products (e.g., fruits, vegetables) that are frequently consumed without heating. The common practice of washing/rinsing raw poultry before cooking has been questioned since this step fails to markedly reduce microbial populations on poultry skin and also leads to increased contamination of kitchen sinks, faucets, and other food preparation areas (79). Since all foodborne pathogens commonly associated with raw poultry (including *L. monocytogenes*) are readily susceptible to heat, thorough cooking appears to be the best means of assuring that such products are free of hazardous microorganisms.

As you will recall from Chapter 8, an Oklahoma breast cancer patient contracted listeriosis in December of 1988 after consuming *Listeria*-contaminated turkey frankfurters. Thus producers of processed poultry products (e.g., turkey/chicken frankfurters, rolls) need to take precautions similar to those previously described for manufacture of roast beef, corned beef, frankfurters, link sausage, and luncheon meats with special attention given to cleanliness of rebagging operations and sausage peelers.

Egg Industry

As stated earlier, contents of intact whole eggs are normally sterile, unless the laying hen infects the yolk with *Salmonella enteritidis*. Foodborne pathogens including *L. monocytogenes* and *S. enteritidis* have frequently been isolated from commercially broken, raw liquid whole egg, with contamination most likely resulting from presence of the organisms in the manufacturing environment or on egg shells. While pasteurization as required for commercially broken, raw liquid whole egg is likely sufficient to eliminate normally encountered populations of *L. monocytogenes* and salmonellae in raw liquid egg, all egg-breaking operations need to be well isolated from pasteurization and filling/packaging areas to minimize recontamination of finished product. Since *L. monocytogenes* and other foodborne pathogens probably enter egg-processing facilities as egg shell contaminants, egg receiving and washing sections of the factory also should be segregated from other processing areas. Considering the potential for postpasteurization contamination, many of the previously described guidelines for cleaning and sanitizing dairy factories also appear applicable to manufacturers of pasteurized liquid egg products.

Fish and Seafood Industry

In 1988 approximately 250,000 Americans used over 100,000 boats to harvest approximately 4 billion pounds of edible fish and seafood (43). However, as of June 1990, the United States government has not yet instituted a mandatory inspection program for fish and seafood. With recent isolations of *L. monocytogenes* and/or various other foodborne pathogens such as *Vibrio*, *Salmonella*, *Shigella*, *Staphylococcus aureus*, *Clostridium botulinum*, *Aeromonas hydrophila*, and certain strains of *Escherichia coli* from raw and/or cooked finfish, shrimp, crab, lobster, oysters, and scallops, the seafood industry faces a major challenge. An integrated approach to product safety is needed to minimize contamination of seafood from harvest to the time of consumption.

Limiting postharvest contamination of freshly caught fish and seafood is the first step toward producing a safe, high quality end product. Adherence to good sanitation and hygienic practices aboard fishing vessels is imperative. Contact between freshly caught seafood and water fowl such as pelicans and seagulls should be minimized because these birds are intestinal carriers of *L. monocytogenes* and other foodborne pathogens. All seafood should be either frozen or refrigerated immediately after harvest to stop or retard growth of microbial contaminants, including spoilage organisms.

Two observations, namely, (a) routine recovery of healthy rather than thermally or otherwise injured listeriae from processed seafood and (b) discovery of *L. monocytogenes* in the manufacturing environment of all American factories that have been involved in *Listeria*-related recalls, indicate that this pathogen enters the product primarily after processing through improper handling. Inadequate separation between raw and finished product resulting from faulty factory design and indifferent attitudes of employees toward proper sanitation have been most frequently cited as factors that promote postprocessing contamination.

The general guidelines that were discussed previously regarding factory design, processing environment, proper cleaning/sanitizing, traffic patterns, and personnel cleanliness also are valid for the seafood industry. In addition to these recommendations, seafood processors also are urged to (a) eliminate processing waste, pooled water, and condensate from walls, floors, and ceilings as well as from processing and refrigerated areas, (b) eliminate use of high pressure sprays, (c) reduce airborne contamination, (d) cover outside dumpsters to decrease problems involving seagulls and other wildlife, (e) assign specific equipment (i.e., product totes) for use in either raw or cooked product areas of the factory, and (f) if possible, replace wooden totes with fiber totes, which can be readily cleaned and sanitized.

Listeria spp., including *L. monocytogenes*, have been isolated most frequently from crabmeat and cooked/peeled shrimp (see Table 13.4). This observation is not surprising if one considers how these products are processed and packaged for the consumer. Processing of Dungeness crab generally begins by immersing and cooking either sections of or the entire crab in boiling water for approximately 7–9 or 17–20 minutes, respectively. While current information indicates that such a heat treatment is sufficient to destroy listeriae (43), underprocessing may lead to survivors. After cooking, the crab is cooled in a water bath and either "picked" immediately or iced and refrigerated in a walk-in cooler until the meat can be hand-picked from the shell. Extensive handling of the product by workers during picking, subsequent inspection, and packaging affords many opportunities for postprocessing contamination. Although lactic acid dips appear to be somewhat useful in reducing populations of *L. monocytogenes* and other microorganisms on the surface of crabmeat as well as fresh and frozen shrimp, such treatments will not completely eliminate listeriae from the finished product (43). Therefore, strict adherence to Good Manufacturing Practices, which include proper employee hygiene and cleaning/sanitizing of picking equipment, must be observed in and among picking areas to avoid negating the benefits of cooking.

Unfortunately, crab processing varies widely with the species of crab—Dungeness, blue, stone, King, and golden crab. Hence, some of the critical control points discussed for Dungeness crab are not applicable to other species. For example, blue crabmeat is typically removed from the animal in the raw state, placed in sealed containers, and then pasteurized (85°C/1 min) to eliminate *L. monocytogenes* and other microbial pathogens. Since pasteurization of blue crabmeat thus becomes a critical point in processing, it may be prudent to certify and/or license crabmeat pasteurization operators or their supervisors, as has been required for operators of retorts in the canning industry for many years.

Problems regarding postprocessing contamination also are encountered during production of cooked/peeled shrimp. After shrimp are cooked, those destined for breading are mechanically peeled and sometimes deveined by splitting and removing the vein-like intestine. Unfortunately, many mechanical shrimp peelers have design flaws which necessitate almost continuous movement of the operator between both raw and cooked sides of the equipment, thus affording ample opportunity for postprocessing contamination. Proper cleaning and sanitizing of the equipment (particularly protective covers over flumes and gutters) and the surrounding area are essential for producing high quality microbiologically safe products.

Even when handled under the best possible conditions, raw seafood such as crab, shrimp, lobster, clams, oysters, and the myriad of finfish currently available to consumers probably will never be completely free of *L. monocytogenes* or other foodborne pathogens. Considering that many individuals are not "seafood-smart," processors and marketers of seafood have an obligation to educate the general public and provide consumers with proper handling and cooking instructions. Individuals who insist on consuming unprocessed fish (e.g., sushi) and seafood (e.g., oysters) also should be made aware of potential health problems associated with consumption of such products.

Fruit and Vegetable Industry

Despite a lack of information concerning incidence of *L. monocytogenes* in raw fruits, the pathogen has been recovered from raw vegetables including cabbage, cucumbers, mushrooms, potatoes, and radishes. Other than the 1981 Canadian listeriosis outbreak involving coleslaw and one isolated case in Finland linked to consumption of raw salted mushrooms, no additional confirmed cases of vegetableborne listeriosis have been documented in the literature. Thus the scientific community and the public at large have been somewhat less concerned about *Listeria* contamination in vegetables than in dairy, meat, poultry, and seafood products.

Routine examination of raw vegetables for *L. monocytogenes* and other foodborne pathogens is unlikely to reduce the risk of foodborne illness to any great extent. However, since raw sheep manure was the probable source of *L. monocytogenes* in the Canadian coleslaw outbreak, vegetable processors should have some assurance that incoming raw vegetables have been grown, irrigated, fertilized, harvested, packaged, and transported to the firm using hygienically sound agricultural practices. Vegetable processors should consider rejecting raw vegetables that probably will be consumed without cooking if the grower fails to clearly demonstrate use of good agricultural practices.

Consumption of vegetables that will be adequately cooked before eating is of little concern since *L. monocytogenes* and other non–spore-forming pathogens are destroyed during cooking. While routine washing of raw vegetables in potable water is recommended for commercial establishments and homes, this practice generally fails to reduce the microbial load on raw vegetables by more than 10-fold. Therefore, persons handling and preparing raw produce and salad vegetables should follow good hygienic practices during slicing, dicing, chopping, and grating operations to prevent the spread of potentially hazardous microorganisms to other foods. Finally, all knives, cutting boards, and other food-contact surfaces should be thoroughly cleaned and sanitized after use to inactivate organisms inadvertently introduced into the kitchen environment during preparation of raw produce.

PRACTICAL APPROACHES TO FOOD SAFETY

Traditional Approach

The traditional approach to controlling microbiological hazards associated with food products involves simultaneous use of employee education and training programs, frequent inspection of facilities and operations, and extensive microbiological testing. Employee education and training programs should be directed toward a thorough understanding of food hygiene, factory cleaning/sanitation requirements, and various causes of microbial contamination, including growth and survival patterns of potential contaminants such as listeriae. Trained employees also should be able to select and apply methods that will provide consumers with safe, high quality products.

The second means of controlling microbiological hazards, frequent inspection of facilities and operations, is necessary to ensure that Good Manufacturing Practices (GMPs) (i.e., procedures that consistently yield safe products of acceptable quality) are being followed. Good manufacturing practices to produce specific foods have been outlined in both advisory and regulatory documents such as GMP guidelines and the various codes of hygienic practice developed by the Codex Alimentarius Committee on Food Hygiene. The final means of controlling microbial hazards in finished products is through rigorous microbiological testing of ingredients as well as unfinished and finished product. Analysis of samples for pathogens or, more commonly, indicator (coliforms, fecal streptococci) or spoilage organisms is crucial to ascertaining that good manufacturing, handling, and distribution practices are being followed.

Hazard Analysis Critical Control Point (HACCP) Approach

Although the traditional approach for controlling microbial contaminants has and is still being used by much of the food industry, numerous cases of foodborne illnesses still occur annually in developed countries. This shortcoming of the traditional approach along with a need to reduce costs associated with ensuring the safety and quality of foods have led to development of the Hazard Analysis Critical Control Point (HACCP) approach to minimize microbiological hazards in food.

The HACCP system, first presented to the scientific community at the 1971 National Conference on Food Protection (3), was originally established to control microbial hazards (e.g., *Clostridium botulinum*) associated with canning of mushrooms and other low acid foods. However, this approach to food safety is now being adopted by other segments of the food industry. The HACCP approach for controlling microbiological hazards in food is based on three important considerations: (a) assessment of hazards (i.e., unacceptable levels of foodborne pathogens and/or spoilage organisms) associated with growing, harvesting, processing/manufacturing, distribution, marketing, preparation, and/or use of a given raw material, ingredient, or food product, (b) determination of critical control points (i.e., hazardous locations or processes) required to control any identified hazard, and (c) establishment of methods to verify that all processing and/or handling procedures at critical control points are being done properly. Such an approach to food safety provides far better control of microbiological hazards than can be obtained using the previously described traditional approach. Since a detailed discussion of the HACCP system is beyond the scope of this book, interested readers are referred to a 1986 publication by the International Commission on Microbiological Specification for Food (ICMSF) (52) for more specific information regarding implications of HACCP principles in various segments of the food industry. However, since this approach is now being recommended for controlling *L. monocytogenes* and other contaminants in dairy (70), meat (1), poultry, and seafood products (24,29,45), a review of basic information regarding the HACCP approach to food safety is appropriate.

Identification of microbiological hazards associated with food production and distribution practices is the first step toward developing an effective HACCP program. According to the ICMSF (52), any properly conducted hazard analysis should (a) identify potentially hazardous raw materials and foods that may contain poisonous substances, pathogens, or large numbers of spoilage organisms and that can support microbial growth (e.g., *L. monocytogenes* in soft, surface-ripened cheese), (b) find sources and specific points of contamination by observing each step in the food chain, and (c) determine the potential for microorganisms to survive and multiply during production, processing, distribution, storage, and preparation of food for consumption.

It is important that food processors conduct a hazard analysis on all existing and any new products to be manufactured since ultimate microbiological safety of nonthermally processed foods is directly related to the quality of raw materials. Any hazard analysis must begin with identification of hazards associated with raw materials, with particular attention given to raw products of animal origin (i.e., milk, meat, poultry, and seafood), all of which may harbor *L. monocytogenes* and other foodborne pathogens. While heat treatments, acidulation, fermentation, salting, and drying are designed to destroy or inhibit growth of pathogenic and spoilage microorganisms, other operations such as slicing/dicing, cooling of cooked products, and filling/packaging may allow both pathogenic and spoilage organisms to contaminate the final product. Therefore, all hazards associated with manufacturing procedures and postprocessing contamination, as previously discussed, must be fully understood along with the consequences of processing failures and/or errors. Food processors also should be familiar with the effect of various physicochemical factors (i.e., pH, water activity, preservatives, type of packaging with or without modified atmosphere) on behavior of spoilage and pathogenic organisms including *L. monocytogenes* in the product during processing, distribution, storage, and use by the consumer. Finally, any change in raw materials, product formulation, processing, packaging, distribution, or intended use of the product should prompt an immediate reassessment of hazards since such changes have the potential to adversely affect both product safety and shelf life.

After identifying all possible hazards associated with food production, manufacturers need to determine all critical control points—locations, practices, procedures, and/or processes where microbiological control can be exercised to minimize or prevent hazardous situations from developing. Specific critical control points important to food processors include (a) raw materials where normal commercial or consumer processing techniques cannot be depended upon to eliminate all pathogenic microorganisms, (b) processing treatments (e.g., heat, fermentation), (c) time/temperature relationships during cooling and freezing, (d) filling/packaging operations, and (e) any other point at which the product is exposed to postprocessing contamination. Repeated microbiological sampling of raw materials and all food contact surfaces encountered at various stages of manufacture are of vital importance in identifying proper critical control points. While most of the potential critical control points associated with postprocessing contamination and pasteurization of milk have been identified elsewhere in this chapter, inherent differences between all food-processing facilities make it necessary for each firm to independently determine the hazards and critical control points associated with manufacture of each item being produced.

No HACCP program is complete without a routine monitoring program to ensure manufacturers that all identified hazards and critical control points are actually under control. The type of monitoring program varies with the particular critical control point under consideration. Microbiological specifications, including statistically based sampling plans and limits, should be developed for all raw materials previously defined as hazardous. While suppliers of such materials should ideally do the required tests to ensure that all materials comply with the manufacturer's specifications upon delivery, receiving firms should occasionally verify that their own specifications are being met by the supplier. After receipt, raw material storage conditions should be monitored to maintain satisfactory product quality until time of actual use. Monitoring of process critical control points (i.e., heating, fermentation, filling/packaging) may include microbiological tests; however, physical and chemical tests are often more helpful since results from these tests are rapidly available. Nonetheless, results from microbiological tests are important in verifying the adequacy of cleaning/sanitation programs. Although product specifications along with microbiological, physical, and chemical testing all are important in any HACCP monitoring program, routine visual inspection is the most important means of monitoring critical control points in the factory environment. Hence, all employees must be trained to recognize and correct potential problems before they compromise product safety or quality. Since the HACCP system is designed to readily identify and correct potentially hazardous situations that might occur during manufacture, microbiological analysis of finished product is very limited and generally confined to high risk foods that will be consumed by individuals who are particularly vulnerable to foodborne illnesses. Assuming that all other requirements of the HACCP program have been properly enforced, information concerning pH, water activity, preservative level, and salt content is often more useful than results from microbiological tests in assessing safety and stability of the final product.

SAMPLING PLANS FOR *L. MONOCYTOGENES* IN FOODS

Prevention of microbiological hazards is clearly of considerable importance when one considers the serious health problems that may develop in certain individuals who consume *Listeria*-contaminated foods. Consequently, the International Commission on Microbiological Specifications for Foods (ICMSF) proposed that *L. monocytogenes* be placed in the same category with *Brucella, Clostridium botulinum, Clostridum perfringens* type C, *Salmonella typhi, Shigella dysenteriae, Vibrio cholera,* and hepatitis A virus (12), all of which pose severe health hazards.

In February 1988, the ICMSF considered application of its sampling plans to assess acceptability of foods with respect to *L. monocytogenes*. (The reader must be cautioned from the start that no microbiological sampling plan other than one which involves total destructive sampling of all products manufactured can ever provide complete consumer protection.) According to terminology developed previously by the ICMSF, sampling plans for *L. monocytogenes* would follow the recommendations made for cases 13, 14, and 15 (52). Case 13 applies when conditions under which the product is normally handled and consumed after sampling reduce the degree of hazard associated with the product, whereas cases 14 and 15 refer to situations in which hazard levels remain constant or increase, respectively. Using a statistically based two-class attribute sampling plan, n (i.e., number of sample units to be examined from a particular lot) would equal 15, 30, or 60 for cases 13, 14, and 15, respectively, and c (i.e., the maximum allowable number of sample units containing *L. monocytogenes*) would equal 0 for all three cases.

A three-class attribute sampling plan also was proposed in the United States by a working group of the National Advisory Committee on Microbiological Criteria for Foods (22). According to this plan, which was developed for ready-to-eat shrimp and crabmeat, n (i.e., number of samples for foods produced in facilities employing HACCP and GMP systems) would equal 10, whereas c (i.e., mandatory standard for *L. monocytogenes* that should not be exceeded) would equal 0. Thus, with the exception of n, this plan is similar to the two-class attribute plan proposed by the ICMSF.

Before recommending any *Listeria*-sampling plan, there must be good epidemiological evidence indicating that the product or product group to be sampled has been implicated in foodborne listeriosis. In addition, there must be good reason to believe that introduction of a sampling program will substantially reduce the risk of contracting listeriosis from consumption of such products.

Based on information available as of February 1988, the ICMSF made a series of recommendations concerning sampling plans for listeriae in milk, soft cheeses, and vegetables (12). Although *L. monocytogenes* is commonly found in raw milk, minimum required pasteurization (71.7°C/15 sec) should eliminate this hazard. Therefore, the ICMSF recommended that manufacturers institute monitoring programs to prevent postpasteurization contamination rather than routine sampling plans of pasteurized end products as the most appropriate means of protecting the consumer.

Many varieties of *Listeria*-contaminated cheese also have been identified since 1985, with contamination most frequently reported in surface-ripened cheeses. Since *L. monocytogenes* can grow rapidly in Brie and Camembert cheese during the late stages of ripening, a two-class attribute sampling program should be considered if such cheeses are destined for consumption by pregnant women, immunocompromised adults, or the elderly. However, since no sampling program can ensure that such products are completely free of *L. monocytogenes*, public health interests are far better served by application of HACCP principles during cheese manufacture and ripening. While the ICMSF recognized that raw vegetables also may become contaminated with *L. monocytogenes*, routine testing of raw vegetables is unlikely to markedly reduce the risk of contracting listeriosis. Hence, consumers of raw vegetables are urged to vigorously wash all such products before consumption.

Following this 1988 report by the ICMSF, several additional cases of listeriosis have been linked to consumption of processed meat and poultry, with undercooked fish also directly responsible for one adult case of human listeriosis in Italy (42). Given the incidence of *L. monocytogenes* in raw and ready-to-eat seafoods, consumption of such products also appears to constitute a potential risk to some consumers. Therefore, the federal government requested that the FDA, National Marine Fisheries Service, and USDA-FSIS (20,27) develop and submit to the United States Congress a comprehensive seafood inspection program based on the HACCP approach (23,26). The previously described three-class attribute sampling plan (14,22,31,69) has been recommended for cooked/ready-to-eat shrimp and crabmeat. In April 1988 the National Advisory Committee also requested that USDA officials develop microbiological criteria for frankfurters (11). These efforts were later expanded to include cooked and/or assembled meat products as well as raw meat and poultry (78). The American Meat Institute, in December of 1987, published interim guidelines for controlling listeriae in ready-to-eat meat products (2). Although USDA officials favor the HACCP approach for controlling listeriae in the meat and poultry industry (23), specific details concerning monitoring of critical control points, sampling plans, and methodology are still open to debate.

In conclusion, end-product–sampling programs are not the complete answer to protecting consumers from listeriosis or other types of foodborne illness. However, microbiological sampling is recommended by many regulatory agencies and the World Health Organization as part of the HACCP approach to prevent opportunities for contamination by, survival, and growth of *L. monocytogenes* as well as other microbial pathogens and spoilage organisms in raw materials, factory environments, and food products during manufacture, storage, distribution, sale, and use. Above all, manufacturers need to promote good manufacturing and good food hygiene practices in the workplace and instill in each employee a sense of public responsibility for producing safe, wholesome foods. Such attitudes will go a long way toward reducing the incidence of *L. monocytogenes* in the food supply, which in turn will decrease the incidence of foodborne listeriosis.

REFERENCES

1. Adams, C. E. 1990. Use of HACCP in meat and poultry inspection. *Food Technol. 44*(5):169–170.
2. American Meat Institute. 1987. Interim guideline: Microbial control during production of ready-to-eat meat products. Controlling the incidence of *Listeria monocytogenes*. American Meat Institute, Washington, DC.
3. Anonymous. 1971. Workshop 2, Prevention of contamination of commercially processed foods. In *Proc. of the 1971 National Conference on Food Protection*, U.S. Govt. Print. Office, Washington, DC, p. 56.
4. Anonymous. 1986. Food and Drug Administration dairy product safety initiatives—Preliminary status report. FDA Center for Food Safety and Applied Nutrition—Milk Safety Branch. Washington, DC, September 22.
5. Anonymous. 1987. FDA continues to find *Listeria* during dairy plant inspections. *Food Chem. News 29*(1):47–48.
6. Anonymous. 1987. FDA convinced dairy industry can avoid *Listeria* contamination. *Food Chem. News 29*(39):3–4.
7. Anonymous. 1987. FSIS to give firms 5 days for clean-up before resampling for *Listeria*. *Food Chem. News 29*(32):7–9.
8. Anonymous. 1987. Ice cream industry seeks parity with meat industry on *Listeria* policy. *Food Chem. News 29*(23):15.
9. Anonymous. 1987. Meat industry research shows *Listeria* widespread, control difficult. *Food Chem. News 29*(17):27–29.
10. Anonymous. 1988. FDA regional workshops to discuss microbial concerns in seafoods. *Food Chem. News 30*(43):27–31.
11. Anonymous. 1988. Hot dogs, shrimp, crab targeted for microbiological criteria. *Food Chem. News 30*(6):43–45.
12. Anonymous. 1988. International Dairy Federation: Group E64—Detection of *Listeria monocytogenes*—sampling plans for *Listeria monocytogenes* in foods, Feb. 9. IDF, Brussels.
13. Anonymous. 1988. *Listeria* destruction in cooked meat products ineffective: Hormel. *Food Chem. News 30*(15):32–34.
14. Anonymous. 1988. Micro criteria for crabmeat, shrimp would have 3-class attributes. *Food Chem. News 30*(24):25–27.
15. Anonymous. 1988. Meat industry workshop warned about *Listeria* threat. *Food Chem. News 29*(47):54–56.
16. Anonymous. 1988. Meat scientists exchange views in Wyoming. *National Provisioner 199*(11):6–10.
17. Anonymous. 1988. Recommandations pour la lutte contre la contamination dans les laiteries. *Rev. Lait. Franc. 473*:57–62.
18. Anonymous. 1988. Recommended guidelines for controlling environmental contamination in dairy plants. *Dairy Food Sanit. 8*:52–56.
19. Anonymous. 1988. USDA to check chicken process changes to lower contamination levels. *Food Chem. News 29*(49):34–35.
20. Anonymous. 1989. Appropriations committee tells USDA to draft fish inspection plan. *Food Chem. News 31*(22):45–46.
21. Anonymous. 1989. Controlling *Listeria*—the Danish solution. *Dairy Ind. Intern. 54*(5):31–32, 35.

22. Anonymous. 1989. HACCP programs are in new draft for micro criteria meeting. *Food Chem. News 30*(47):53–55.
23. Anonymous. 1989. HACCP "working definition" assignment taken on by micro subgroup. *Food Chem. News 30(49):55–57.*
24. Anonymous. 1989. Micro committee approves HACCP scheme: First major document. *Food Chem. News 31*(40):45–47.
25. Anonymous. 1989. Monitoring of changes leading to listeriosis problem urged. *Food Chem. News 31*(20):13–17.
26. Anonymous. 1989. NFI board votes to seek HACCP-type seafood inspection legislation. *Food Chem. News 31*(9):34–35.
27. Anonymous. 1989. Three agencies woo Congress on fish inspection. *Food Chem. News 31*(29):53–54.
28. Anonymous. 1990. Changes in *Listeria* regulatory strategy recommended by AMI. *Food Chem. News 32*(2):58–59.
29. Anonymous. 1990. Fish inspection bill by end of year predicted by NFI's Weddig. *Food Chem. News 31*(48):50–51.
30. Anonymous. 1990. USDA monitoring finds *Listeria* in ready-to-eat products at 78 plants. *Food Chem. News 32*(7):71–73.
31. Ball, H. R., M. Hamid-Samimi, P. M. Foegeding, and K. R. Swartzel. 1987. Functionability and microbial stability of ultrapasteurized, aseptically packaged refrigerated whole egg. *J. Food Sci. 52*:1212–1218.
32. Barnier, E., J. P. Vincent, and M. Catteau. 1988. *Listeria* et environnement industriel. *Sci. Aliment. 8*:239–242.
33. Best, M., M. E. Kennedy, and F. Coates. 1990. Efficacy of a variety of disinfectants against *Listeria* spp. *Appl. Environ. Microbiol. 56*:377–380.
34. Boyle, D. L., J. N. Sofos, and G. R. Schmidt. 1990. Growth of *Listeria monocytogenes* inoculated in waste fluids collected from a slaughterhouse. *J. Food Prot. 53*:102–104, 118.
35. Boyle, D. L., G. R. Schmidt, and J. N. Sofos. 1990. Growth of *Listeria monocytogenes* inoculated in waste-fluids from clean-up of a meat grinder. *J. Food Sci. 55*:277–278.
36. Bradley, R. L., Jr. 1986. The hysteria of *Listeria. Dairy Field 169*(11):37, 57.
37. Breer, C. 1988. Occurrence of *Listeria* spp. in different foods. WHO Working Group on Foodborne Listeriosis, Geneva, Switzerland, Feb. 15–19.
38. Charlton, B. R., H. Kinde, and L. H. Jensen. 1990. Environmental survey for *Listeria* species in California milk processing plants. *J. Food Prot. 43*:198–201.
39. Cox, L. J. 1988. *Listeria monocytogenes*—a European viewpoint. General Assembly of IOCCC, Hershey, PA, April 28–30.
40. Cox, L. J. 1988. Prevention of foodborne listeriosis—the role of the food processing industry. WHO Informal Working Group on Foodborne Listeriosis, Geneva, Switzerland, February 15–19.
41. Cox, L. J., T. Kieiss, J. L. Cordier, C. Cordellana, P. Konkel, C. Pedrazzini, R. Beumer, and A. Siebenga. 1989. *Listeria* spp. in food processing, non-food and domestic environments. *Food Microbiol. 6*:49–61.
42. Facinelli, B., P. E. Varaldo, M. Toni, C. Casolari, and V. Fabio. 1989. Ignorance about *Listeria. Brit. Med. J. 299*:738.
43. Food and Drug Administration. 1988. *Proceedings of the National Meeting on Cooked/Processed Seafood*, Food and Drug Administration, Center for Food Safety and Applied Nutrition, Washington, DC, December 16.
44. Gabis, D. A., R. S. Flowers, D. Evanson, and R. E. Faust. 1989. A survey of 18 dry dairy product processing plant environments for *Salmonella, Listeria* and *Yersinia. J. Food Prot. 52*:122–124.
45. Garrett, S. E., and M. Hudak-Roos. 1990. Use of HACCP for seafood surveillance and certification. *Food Technol. 44*(5):159–165.
46. Genigeorgis, C. A., D. Dutulescu, and J. F. Garayzabal. 1989. Prevalence of *Listeria* spp. in poultry meat at the supermarket and slaughterhouse level. *J. Food Prot. 52*:618–624, 630.

47. Genigeorgis, C. A., P. Oanca, and D. Dutulescu. 1990. Prevalence of *Listeria* spp. in turkey meat at the supermarket and slaughterhouse level. *J. Food Prot.* 53:282–288.
48. Gilbert, R. J. 1990. Personal communication.
49. Goff, H. D. 1988. Hazard analysis and critical control point identification in ice cream plants. *Dairy Food Sanit.* 8:131–135.
50. *HTST Pasteurizer Operation Manual.* 1987. Oregon Association of Milk, Food and Environmental Sanitarians, Oregon State University, Corvallis, OR.
51. Hudson, W. R., and G. C. Mead. 1989. *Listeria* contamination at a poultry processing plant. *Lett. Appl. Microbiol.* 9:211–214.
52. International Commission on Microbiological Specifications for Foods. 1986. *Microorganisms in Foods. 2-Sampling for Microbiological Analysis: Principles and Specific Applications*, 2nd ed., University of Toronto Press, Toronto.
53. Jacobs, M. 1988. Personal communication.
54. Kang, Y.-J., and J. F. Frank. 1989. Biological aerosols: A review of airborne contamination and its measurement in dairy processing facilities. *J. Food Prot.* 52:512–524.
55. Kang, Y.-J., and J. F. Frank. 1990. Characteristics of biological aerosols in dairy processing plants. *J. Dairy Sci.* 73:621–626.
56. Klausner, R., and C. W. Donnelly. 1989. Personal communication.
57. Kozak, J. J. 1986. FDA's dairy program initiatives. *Dairy Food Sanit.* 6:184–185.
58. Lacey, R. W., and K. G. Kerr. 1989. Listeriosis—the need for legislation. *Lett. Appl. Microbiol.* 8:121–122.
59. Lecos, C. 1986. Of microbes and milk: Probing America's worst *Salmonella* outbreak. *FDA Consumer* 20(1):18–21.
60. Llabrés, C. M., and B. E. Rose. 1989. Antibacterial properties of retail sponges. *J. Food Prot.* 52:49–50, 54.
61. Lopes, J. A. 1986. Evaluation of dairy and food plant sanitizers against *Salmonella typhimurium* and *Listeria monocytogenes*. *J. Dairy Sci.* 69:2791–2796.
62. Netten, P. van, and D. A. A. Mossel. 1981. The ecological consequences of decontaminating raw meat surfaces with lactic acid. *Arch. Lebensmittelhyg.* 31:190–191.
63. Notermans, S., R. J. Terbijhe, and M. van Schothorst. 1980. Removing faecal contamination of broilers by spray-cleaning during evisceration. *Brit. Poultry Sci.* 21:115–121.
64. Notermans, S., J. Dufrenne, and W. J. van Leeuwen. 1982. Contamination of broiler chickens by *Staphylococcus aureus* during processing; incidence and origin. *J. Appl. Bacteriol.* 52:275–280.
65. Orth, R., and H. Mrozek. 1989. Is the control of *Listeria*, *Campylobacter*, and *Yersinia* a disinfection problem? *Fleischwirtschaft* 69:1575–1576.
66. Petran, R., and E. A. Zottola. 1988. Survival of *Listeria monocytogenes* in simulated milk cooling systems. *J. Food Prot.* 51:172–175.
67. Prentice, G. A. 1989. Living with *Listeria*. *J. Soc. Dairy Technol.* 42:55–58.
68. Radmore, K., W. H. Holzapfel, and H. Lück. 1988. Proposed guidelines for maximum acceptable air-borne microorganism levels in dairy processing and packaging plants. *Intern. J. Food Microbiol.* 6:91–95.
69. Rank, R. J. 1989. Liquid eggs deviating from the standard of identity; temporary permit for market testing. *Fed. Reg.* 54:1794–1795.
70. Shapton, N. 1988. Hazard analysis applied to control of pathogens in the dairy industry. *J. Soc. Dairy Technol.* 41:62–63.
71. Spurlock, A. T., E. A. Zottola, and R. K. L. Petran. 1989. The survival of *Listeria monocytogenes* in aerosols. *J. Food Prot.* 52:751 (Abstr.).
72. Stanfield, J. T., C. R. Wilson, W. H. Andrews, and G. J. Jackson. 1987. Potential role of refrigerated milk packaging in the transmission of listeriosis and salmonellosis. *J. Food Prot.* 50:730–732.
73. Surak, J. G., and S. F. Barefoot. 1987. Control of *Listeria* in the dairy plant. *Vet. Hum. Toxicol.* 29:247–249.

74. Terplan, G. 1988. *Listeria* in the dairy industry—situation and problems in the Federal Republic of Germany. *Foodborne Listeriosis—Proceedings of a Symposium*, Wiesbaden, West Germany, Sept. 7, pp. 52–70.
75. United States Food and Drug Administration and Milk Industry Foundation—International Ice Cream Association. 1988. Recommended guidelines for controlling environmental contamination in dairy plants. *Dairy Food Sanit. 8*:52–56.
76. Venables, L. J. 1989. *Listeria monocytogenes* in dairy products—the Victorian experience. *Food Australia 41*:942–943.
77. Wagner, L. R. Van. 1989. FDA takes action to combat seafood contamination. *Food Proc. 50*(2):8–12.
78. Wimpfeimer, L., N. S. Altman, and J. H. Hotchkiss. 1990. Growth of *Listeria monocytogenes* Scott A, serotype 4 and competitive spoilage organisms in raw chicken packaged under modified atmospheres and in air. *Intern. J. Food Microbiol. 11*:205–214.
79. Woodburn, M. 1989. Myth: Wash poultry before cooking. *Dairy Food Environ. Sanit. 9*:65–66.

APPENDIX I

Media to Isolate and Cultivate *Listeria monocytogenes* and *Listeria* spp.

A. FLUID MEDIA FOR ENRICHMENT OF *LISTERIA* SPP.

Fraser broth

Proteose peptone	5 g
Tryptone	5 g
Lab-Lemco powder	5 g
Yeast extract	5 g
NaCl	20 g
KH_2PO_4	12 g
Na_2HPO_4	12 g
Esculin	1 g
Nalidixic acid	20 mg
Lithium chloride	3 g
Acriflavine	25 mg
Ferric ammonium citrate	0.5 g
Distilled H_2O	1000 ml

Holman medium

Lab-Lemco powder	10 g
Peptone	10 g
NaCl	5 g
Defibrinated sheep blood	50 ml
Distilled H_2O	1000 ml

Steam ingredients at 100°C for 1 hour. Filter and adjust filtrate to pH 7.4–7.6. Put minced meat into tubes to a height of 1.5–2.0 cm and add 7–8 ml of filtrate to each tube. Autoclave at 121°C/20 min.

HPB enrichment broth

Tryptone soy broth	27.5 g
Yeast extract	6 g
Lithium chloride	5 g
Nalidixic acid	30 mg
Acriflavine · HCl	20 mg
Distilled H_2O	1000 ml

IDF pre-enrichment broth
    Peptone   10 g
    NaCl   5 g
    $Na_2HPO_4 \cdot 12 H_2O$ 9 g
    K_2HPO_4 1.5 g
    Distilled H_2O 1000 ml

IDF enrichment broth
    Tryptone soy broth   30 g
    Yeast extract   6 g
    Acriflavine · HCl   10 mg
    Nalidixic acid   40 mg
    Cycloheximide   50 mg
    Distilled H_2O 1000 ml

L-PALCAMY broth
    Special peptone (Oxoid)   23 g
    Yeast extract   5 g
    Lab-Lemco powder   5 g
    Peptonized milk (Oxoid)   5 g
    NaCl   5 g
    D-Mannitol   5 g
    Esculin   0.8 g
    Ferric ammonium citrate   0.5 g
    Phenol red   80 mg
    Polymyxin B   100,000 IU
    Acriflavine · HCl   5 mg
    Lithium chloride   10 g
    Ceftazidime, Latamoxef, or Moxalactam   30 mg
    Egg yolk emulsion   25 ml
    Distilled H_2O 1000 ml

Levinthal broth + nalidixic acid + trypaflavine
    Peptone   10 g
    Lab-Lemco powder   10 g
    NaCl   5 g
    Defibrinated sheep blood   50 ml
    Distilled H_2O 1000 ml

Steam ingredients at 100°C for 1 hour. Filter and adjust filtrate to pH 7.4. Autoclave at 121°C/15 min. Add 2.0 ml of 1% trypaflavine and 20 ml of 0.2% nalidixic acid.

Listeria test broth
    Trypticase soy broth   30 g
    Yeast extract   6 g
    Na_2HPO_4 9.6 g
    Tween 80   10 mg
    Esculin   1 g
    Glucose   1 g
    Acriflavine   12 mg
    Moxalactam   20 mg
    Horse serum   20 ml
    Distilled H_2O 1000 ml

Rodriguez collection medium A
    Peptone   5 g
    Neopeptone   5 g
    Trehalose dihydrate   3 g
    NaCl   10 g
    Disodium phosphate-2-hydrate   12 g
    Potassium phosphate, monobasic   1 g
    Distilled H_2O 1000 ml

Rodriguez collection medium B
    Peptone   10 g
    Rhamnose   2 g
    NaCl   10 g
    Disodium phosphate-2-hydrate   12 g
    Potassium phosphate, monobasic   3 g
    Potassium phosphate, dibasic   1.5 g
    Distilled H_2O 1000 ml

Rodriguez collection medium C
    Peptone   5 g
    Neopeptone   5 g
    Esculin   1 g
    NaCl   8 g
    Dipotassium phosphate-2-hydrate   12 g
    Potassium phosphate, monobasic   2 g
    Ferric ammonium citrate   1 g
    Agar   1.5 g
    Distilled H_2O 1000 ml

Rodriguez enrichment medium 1

Peptone	5 g
Neopeptone	5 g
Lab-Lemco powder	10 g
Yeast extract	5 g
Glucose	5 g
NaCl	50 g
Disodium phosphate-2-hydrate	53.22 g
Potassium phosphate, monobasic	1.35 g
Nalidixic acid	50 mg
Polymyxin B	8×10^5 IU
Trypan blue	80 mg
Distilled H_2O	1000 ml

Rodriguez enrichment medium 2

Peptone	5 g
Neopeptone	5 g
Lab-Lemco powder	10 g
Rhamnose	2 g
NaCl	50 g
Disodium phosphate-2-hydrate	53.22 g
Potassium phosphate, monobasic	1.35 g
Nalidixic acid	50 mg
Trypan blue	80 mg
Distilled H_2O	1000 ml

Rodriguez enrichment medium 3

Protease peptone	5 g
Tryptone	5 g
Lab-Lemco powder	5 g
Yeast extract	5 g
Esculin	1 g
NaCl	20 g
Disodium phosphate-2-hydrate	24 g
Potassium phosphate, monobasic	1.35 g
Ferric ammonium citrate	1 g
Nalidixic acid	30 mg
Trypan blue	40 mg
Agar	3 g
Distilled H_2O	1000 ml

University of Montana broth
    Proteose peptone   5 g
    Phytone peptone   5 g
    Dextrose   5 g

University of Montana broth	
Proteose peptone	5 g
Phytone peptone	5 g
Dextrose	5 g
NaCl	5 g
Yeast extract	1 g
Na pyruvate	1 g
Na_2HPO_4	2.5 g
Distilled H_2O	1000 ml

University of Vermont medium	
Proteose peptone	5 g
Tryptone	5 g
Lab-Lemco powder	5 g
Yeast extract	5 g
NaCl	20 g
Disodium phosphate-7-hydrate	12 g
Potassium phosphate, monobasic	1.35 g
Esculin	1 g
Nalidixic acid	40 mg
Acriflavine · HCl	12 mg
Distilled H_2O	1000 ml

B. SOLID MEDIA TO ISOLATE OF *LISTERIA* SPP.

ALPAMY agar	
Columbia blood agar base (Oxoid)	39 g
Lithium chloride	15 g
D-Mannitol	10 g
2-Phenylethanol	2.5 g
Ferric ammonium citrate	0.5 g
Esculin	0.5 g
Acriflavine	10 mg
Phenyl red	80 mg
Egg yolk emulsion (Oxoid)	25 ml
Distilled H_2O	1000 ml

ARS—modified MMLA	
Phenylethanol agar (Difco)	35.5 g
Lithium chloride	0.5 g
Glycine anhydride	10 g
Cycloheximide	0.2 g
Nalidixic acid	50 mg
Moxalactam	5 mg
Bacitracin	20 mg
Distilled H_2O	1000 ml

Basal medium + antibiotics
    Proteose peptone   10 g
    NaCl   5 g
    Beef extract   10 g
    $Na_2HPO_4 \cdot 12\ H_2O$ 4 g
    Glucose   10 g
    Agar   10 g
    Nalidixic acid   40 mg
    Rivanol   25 mg
    Indigo-carmine   0.1 g
    Tartrazin   0.1 g
    Twice inactivated beef serum   50 ml
    Distilled H_2O 1000 ml

Bind's acriflavine agar
    Heart infusion agar (Difco)   40 g
    Potassium thiocyanate   50 mg
    Nalidixic acid   30 mg
    Colimycin   20 mg
    Acriflavine, neutral   25 mg
    Distilled H_2O 1000 ml

Brackett and Beuchat selective enrichment agar
    Nonfat dry milk   100 g
    Ferric citrate   20 mg
    Phenylethanol   2.5 g
    Nalidixic acid   40 mg
    Cycloheximide   200 mg
    Polymyxin B   16,000 IU
    Agar   15 g
    Distilled H_2O 1000 ml

CNPA agar
    Tryptose   20 g
    NaCl   10 g
    Glucose   5 g
    Yeast extract   2 g
    Tris   7 g
    Agar   15 g
    1,2-Cyclohexanedione   3 g
    Nalidixic acid   45 mg
    Phenylethanol   1 ml
    Distilled H_2O 1000 ml

Farber agar
    Phenylethanol agar (Difco)   35.5 g
    Lithium chloride   3 g
    Glucose   1 g
    Moxalactam   10 mg
    Oxolinic acid   15 mg
    Thallium acetate   5 mg
    Distilled H_2O 1000 ml

FDA-modified McBride *Listeria* agar (FDA-MMLA)
    Phenylethanol agar   35.5 g
    Glycine anhydride   10 g
    Lithium chloride   0.5 g
    Cycloheximide   0.2 g
    Distilled H_2O 1000 ml

Gum base nalidixic acid medium
    Tryptone broth (Oxoid)   10 g
    Nalidixic acid   50 mg
    $MgCl_2 \cdot 6\ H_2O$ 0.7 g
    Hydrocolloid gum (Merck-Gellan Gum KA40)   8 g
    Distilled H_2O 1000 ml

Lithium chloride-ceftazidime agar
    Brain–heart infusion agar   52 g
    Lithium chloride   5 g
    Glycine anhydride   10 g
    Ceftazidime pentahydrate   2.5 ml
    Distilled H_2O 1000 ml

Modified Desperries agar
    Brain–heart infusion broth   37 g
    Peptone   10 g
    NaCl   5 g
    Rhamnose   1 g
    Methylene blue   10 mg
    Nalidixic acid   40 mg
    Polymyxin B   16,000 IU
    Acriflavine   2.5 mg
    Agar   15 g
    Distilled H_2O 1000 ml

Modified Doyle/Schoeni selective agar II
    Tryptose   9 g
    Dextrose   5 g
    K_2HPO_4 1.5 g
    Ferric citrate   5 mg
    Defibrinated sheep blood   50 ml
    Polymyxin B   16,000 IU
    Nalidixic acid   40 mg
    Acriflavine · HCl   10 mg
    Agar   15 g
    Distilled H_2O 1000 ml

Modified LPM agar
    Brain–heart infusion agar   52 g
    Lithium chloride   5 g
    Glycine anhydride   10 g
    Ceftazidime   50 mg
    Distilled H_2O 1000 ml

Modified Oxford agar
    Columbia blood agar base   39 g
    Esculin   1 g
    Ferric ammonium citrate   0.5 g
    Lithium chloride   15 g
    1% Colistin solution   1 ml
    1% Moxalactam solution   1 ml
    Agar   2 g
    Distilled H_2O 1000 ml

Modified Vogel-Johnson agar
    Vogel-Johnson agar base   60 g
    Nalidixic acid   50 mg
    Bacitracin   20 mg
    Moxalactam   5 mg
    1% Potassium tellurite solution   20 ml
    Distilled H_2O 980 ml

Oxford *Listeria* agar

Columbia agar base	39 g
Esculin	1 g
Ferric ammonium citrate	0.5 g
Lithium chloride	15 g
Cycloheximide	400 mg
Colistin sulfate	20 mg
Acriflavine	5 mg
Cefotetan	2 mg
Fosfomycin	10 mg
Distilled H_2O	1000 ml

PALCAM agar

Columbia agar base	39 g
D-Glucose	0.5 g
D-Mannitol	10 g
Esculin	0.8 g
Ferric ammonium citrate	0.5 g
Phenol red	80 mg
Polymyxin B	100,000 IU
Acriflavine · HCl	5 mg
Lithium chloride	15 g
Ceftazidime, Latamoxef, or Moxalactam	20 mg
Distilled H_2O	1000 ml

RAPAMY agar

Columbia blood agar base	39 g
D-Mannitol	10 g
2-Phenylethanol	2.5 g
D-Glucose	1 g
Ferric ammonium citrate	0.5 g
Esculin	0.5 g
Nalidixic acid	40 mg
Acriflavine	10 mg
Phenol red	80 mg
Egg yolk emulsion (Oxoid)	25 ml
Distilled H_2O	1000 ml

Rodriguez isolation medium I
Peptone	5 g
Neopeptone	5 g
Lab-Lemco powder	7 g
Glucose	1 g
NaCl	5 g
Disodium phosphate-2-hydrate	11.83 g
Potassium phosphate, monobasic	1.35 g
Nalidixic acid	40 mg
Acriflavine · HCl	12 mg
Defibrinated sheep blood	50 ml
Agar	15 g
Distilled H_2O	1000 ml

Rodriguez isolation medium II
Peptone	5 g
Neopeptone	5 g
Lab-Lemco powder	10 g
Yeast extract	5 g
Glucose	5 g
NaCl	40 g
Disodium phosphate-2-hydrate	1.83 g
Potassium phosphate, monobasic	1.35 g
Nalidixic acid	40 mg
Polymyxin B	3×10^4 IU
Acriflavine · HCl	18.7 mg
Defibrinated sheep blood	50 ml
Agar	15 g
Distilled H_2O	1000 ml

Rodriguez isolation medium III
Peptone	3 g
Neopeptone	5 g
Proteose peptone	3 g
Esculin	1 g
NaCl	5 g
Disodium phosphate-2-hydrate	12 g
Ferric ammonium citrate	1 g
Nalidixic acid	40 mg
Acriflavine · HCl	12 mg
Defibrinated sheep blood	50 ml
Agar	15 g
Distilled H_2O	1000 ml

Trypaflavine nalidixic acid serum agar

Peptone	10 g
Lab-Lemco powder	10 g
NaCl	5 g
Inactivated bovine serum	50 ml
Trypaflavine	20 mg
Nalidixic acid	40 mg
Polymyxin B	3 mg
Agar	15 g
Distilled H_2O	1000 ml

University of Montana agar

Protease peptone	5 g
Phytone peptone	5 g
Dextrose	5 g
Yeast extract	1 g
Na pyruvate	2.5 g
Na_2HPO_4	2.5 g
Esculin	1 g
Ferric citrate	0.5 g
Acriflavine	40 mg
Lithium chloride	10 g
Glycine anhydride	5 g
Tween 80	1 g
Ceftazidime	25 mg
Nalidixic acid	20 mg
Polymyxin B	10 mg
Phosphomycin	20 mg
Agar	15 g
Distilled H_2O	1000 ml

University of Vermont agar

Proteose peptone	5 g
Tryptone	5 g
Lab-Lemco powder	5 g
Yeast extract	5 g
NaCl	20 g
Disodium phosphate-7-hydrate	12 g
Potassium phosphate, monobasic	1.35 g
Esculin	1 g
Nalidixic acid	40 mg
Acriflavine · HCl	12 mg
Agar	15 g
Distilled H_2O	1000 ml

APPENDIX II

Additional References

INTRODUCTION

After the manuscript of a scientific book is prepared, at least nine months elapse before the book is available to the public. During that interval additional publications on the topic of the book will appear in the scientific literature. This is particularly true in a fast-moving field, and currently "*Listeria*, Listeriosis and Food Safety" is such a field. Thus this list of references not cited in the text of the book was compiled to provide the reader with access to the literature as current as possible. Included are references that appeared after the text was completed but before the publication process for this book was completed. In addition, a few older references that were not available when various sections of the book were written are included.

The references are arranged to correspond with chapters in the book. However, all references related to methods or milk and milk products are grouped into a single list. Sometimes a reference discusses research on two topics (e.g., beef and chicken meat). In such instances the reference is listed only under one of the topics.

LISTERIA MONOCYTOGENES: CHARACTERISTICS AND CLASSIFICATION

Adams, T. J., S. Vartivarian, and R. E. Cowart. 1990. Iron acquisition systems of *Listeria monocytogenes*. *Infect. Immun. 58*:2715–2718.

Adams, T., S. Vartivarian, and R. Cowart. 1990. Iron transport in *Listeria monocytogenes*. Ann. Mtg. Amer. Soc. Microbiol., Anaheim, CA, May 13–17. Abstr. I-9.

Alexander, J. E., P. W. Andrew, D. Jones, and I. S. Roberts. 1990. Development of an optimized system for electroporation of *Listeria* species. *Lett. Appl. Microbiol. 10*:179–181.

Anonymous. 1990. Microbial contamination computer program attracts 300 companies. *Food Chem. News 32*(12):20.

Arrieta, E. 1989. *Listeria monocytogenes*, contaminante de alimentos de importancia emergente. *Alimentos 14*:85–88.

Aseptic Processing Association. 1991. Proceedings of the Intern. Conf. on *Listeria* and Food Safety, Laval, France, June 13–14.

Ashton, F. E., E. P. Ewan, and J. M. Farber. 1989. Evidence for *Listeria* transmission by food. *Can. Dis. Weekly Rep. 15*:218–220.

Barclay, R., D. R. Threlfall, and I. Leighton. 1989. Haemolysins and extracellular enzymes of *Listeria monocytogenes* and *L. ivanovii*. *J. Med. Microbiol. 30*:111–118.

Barclay, R., D. R. Threlfall, and I. Leighton. 1989. Separation and properties of the haemolysins and extracellular enzymes of *Listeria monocytogenes* and *L. ivanovii*. *J. Med. Microbiol. 30*:119.

Beattie, I. A., B. Swaminathan, and H. K. Ziegle. 1990. Cloning and characterization of T-cell reactive protein antigens from *Listeria*. *Infect. Immun. 58*:2792–2803.

Bernth, S., and M. Pitron. 1989. Haemolysin producing capacity and mouse pathogenicity of *Listeria monocytogenes*. *Acta Microbiol. Hung. 36*:373–376.

Bielecki, J., and D. A. Portnoy. 1990. Expression of *Listeria monocytogenes* hemolysin by *Bacillus subtilis* is sufficient for intracellular growth in a macrophage cell line. Ann. Mtg. Amer. Soc. Microbiol., Anaheim, CA. May 13–17, Abstr. B-167.

Bielecki, J., P. Youngman, P. Connelly, and D. A. Portnoy. 1990. *Bacillus subtilis* expressing a haemolysin gene from *Listeria monocytogenes* can grow in mammalian cells. *Nature 345*:175–176.

Boisvon, A., C. Guiomar, and C. Carbon. In vitro bactericidal activity of amoxicillin, gentamicin, rifampicin, ciprofloxain and trimethoprim-sulfamethoxazole alone or in combination against *Listeria monocytogenes*. *Eur. J. Clin. Microbiol. Infect. Dis. 9*:206–209.

Boland, J. V., L. Dominguez, E. R. Ferri, J. F. Garayzabal, and G. Suarez. 1989. Preliminary evidence that different domains are involved in cytolytic activity and receptor (cholesterol) binding in listeriolysin O, the *Listeria monocytogenes* thiol-activated toxin. *FEMS Microbiol. Lett. 65*:95–100.

Boland, J. V., L. Dominguez, E. R. Ferri, and G. Suarez. 1989. Purification and characterization of two *Listeria ivanovii* cytolysins, a sphingomyelinase C and a thiol-activated toxin (ivanolysin O). *Infect. Immun. 57*:3928–3935.

Boland, J. A., L. Dominguez, J. F. Garayzabal, V. Briones, J. A. Garcia, and G. Suarez. 1990. O antigenic structure of *Listeria grayi* and *Listeria murrayi*. *Acta Microbiol. Hung. 37*:93–96.

Boneberger, W., M. Albrecht, and M. Busse. 1989. Nutrient restricted growth of *Listeria*. pp. 387–388. *In* Proceedings of the International Seminar on Modern Microbiological Methods for Dairy Products, Santander, Spain, May 22–24.

Bosgiraud, C., A. Menudier, M. J. Cornuejols, N. Hangard-Vidaud, and J. A. Nicolas. 1989. Etude de la virulence de *Listeria monocytogenes* isolées d'aliments de l'homme. *Microbiol. Aliment. Nutr. 7*:413–420.

Brunt, L. M., D. A. Portnoy, and E. R. Unanue. 1990. Presentation of *Listeria monocytogenes* to CD8+-cells require secretion of hemolysin and intracellular bacterial growth. *J. Immunol. 145*:3540–3546.

Chou, S., Kasatiya, and N. Irvine. 1990. Cellular fatty acid composition of *Oerskovia* species, CDC coryneform groups A-3, A-4, A-5, *Corynebacterium aquaticum*, *Listeria denitrificans* and *Brevibacterium acetylicum*. *Anton. Leeuwenh. Int. J. Gen. Molecular Microbiol. 58*:115–120.

Cluff, C. W., M. Garcia, and H. K. Ziegler. 1990. Intracellular hemolysin-producing *Listeria monocytogenes* strains inhibit macrophage-mediated antigen processing. *Infect. Immun. 58*:3601–3612.

Conner, D. E., V. N. Scott, S. S. Sumner, and D. T. Bernard. 1989. Pathogenicity of foodborne, environmental and clinical isolates of *Listeria monocytogenes* in mice. *J. Food Sci. 54*:1553–1556.

Corral, F. del, R. L. Buchanan, M. M. Bencivengo, and P. H. Cooke. 1990. Quantitative comparison of selected virulence associated characteristics in food and clinical isolates of *Listeria*. *J. Food Prot. 53*:1003–1009.

Cossart, P., and J. Mengaud. 1990. *Listeria monocytogenes*—A model system for the molecular study of intracellular parasitism. *Mol. Biol. Med. 6*:463–474.

Cossart, P., M. F. Vicente, J. Mengaud, F. Baquero, J. C. Perez-Diaz, and P. Berche. Listeriolysin O is essential for virulence of *Listeria monocytogenes*: Direct evidence obtained by gene complementation. *Infect. Immun. 57*:3629–3636.

Czuprynski, C., and J. Roll. 1990. Intragastric inoculation of nonhemolytic *Listeria monocytogenes* does not cause invasive infection in mice. Ann. Mtg. Amer. Soc. Microbiol., Anaheim, CA, May 13–17. Abstr. B-165.

Czuprynski, C. J., J. F. Brown, and J. T. Roll. 1989. Growth at reduced temperatures increases the virulence of *Listeria monocytogenes* for intravenously but not intragastrically inoculated mice. *Microbial Pathogen 7*:213–223.

Dabiri, G. A., J. M. Sanger, D. A. Portnoy, and F. S. Southwick. 1990. *Listeria monocytogenes* moves rapidly through the host-cell cytoplasm by inducing directional actin assembly. *Proc. Nat. Acad. Sci. 87*:6068–6072.

Dallmier, A. W., and S. E. Martin. 1990. Catalase, superoxide dismutase, and hemolysin activities and heat susceptibility of *Listeria monocytogenes* after growth in media containing sodium chloride. *Appl. Environ. Microbiol. 56*:2807–2810.

Denis, M., and E. O. Gregg. 1990. Studies on cytokine activation of listericidal activity in murine macrophages. *Can. J. Microbiol. 36*:671–675.

Domann, E., M. Leimeisterwachter, W. Goebel, and T. Chakraborty. 1991. Molecular cloning, sequencing and identification of a metalloprotease gene from *Listeria monocytogenes* that is species specific and physically linked to the listeriolysin gene. *Infect. Immun. 59*:65–72.

Egan, P., and C. Cheers. 1990. Relationship between colony-stimulating activity and interferon production during infection. *Immunology 70*:191–196.

Espaze, E. P. 1989. La taxonomie de *Listeria*: implication dans l'identification de *Listeria* et l'épidémiologie de la listériose. *Sci. Aliment. 9*:57–63.

Galsworthy, S. B., S. Girdler, and S. F. Koval. 1990. Chemotaxis in *Listeria monocytogenes*. *Acta Microbiol. Hung. 37*:81–86.

Garcia, J. A., L. Dominguez, V. Briones, M. Blanco, J. F. F. Garayzabal, and G. Suarez. 1990. Revision of the antigenic structure of genus *Listeria*. *FEMS Microbiol. Lett. 55*:113–120.

Garcia, J. A., L. Dominguez, V. Briones, J. F. F. Garayzabal, J. V. Boland, and G. Suarez. 1990. Revision of the O antigenic scheme of *Listeria*. *Acta Microbiol. Hung. 37*:87–92.

Geoffroy, C., J. Mengaud, J. E. Alouf, and P. Cossart. 1990. Alveolysin, the thiol-activated toxin of *Bacillus alvei*, is homologous to Listeriolysin-O, Perfringolysin-O, Pneumolysin, and Strep-tolysin-O and contains a single cysteine. *J. Bacteriol. 172*:7301–7305.

Geoffroy, C., J.-L. Gaillard, J. E. Alouf, and P. Berche. 1989. Production of thiol-dependent haemolysins by *Listeria monocytogenes* and related species. *J. Gen. Microbiol. 135*:481–487.

Gormley, E., J. Mengaud, and P. Cossart. 1989. Sequences homologous to the listeriolysin O gene region of *Listeria monocytogenes* are present in virulent and avirulent haemolytic species of the genus *Listeria*. *Res. Microbiol. 140*:631–643.

Gutekunst, K. A., L. Pine, S. Kathariou, J. Pohl, B. Holloway, and G. M. Carlone. 1990. Genetic characterization and the potential role in virulence of a 60-kilodalton extracellular protein of *Listeria monocytogenes*. Ann. Mtg. Amer. Soc. Microbiol., Anaheim, CA, May 13–17. Abstr. B-171.

Heil, G., and A. Weber. 1990. Investigations on the pathogenicity of *Listeria* strains by use of a continuous cell line as a replacement of animal experiment. *Zbl. Veterinärmed. B37*:707–711.

Helsel, L., S. Johnson, W. Dewitt, and W. Bibb. 1990. Characterization of monoclonal antibodies to the hemolysin of *Listeria monocytogenes* and use of the antibodies in affinity purification of the protein. Ann. Mtg. Amer. Soc. Microbiol., Anaheim, CA, May 13–17. Abstr. B-168.

Holdt, E. 1989. *Listeria*, prøvestørrelser, infektionsniveauer, o.a. *Mælkeritidende 102*:393–396.

Johnson, S., W. Dewitt, B. Swaminathan, and J. Wenger. 1990. Reactivity profile of a monoclonal antibody to β-hemolysin of *Listeria monocytogenes* serotype 4b. Ann. Mtg. Amer. Soc. Microbiol., Anaheim, CA, May 13–17. Abstr. B-169.

Julak, J., M. Ryska, I. Koruna, and E. Mencikova. 1989. Cellular fatty acids and fatty aldehydes of *Listeria* and *Erysipelothrix*. *Zbl. Bakteriol. 272*:171–180.

Kathariou, S., L. Pine, V. George, G. M. Carlone, and B. P. Holloway. 1990. Nonhemolytic *Listeria monocytogenes* mutants that are also noninvasive for mammalian cells in culture—evidence for coordinate regulation of virulence. *Infect. Immun. 58*:3988–3995.

Kroll, R. G., and R. A. Patchett. 1990. Induced acid resistance in *Listeria monocytogenes.* Soc. Appl. Microbiol. Summer Conf., Leeds, England, July 16–20, poster 6.

Kuhn, M., and W. Goebel. 1989. Identification of an extracellular protein of *Listeria monocytogenes* possibly involved in intracellular uptake by mammalian cells. *Infect. Immun. 57*:55–61.

Kuhn, M., M. C. Prevost, J. Mounier, and P. J. Sansonetti. 1990. A nonvirulent mutant of *Listeria monocytogenes* does not move intracellularly but still induces polymerization of actin. *Infect. Immun. 58*:3477–3486.

Lammerding, A. M., K. A. Glass, A. Gendron-Fitzpatrick, and M. P. Doyle 1990. Virulence of *Listeria monocytogenes* in a pregnant animal model. *J. Food Prot. 53*:902. (Abstr.)

Langley-Danysz, P. 1989. Les substances anti-*Listeria*. *R.I.A. 433*:41–42.

Leimeister-Wächter, M. L., W. Goebel, and T. Chakraborty. 1989. Mutations affecting hemolysin production in *Listeria monocytogenes* located outside the listeriolysin gene. *FEMS Microbiol. Lett. 65*:23–30.

Leimeister-Wächter, M., C. Haffner, E. Domann, W. Goebel, and T. Chakraborty. 1990. Identification of a gene that positively regulates expression of listeriolysin, the major virulence factor of *Listeria monocytogenes*. *Proc. Nat. Acad. Sci. 87*:8336–8340.

Lucas, R. D., and R. E. Levin. 1989. Genetic transformation between strains of *Listeria monocytogenes*. *Lett. Appl. Microbiol. 9*:215–218.

MacGowan, A. P., D. S. Reeves, and J. McLauchlin. 1990. Antibiotic resistance of *Listeria monocytogenes*. *Lancet ii*:513–514.

MacGowan, A. P., H. A. Holt, and D. S. Reeves. 1990. In-vitro synergy testing of nine antimicrobial combinations against *Listeria monocytogenes*. *J. Antimicrob. Chemother. 25*:561–566.

MacGowan, A. P., H. A. Holt, M. J. Bywater, and D. S. Reeves. 1990. In-vitro antimicrobial susceptibility of *Listeria monocytogenes* and other *Listeria* species isolated in the UK. *Eur. J. Clin. Microbiol. Infect. Dis. 9*:767–769.

Mazing, Y. A., M. A. Danilova, V. N. Kokryakov, V. G. Seliverstova, V. E. Pigarevskii, S. Voros. M. Kerenyi, and B. Ralovich. 1990. Haematological reactions of rabbits infected intravenously with *Listeria* strains of different virulence. *Acta Microbiol. Hung. 37*:135–144.

McCardell, B. A., and C. E. Coffman. 1990. Purification of a cytotonic toxin produced by *Listeria monocytogenes*. Ann. Mtg. Amer. Soc. Microbiol., Anaheim, CA, May 13–17. Abstr. B-170.

McLauchlin, J., and A. G. Taylor. 1989. The use of monoclonal antibodies in the characterization and purification of cell surface antigens of *Listeria monocytogenes* serogroup 4. *Acta Microbiol. Hung. 36*:459–466.

Menčíková, E., and B. Korych. 1990. Cytotoxic activity of listeriae in cell cultures. *Folia Microbiol. 35*: 525. (Abstr.)

Meyer, D. H., M. Bunduki, C. M. Beliveau, and C. W. Donnelly. 1990. Differences in association of *Listeria* spp. with mammalian gut cells. Ann. Mg. Amer. Soc. Microbiol., Anaheim, CA, May 13–17. Abstr. P-59.

Mira-Gutiérrez, J., C. Perez de Lara, and M. A. Rodriguez-Iglesias. 1990. Identification of species of the genus *Listeria* by fermentation of carbohydrates and enzymatic patterns. *Acta Microbiol. Hung. 37*:123–130.

Nicolas, J. A., M. J. Cornuejols, N. Hangard-Vidaud, C. Bosgiraud, and A. Menudier. 1989. Etude de la virulence de *Listeria monocytogenes* isolées des aliments. *Sci. Aliment. 9*:31–37.

Nocera, D., E. Bannerman, J. Rocourt, K. Jaton-Ogay, and J. Bille. 1990. Characterization by DNA restriction endonuclease analysis of *Listeria monocytogenes* strains related to the Swiss epidemic of listeriosis. *J. Clin. Microbiol. 28*:2259–2263.

Paolo, B. A. A. 1989. Some aspects of virulence in *Listeria monocytogenes*. II. *Latte 14*:975–977.

Payne, K. D., P. M. Davidson, S. P. Oliver, and G. L. Christen. 1990. Influence of bovine lactoferrin on the growth of *Listeria monocytogenes*. *J. Food Prot. 53*:468–472.

Peterkin, P. I., E. S. Idziak, and A. N. Sharpe. 1990. Virulence of *Listeria monocytogenes* hemolysins. *J. Food Prot. 53*:902. (Abstr.)

Pine, L., G. B. Malcolm, and B. D. Plikaytis. 1990. Comparison of intraperitoneal and intragastric mouse LD$_{50}$'s of *Listeria monocytogenes*. Ann. Mtg. Amer. Soc. Microbiol., Anaheim, CA, May 13–17. Abstr. B-164.

Pine, L., G. B. Malcolm, and B. D. Plikaytis. 1990. *Listeria monocytogenes* intragastric and intraperitoneal approximate 50% lethal doses for mice are comparable, but death occurs earlier by intragastric feeding. *Infect. Immun.* 58:2940–2945.

Rocourt, J. 1989. Taxonomie des *Listeria-Intérêt en microbiologie alimentare. Microbiol. Aliment. Nutr.* 7:325–328.

Roll, J. T., and C. J. Czuprynski. 1990. Hemolysin is required for extraintestinal dissemination of *Listeria monocytogenes* in intragastrically inoculated mice. *Infect. Immun.* 58:3147–3150.

Schultz, F., R. Benedict, and P. Cooke. 1990. Localization and characterization of catalase from *Listeria monocytogenes*. Ann. Mtg. Amer. Soc. Microbiol., Anaheim, CA, May 13–17. Abstr. P-53.

Seeliger, H. P. R., and J. Rocourt. 1989. Les grandes etapes de la connaissance de *Listeria. Microbiol. Aliment. Nutr.* 7:319–323.

Siragusa, G. R., and M. G. Johnson. 1990. Monoclonal antibody specific for *Listeria monocytogenes, Listeria innocua* and *Listeria welshimeri. Appl. Environ. Microbiol.* 56:1897–1904.

Siragusa, G. R., S. M. Haefner, and M. G. Johnson. 1990. β-Glucosidase activity and pathogenicity of petite *Listeria* colony isolates. Ann. Mtg. Amer. Soc. Microbiol., Anaheim, CA, May 13–17. Abstr. P-58.

Siragusa, G. R., L. A. Elphingstone, P. L. Wiese, S. M. Haefner, and M. G. Johnson. 1990. Petite colony formation by *Listeria monocytogenes* and *Listeria* species grown on esculin-containing agar. *Can. J. Microbiol.* 36:697–703.

Slade, P. J., and D. L. Collins-Thompson. 1990. *Listeria*, plasmids, antibiotic resistance, and food. *Lancet ii*:1004.

Sokolovic, Z., A. Fuchs, and W. Goebel. 1990. Synthesis of species-specific stress proteins by virulent strains of *Listeria monocytogenes. Infect. Immun.* 58:3582–3587.

Sun, A. N., A. Camilli, and D. A. Portnoy. 1990. Isolation of *Listeria monocytogenes* small-plaque mutants defective for intracellular growth and cell-to-cell spread. *Infect. Immun.* 58:3770–3778.

Szabo, E. A., and P. M. Desmarchelier. 1990. A comparative study of clinical and food isolates of *Listeria monocytogenes* and related species. *Epidemiol. Infect.* 105:245–254.

Tabouret, M. 1991. Etude des proteines de surface de *Listeria*, relation avec l'espèce, le serotype et la virulence. Soc. Francaise Microbiol. Colloques, Paris, France, March 13–14.

Tilney, L. G., and D. A. Portnoy. 1989. Actin filaments and the growth, movement and spread of the intracellular parasite, *Listeria monocytogenes. J. Cell Biol.* 109:1597–1608.

Vicente, M. F., J. Berenguer, M. A. Depedro, J. C. Perez-Diaz, and F. Baquero. 1990. Penicillin binding proteins in *Listeria monocytogenes. Acta Microbiol. Hung.* 37:227–232.

Vicente, M. F., J. C. Pieraz-Diaz, F. Baquero, M. A. de Pedro, and J. Berenguer. 1990. Penicillin-binding protein 3 of *Listeria monocytogenes* as the primary lethal target for beta-lactams. *Antimicrob. Agents Chemother.* 34:539–542.

Vogt, R. L., C. Donnelly, B. Gellin, W. Bibb, and B. Swaminathan. 1990. Linking environmental and human strains of *Listeria monocytogenes* with isoenzyme and ribosomal RNA typing. *Eur. J. Epidemiol.* 6:229.

nocytogenes located outside the listeriolysin gene. *FEMS Microbiol. Lett.* 65:23–30.

Walencka, M., and T. Goscicka. 1990. Effect of *Listeria* infection on the allotransplantation reaction in cyclosporin A treated mice. *Acta Microbiol. Hung.* 37:113–118.

Wesley, I. V. 1990. Current studies on *Listeria monocytogenes. J. Food Prot.* 53:908. (Abstr.)

Wesley, I., R. Ruby, J. Heisick, and F. Ashton. 1990. Restriction enzyme analysis of epidemic strains of *Listeria monocytogenes*. Ann. Mtg. Amer. Soc. Microbiol., Anaheim, CA, May 13–17. Abstr. P-54.

Wesley, I. V., R. D. Wesley, J. Heisick, F. Harrell, and D. Wagner. 1990. Characterization of *Listeria monocytogenes* isolates by southern blot hybridization. *Vet. Microbiol.* 24:341–354.

OCCURRENCE IN NATURAL ENVIRONMENTS

Barnier, E., J. P. Vincent, and M. Catteau. 1988. *Listeria* et environment industriel. *Sci. Aliment.* 8:239–242.

Colburn, K. G., C. A. Kaysner, C. Abeyta, Jr., and M. W. Wekell. 1990. *Listeria* species in a California coast estuarine environment. *Appl. Environ. Microbiol. 56*:2007–2011.

Tiwari, N. P., and S. G. Aldenrath. 1990. Occurrence of *Listeria* species in food and environmental samples in Alberta. *Can. Inst. Food Sci. Technol. J. 23*:109–111.

LISTERIOSIS—ANIMALS

Barley, J. 1989. *Listeria* and listeriosis. *Goats Today 82*:145.

Dijkstra, R. G. 1989. Ecology of *Listeria*. Epidemiological studies on listeriosis in animals and its relationship to food and man. *Microbiol. Aliment. Nutr. 7*:353–359.

Dijkstra, R. G. 1989. Prophylactic measures to prevent listeriosis in animals and in consequence to man. *Microbiol. Aliment. Nutr. 7*:361–366.

Dirksen, G. 1989. Listeriosis in cattle: experiences with diagnosis and therapy. *Rev. Med. Vet. 140*:681.

Farber, J. M., J. Fournier, E. Daley, and K. Dodds. 1990. Feeding trials of *Listeria monocytogenes* using a non-human primate model. Ann. Mtg. Amer. Soc. Microbiol., Anaheim, CA, May 13–17. Abstr. P-57.

Flatscher, J., E. Stastny, H. Schnabl, M. Mikula, W. Schuller, and A. Schonberg. 1990. Isolation of *Listeria* out of brains of ruminants suspicious for rabies. *Wiener tierär. Monatssch. 77*:291–296.

Gitter, M. 1989. Veterinary aspects of listeriosis. *Public Health Laboratory Service Digest 6*:38–43.

Harwood, D. G. 1989. Listeriosis in goats. *Goat Vet. Soc. J. 10*:1–4.

Husu, J. R. (1990. Epidemiological studies on the occurrence of *Listeria monocytogenes* in the feces of dairy cattle. *Zbl. Veterinärmed. Reihe B 37*:276–282.

Husu, J. R., J. T. Beery, E. Nurmi, and M. P. Doyle. 1990. Fate of *Listeria monocytogenes* in orally dosed chicks. *Intern. J. Food Microbiol. 11*:259–270.

Jeffrey, M., W. G. Halliday, and K. C. Taylor. 1990. Listeriosis confusion. *Vet. Rec. 127*:459.

Kobayashi, M., Y. Okawa, S. Suzuki, and M. Suzuki. 1990. Protective effect of baker's yeast mannan against *Listeria monocytogenes* and *Pseudomonas aeruginosae* infection in mice. *Chem. Pharmaceut. Bull. 38*:807–809.

Kovincic, I., B. Stajner, I. F. Vujicic, M. Svabic-Vlahovic, M. Mrdjen, M. Galic, M. Gagic, and J. H. Bryner. 1990. Comparison of allergenic skin test with serological and bacteriological examination of cattle for *Listeria monocytogenes*. *Acta Microbiol. Hung. 37*:131–134.

Lopez, A., and R. Bildfell. 1989. Neonatal porcine listeriosis. *Can. Vet. J. 30*:828–829.

Miettinen, A., J. Husu, and J. Toumi. 1990. Serum antibody response to *Listeria monocytogenes*, listerial excretion, and clinical characteristics in experimentally infected goats. *J. Clin. Microbiol. 28*:340–343.

Oni, O. O., A. A. Adesiyun, J. O. Adekeye, and S. N. A. Saidu. 1989. Prevalence and some characteristics of *Listeria monocytogenes* isolated from cattle and milk in Kaduna State, Nigeria. *Israel J. Vet. Med. 45*:12–17.

Seaman, J. T., M. J. Carrigan, F. A. Cockram, and G. I. Carter. 1990. An outbreak of listerial myelitis in sheep. *Austral. Vet. J. 67*:142–143.

Wesley, I. V., M. Vandermaaten, and J. Bryner. 1990. Antibody response of dairy cattle experimentally infected with *Listeria monocytogenes*. *Acta Microbiol. Hung. 37*:105–112.

Wesley, I. V., J. H. Bryner, M. J. Van Der Maaten, and M. Kehrli. 1989. Effects of dexamethazone on shedding of *Listeria monocytogenes* in dairy cattle. *Am. J. Vet. Res. 50*:2009–2013.

LISTERIOSIS—HUMAN

Alford, C. E., E. Amaral, and P. A. Campbell. 1990. Listericidal activity of human neutrophil cathepsin G. *J. Gen. Microbiol. 136*:997–1000.

Algan, M., B. Jonon, J. L. George, C. Lion, M. Kessler, and J. C. Burdin. 1990. *Listeria monocytogenes* endopthalmitis in a renal transplant patient receiving cyclosporin. *Opthalmologica 201*:23–27.

Anonymous. 1990. Annual costs of listeriosis cases put at $480 million by USDA, CDC. *Food Chem. News 32*(2):10.

Aseptic Processing Association. 1991. Proceedings of the Intern. Conf. on *Listeria* and Food Safety, Laval, France, June 13–14.

Baldridge, J. R., R. A. Barry, and D. J. Hinrichs. 1990. Expression of systemic protection and delay-type hypersensitivity to *Listeria monocytogenes* is mediated by different T-cell subunits. *Infect. Immun. 58*:654–668.

Booth, L. V., M. T. Walters, A. C. Tuck, R. A. Luqmani, and M. I. Cawley. 1990. *Listeria monocytogenes* infection in a prosthetic knee joint in rheumatoid arthritis. *Ann. Rheum. Dis. 49*:58–59.

Bottone, E. J., H. Namdari, and G. Sellers. 1990. *Listeria monocytogenes*: Investigation of an unexpected increased incidence of infection by plasmid profiling. Ann. Mtg. Amer. Soc. Microbiol., Anaheim, CA, May 13–17. Abstr. C-358.

Buchdahl, R., M. Hird, H. Gamsu, A. Tapp, D. Gibb, and C. Tzannatos. 1990. Listeriosis revisited: The role of the obstetrician. *Brit. J. Obstet. Gynecol. 97*:186–189.

Calubiran, O. V., J. Horiuchi, N. C. Klein, and B. A. Cunha. 1990. *Listeria monocytogenes* meningitis in a human immunodeficiency virus-positive patient undergoing hemodialysis. *Heart Lung 19*:21–23.

Campbell, D. M. 1990. Human listeriosis in Scotland 1967–1988. *J. Infect. 20*:241–250.

Crellin, A. M., D. S. Shareef, and E. J. Maher. 1990. Opportunistic *Listeria* pericardial effusion. *Postgrad. Med. J. 66*:203–204.

Dempster, J. F. 1989. Listeriosis: Much yet to be heard. *Food Ireland 10*:71–73.

Eiferman, R. A., K. T. Flaherty, and A. K. Rivard. 1990. Persistent corneal defect cause by *Listeria monocytogenes. Amer. J. Opthalmol. 109*:97–98.

Friedrich, L. V., R. L. White, and A. C. Reboli. 1990. Pharmacodynamics of trimethoprim-sulfamethoxazole in *Listeria* meningitis: A case report. *Pharmacotherapy 10*:301–304.

Galsworthy, S. B. 1990. Monocytosis producing activity from virulent and avirulent strains of *Listeria. Acta Microbiol. Hung. 37*:97–100.

Gilbert, R. J., S. M. Hall, and A. G. Taylor. 1989. Listeriosis update. *Pub. Health Lab. Service Dig. 6*:33–37.

Heidemann, D. G., M. Trese, S. F. Murphy, D. Bradford, M. Lewis, and S. P. Dunn. 1990. Endogenous *Listeria monocytogenes* endophthalmitis presenting as keratouveitis. *Cornea 9*:179–180.

Hof, H. 1990. Pathogenesis and treatment of listeriosis. *Deut. Med. Wochenschrift 115*:1639–1646.

Huang, J. C., H. S. Huang, M. Jurima-Romet, F. Ashton, and B. H. Thomas. 1990. Hepatocidal toxicity of *Listeria* species. *FEMS Microbiol. Lett. 72*:249–252.

Kalckreuth, G. von, D. Staab, F. Haverkamp, E. Molitor, and G. Marklein. 1990. *Listeria* meningioencephalitis in a 2-year-old boy. *Monatsschrift Kinderheilkunde 138*:351–353.

Kales, C. P., and R. S. Holzman. 1990. Listeriosis in patients with HIV infection: Clinical manifestations and response to therapy. *J. Acquired Immune Deficiency Syndromes 3*:139–143.

Kellner, M., A. Sonntag, and F. Strian. 1990. Psychiatric sequelae of listeriosis. *Brit. J. Psychiat. 157*:299.

Khardori, N., P. Berkey, S. Hayat, B. Rosenbaum, and G. P. Bodey. 1989. Spectrum and outcome of microbiologically documented *Listeria monocytogenes* infections in cancer patients. *Cancer 64*:1968–1970.

Kluge, R. M. 1990. Listeriosis problems and therapeutic options. *J. Antimicrob. Agents Chemother.* *25*:887–890.

Kuroki, H., K. Sugimoto, Y. Kohri, and T. Toba. 1990. Three cases of meningitis due to *Listeria monocytogenes* type 16b. *Kansenshogaku Zasshi 64*:249–256.

Larner, A. J., M. A. Conway, R. G. Mitchell, and J. C. Forfar. 1989. Recurrent *Listeria monocytogenes* meningitis in a heart transplant patient. *J. Infect. 19*:263–266.

Louria, D. B., J. Skurnick, and B. Holland. 1990. *Listeria* epidemic overinterpreted. *J. Infect. Dis. 162*:274–275.

Louthrenoo, W., and H. R. Schumacher, Jr. 1990. *Listeria monocytogenes* osteomyelitis complicating leukemia: Report and literature review of *Listeria* osteoarticular infections. *J. Rheumatol. 17*:107–110.

Ly, T. M. C., and H. E. Müller. 1990. Ingested *Listeria monocytogenes* survive and multiply in protozoa. *J. Med. Microbiol. 33*:51–54.

MacGowan, A. P. 1990. Listeriosis—The therapeutic options. *J. Antimicrobial Chemotherapy 26*:721.

Massarotti, E. M., and H. Dinerman. 1990. Septic arthritis due to *Listeria monocytogenes*: Report and review of the literature. *J. Rheumatol. 17*:111–113.

McLauchlin, J. 1990. Distribution of serovars of *Listeria monocytogenes* isolated from different categories of patients with listeriosis. *Eur. J. Clin. Microbiol. Infect. Dis. 9*:210–213.

McLauchlin, J. 1990. Human listeriosis in Britain, 1967–85, a summary of 722 cases. 1. Listeriosis during pregnancy and in the newborn. *Epidemiol. Infect. 104*:181–189.

McLauchlin, J. 1990. Human listeriosis in Britain, 1967–85, a summary of 722 cases. 2. Listeriosis in non-pregnant individuals, a changing pattern of infection and seasonal incidence. *Epidemiol. Infect. 104*:191–201.

Müller, H. E. 1990. *Listeria* isolations from feces of patients with diarrhea and from healthy food handlers. *Infection 18*:97–100.

Nau, R., W. Bruck, E. Bollensen, and H. W. Prange. 1990. Meningioencephalitis with septic intracerebral infarction: A new feature of CNS listeriosis. *Scand. J. Infect. Dis. 22*:101–103.

Peetermans, W. E., H. P. Endtz, A. R. Janssens, and P. J. van den Brock. 1990. Recurrent *Listeria monocytogenes* bacteraemia in a liver transplant patient. *Infection 18*:107–108.

Raps, E. C., D. H. Gutmann, J. R. Brorson, M. O'Connor, and H. I. Hurtig. 1989. Symptomatic hydrocephalus and reversible spinal cord compression in *Listeria monocytogenes* meningitis. *J. Neurosurg. 71*:620–622.

Renneberg, J., K. Persson, and P. Christensen. 1990. Western blot analysis of the antibody response in patients with *Listeria monocytogenes* meningitis and septicemia. *Eur. J. Clin. Microbiol. Infect. Dis. 9*:659–663.

Ribiere, O., P. Coutarel, V. Jarlier, O. Bousquet, V. Balderacchi, J. P. Lecouturier, and F. Thervet. 1990. Liver abscess due to *Listeria monocytogenes* in a diabetic patient. *Presse Med. 19*:1538–1540.

Rocourt, J. 1989. Listeriose humaine: Aspects cliniques et epidemiologiques. Role de l'alimentation. *Biologiste 179*:29–40.

Samuelsson, S., N. P. Rothgardt, A. Carvajal, and W. Frederickson. 1990. Human listeriosis in Denmark 1981–1987 including an outbreak November 1985–March 1987. *J. Infect. 20*:251–259.

Siegfried, C., and T. T. Schubert. 1990. Secondary bacterial peritonitis due to *Listeria monocytogenes* after paracentesis. *Southern Med. J. 83*:213–214.

Stamm, A. M., S. H. Smith, J. K. Kirklin, and D. C. McGiffin. 1990. Listerial myocarditis in cardiac transplantation. *Rev. Infect. Dis. 12*:820–823.

Schwarz, M. A., D. F. Welch, S. L. Harris, and R. A. Greenfield. 1990. Meningitis due to catalase-negative *Listeria monocytogenes*. Ann. Mtg. Amer. Soc. Microbiol., Anaheim, CA, May 13–17. Abstr. C-372.

Takeda, Y., Y. Yoshikai, S. Ohga, and K. Nomoto. 1990. Augmentation of host defense against *Listeria monocytogenes* infection by oral administration with polysaccharide RBS (RON). *Int. J. Immunopharmacol. 12*:373–383.

Thangkhiew, I., M. K. Ghosh, N. K. Kar, and P. J. Robinson. 1990. Septic arthritis due to *Listeria monocytogenes*. *J. Infect. 21*:324.

Tosca, M. L., P. Mshar, and M. Cartter. 1990. Incidence of listeriosis in Connecticut. *Conn. Med. 54*:303–304.

Varughese, P. 1989. Human listeriosis in Canada—1988. *Can. Dis. Weekly Rep. 15*:213–217.

Weiler, P. J., and D. E. Hastings. 1990. *Listeria monocytogenes*—An unusual cause of late infection in a prosthetic hip joint. *J. Rheumatol. 17*:705–707.

Zaidman, G. W., P. Coudron, and J. Pires. 1990. *Listeria monocytogenes* keratitis. *Amer. J. Ophthamol. 109*:334–339.

CHARACTERISTICS OF *LISTERIA MONOCYTOGENES* IMPORTANT TO FOOD PROCESSORS

Ahamad, N., and E. H. Marth. 1990. Acid-injury of *Listeria monocytogenes*. *J. Food Prot. 53*:26–29.

Aseptic Processing Association. 1991. Proceedings of the Intern. Conf. on *Listeria* and Food Safety, Laval, France, June 13–14.

Asperger, H., and B. Url. 1990. In vitro and in vivo efficiency of bacteriocins on *Listeria*. *FEMS Microbiol. Rev. 87*:85. (Abstr. E4)

Buchanan, R. L., and L. A. Klawitter. 1990. Effect of temperature and oxygen on the growth of *Listeria monocytogenes* at pH 4.5. *J. Food Sci. 57*:1754–1756.

Buchanan, R. L., and L. A. Klawitter. 1990. Effect of temperature history on growth of *Listeria monocytogenes* at refrigeration temperatures. Ann. Mtg. Inst. Food Technol., June 16–20. Abstr. 388.

Buchanan, R. L., and J. G. Phillips. 1990. Response surface model for predicting the effects of temperature, pH, sodium chloride content, sodium nitrite concentration and atmosphere on the growth of *Listeria monocytogenes*. *J. Food Prot. 53*:370–376, 381.

Bunning, V. K., J. T. Peeler, J. T. Tierney, and R. G. Crawford. 1990. Thermal resistance of heat-shocked *Listeria monocytogenes* exposed to high temperature–short time (HTST) pasteurization. Ann. Mtg. Amer. Soc. Microbiol., Anaheim, CA, May 13–17. Abstr. Q-90.

Bunning, V. K., R. G. Crawford, J. T. Tierney, and J. T. Peeler. 1990. Thermotolerance of *Listeria monocytogenes* and *Salmonella typhimurium* after sublethal heat shock. *Appl. Environ. Microbiol. 56*:3216–3219.

Busch, S. V., and C. W. Donnelly. 1990. Repair of heat-injured *Listeria monocytogenes* F 5069 as affected by yeast extract, lactose and sucrose. Ann. Mtg. Amer. Soc. Microbiol., Anaheim, CA, May 13–17. Abstr. P-50.

Carminati, D., and S. Carini. 1989. Antimicrobial activity of lysozyme against *Listeria monocytogenes* in milk. *Microbiol. Aliment. Nutr. 7*:49–56.

Carminati, D., G. Giraffa, and S. Carini. 1989. Comportement de *Listeria monocytogenes* en présence de *Streptococcus lactis* producteurs de substances de type bactériocine. *Microbiol. Aliment. Nutr. 7*:293–301.

Catteau, M. 1991. Système lactoperoxydas et *Listeria*. Soc. Francaise Microbiol. Colloques, Paris, France. March 13–14.

Chaudhary, V., P. Jhons, R. P. Gupta, and R. P. Sinha. 1990. Lethal effects of pulsed high electric fields on food-borne pathogens. *J. Dairy Sci. 73*(Suppl. 1):99. Abstr. D92.

Cole, M. B., M. V. Jones, and C. Holyoak. 1990. The effect of pH, salt concentration and temperature on the survival and growth of *Listeria monocytogenes*. *J. Appl. Bacteriol. 69*:63–72.

Comi, G., S. D'Aubert, and M. Valenti. 1990. Attivita inibente di acidi grassi alimentari nei confronti di *Listeria monocytogenes*. *Ind. Aliment. 29*:358–361.

Conner, D. E., V. N. Scott, and D. T. Bernard. 1990. Growth, inhibition, and survival of *Listeria monocytogenes* as affected by acidic conditions. *J. Food Prot. 53*:652–655.

Denis, F., and J. P. Ramet. 1989. Antibacterial activity of the lactoperoxidase system on *Listeria monocytogenes*. *Microbiol. Aliment. Nutr. 7*:25–30.

Doores, S., J. Amelang, and R. A. Wilson. 1990. Heat resistance of *Listeria monocytogenes* in phagocytized macrophages and neutrophils. Ann. Mtg. Amer. Soc. Microbiol., Anaheim, CA, May 13–17. Abstr. P-51.

Farag, M. D. E. H., K. Shamsuzzaman, and J. Borsa. 1990. Radiation sensitivity of *Listeria monocytogenes* in phosphate buffer, trypticase soy broth and poultry feed. *J. Food Prot. 53*:648–651.

Farber, J. M., and B. E. Brown. 1990. Effect of prior heat shock on heat resistance of *Listeria monocytogenes* in meat. *Appl. Environ. Microbiol. 56*:1584–1587.

Farber, J. M., G. W. Sanders, S. Dunfield, and R. Prescott. 1989. The effects of various acidulants on the growth of *Listeria monocytogenes. Lett. Appl. Microbiol. 9*:181–183.

Faxholm, H. 1989. Can *Listeria monocytogenes* survive pasteurization at 72°C in a plate heat exchanger? *Maelkeritidende 102*:174–175.

Fedio, W. M., and H. Jackson. 1989. Effect of tempering on the heat resistance of *Listeria monocytogenes. Lett. Appl. Microbiol. 9*:157–160.

Fenlon, D. R. 1989. The influence of gaseous environment and water availability on the growth of *Listeria. Microbiol. Aliment. Nutr. 7*:165–169.

Foegeding, P. M., and N. W. Stanley. 1990. *Listeria innocua* or an antibiotic-resistant transformant as thermal resistance indicators for *Listeria monocytogenes.* Ann. Mtg. Inst. Food Technol., Anaheim, CA, June 16–20. Abstr. 410.

Galuska, P. J., R. W. Kolarik, P. C. Vasavada, and E. H. Marth. 1989. Inactivation of *Listeria monocytogenes* by microwave treatment. *J. Dairy Sci. 72*(Suppl. 1):139. (Abstr.)

Gaze, J. E., G. D. Brown, D. E. Gaskell, and J. G. Banks. 1989. Heat resistance of *Listeria monocytogenes* in homogenates of chicken, beef steak and carrot. *Food Microbiol. 6*:251–259.

Giraffa, G., D. Carminati, M. G. Bossi, E. Neviani, L. Cilano, and M. Lion. 1990. Role of bacteriocins from lactic acid bacteria on microbial ecology. *FEMS Microbiol. Rev. 87*:84. (Abstr.)

Gueguen, M. 1991. Inhibition de *Listeria monocytogenes* par *Geotrichum candidum.* Soc. Francaise Microbiol. Colloques, Paris, France, March 13–14.

Harding, C. D., and B. G. Shaw. 1990. Antimicrobial activity of *Leuconostoc gelidum* against closely related species and *Listeria monocytogenes. J. Appl Bacteriol. 69*:648–654.

Hastings, J. W., and M. E. Stiles. 1990. Antibiosis of a *Leuconostoc* sp. isolated from meat. *FEMS Microbiol. Rev. 87*:86. (Abstr.)

Hechard, Y., M. Dherbomez, Y. Centiempo, and F. Letellier. 1990. Antagonism of lactic acid bacteria from goat's milk against pathogenic strains assessed by the "sandwich method." *Lett. Appl. Microbiol. 11*:185–188.

Hoover, D. G., K. J. Dishart, and M. A. Hermes. 1989. Antagonistic effect of *Pediococcus* spp. against *Listeria monocytogenes. Food Biotechnol. 3*:183–196.

Hug-Michel, C., S. Barben, and U. Kaufmann. 1989. Hemmung von *Listeria* spp. durch Microorganismen aus der Rinde von Rotschmiereweichkäse. *Schweiz. milchwirtsch. Forsch. 18*:46–49.

Ita, P. S., and R. W. Hutkins. 1991. Intracellular pH and survival of *Listeria monocytogenes* Scott A in tryptic soy broth containing acetic, lactic, citric and hydrochloric acids. *J. Food Prot. 54*:15.

Kamau, D. N., S. Doores, and K. M. Pruitt. 1990. Antibacterial activity of the lactoperoxidase system against *Listeria monocytogenes* and *Staphylococcus aureus* in milk. *J. Food Prot. 53*:1010–1014.

Kamau, D. N., S. Doores, and K. M. Pruitt. 1990. Enhanced thermal destruction of *Listeria monocytogenes* and *Staphylococcus aureus* by the lactoperoxidase system. *Appl. Environ. Microbiol. 56*:2711–2716.

Laemaire, V., O. Cerf, and A. Audurier. 1989. Thermal resistance of *Listeria monocytogenes. Ann. Rech. Vet. 20*:493–500.

Lee, S. H., and J. F. Frank. 1990. Effects of growth temperature and media on inactivation of *Listeria monocytogenes* by chlorine. *J. Dairy Sci. 73*(Suppl. 1):98. (Abstr.)

Linton, R. H., M. D. Pierson, and J. R. Bishop. 1990. Increase in heat resistance of *Listeria monocytogenes* Scott A by sublethal heat shock. *J. Food Prot. 53*:924–927.

Linton, R. H., M. D. Pierson, and J. R. Bishop. 1990. Increased heat resistance of *Listeria monocytogenes* due to heat shock response. Ann. Mtg. Inst. Food Technol., Anaheim, CA, June 16–20. Abstr. 445.

Lovett, J., I. V. Wesley, M. J. Vandermaaten, J. G. Bradshaw, D. W. Francis, R. G. Crawford, C. W. Donnelly, and J. W. Messer. 1990. High-temperature short-time pasteurization inactivates *Listeria monocytogenes*. *J. Food Prot.* *53*:734–738.

Lücke, F.-K., and U. Schillinger. 1990. Possible use of bacteriocin-producing lactobacilli in meats. *FEMS Microbiol. Rev.* *87*:85. (Abstr.)

Mackey, B. M., C. Pritchet, A. Norris, and G. C. Mead. 1990. Heat resistance of *Listeria*: strain differences and effects of meat type and curing salts. *Lett. Appl. Microbiol.* *10*:251–256.

McClure, P. J., T. A. Roberts, and P. O. Oguru. 1989. Comparison of the effects of sodium chloride, pH and temperature on the growth of *Listeria monocytogenes* on gradient plates and in liquid medium. *Lett. Appl. Microbiol.* *9*:95–99.

McKay, A. M. 1990. Antimicrobial activity of *Enterococcus faecium* against *Listeria* spp. *Lett. Appl. Microbiol.* *11*:15–17.

Nabrdalik, M., and R. Skarbek. 1974. Inhibitory properties of bee's honey. *Medycyna Weterynaryjna* *30*:669–670.

Nielsen, J. W., J. S. Dickson, and J. D. Crouse. 1990. Use of a bacteriocin produced by *Pediococcus acidilactici* to inhibit *Listeria monocytogenes* associated with fresh meats. *Appl. Environ. Microbiol.* *56*:2142–2145.

Oscroft, A. A. 1989. Effects of freezing on the survival of *Listeria monocytogenes*. Technical Memorandum No. 535, Campden Food and Drink Research Association.

Palumbo, S. A., and A. C. Williams. 1990. Effect of temperature, relative humidity and suspending menstrua on the resistance of *Listeria monocytogenes* to drying. *J. Food Prot.* *53*:377–381.

Peterkin, P. I., E. S. Idziak, and A. N. Sharpe. 1990. The potential for use of diacetyl as a bacteriostatic agent in food systems. *J. Food Prot.* *53*:903. (Abstr.)

Quintavalla, S., and S. Barbuti. 1989. Caractérisation microbiologique et résistance thermique de *Listeria* isolée de produits de viande. *Sci. Aliment.* *9*:125–128.

Quintavalla, S., and S. Barbuti. 1989. Resistenza termica di *Listeria innocua* e di *Listeria monocytogenes* islate da carne suina. *Ind. Censerve* *64*:8–12.

Schillinger, U., and W. H. Holzapfel. 1990. Bacteriocin production within the genus carnobacterium. *FEMS Microbiol. Rev.* *87*:87. (Abstr.)

Siragusa, G. R., and M. G. Johnson. 1989. Inhibition of *Listeria monocytogenes* growth by the lactoperoxidase-thiocyanate-H_2O_2 antimicrobial system. *Appl. Environ. Microbiol.* *55*:2802–2805.

Skoog, J. A., and S. R. Tatini. 1990. The potential for use of diacetyl as a bacteriostatic agent in food systems. *J. Food Prot.* *53*:903. (Abstr.)

Skoog, J. A., S. R. Tatini, and E. A. Zottola. 1990. Influence of added diacetyl on heat inactivation of *Listeria monocytogenes*. *J. Dairy Sci.* *73*(Suppl. 1):87. (Abstr.)

Smith, J. L. 1990. Temperature shift effects on injury and death in *Listeria monocytogenes*. *J. Food Prot.* *53*:902. (Abstr.)

Smith, J. L., B. Marmer, and R. C. Benedict. 1990. Influence of growth temperature on injury and death in *Listeria monocytogenes*, Scott A strain. Ann. Mtg. Amer. Soc. Microbiol., Anaheim, CA, May 13–17. Abstr. P-49.

Sorrells, K. M., and D. C. Enigl. 1990. Effect of pH, acidulant, sodium chloride and temperature on the growth of *Listeria monocytogenes*. *J. Food Safety* *11*:31–37.

Tarjan, V. 1990. Sensitivity of *Listeria monocytogenes* to irradiation. *Acta Microbiol. Hung.* *37*:101–104.

Vanderbergh, P. A., M. J. Pucci, B. S. Kunka, and E. R. Vedamuthu. 1990. Method for inhibiting *Listeria monocytogenes* using a bacteriocin. United States Patent 4929445.

Walker, S. J., P. A. Archer, and J. G. Banks. 1989. Growth of pathogenic bacteria at chill temperatures: *Listeria monocytogenes, Bacillus cereus*. Technical Memorandum No. 549, Campden Food and Drink Research.

Walker, S. J., J. Bows, P. Richardson, and J. G. Banks. 1989. Effect of recommended microwave cooking on the survival of *Listeria monocytogenes* in chilled retail products. Technical Memorandum No. 548, Campden Food and Drink Research Association.

Williams, D. J., and S. R. Tatini. 1990. Behavior of *Listeria monocytogenes* in associative growth with nisin producing starter cultures. *J. Dairy Sci. 73*(Suppl. 1):87. (Abstr.)

Young, K. M., and P. Foegeding. 1990. Organic acid and pH inhibition of growth of *Listeria monocytogenes.* Ann. Mtg. Amer. Soc. Microbiol., Anaheim, CA, May 13–17. Abstr. P-55.

METHODS—CONVENTIONAL AND RAPID

Al-Zoreky, N., and W. E. Sandine. 1990. Highly selective medium for isolation of *Listeria monocytogenes* from food. *Appl. Environ. Microbiol. 56*:3154–3157.

Aseptic Processing Association. 1991. Proceedings of the Intern. Conf. on *Listeria* and Food Safety, Laval, France, June 13–14.

Back, J. P., M. D. Collins, and R. G. Kroll. 1990. Fluorescent oligonucleotide probes for *Listeria* spp. Soc. Appl. Bacteriol. Summer Conference, Leeds, England, July 17–20. Poster 5.

Bailey, J. S., and N. A. Cox. 1990. Preenrichment broth for the simultaneous sampling of foods for *Salmonella* and *Listeria.* Ann. Mtg. Amer. Soc. Microbiol., Anaheim, CA, May 13–17. Abstr. P-38.

Bailey, J. S., D. L. Fletcher, and N. A. Cox. 1990. Effect of enrichment media and sampling protocol on recovery of *Listeria monocytogenes. J. Food Prot. 53*:505–507.

Bailey, J. S., D. L. Fletcher, and N. A. Cox. 1990. Efficacy of enrichment media for recovery of heat injured *Listeria monocytogenes. J. Food Prot. 53*:473–477.

Bailey, J. S., M. D. Pratt, and R. W. Johnston. 1990. Rapid method for *Listeria* speciation. Ann. Mtg. Amer. Soc. Microbiol., Anaheim, CA, May 13–17. Abstr. P-46.

Bernard, K. A., M. Bellefeuille, and E. P. Ewan. 1991. Cellular fatty acid composition as an adjunct to the identification of asporogenous, aerobic gram-positive rods. *J. Clin. Microbiol. 29*:83–89.

Bessesen, M. T., Q. Luo, H. A. Rotbart, M. J. Blaser, and R. T. Ellison III. 1990. Detection of *Listeria monocytogenes* by using the polymerase chain reaction. *Appl. Environ. Microbiol. 56*:2930–2932.

Beumer, R. R., and E. Brinkman. 1989. Detection of *Listeria* spp. with a monoclonal antibody-based enzyme-linked immunosorbent assay (ELISA). *Food Microbiol. 6*:171–177.

Beumer, R. R., E. Brinkman, and I. Stoelhort. 1989. Aantonen van *Listeria* met behulp van een enzyme-linked immunosorbent assay (ELISA). *Voedingsm. Technol. 22*:13–16.

Bhunia, A. K., P. H. Ball, G. R. Siragusa, and M. G. Johnson. 1990. Detection of *Listeria monocytogenes* by agglutination dot blotting. Ann. Mtg. Amer. Soc. Microbiol., Anaheim, CA, May 13–17. Abstr. P-45.

Bhunia, A. K., P. H. Ball, G. R. Siragusa, and M. G. Johnson. 1990. Microcolony-immunoblot method to detect *Listeria monocytogenes* in food in 18 h. Ann. Mtg. Amer. Soc. Microbiol., Anaheim, CA, May 13–17. Abstr. P-44.

Bibb, W. F., B. G. Gellin, R. Weaver, B. Schwartz, B. D. Plikaytis, M. W. Reeves, R. W. Pinner, and C. V. Broome. 1990. Analysis of clinical and food-borne isolates of *Listeria monocytogenes* in the United States by multilocus enzyme electrophoresis and application of the method to epidemiologic investigations. *Appl. Environ. Microbiol. 567*:2133–2141.

Boland, J. A., L. Dominguez, J. F. Fernandez, E. F. Ferri, V. Briones, M. Blanco, and G. Suarez. 1990. Revision of the validity of CAMP tests for *Listeria* identification—Proposal of an alternative method for the determination of haemlytic activity by *Listeria* strains. *Acta Microbiol. Hung. 37*:201–206.

Border, P. M., J. J. Howard, G. S. Plastow, and K. W. Siggens. 1990. Detection of *Listeria* species and *Listeria monocytogenes* using polymerase chain reaction. *Lett. Appl. Microbiol. 11*:158–162.

Brzin, B., N. Kuhar, B. Naverznik, and A. Vadnjal. 1990. Functional similarity of *Listeria ivanovii* and *Staphylococcus aureus* in CAMP test. *Int. J. Med. Microbiol. 273*:179–183.

Cantoni, C., M. Valenti, and S. D'Aubert. 1990. Confronto tra il terreno Oxford e il terreno PALCAM per l'isolamento di listerie. *Indust. Aliment.* 29:117–118.

Carozzi, F., and M. Motta. 1990. Sonde di DNA per la determinazione colorimetrica di *Salmonella, Listeria* ed *E. coli* nei campioni alimentari. *Latte 15*:588–591.

Casolari, C., B. Facinelli, V. Fabio, J. Rocourt, and P. E. Varaldo. 1990. Restriction endonuclease analysis of chromosomal DNA from *Listeria monocytogenes* strains. *Eur. J. Epidemiol. 6*:319–322.

Cassiday, P. K., L. M. Graves, and B. Swaminathan. 1990. Replica plating of colonies from *Listeria*-selective agars to blood agar to improve the isolation of *Listeria monocytogenes* from foods. *Appl. Environ. Microbiol. 56*:2274–2275.

Cirigliano, M. C., and R. T. McKenna. 1990. Comparison of four media for the preservation and transport of *Listeria* in environmental samples. Ann. Mtg. Amer. Soc. Microbiol., Anaheim, CA, May 13–17. Abstr. P-37.

Comi, G., C. Cantoni, and M. Valenti. 1990. Evaluation of an enzymatic method for rapid detection of *Listeria* spp. in cheese. *Ind. Aliment. 29*:231–236.

Corral, F. del, and R. L. Buchanan. 1990. Evaluation of the API-ZYM system for identification of *Listeria. Food Microbiol. 7*:99–106.

Cotton, L. N., and C. H. White. 1990. Predictive tests for the presence of environmental pathogens. *J. Dairy Sci. 73*(Suppl. 1):260. (Abstr.)

Cotton, L. N., C. H. White, and K. Farooq. 1990. Microbiological tests and plant inspection scores as predictors of environmental pathogen presence. *J. Dairy Sci. 73*(Suppl. 1):99. (Abstr.)

Cox, L. J., and C. Pedrazzini. 1989. Enrichment procedures for *Listeria* spp. p. 390. *In* Proceedings of the International Seminar on Modern Microbiological Methods for Dairy Products, Santander, Spain, May 22–24.

Curialie, M. S., T. Sons, M. T. Knight, J. R. Agin, J. F. Black, H. Geers, C. P. Cunningham, and B. J. Robinson. 1990. Enzyme immunoassay (ELISA) for detection of *Listeria* in foods: precollaborative study. Ann. Mtg. AOAC, New Orleans, LA. Sept. 10–13. Abstr.

Dallas, H. L., T. T. Tran, C. Poindexter, and A. D. Hitchins. 1990. Competition of food bacteria with *Listeria monocytogenes* during enrichment. Ann. Mtg. Amer. Soc. Microbiol., Anaheim, CA, May 13–17. Abstr. P-40.

Deneer, H. G., and I. Boychuk. 1991. Species specific detection of *Listeria monocytogenes* by DNA amplification. *Appl. Environ. Microbiol. 57*:606–609.

Dickson, J. S. 1990. Comparison of homogenization by blending or stomaching on the recovery of *Listeria monocytogenes* from beef tissues. *J. Food Sci. 55*:655–657.

Dominguez, L., J. F. Garayzabal, M. del Mar Blanco, V. Briones, J. A. Boland, J. L. Blanco, and G. Suarez. 1990. Overlay technique for direct detection and identification of haemolytic *Listeria* on selective plating medium. Comparison of five media. *Z. Lebensm.-Unters. Forsch. 191*:16–19.

Eley, A. 1990. New rapid detection methods for *Salmonella* and *Listeria. Br. Food J. 92*:28–31.

Espaze, E. P. 1989. Identification et caractérisation bactériologique de *Listeria* aspects actuels et perspectives. *Microbiol. Aliment. Nutr. 7*:329–336.

Evanson, D. J., M. J. Klatt, T. P. DonLevy, and R. S. Flowers. 1990. Agar based 24 hr method for presumptive identification of *Listeria monocytogenes*. Ann. Mtg. Inst. Food Technol., Anaheim, CA, June 16–20. Abstr. 443A.

Garayzabal, J. F., and C. Genigeorgis. 1990. Quantitative evaluation of three selective enrichment broths and agars used in recovering *Listeria* microorganisms. *J. Food Prot. 53*:105–110.

Groody, E. P. 1991. Detection of foodborne pathogens using DNA probes. *Food Austral. 43*:28–34.

Guinet, R., and I. Emery. 1989. Détection immunoenzymatique rapide de *Listeria monocytogenes. Sci. Aliment. 9*:39.

Hahn, G., P. Hammer, and W. Heeschen. 1988. Immunological detection of *Listeria*. pp. 389–397. *In* 29th Arbeitstagung des Arbeitsgebietes "Lebensmittelhygiene." Leitthema: Qualitätssicherung und Lebensmittelhygiene. Garmisch-Partenkirchen, Federal Republic of Germany, September 13–16.

Haines, S. D., and P. D. Patel. 1989. Evaluation of the Listeria-Tek kit for the rapid detection of *Listeria* spp. in foods. *J. Appl. Bacteriol. 67*(6):xxxiii.

Hale, K. A., and S. Doores. 1990. A qualitative isolation procedure for *Listeria monocytogenes*. Ann. Mtg. Inst. Food Technol., Anaheim, CA, June 16–20. Abstr. 402.

Hale, K. A., S. Doores, and R. A. Walsh. 1990. An enzyme surfactant treatment and filtration technique for the retrieval of *Listeria monocytogenes* from ice cream mix. *Food Structure 9*:61–67.

Haltzer, A., H. Asperger, and B. Uri. 1989. Detection of *Listeria* in brine and smear: Improvement of sample preparation. pp. 392–393. *In* Proceedings of the International Seminar on Modern Microbiological Methods for Dairy Products, Santander, Spain, May 22–24.

Hammer, P., G. Hahn, H. Kirchhoff, and W. Heeschen. 1990. Vergleich der Eignung von Oxford- und PALCAM-Medium zur Isolierung von *Listeria monocytogenes* aus Weichkäse. *Dtsch. Milchwirtsch. 41*:334–336.

Hayes, P. S., L. M. Graves, G. W. Ajello, B. Swaminathan, and the *Listeria* study group. 1990. Comparison of two methods for isolating *Listeria monocytogenes* from foods. Ann. Mtg. Inst. Food Technol., Anaheim, CA, June 16–20. Abstr. 406.

Henzler, B., G. Sulzer, and M. Busse. 1989. A tube test for hemolysis in *Listeria.* pp. 395–397. *In* Proceedings of the International Seminar on Modern Microbiological Methods for Dairy Products, Santander, Spain, May 22–24.

Hitchins, A. D., and T. Tran. 1990. Initial cell concentration and selective media effects on the isolation of *Listeria monocytogenes* from enrichment cultures of inoculated foods. *J. Food Prot. 53*:502–504.

Jatisatienr, Ch., and M. Busse. 1989. Comparison of selective media for *Listeria.* pp. 399–400. *In* Proceedings of the International Seminar on Modern Microbiological Methods for Dairy Products, Santander, Spain, May 22–24.

Jemmi, T., P.-F. Gobart, and S. Guyer. 1990. Praktische Erfahrungen mit den Selektivmedien Oxford und Palcam zum Nachweis von *Listeria monocytogenes* aus kontaminierten Materialien. *Mitt. Gebiete Lebensm. 81*:559–564.

Kajioka, R., and M. Noble. 1990. Analysis of *Listeria monocytogenes* by pyrolysis mass spectrometry. Ann. Mtg. Amer. Soc. Microbiol., Anaheim, CA, May 13–17. Abstr. C-354.

Kathariou, S., L. Pine, F. D. Quinn, K. Birkness, and V. George. 1990. Cell culture model system for the differentiation of virulent from avirulent strains of *Listeria monocytogenes*. Ann. Mtg. Amer. Soc. Microbiol., Anaheim, CA, May 13–17. Abstr. B-166.

Kerr, K. G., N. A. Rotowa, P. M. Hawkey, and R. W. Lacey. 1990. Four hour identification and speciation of *Listeria* spp. using the Rosco System. Ann. Mtg. Amer. Soc. Microbiol., Anaheim, CA, May 13–17. Abstr. C-316.

Kerr, K. G., N. A. Rotowa, P. M. Hawkey, and R. W. Lacey. 1990. Evaluation of the Mast ID and API 50CH Systems for identification of *Listeria* spp. *Appl. Environ. Microbiol. 56*:657–660.

Kim, C., L. M. Graves, B. Swaminathan, L. W. Mayer, and R. E. Weaver. 1991. Evaluation of hybridization characteristics of a cloned pRF106 probe for *Listeria monocytogenes* detection and development of a nonisotopic colony hybridization assay. *Appl. Environ. Microbiol. 57*:289–294.

Kim, C., B. Swaminathan, B. Holloway, R. Pinner, and V. A. Varma. 1990. Detection of *Listeria monocytogenes* in formalin-fixed paraffin-embedded tissues using a 2-stage nested polymerase chain reaction. Ann. Mtg. Amer. Soc. Microbiol., Anaheim, CA, May 13–17. Abstr. D-54.

Kim, C., B. Swaminathan, P. K. Cassiday, L. W. Mayer, and B. P. Holloway. 1990. Rapid detection and quantitation of *Listeria monocytogenes* in foods by a nonradioactive colony blot assay. Ann. Mtg. Inst. Food Technol., Anaheim, CA, June 16–20. Abstr. 400.

Knight, M. T., J. R. Black, D. Wood, and J. R. Agin. 1990. Identification of *Listeria* sp. using Vitek GNI and GPI cards versus a GPI and off-line biochemicals. Ann. Mtg. AOAC, New Orleans, LA, Sept. 10–13, Abstr.

Köhler, S., M. Leimeister-Wächter, T. Charkraborty, F. Lottspeich, and W. Goebel. 1990. The gene coding for protein p^{60} of *Listeria monocytogenes* and its use as a specific probe for *Listeria monocytogenes*. *Infect. Immun. 58*:1943–1950.

Lachica, R. V. 1990. Same-day identification scheme for colonies of *Listeria monocytogenes*. *Appl. Environ. Microbiol. 56*:1166–1168.

Lachica, R. V. 1990. Simplified Henry technique for initial recognition of *Listeria* colonies. *Appl. Environ. Microbiol. 56*:1164–1165.

Lammerding, A. M., and M. P. Doyle 1989. Evaluation of enrichment procedures for recovering *Listeria monocytogenes* from dairy products. *Int. J. Food Microbiol. 9*:249–268.

Leasor, S. B., C. A. Abbas, and R. Firstenberg-Eden. 1990. Evaluation of UVM as a growth medium for *Listeria monocytogenes*. Ann. Mtg. Amer. Soc. Microbiol., Anaheim, CA, May 13–17. Abstr. P-39.

Lieval, F., J. Tache, and J. Poumeyrol. 1989. Qualité microbiologique et *Listeria* sp. dans les produits de la restauration rapide. *Sci. Aliment. 9*:111–115.

Loessner, M. J., and M. Busse. 1990. Bacteriophage typing of *Listeria* species. *Appl. Environ. Microbiol. 56*:1912–1918.

Loessner, M. J., and M. Busse. 1990. Phagentypisierung von *Listerien* als Instrument zur Anlagensanierung. *Dtsch. Milchwirtsch. 41*:1115–1118.

Loesner, M., H. Schirmer, and M. Busse. 1989. Phage typing of *Listeria*. pp. 402–404. *In* Proceedings of the International Seminar on Modern Microbiological Methods for Dairy Products, Santander, Spain, May 22–24.

Lowry, P. D., and I. Tiong. 1989. Evaluation of isolation and identification techniques for *Listeria monocytogenes* on meat. *Food Australia 41*:1084–1087.

Lund, A. M., E. A. Zottola, and D. J. Pusch. 1990. Comparison of methods for the isolation of *Listeria* from raw milk. *J. Dairy Sci. 73*(Suppl. 1):87. (Abstr.)

MacGowan, A. P., R. J. Marshall, and D. S. Reeves. 1989. Evaluation of API 20 STREP system for identifying *Listeria* species. *J. Clin. Pathol. 45*:518–550.

McCarthy, S. A. 1990. Determination of heat-stressed and resuscitated heat-stressed cells of *Listeria monocytogenes*. Ann. Mtg. Amer. Soc. Microbiol., Anaheim,CA, May 13–17. Abstr. Q-92.

McKay, T., J. Wilson, D. R. Fenlon, and B. Seddon. 1989. Viablue 2 distinguishes between viable and dead bacterial cells. *J. Appl. Bacteriol. 67*(6):xli.

McLauchlin, J. 1989. Rapid non-cultural methods for the detection of *Listeria* in food—A review. *Microbiol. Aliment. Nutr. 7*:279–284.

McLauchlin, J., A. M. Ridley, and A. G. Taylor. 1990. The use of monoclonal antibodies against *Listeria monocytogenes* in a direct immunofluorescence technique for the rapid presumptive identification and direct demonstration of *Listeria* in food. *Acta Microbiol. Hung. 36*:467.

Miller, K. L. 1989. A comparison of two methods for the isolation of *Listeria monocytogenes* from soft cheese. *J. Appl. Bacteriol. 67*(6):xix-xx.

Mohamood, A., B. Wentz, A. Datta, and B. Eribo. 1990. Application of a synthetic listeriolysin O gene probe to the identification of β-hemolytic *Listeria monocytogenes* in retail ground beef. Ann. Mtg. Amer. Soc. Microbiol., Anaheim, CA, May 13–17. Abstr. P-10.

Northolt, M. D. 1989. Recovery of *Listeria monocytogenes* from dairy products using the TNCB-TNSA method and the draft IDF methods. *Neth. Milk Dairy J. 43*:299–310.

Okwumabua, O., C. Kim, B. Swaminathan, and P. Edmonds. 1990. Rapid detection of *Listeria monocytogenes* by a chemiluminescent hybridization assay in microtiter plates. Ann. Mtg. Amer. Soc. Microbiol., Anaheim, CA, May 13–17. Abstr. D-55.

Olander, A., S. Harlander, and B. Swaminathan. 1990. DNA fingerprinting and ribosomal RNA typing of *Listeria monocytogenes* implicated in foodborne illness outbreaks. Ann. Mtg. Amer. Soc. Microbiol., Anaheim, CA, May 13–17. Abstr. P-47.

Ottaviani, F., G. Arvati, D. Spolaor, L. dal Santo, and F. Zilio. 1990. Impiego dei metodi di ibridazione nel controllo microbiologico degli alimenti. Esperienze con sonde marcate con enzimi. *Ind. Aliment. 29*:541–549.

Peterkin, P. I., E. S. Idziak, and A. N. Sharp. 1991. Detection of *Listeria monocytogenes* by using direct colony hybridization on hydrophobic grid-membrane filters by using a chromogen-labeled DNA probe. *App. Environ. Microbiol. 57*:586–591.

Poda, G., D. Cesaroni, E. Ponti, A. Andreucci, and B. Bragaglia. 1989. Ricerca di *Listeria* con la tecnica del prearricchimento a freddo e con quella F.D.A. in campioni di carne cruda alla vendita. *Riv. Soc. Ital. Sci. Aliment. 18*:263–270.

Poumyrol, M. 1991. Numération des *Listeria* dans les viandes hâchées. Soc. Francaise Microbiol. Colloques, Paris, France, March 13–14.

Pritchard, T. J., and C. W. Donnelly. 1990. Plasmid profile analysis of *Listeria innocua* for use in tracing sources of environmental contamination. Ann. Mtg. Amer. Soc. Microbiol., Anaheim, CA, May 13–17. Abstr. P-48.

Robison, B. J., and S. J. Walker. 1990. Comparison of cultural and ELISA procedures for detection of *Listeria* in foods. Ann. Mtg. Inst. Food Technol., Anaheim, CA, June 16–20. Abstr. 405.

Robison, B.,D. Kronish, L. Beck, and C. Brown. 1990. Identification of *Listeria* species using MICRO-ID *Listeria*. Ann. Mtg. Amer. Soc. Microbiol., Anaheim, CA, May 13–17. Abstr. P-43.

Schiemann, D. A., S. R. Shope, and M. J. Brown. 1990. Development of new enrichment broths and plating agars for isolation of hemolytic species of *Listeria*. *J. Food Safety 10*:233–252.

Skjerve, E., L. M. Rorvik, and O. Olsvik. 1990. Detection of *Listeria monocytogenes* in food by immunomagnetic separation. *Appl. Environ. Microbiol. 56*:3478–3481.

Slade, P. J., and D. L. Collins-Thompson. 1990. Identification of *Listeria* spp. and closely related gram-positive bacteria using low molecular weight RNA profiles. Ann. Mtg. Inst. Food Technol., Anaheim, CA, June 16–20. Abstr. 444.

Smith, J. L., and R. L. Buchanan. 1990. Identification of supplements that enhance the recovery of *Listeria monocytogenes* on Modified Vogel Johnson Agar. *J. Food Safety 10*:155–164.

Sorin, M. L., M. Garnier, M. Bonneau, and R. Robinson. 1988. Test de detection rapide des *Listeria* dans les produits laitiers. *Sci. Aliment. 8*:229–234.

Szemeredi, G. 1990. New method for the isolation of *Listeria monocytogenes* from contaminated samples. *Acta Microbiol. Hung. 37*:165–170.

Terplan, G., K. Friedrich, and S. Steinmaier. 1991. Ricerca Analitica delle Listerie. *Latte 16*:66–69.

Tiwari, N. P., and S. G. Aldenrath. 1990. Isolation of *Listeria monocytogenes* from food products on four selective plating media. *J. Food Prot. 53*:382–385.

Tran, T. T., P. Stephenson, and A. D. Hitchins. 1990. The effect of aerobic mesophilic microflora levels on the isolation of inoculated *Listeria monocytogenes* strain LM82 from selected foods. *J. Food Safety 10*:267–276.

Url, B., H. Asperger, and A. Haltzer. 1989. Detection of *Listeria*: Comparison of selective enrichment procedures. pp. 406–408. *In* Proceedings of the international seminar on modern microbiological methods for dairy products, Santander, Spain, May 22–24.

Vanderkelen, D., and J. A. Lindsay. 1990. Differential hemolytic response of *Listeria monocytogenes* strains on various blood agars. *J. Food Safety 11*:9–12.

Vanrolleghem, P., X. Patigny, J. F. Richard, J. Fache, and D. Van Dijck. 1989. A comparative study of different enrichment and direct plating methods for isolation and enumeration of pathogenic *Listeria* from foods and other materials. *Meded. Fac. Landbouwwet. Rijksuniv. Gent 54*:1393–1400.

Walker, J. S., P. Archer, and J. Appleyard. 1989. Comparison of cultural procedures with the *Listeria*-Tek ELISA kit for the rapid detection of *Listeria* species in foods. Technical Memorandum No. 572, Campden Food and Drink Research Association.

Werner, B. S., and D. V. Lim. 1990. Growth of *Listeria monocytogenes* in different media. Ann. Mtg. Amer. Soc. Microbiol., Anaheim, CA, May 13–17. Abstr. P-41.

Yu, L. S. L., and D. Y. C. Fung. 1990. Evaluation of FDA and USDA procedures for enumeration of *Listeria monocytogenes*. Ann. Mtg. Amer. Soc. Microbiol., Anaheim, CA, May 13–17. Abstr. P-42.

FOODBORNE LISTERIOSIS

Aseptic Processing Association. 1991. Proceedings of the Intern. Conf. on *Listeria* and Food Safety, Laval, France, June 13–14.

Engel, R. E., C. E. Adams, and L. M. Crawford. 1990. Foodborne listeriosis: risk from meat and poultry. *Food Control 1*:27–31.

Jones, D. 1990. Foodborne listeriosis. *Lancet ii*:1171–1174.

Katsube, Y., and S. Maruyama. 1989. Listeriosis and food hygiene. *Shokuhin Elseigaku Zasshi 30*:479–490.

Lund, B. M. 1990. The prevention of foodborne listeriosis. *Br. Food J. 92*:13–22.

Ridgway, E. J., and J. M. Brown. 1989. *Listeria monocytogenes* meningitis in the acquired immune deficiency syndrome—limitations on conventional typing methods in tracing a foodborne source. *J. Infect. 19*:167–171.

Steinmeyer, S., and G. Terplan. 1990. Listerien in Lebensmitteln—eine aktuelle Übersicht zu Vorkommen, Bedeutung als Krankheitserreger, Nachweis und Bewertung. Teil II. *DMZ Lebensm. Milchwirtsch. 111*:179–183.

Stubbs, A. 1989. Listeriosis and food products. *Goat Vet. Soc. J. 10*:5–9.

Upton, M. 1989. *Listeria monocytogenes*—How real is the problem? *Food Ireland 3*:31–35.

Vlayen, P. 1987. Listeriose et fromages. *Aliment. Diet. Hyg. 6*:26–29.

Witting, Ö. 1988. *Listeria monocytogenes*: ett problem for livsmedelsindustrin. *Mejeritidskrift för Finlands Svenskbygd 50*:4–7.

MILK AND MILK PRODUCTS

Ahmed, A. A. H. 1989. Behavior of *Listeria monocytogenes* during preparation and storage of yoghurt. *Assiut Vet. Med. J. 22*:76–80.

Ahmed, A. A. H., S. H. Ahmed, M. K. Moustafa, and N. M. Saad. 1989. Growth and survival of *Listeria monocytogenes* during manufacture and storage of Domiata cheese. *Assiut Vet. Med. J. 22*:88–94.

Anonymous. 1989. *Listeria monocytogenes* in Dutch cheese? *Voedingsm. Technol. 22*(5):25.

Anonymous. 1990. Frozen confection bars recalled because of *Listeria. Food Chem. News 32*(9):15.

Anonymous. 1990. Ice cream bars recalled. FDA Enforcement Rep., April 25.

Anonymous. 1990. Ice milk bars recalled. FDA Enforcement Rep., April 25.

Anonymous. 1990. Italian soft ripened and semi-soft cheese recalled. FDA Enforcement Report, Nov. 7.

Anonymous. 1990. Vanilla ice cream recalled. FDA Enforcement Rep., Nov. 7.

Aseptic Processing Association. 1991. Proceedings of the Intern. Conf. on *Listeria* and Food Safety, Laval, France, June 13–14.

Asperger, H. 1989. *Listeria* detection in cheese factories. pp. 324–327. *In* 30th Arbeitstagung des Arbeitsgebietes "Lebensmittelhygiene." Leitthema: Verbraucherschutz in den 90er Jahren. Garmisch-Partenkirchen, Federal Republic of Germany, Sept. 25–28.

Asperger, H., B. Url, and E. Brandl. 1989. Interactions between *Listeria* and the ripening flora of cheese. *Neth. Milk Dairy J. 43*:287–298.

Barnier, E., J. P. Vincent, and M. Catteau. 1988. Survie de *Listeria monocytogenes* dans les saumures et le serum de fromagerie. *Sci. Aliment. 8*:175–188.

Beumer, R. R., L. J. Cox, I. Stoelhorst, and M. Sherbini. 1989. Detection of *Listeria* species in cheese. p. 349. *In* Proceedings of the International Seminar on Modern Microbiological Methods for Dairy Products, Santander, Spain, May 22–24.

Bibi, W., and M. R. Bachmann. 1990. Antibacterial effect of the lactoperoxidase-thiocyanate-hydrogen peroxide system on the growth of *Listeria* spp. in skim milk. *Milchwissenschaft 45*:26–28.

Bradshaw, J. G., J. T. Peeler, and R. M. Twedt. 1991. Thermal resistance of *Listeria* spp. in milk. *J. Food Prot. 54*:12.

Brindani, F., and E. Freshchi. 1988/1989. *Listeria monocytogenes* in sheep and goat milk, and in various cheeses. *Annali della Facoltà di Medicina Veterinaria, Università di Parma 8–9*:205–219.

Buldrini, A., C. Maini, and G. Sanavio. 1990. Isolamento di *Listeria* spp. da prodotti lattiero-caseari e da alimenti carnei. *Ind. Aliment. 29*:550–552.

Cantoni, C., S. D'Aubert, M. Valenti, and G. Comi. 1989. *Listeria* spp. in formaggi ed insaccati crudi. *Ind. Aliment. 28*:1068–1070.

Chiu, I., J. A. Skoog, S. R. Tatini, and L. L. McKay. 1989. Inhibition of *Listeria monocytogenes* by associative growth of nisin producing *Lactococcus lactis* subsp. *lactis* in fermented milk. *J. Dairy Sci. 72*(Suppl. 1):138. (Abstr.)

Cloet, P. R., L. Florant, and A. Millet. 1989. Enquête sur la contamination d'un lait de tank d'une exploitation par *Listeria monocytogenes*. *Bull. G.T.V. 5*:79–85.

Cogan, T. M., and M. Rea. 1988. *Listeria* in dairy products. What are they and how widespread? *Farm Food Res. 19*:31–32.

Comi, G., S. D'Aubert, and M. Valenti. 1990. Attivita inibente di acidi grassi alimentari nei confronti di *Listeria monocytogenes*. *Mondo Latte 44*:422–426.

Cottoin, J., F. Picard-Bonnaud, and B. Carbonnelle. 1990. Study of *Listeria monocytogenes* survival during the preparation and the conservation of two kinds of dairy products. *Acta Microbiol. Hung. 37*:119–122.

Daeschel, M. A., D.-S. Jung, and F. W. Bodyfelt. 1990. Influence of fat on the efficacy of nisin in inhibiting *Listeria monocytogenes* in fluid milk. *J. Dairy Sci. 73*(Suppl. 1):86. (Abstr.)

D'Errico, M. M., P. Villari, G. M. Grasso, F. Romano, and I. F. Angelillo. 1990. Isolamento di *Listeria* spp. da latte e formaggi. *Riv. Soc. Ital. Sci. Aliment. 19*:47–52.

Dumur, P., J.-L. Bind, and A. Audurier. 1989. Ecologie des *Listeria* dans les aliments autres que les produits laitiers. *Sci. Aliment. 9*:97–102.

Farber, J. M., G. W. Sanders, and J. I. Speirs. 1990. Growth of *Listeria monocytogenes* in naturally-contaminated raw milk. *Lebensm.-Wiss. Technol. 23*:252–254.

Gelosa, L. 1990. Survey on *Listeria monocytogenes* contamination of milk and cheese. *Indust. Aliment. 29*:137–139.

Griffith, M., and K. E. Deibel. 1990. Survival of *Listeria monocytogenes* in yogurt with varying levels of fat and solids. *J. Food Safety 10*:219.

Hammer, P., and G. Hahn. 1989. Bedeutung, Nachweis und Vorkommen von Listerien in Käse. *Welt Milch 43*:670–673.

Hammer, P. von, G. Hahn, and W. Heeschen. 1989. Vergleichende Untersuchungen zum Nachweis von *Listeria monocytogenes* in Weichkäse. *Kieler Milchwirtschaftliche Forschungsberichte 41*:175–210.

Hartmann, V. 1989. Occurrence and detection of *Listeria* in cheese factories. Thesis. Ludwig-Maximilians Universität, Munich, Germany.

Hashisaka, A. E., S. D. Weagant, and F. M. Dong. 1989. Survival of *Listeria monocytogenes* in Mozzarella cheese and ice cream exposed to gamma irradiation. *J. Food Prot. 52*:490–492.

Hechard, Y., M. Dherbomez, Y. Cenatiempo, and F. Letellier. 1990. Antagonism of lactic acid bacteria from goat's milk against pathogenic strains assessed by the "sandwich method." *Lett. Appl. Microbiol. 11*:185–188.

Heeschen, W. 1988. Hygienische Risken von Rohmilchkaese. *Dtsch. Milchwirtsch. 39*:145–149.

Holdt, E. 1989. Some practical hints for detecting contamination by *Listeria*. *Maelkeritidende 102*:234–236.

Husu, J. R., J. T. Seppänen, S. K. Sivelä, and A. L. Rauramaa. 1990. Contamination of raw milk by *Listeria monocytogenes* on dairy farms. *Zbl. Veterinärmed. Reihe B 37*:268–275.

Jacquet, C., J. Rocourt, and A. Reynaud. 1991. Produits laitiers et *Listeria monocytogenes*: étude des sites de contamination d'une fromagerie. Soc. Francaise Microbiol. Colloques, Paris, France, March 13–14.

Johnson, E. A., J. H. Nelson, and M. Johnson. 1990. Microbiological safety of cheese made from heat-treated milk. Part I. Executive summary, introduction and history. *J. Food Prot. 53*:441–452.

Johnson, E. A., J. H. Nelson, and M. Johnson. 1990. Microbiological safety of cheese made from heat-treated milk. Part II. Microbiology. *J. Food Prot. 53*:519–540.

Johnson, E. A., J. H. Nelson, and M. A. Johnson. 1990. Microbiological safety of cheese made from heat-treated milk. Part III. Technology, discussion, recommendations, bibliography. *J. Food Prot. 53*:610–623.

Lausseger, I., and H. Asperger. 1989. Screening for presence of *Listeria* in raw milk by examining centrifuge sludge. pp. 150–151. *In* Proceedings of the international seminar on modern microbiological methods for dairy products, Santander, Spain, May 22–24.

Lund, A. M., and E. A. Zottola. 1990. Inhibition of *Listeria* species by *Bacillus* in raw milk. *J. Food Prot. 53*:903. (Abstr.)

Maisnier-Patin, S., N. Deschamps, and J. Richard. 1991. Comportement de *Listeria monocytogenes* en présence de bacteries lactiques productrices de nisine au cours de la fabrication et de lafinage de camemberts. Soc. Francaise Microbiol. Colloques, Paris, France, March 13–14.

Malaspina, P., and R. Lodi. 1990. Rassegna delle osservazioni emerse su *L. monocytogenes* nel settore lattiero-caseario. *Latte 15*:516–520.

Michard, J., N. Jardy, and J. L. Gey. 1989. Dénombrement et localisation de *Listeria monocytogenes* dans des fromages à pâte molle et à croûte lavée fabriqués avec du lait cru en provenance d'une enterprise fromagère. *Microbiol. Aliment. Nutr. 7*:131–137.

Michard, J., N. Jardy, and K. Laine. 1989. Croissance des *Listeria* dans des jus de laitue. Effets de la température et de la microflore associée. *Microbiol. Aliment. Nutr. 7*:31–42.

Northolt, M. D., and L. Toepel. 1988. *Listeria monocytogenes* in melk en zuivel produkten. *Voedingsm. Technol. 21*:19–21.

Renterghem, R. van, G. Waes, and H. de Ridder. 1990. Detection of *Listeria monocytogenes* in cheese by DNA-colony hybridization. *Milchwissenschaft 45*:426–427.

Rousset, A., and M. Rousset. 1989. *Listeria monocytogenes* isolées de fromages prélevés au niveau de différents points de vente. *Sci. Aliment. 9*:129–131.

Roy, R. 1990. Competitive survival of *Yersinia enterocolitica* and *Listeria monocytogenes* in UHT milk stored at 4°C. *J. Dairy Sci. 73*(Suppl. 1):88. (Abstr.)

Seiler, H. von, and M. Busse. 1989. Biochemical differentiation of *Listeria* spp. from cheese. Berl. Münch. tierärztl. Wschr. 102:166–170.

Singh, R. S., and H. Chander. 1990. Detection, identification and control of *L. monocytogenes* in milk and milk products. *Indian Dairyman 42*:243–247.

Suaudeau, H. 1989. Produits laitiers. Pâtes pressées cuites: La qualité en question. *Libre Serv. Actual. 32*:45.

Takai, S., F. Orii, K. Yasuda, S. Inoue, and S. Tsubaki. 1990. Isolation of *Listeria monocytogenes* from raw milk and its environment at dairy farms in Japan. *Microbiol. Immunol. 34*:631–634.

Terplan, G. 1989. Bedeutung der Listerien für die Milchwirtschaft. Eine aktuelle Übersicht. *Dtsch. Milchwirtsch. 41*:168–169.

Terplan, G., and H. Becker. 1989. Salmonellen, *E. coli*, Stapylokokken und Listerien in Trockenmilchprodukten. *Molkereitechnik 82/83*:71–75.

Terplan, G., S. Steinmeyer, H. Becker, and K. Friedrich. 1990. Detection of *Listeria* in milk and dairy products—A contribution to the situation in 1990. *Arch. Lebensmittelhyg. 41*:102–106.

Valdes-Stauber, N., R. Braatz, H. Gotz, G. Sulzer, and M. Busse. 1990. Der Einfluss die Mikroflora von Käse auf die *Listeria*. Entwicklung Dtsch. Milchwirtsch. 41:1126–1130.

Vanrenterghem, R., G. Waes, and H. Deridder, 1990. Detection of *Listeria monocytogenes* in cheese by DNA-colony hybridization. *Milchwissenschaft 45*:426–427.

Wenzel, J.M., and E. H. Marth. 1990. Behavior of *Listeria monocytogenes* at 4 and 7°C in raw milk inoculated with a commercial culture of lactic acid bacteria. *Milchwissenschaft 45*:772–774.

Wenzel, J. M., and E. H. Marth. 1990. Behavior of *Listeria monocytogenes* in the presence of lactic acid bacteria in a medium with internal pH control requiring agitation (IPCM-2). *J. Food Prot. 53*:902. (Abstr.)

Wenzek, J. M., and E. H. Marth. Changes in populations of *Listeria monocytogenes* in a medium with internal pH control containing *Streptococcus cremoris. J. Dairy Sci. 73*:3357–3365.

Williams, D. J., and S. R. Tatini. 1990. Behavior of *Listeria monocytogenes* in associative growth with nisin producing starter cultures. *J. Dairy Sci. 73*(Suppl. 1):87. (Abstr.)

Wnorowski, T. 1990. The prevalence of *Listeria* species in raw milk from the Transvaal region. *Suid-Afrikaanse Tydskrif vir Suiwelkunde 22*:15–21.

Yousef, A. E., and E. H. Marth. 1990. Fate of *Listeria monocytogenes* during the manufacture and ripening of parmesan cheese. *J.D.S. 72*:3351.

MEAT AND MEAT PRODUCTS

Anonymous. 1990. Prepared sandwiches recalled. FDA Enforcement Report, Nov. 14.

Aseptic Processing Association. 1991. Proceedings of the Intern. Conf. on *Listeria* and Food Safety, Laval, France, June 13–14.

Barbuti, S., M. Ghisi, and M. Campanini. 1989. *Listeria* in prodotti carnei: Isolamento, incidenza e caratteristiche di sviluppo. *Ind. Conserve 64*:221–224.

Bergann, T. 1990. Studies into occurrence of *Listeria* spp. in foodstuff. *Monat. Veterinarmed. 45*:801–802.

Billaux, F. 1990. *Listeria monocytogenes*: Recouvrement dans les produits carnés. *Viandes Produits Carnes 9*:254–256.

Boonmasiri, N., J. N. Sofos, and G. R. Schmidt. 1990. Thermal destruction of *Listeria monocytogenes* in ground pork with different fat levels. Ann. Mtg. Inst. Food Technol., Anaheim, CA, June 16–20. Abstr. 387.

Brown, W. L. 1990. Guidelines for *Listeria monocytogenes* inactivation studies for extended shelf-life pre-cooked refrigerated foods. Ann. Mtg. Inst. Food Technol., Anaheim, CA, June 16–20. Abstr. 542.

Brown, W. L. 1990. The fate of *Clostridium botulinum* and *Listeria monocytogenes* in a refrigerated, meat-filled ravioli. Ann. Mtg. Amer. Soc. Microbiol., Anaheim, CA, May 13–17. Abstr. P-33.

Carter, P. T., and M. F. Patterson. 1990. The survival and growth of *Listeria monocytogenes* in irradiated meat. Soc. Appl. Bacteriol. Summer Conference, Leeds, England, July 15–20, Poster 7.

Dealler, S., N. Rotowa, and R. Lacey. 1990. Microwave reheating of convenience meals. *Br. Food J. 92*:19–21.

Dickson, J. S. 1990. Survival and growth of *Listeria monocytogenes* on beef tissue surfaces as affected by simulated processing conditions. *J. Food Safety 10*:165–174.

Gildemeister, B. D., J. N. Sofos, and G. R. Schmidt. 1990. Survival of *Listeria monocytogenes* in aqueous solutions of meat curing ingredients. Ann. Mtg. Inst. Food Technol., Anaheim, CA, June 16–20. Abstr. 384.

Gill, C. O., and M. P. Reichel. 1989. Growth of cold-tolerant pathogens *Yersinia enterocolitica*; *Aeromonas hydrophila* and *Listeria monocytogenes* on high-pH beef packaged under vacuum or carbon dioxide. *Food Microbiol. 6*:223–230.

Glenn, E., R. Geisen, and L. Leistner. 1989. Control of *Listeria monocytogenes* in mould-ripened raw sausages by strains of *Penicillium nalgiovense. Mitteil. Bundes. Fleischfor., Kulmbach 105*:317–324.

Grau, F. H., and P. B. Vanderlinde. 1990. Growth of *Listeria monocytogenes* on vacuum-packaged beef. *J. Food Prot. 53*:739–741.

Hunter, P. R., H. Hornby, and I. Green. 1990. The microbiological quality of pre-packed sandwiches. *Br. Food J. 92*:15–18.

Kaya, M., and U. Schmidt. 1990. Behavior of *Listeria monocytogenes* in vacuum packaged beef. *Mitteil. Bundes. Fleischfor., Kulmbach 107*:29–37.

Kaya, M., and U. Schmidt. 1989. Multiplication of *Listeria monocytogenes* on meat surfaces. *Mitteil. Bundes. Fleischfor., Kulmbach 106*:440–449.

Lowry, P. D. 1990. The hysteria over *Listeria*. In Proc. 25th Meat Industry Research Conf., pp. 176–180, Hamilton, New Zealand, July 12–14.

Nitcheva, L., V. Yonkova, V. Popov, and C. Manev. 1990. *Listeria* isolation from foods of animal origin. *Acta Microbiol. Hung. 37*:223–226.

Ozari, R., and F. A. Stolle. 1990. Occurrence of *Listeria monocytogenes* in meat, meat products and poultry. *Arch. Lebensmittelhyg. 41*:47.

Schmidt, U., and M. Kaya. 1990. Verhalten von *Listeria monocytogenes* in vakuumverpacktem Brühwurstaufschnitt. *Fleischwirtschaft 70*:236–240.

Seneviratna, P., J. Robertson, I. D. Robertson, and D. J. Hampson. 1990. *Listeria* species in foods of animal origin. *Austral. Vet. J. 67*:384.

Tran, T. T., P. Stephenson, and A. O. Hitchins. 1990. The effect of aerobic mesophilic microfloral levels on the isolation of inoculated *Listeria monocytogenes* strain LM82 from selected foods. *J. Food Safety 10*:267–275.

Unda, J. R., R. A. Molins, and H. W. Walker. 1990. *Clostridium sporogenes* and *Listeria monocytogenes*: Survival and inhibition in microwave-ready beef roasts containing selected antimicrobials. Ann. Mtg. Inst. Food Technol., Anaheim, CA, June 16–20. Abstr. 381.

Wimpfheimer, L., N. S. Altman, and J. H. Hotchkiss. 1990. Growth of *Listeria monocytogenes* Scott A, serotype-4 and competitive spoilage organisms in raw chicken packaged under modified atmospheres and in air. *Intern. J. Food Microbiol. 11*:205–214.

Wong, H.-C., W.-L. Chao, and S.-J. Lee. 1990. Incidence and characterization of *Listeria monocytogenes* in foods available in Taiwan. *Appl. Environ. Microbiol. 56*:3101–3104.

Yen, L., J. N. Sofos, and G. R. Schmidt. 1990. Effect of sodium chloride on thermal destruction of *Listeria monocytogenes* in ground pork. Ann. Mtg. Inst. Food Technol., Anaheim, CA, June 16–20. Abstr. 385.

POULTRY AND EGG PRODUCTS

Bartlett, F. M., J. M. Laird, and R. C. McKellar. 1990. Survival of *Listeria monocytogenes* in synthetic egg washwater. *J. Food Prot. 53*:903. (Abstr.)

Hart, C. D., G. C. Mead, and A. P. Norris. 1991. Effects of gaseous environment and temperature on the storage behavior of *Listeria monocytogenes* on chicken breast meat. *J. Appl. Bacteriol. 70*:40–46.

Kerr, K. G., N. A. Rotowa, P. M. Hawkey, and R. W. Lacey. 1990. Incidence of *Listeria* spp. in pre-cooked, chilled chicken products as determined by culture and enzyme-linked immunoassay (ELISA). *J. Food Prot. 53*:606–607, 629.

Shelef, L. A., and Q. Yang. 1990. Growth suppression of *Listeria monocytogenes* by sodium or potassium lactate in cooked chicken or beef. *J. Food Prot. 53*:903. (Abstr.)

Varabioff, Y. 1990. Incidence and recovery of *Listeria* from chicken with a pre-enrichment technique. *J. Food Prot. 53*:555–557, 624.

Wang, C., and L. A. Shelef. 1990. Factors contributing to growth inhibition of *Listeria monocytogenes* in raw egg albumin. *J. Food Prot. 53*:902–903. (Abstr.)

Wenger, J. D., B. Swaminathan, P. S. Hayes, S. S. Green, M. Pratt, R. W. Pinner, A. Schuchat, and C. V. Broome. 1990. *Listeria monocytogenes* contamination in turkey franks: Evaluation of a production facility. *J. Food Prot. 53*:1015–1019.

FISH AND SEAFOOD

Anonymous. 1990. Cold smoked salmon recalled. FDA Enforcement Rep., July 11.

Anonymous. 1990. Smoked salmon recalled. FDA Enforcement Rep., July 11.

Anonymous. 1990. Smoked salmon recalled. FDA Enforcement Rep., Aug. 8.

Anonymous. 1990. Smoked salmon recalled. FDA Enforcement Rep., Oct. 31.

Brackett, R. E., and L. R. Beuchat. 1990. Pathogenicity of *Listeria monocytogenes* grown on crabmeat. *Appl. Environ. Microbiol. 56*:1216–1220.

Figueroa, G., H. Galeno, M. Troncoso, and J. M. Aguilera. 1990. Analysis of the microbial flora of jack mackerel (*Trachurus murphyi*) minced products. *Sci. Aliments 10*:907–912.

Hangard-Vidaud, N., J. A. Nicolas, C. Bosgiraud, and M. J. Cornuejols. 1989. Recherche de *Listeria* chez les poissons d'eau douce. *Microbiol. Aliment. Nutr. 7*:421–423.

Harrison, M. A., and Y. W. Huang. 1990. Thermal death times for *Listeria monocytogenes* in crab meat. Ann. Mtg. Inst. Food Technol., Anaheim, CA, June 16–20. Abstr. 363.

Harrison, M. A., and Y. W. Huang. 1990. Thermal death times for *Listeria monocytogenes* (Scott A) in crabmeat. *J. Food Prot. 53*:878–880.

Hofer, E., and R. Riberio. 1990. Occurrence of *Listeria* species in frozen shrimp. *Rev. Microbiol.* *21*:207–213.

Jemmi, T. 1990. Occurrence of *Listeria monocytogenes* in imported smoked and fermented fish. *Arch. Lebensmittelhyg.* *41*:107–108.

Jemmi, T. 1990. Stand der Kenntnisse über Listerien bei Fleisch- und Fischprodukten. *Mitt. Geb. Lebensmittelunter. Hyg.* *81*:144–157.

Lovett, J., D. W. Francis, J. T. Peeler, and R. M. Twedt. 1991. Quantitative comparison of two encirclement methods for isolating *Listeria monocytogenes* from seafood. *J. Food Prot.* *54*:7.

McCarthy, S. A., M. L. Motes, and R. M. McPhearson. 1990. Recovery of heat-stressed *Listeria monocytogenes* from experimentally and naturally contaminated shrimp. *J. Food Prot.* *53*:22–25.

Nicolas, J. A., M. J. Cornuejols, N. Hangard-Vidaud, and C. Bosgiraud. 1989. Etude de la contamination par *Listeria* des aliments destinés à la consommation humaine: Viandes, fromages, poissons. *Biologiste 179*:41–45.

PLANT PRODUCTS

Al-Ghuzali, M. R., and S. K. Al-Azawi. 1990. *Listeria monocytogenes* contamination of crops grown on soil treated with sewage sludge cake. *J. Appl. Bacteriol.* *69*:642–647.

Anonymous. 1990. Cheese spreads, cole slaw and various salads recalled. FDA Enforcement Rep., Jan. 17.

Anonymous. 1990. Hot jalapeno spread recalled. FDA Enforcement Rep., Nov. 14.

Anonymous. 1990. Potato salad recalled. FDA Enforcement Rep., Aug. 8.

Barnes, P. 1989. *Listeria*—a threat to margarine? *Lipid Technol.* *1*:46–47.

Beuchat, L. R., and R. E. Brackett. 1990. Inhibiting effects of raw carrots on *Listeria monocytogenes*. *Appl. Environ. Microbiol.* *56*:1734–1742.

Beuchat, L. R., and R. E. Brackett. 1990. Survival and growth of *Listeria monocytogenes* on lettuce as influenced by shredding, chlorine treatment, modified atmosphere packaging and temperature. *J. Food Sci.* *55*:755–758, 870.

Catteau, M. 1991. Croissance de *Listeria* sur des produits végétaux en sachets. Soc. Francaise Microbiol. Colloques, Paris, France, March 13–14.

Chung, K.-T., W. R. Thomasson, and C. D. Wu-Yuan. 1990. Growth inhibition of selected food-borne bacteria, particularly *Listeria monocytogenes*, by plant extracts. *J. Appl. Bacteriol.* *69*:498–503.

El-Gazzar, F. E., and E. H. Marth. 1990. Survival of *Listeria monocytogenes* in a food colorant derived from red beets. *J. Dairy Sci.* *73*(Suppl. 1):99. (Abstr.)

Fenlon, D. R. 1989. Silage as a potential source of *Listeria monocytogenes* in the food chain. *Microbiol. Aliment. Nutr.* *7*:171–173.

Forbes, G. 1989. Listeriosis—a possible association with margarine. *Commun. Dis. Scotland Weekly Rep. 23*:34.

George, A. E., and P. N. Levett. 1989. The effect of temperature and pH on the survival of *Listeria monocytogenes* in coleslaw. *Intern. J. Food Microbiol.* *11*:345–350.

Gola, S., M. P. Previdi, P. Mutti, and S. Belloli. 1990. Microbiological investigation of frozen vegetables, incidence of *Listeria* and other psychrotrophic pathogens. *Industria Conserve 65*:36–38.

Husu, J. R., S. K. Sivela, and A. L. Raurama. 1990. Prevalence of *Listeria* species as related to chemical quality of farm-ensiled grass. *Grass Forage Sci.* *45*:309–314.

Laine, K., and J. Michard. 1988. Fréquence et abondance des *Listeria* dans les légumes frais découpés prêts a l'emploi. *Microbiol. Aliment. Nutr.* *6*:329–335.

Magnuson, J. A., A. D. King, and T. Torok. 1990. Microflora of partially processed lettuce. *Appl. Environ. Microbiol.* *56*:3851–3854.

Perry, C. M., and C. W. Donnelly. 1990. Incidence of *Listeria monocytogenes* in silage and its subsequent control by specific and nonspecific antagonism. *J. Food Prot.* *53*:642–647.

CONTROL IN FOOD FACTORIES

Amgar, A. 1990. Are there any anti-*Listeria* disinfectants? *Process 1048*:23–24.

Anonymous. 1991. Meat hygiene guidance for local authorities. *Vet. Rec. 128*:24.

Aseptic Processing Association. 1991. Proceedings of the Intern. Conf. on *Listeria* and Food Safety, Laval, France, June 13–14.

Best, M., M. E. Kennedy, and F. Coates. 1990. Efficacy of a variety of disinfectants against *Listeria* spp. *Appl. Environ. Microbiol. 56*:377–380.

Busse, M. 1990. Preventive measures against *Listeria. Eur. Dairy Mag. 1*:66–68, 70–77.

Buyser, M. L. de. 1991. Evaluation du niveau de contamination de produits de charcuterie et salaisons par *Listeria*. Soc. Francaise Microbiol. Colloques, Paris, France, March 13–14.

Cotton, L. N., C. H. White, and K. Farooq. 1990. Microbiological tests and plant inspection scores as predictors of environmental pathogen presence. *J. Dairy Sci. 73* (Suppl. 1):99. (Abstr.)

Daly, C. 1987. *Listeria*: A new quality control problem for the food industry. *Food Ireland 9/10*:41–43.

Disegna, L., F. Ottaviani, D. Giacon, and A. Loddo. 1989. Technology and microbial ecology in the prevention of sanitary risks in products of animal origin with *Listeria monocytogenes. Latte 14*:140–151.

Frank, J. F. 1990. Microbial ecology of listeriae-containing biofilms. *J. Food Prot. 53*:901. (Abstr.)

Frank, J. F., and R. A. Koffi. 1990. Surface-adherent growth of *Listeria monocytogenes* is associated with increased resistance to surfactant sanitizers and heat. *J. Food Prot. 53*:550–554.

Frank, J. F., and R. A. N. Gillett. 1990. Microbial content of *Listeria*—contaminated surfaces of dairy processing plants. *J. Dairy Sci. 73*(Suppl. 1):261. (Abstr.)

Frank, J. F., R. A. N. Gillett, and G. O. Ware. 1990. Association of *Listeria* spp. contamination in the dairy processing plant environment with the presence of staphylococci. *J. Food Prot. 53*:928–932.

Frank, J. F., R. A. N. Gillett, and G. O. Ware. 1990. Staphylococci are an indicator group for the presence of listeriae in the dairy processing plant environment. *J. Dairy Sci.* (Suppl. 1):98. Abstr. D89.

Gasparrolle, M. N., R. Bishop, and M. D. Pierson. 1990. Attachment of *Pseudomonas fragi*, *Listeria monocytogenes*, and *Bacillus cereus* to gasket materials. Ann. Mtg. Inst. Food Technol., Anaheim, CA, June 16–20. Abstr. 413.

Gobat, P.-F., and T. Jemmi. 1990. Epidemiological studies on *Listeria* spp. in slaughterhouses. *Fleischwirtschaft 70*:1448–1450.

Goff, H. D., and P. J. Slade. 1990. Transmission of a *Listeria* sp. through a cold-air wind tunnel. *Dairy Food Environ. Sanit. 10*:340–343.

Gorden, J. 1990. 1991 and the Food Safety Act. *Dairy Ind. Intern. 55*(12):26.

Holdt, E. 1989. Nogle synspunkter og forslag praktiske hjælpemidler ved sporing af *Listeria*-infektioner. *Maelkeritidende 102*:234–236.

Hsu, J. C. 1990. Effective control of *Listeria monocytogenes* in a dairy processing and packaging plant by isothiazolone microbicide. *J. Food Prot. 53*:902. (Abstr.)

Lee, S.-H., and J. F. Frank. 1991. Inactivation of surface adherent *Listeria monocytogenes* hypochlorite and heat. *J. Food Prot. 54*:4.

Mafu, A. A., D. Roy, J. Goulet, and P. Magny. 1990. Attachment of *Listeria monocytogenes* to stainless steel, glass, polypropylene and rubber surfaces after short contact time. *J. Food Prot. 53*:742–746.

Mafu, A. A., D. Roy, J. Goulet, L. Savoie, and R. Roy. Efficiency of sanitizing agents for destroying *Listeria monocytogenes* on contaminated surfaces. *J.D.S. 73*:3428.

Mafu, A. A., D. Roy, L. Savoie, R. Roy, and T. Goulet. 1989. Effect of sanitizing agents on *Listeria monocytogenes* attached to milk contact surfaces at different temperatures. *J. Dairy Sci. 72*(Suppl. 1):172. (Abstr.)

Mosteller, T. M., and J. R. Bishop. 1990. Determination of minimum inhibitory concentrations of sanitizers for attached environmental bacteria. *J. Dairy Sci. 73*(Suppl. 1):116. (Abstr.)

Nelson, J. H. 1990. Where are *Listeria* likely to be found in dairy plants? *Dairy Food Environ. Sanit. 10*:344–345.

Olsen, B. 1990. *Listeria*-problematikkeh. *Mælkeritidene 103*:72–74.

Smola, J. 1990. Possibilities of *Listeria* monitoring in slaughter animals. *Acta Microbiol. 35*:535. (Abstr.)

Spurlock, A. T., and E. A. Zottola. 1990. Persistence and control of *Listeria monocytogenes* in non-food contact areas in a food processing plant. *J. Food Prot. 53*:903. (Abstr.)

Toquin, M. T. 1991. Influence des opérations de nettoyage et de désinfection sur la persistance de *Listeria monocytogenes* dans un abattoir de volailles. Soc. Francaise Microbiol. Colloques, Paris, France, March 13–14.

Waes, G. 1987. Aanwezigheid en controle van *L. monocytogenes* in kaas. *Belg. J. Food Chem. Biotechnol. 42*:184–187.

Weise, E., and P. Teufel. 1989. Listerien in Lebensmitteln—ein ungelöstes problem. *Ärztliche Laboratorium 35*:205–208.

White, C. H. 1990. Relationship of plant cleanliness and routine microbiological testing to finished product quality and presence of environmental pathogens. *J. Dairy Sci. 73*(Suppl. 1):117. (Abstr.)

Index